S0-AIF-949

Introduction to Critical Care Nursing

Introduction to Critical Care Nursing

JEANETTE HARTSHORN, PhD, RN, FAAN
University of Texas Health Science Center
School of Nursing
San Antonio, Texas

MARILYN LAMBORN, PhD, RN
University of Texas Health Science Center
School of Nursing
San Antonio, Texas

MARY LOU NOLL, PhD, RN, CCRN
Visiting Associate Professor
University of Central Florida
Orlando, Florida

W.B. SAUNDERS COMPANY *A Division of Harcourt Brace & Company* Philadelphia London Toronto Montreal Sydney Tokyo

W.B. SAUNDERS COMPANY
A Division of
Harcourt Brace & Company

The Curtis Center
Independence Square West
Philadelphia, Pennsylvania 19106

Library of Congress Cataloging-in-Publication Data

Hartshorn, Jeanette.
Introduction to critical care nursing / Jeanette Hartshorn, Marilyn Lamborn, Mary Lou Noll.
p. cm.
Includes index.

ISBN 0-7216-3526-1

1. Intensive care nursing. I. Lamborn, Marilyn. II. Noll, Mary Lou. III. Title.
[DNLM: 1. Critical Care—nurses' instruction. WY 154 H335i]
RT120.I5H37 1993
610.73'61—dc20
DNLM/DLC 92-22966

Introduction to Critical Care Nursing ISBN 0-7216-3526-1

Printed in the United States of America.

Last digit is the print number: 9 8 7 6 5 4

For Amy, Katie, and Ed, whose constant devotion makes everything possible.

J.C.H.

To my parents, Alberta and George, who gave me life and the desire to enjoy and discover it; and to my sister, Barbara, who has made life that much happier by having her here to share it.

M.L.L

To the "grandmothers" in my life: Lula Falkenstein, R.N., Vera Nolte, and Josephine Ferda. They have been a great source of motivation throughout my life and career.

M.L.N.

About the Authors

Jeanette Hartshorn

Jeanette Hartshorn, Ph.D., R.N., FAAN, is currently Associate Dean for Undergraduate Nursing at the University of Texas Health Science Center at San Antonio School of Nursing. Previously, she was an Associate Professor at the Medical University of South Carolina College of Nursing, where she headed a graduate program in critical care nursing. She received a diploma in nursing from Evanston Hospital, Evanston, Illinois, a B.S.N. from the Medical University of South Carolina, an M.S.N. from the University of South Carolina, and a Ph.D. in nursing from the University of Texas at Austin. She is active in several nursing organizations and is a past president of the American Association of Critical Care Nurses. She has published over 30 articles and book chapters. With 19 years of nursing experience, she has worked as a staff nurse, clinical nurse specialist, and administrator.

Marilyn Lamborn

Marlyn Lamborn, Ph.D., R.N., received a diploma in nursing from Georgia Baptist Hospital School of Nursing, Atlanta, a bachelor's and master's of science in nursing from the Medical College of Georgia, and a Ph.D. in nursing from the University of Texas at Austin. She has been employed as a staff nurse, head nurse, and co-director of patient referral, education, and home health care services; diabetic and cardiac educator, clinical specialist; and academic educator. For two years she was academic assistant to the dean of the University of Texas at Austin School of Nursing. Marilyn has been involved in critical care education and clinical activities for over 18 years. She is currently an Assistant Professor at the University of Texas Health Science Center at San Antonio School of Nursing.

Mary Lou Noll

Mary Lou Noll, Ph.D., R.N., CCRN, has over 17 years of experience in critical care practice, education, and research. She is currently Visiting Associate Professor at the University of Central Florida in Orlando, and she has taught critical care at both graduate and undergraduate levels at the University of Texas Health Science Center at San Antonio School of Nursing. She received a doctorate in nursing from the University of Texas at Austin, a master's degree in nursing from Ohio State University, a BSN from Ohio University, and a diploma from Ohio Valley General Hospital School of Nursing. She is active in the American Association of Critical-Care Nurses (AACN) at both chapter and national levels. She is also actively involved in Sigma Theta Tau and was president of the Delta Alpha Chapter. She is also a member of the American Nurses Association, National League for Nursing, Phi Kappa Phi, and Sigma Xi. She is a 1992 recipient of the Glaxo-AACN Excellence in Critical Care Education Award. She has published extensively in critical care literature and serves as an editorial consultant or board member for three critical care journals: *AACN Clinical Issues in Critical Care Nursing, Dimensions of Critical Care Nursing,* and *Heart & Lung.*

Contributors

Charold L. Baer, PhD, RN, FCCM, CCRN
Professor
School of Nursing
Oregon Health Science University
Portland, Oregon
Acute Renal Failure

Vicki Byers, PhD, RN
Associate Professor
Division of Nursing and Sciences
Incarnate Word College
San Antonio, Texas
Nervous System Injury

Charlotte L. DePew, MSN, RN, CCRN
Captain, US Army Nurse Corps
Burn Intensive Care Unit
US Army Institute of Surgical Research
Fort Sam Houston, Texas
Burns

Deborah J. Duncan, MSN, RN, CCRN
Major, US Army Nurse Corps
Chief of Nursing Education and Staff Development
US Army Institute of Surgical Research
Fort Sam Houston, Texas
Burns

Enid Denise Ebert, MSN, RN
Clinical Education Coordinator
Critical Care Units
Norman Regional Hospital
Norman, Oklahoma
Individual and Family Response to the Critical Care Experience

Phyllis A. Enfanto, MS, RN, CCRN
Critical Care Nurse Educator
St. Elizabeth's Hospital
Boston, Massachusetts
Acute Respiratory Failure

Marsha E. Fonteyn, PhD, RN, CCRN
Assistant Professor
School of Nursing
University of San Francisco
San Francisco, California
Cardiac Alterations

Leslie R. Goddard, PhD, RN
Assistant Professor
School of Nursing
University of Texas Health Science Center, San Antonio
San Antonio, Texas
Nervous System Injury

Jeanette Hartshorn, PhD, RN, FAAN
Associate Dean, Undergraduate Program
School of Nursing
University of Texas Health Science Center, San Antonio
San Antonio, Texas
Introduction; Individual and Family Response to the Critical Care Experience; Nervous System Injury

Anne-Marie Jones, MSN, RN, CCRN
Critical Care Consultant
Layton, Utah
Code Management; Hematology/Immunology

JoAnn M. Krumberger, MSN, RN, CCRN
Critical Care Clinical Nurse Specialist
Veterans Administration Medical Center
Milwaukee, Wisconsin
Gastrointestinal Alterations; Endocrine Crises

Marilyn Lamborn, PhD, RN
Assistant Professor
School of Nursing
University of Texas Health Science Center, San Antonio
San Antonio, Texas
Code Management; Cardiac Alterations

Mary G. McKinley, MSN, RN, CCRN
Clinical Nurse Specialist, Critical Care
Ohio Valley Medical Center
Wheeling, West Virginia
Shock

Nancy C. Molter, MSN, RN, CCRN
Colonel US Army Nurse Corps
Chief Nurse
US Army Institute of Surgical Research
Fort Sam Houston, Texas
Burns

Mary Lou Noll, PhD, RN, CCRN
Visiting Associate Professor
University of Central Florida
Orlando, Florida
Ventilatory Assistance; Code Management

Cynthia Kline O'Sullivan, MSN, RN
Nurse Manager, Surgical Intensive Care Unit
The University Hospital at Boston University Medical Center
Boston, Massachusetts
Introduction to Hemodynamics

Catherine Freismuth Robinson, MS, RN, CEN, CCRN
Clinical Nurse Specialist, Emergency Department
Ohio Valley Medical Center
Wheeling, West Virginia
Shock

Gwenn Arlene Scott, MSN, RN, CCRN
Assistant Administrator for Clinical Services
McKenna Memorial Hospital
New Braunfels, Texas
Individual and Family Response to the Critical Care Experience

Joan M. Vitello-Cicciu, MSN, RN, CCRN, CS
Clinical Nurse
Specialist, Intensive Care Unit
The University Hospital at Boston University Medical Center
Boston, Massachusetts
Introduction to Hemodynamics

Linda Waite, MN, RN, CCRN
Critical Care Consultant/Educator
Milwaukee, Wisconsin
Endocrine Crises

Linda S. Weaver, MSN, RN, CCRN
Captain, US Army Nurse Corp
William Beaumont Medical Center
El Paso, Texas
Individual and Family Response to the Critical Care Experience

Stephanie L. Woods, MSN, RN, CCRN
Manager
Educational Resources
Santa Rosa Hospital Corporation
San Antonio, Texas
Understanding Basic Electrocardiography and Interpreting Dysrhythmias

Susan L. Zorb, MSN, RN, CCRN
Clinical Specialist, Medical
Critical Care
The University Hospital at Boston University Medical Center
Boston, Massachusetts
Acute Respiratory Failure

Preface

The knowledge base of critical care nursing has steadily grown since the specialty emerged in the 1970s. Today, most nurses entering the field of critical care are overwhelmed by the amount of information needed for successful practice. A challenge facing any critical care educator who is responsible for teaching novices is to identify content that is essential to practice.

The purpose of *Introduction to Critical Care Nursing* is to provide essential information to nurses who are new to critical care. The book has been specifically developed to meet the needs of the baccalaureate nursing student or the nurse who is new to critical care nursing. *Introduction to Critical Care Nursing* is not intended to be a complete reference on critical care nursing; rather, it has been developed to provide content essential to entry level practice in critical care. The information presented is believed to be common to all critical care nursing practice, regardless of the specific setting.

The book is organized into three sections. Part I, Fundamental Concepts, includes two chapters with information basic to all types of critical care nursing practice. Part II, Tools for the Critical Care Nurse, includes four chapters with vital information concerning electrocardiography, hemodynamics, ventilation, and management of life-threatening emergencies.

The final nine chapters of the book complete Part III, "Nursing Care During Critical Illness." In each chapter, the nursing process is used as the organizing framework. Nursing Care Plans utilizing nursing diagnosis assist the reader in understanding how the information fits together. An extensive index is provided to facilitate use of the text as a reference.

The challenge of working in a Critical Care Unit is a great one. Our hope is that the information in this text will help both teacher and student to identify essential information for practice. Once this information is mastered, the student will wish to consult other texts to provide depth within specific areas. *Introduction to Critical Care Nursing* will provide the basic content.

J.C.H.
M.L.L.
M.L.N.

Contents in Brief

PART I

FUNDAMENTAL CONCEPTS

PART II

TOOLS FOR THE CRITICAL CARE NURSE

PART III

NURSING CARE DURING CRITICAL ILLNESS

Contents

PART

I

Fundamental Concepts

Chapter

1

Jeanette C. Hartshorn, Ph.D., R.N., FAAN

Introduction

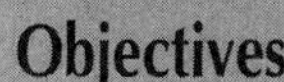

Objectives

- Define critical care nursing.
- Describe the scope of practice of critical care nursing.
- Differentiate between structure, process, and outcome standards for critical care nursing.

To begin the study of critical care nursing, it is necessary to view the specialty within the context of the profession. The purpose of this chapter is to define critical care nursing, describe the scope of practice, and present standards for critical care nursing practice. An understanding of these concepts will facilitate the nurse's ability to practice within a professional framework.

Critical care nursing developed as a specialty in the 1970s. Prior to that decade, most of critical care practice involved care of cardiac patients. Within only a few years critical care evolved to include other areas of practice such as patients with renal, pulmonary, metabolic, and neurological problems. As the practice of critical care nursing evolved and grew, the need for a definition of the practice and standards to guide the practice developed.

Definition

In 1984, the American Association of Critical-Care Nurses' (AACN) defined critical care nursing in the following way:

> In *Nursing, A Social Policy Statement,* the American Nurses' Association defines nursing as "the diagnosis and treatment of human responses to actual or potential health problems." Critical care nursing is that specialty within nursing that deals specifically with human responses to life-threatening problems.

Analysis of this definition reveals several important concepts. The basis of the definition rests with the words *human responses.* Critical care nurses deal with the total human being and his or her response to actual and potential health problems. This suggests that the critical care nurse is involved with prevention as well as cure. Inherent in human response is the notion that the focus of the critical care nurse includes the family and its response in addition to the individual patient's response. Additionally, human response can take the form of a physiological or a psychological phenomenon.

Critical care nursing is specifically concerned with human responses to life-threatening problems. Examples of this, such as trauma or major surgery, seem obvious. However, prevention can also be viewed as appropriate in this definition.

For example, a critical care nurse can teach a patient methods to lower blood cholesterol levels, which may then prevent a life-threatening problem. This definition of critical care nursing helps to guide practice.

Scope of Practice

A scope of practice statement provides a framework within which an individual can provide a particular service. The AACN's *Scope of Critical Care Nursing Practice* statement (AACN, 1986) provides a definition and description of the practice of critical care nursing. The major components of the AACN scope of practice include the critically ill patient, the critical care nurse, and the critical care environment. Central to the scope are nurse-patient interactions.

The Critically Ill Patient

The AACN's scope of practice places the critically ill patient at the center of practice. The patient is "characterized by the presence of, or being at high risk for developing life-threatening problems. The critically ill patient requires constant intensive multidisciplinary assessment and intervention in order to restore stability, prevent complications, and achieve and maintain optimal responses" (AACN, 1986). The critical care nurse is identified as the coordinator for the interventions directed at resolving life-threatening problems.

The Critical Care Nurse

The critical care nurse is a licensed professional who is responsible for ensuring that all critically ill patients receive optimal care. The scope of practice confirms that the critical care nurse practices in accordance with standards and within an ethical framework. The importance of the interaction between the critical care nurse and the critically ill patient is highlighted.

The Critical Care Environment

The critical care environment is viewed from three perspectives. The environment is defined at a primary level by the conditions and circumstances surrounding the direct interaction between the critical care nurse and the critically ill patient. The environment must contain resources that constantly support this interaction, e.g., equipment and supplies.

A second perspective on the critical care environment includes the institution or setting within which critically ill patients receive care. Here critical care management and administrative structure ensure effective care delivery through provision of resources, quality control systems, and maintenance of standards of nursing care.

The third and final perspective on the environment includes all of the factors that influence the provision of care to the critically ill. These include legal, regulatory, social, economic, and political factors.

Standards

A standard has been defined as an optimal level of care against which actual performance is compared (Wright, 1984). Standards serve as guides for clinical practice. They establish goals for patient care and provide mechanisms for nurses to assess achievement of patient goals.

Standards are divided into three categories: structure, process, and outcome. Structure standards present an organizational framework within which care is provided and also reflect the setting in which the process of care takes place. Exam-

Table 1–1. EXAMPLES OF AACN COMPREHENSIVE STRUCTURE AND PROCESS STANDARDS

Structure

1. The critical care unit shall be designed to ensure a safe and supportive environment for critically ill patients and for the personnel who care for them.
2. The critical care unit shall be constructed, equipped, and operated in a manner that protects patients, visitors, and personnel from electrical hazards.

Process Standards

1. Data shall be collected continuously on all critically ill patients wherever they may be located.
2. The identification of patient problems/needs and their priority shall be based upon collected data.

American Association of Critical-Case Nurses. (1989): *Standards for Nursing Care of the Critically Ill*, 2nd ed. Norwalk, CT: Appleton & Lange.

ples of areas included in structure standards are administrative procedures and staffing levels.

Process standards are concerned with nurse performance. Foglesong (1987) defines this as implementation of nursing care, including "assessment, nursing diagnosis, problem identification, plan of intervention, patient education and continuity of care." An example of process standards includes availability of the nursing care plan.

The third type of standards, outcome standards, relate to patient welfare. These standards help to articulate expected patient goals or outcomes. Examples include patient health status and satisfaction with care.

Standards for Critical Care Practice

In 1980, the AACN published the first edition of the *Standards for Nursing Care of the Critically Ill.* A second edition of this work was published in 1989 (AACN, 1989). This volume contains both structure and process standards. Examples of these standards are shown in Table 1-1.

Another publication, *Outcome Standards for Nursing Care of the Critically Ill,* delineates those specific outcomes desired as a result of nursing care delivered (AACN, 1990). The outcome standards suggested by the AACN contain several

Table 1-2. COMPONENTS OF OUTCOME STANDARDS

Nursing Diagnosis

A Nursing diagnosis is "a clinical judgement about an individual, family or community response to actual or potential health problems/life processes which provides the basis for definitive therapy toward achievement of outcomes for which the nurse is accountable" (North American Nursing Diagnosis Association* [NANDA], 1989, p. 6). Each patient problem or condition in the outcome standards is described by using nursing diagnosis terminology.

Specification

Specification of the diagnosis is a differentiation of the diagnosis in areas in which the etiologies or interventions or both are different.

Definition

The definition of the diagnosis, with specification if applicable, expresses the essential nature of the problem or condition and differentiates the diagnosis from other diagnoses.

Defining Characteristics

The defining characteristics are the signs and symptoms that indicate the presence of the problem or condition defined by the nursing diagnosis. They are divided into the traditional subjective (patient reported) and objective (nurse observed) categories for ease of use.

Etiologies/Related Factors

Etiologies and related factors reflect the cause of the problem or condition defined by the nursing diagnosis if it can be determined and/or other factors commonly associated with but not necessarily causative of the problem or condition.

Outcome Standard

The outcome standard is a statement of quality that reflects the desired result for patients with a particular nursing diagnosis.

Outcome Criteria

The outcome criteria are the key physiological and psychosocial measures that determine if the outcome standard has been met.

Interventions

The interventions are nursing actions specifically designed to achieve the desired patient outcome. The interventions listed concentrate on implementation of nursing orders, including patient teaching.

Monitoring

Monitoring is the collection of assessment data on an ongoing basis. Monitoring activities determine the status of the problem or condition defined by the nursing diagnosis and are used to evaluate the effect of the interventions. Evaluation of the status of the problem or condition is the purpose of monitoring activities; monitoring does not include the initial assessment activities performed to make the nursing diagnosis.

Potential Nursing Diagnoses

Potential nursing diagnoses are those problems or conditions that may occur as a result of the problem or condition defined by the original nursing diagnosis.

Selected Related Medical Conditions/Diagnoses

Selected medical conditions/diagnoses are those conditions or diagnoses that commonly are associated with specific nursing diagnoses.

Adapted from American Association of Critical-Care Nurses (1990): *Outcome Standards for Nursing Care of the Critically Ill.* Newport Beach, CA.
* North American Nursing Diagnosis Association (1989). Working definition of nursing diagnosis. *NDX: Nursing Diagnosis Newsletter,* Vol. 16, p. 6.

Table 1–3. EXAMPLES OF OUTCOME STANDARDS

Powerlessness

Definition

The state in which an individual perceives a loss of control over certain events or situations (adapted from Carpenito, L.J. (1987): *Handbook of Nursing Diagnosis.* Philadelphia: J.B. Lippincott. 1987).

Outcome Standard

Sense of control is perceived.

Outcome Criteria

Expresses control over events/situations
Participates in activities of daily living
Participates in decision making

Impaired Skin Integrity

Definition

The state in which an individual's skin is adversely altered or at risk of being adversely altered (North American Nursing Diagnosis Association (1989): *Taxonomy I: With Official Diagnostic Categories (Revised 1989).* St. Louis: C.V. Mosby).

Outcome Standard

Skin is intact, or integrity is improved.

Outcome Criteria

Skin color, texture, turgor, moisture, and temperature normal for patient
Ulcers, lesions, or erythema absent
Tissue epithelialization/granulation at site of impaired skin integrity evident
Mucous membrane intact

Adapted from American Association of Critical-Care Nurses (1990): *Outcome Standards for Nursing Care of the Critically Ill.* Newport Beach, CA.

components. These are listed in Table 1–2. Examples of outcome standards are shown in Table 1–3.

This discussion of outcome standards was designed to be brief and provide an overview of the available resources. The reader is encouraged to review the two above-mentioned publications in some detail to provide a thorough understanding of the topic.

Summary

Definitions of critical care, standards, and scope of practice are important parameters to consider for the nurse entering critical care practice. The reader is challenged to apply the concepts discussed throughout this book to daily practice.

References

American Association of Critical-Care Nurses (1984): *Definition of Critical Care Nursing* (position statement). Newport Beach, CA: Author.

American Association of Critical-Care Nurses (1986): *Scope of Critical Care Nursing Practice* (position statement). Newport Beach, CA: Author.

American Association of Critical-Care Nurses (1989): *Standards for Nursing Care of the Critically Ill,* 2nd ed. Norwalk, CT: Appleton & Lange.

American Association of Critical-Care Nurses (1990): *Outcome Standards for Nursing Care of the Critically Ill.* Newport Beach, CA: Author.

Foglesong, D. (January 1987): Standards promote effective production. *Nursing Management* 18:24–27.

Wright, D. (1984): An introduction to the evaluation of nursing care: A review of the literature. *Journal of Advanced Nursing* 9:457–467.

Chapter 2

Jeanette C. Hartshorn, Ph.D., R.N., FAAN
Denise Ebert, M.S.N., R.N.
Gwenn Scott, M.S.N., R.N., CCRN
Linda Weaver, M.S.N., R.N., CCRN

Individual and Family Response to the Critical Care Experience

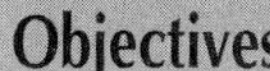

Objectives

- Relate the symptoms of powerlessness and anger in the critically ill to selected nursing interventions.
- Define the causes and treatment of ICU syndrome.
- Discuss the effect of the intensive care environment on circadian rhythm.
- Develop an understanding of the techniques needed for care of the critically ill elderly.
- Define the main needs of the family of the critically ill.
- Discuss techniques that the nurse can use in the development of a career in critical care nursing.

Critical illness is a dramatic event for both the individual and family. In a few situations, some psychological preparation may be possible. For example, patients undergoing open heart surgery frequently schedule the procedure and have an opportunity to learn about the critical care experience before it happens. Many other patients have no warning that a critical illness or injury will strike. Patients who experience trauma and are consequently admitted to the critical care unit have no opportunity to consider the critical care experience. Thus, a major psychological insult is superimposed on a major physiological insult. This psychological insult affects the family as well as the patient. The critical care nurse is in the most important position to not only understand this phenomenon, but to put into operation techniques that will help both patients and families cope with the situation. Psychosocial interventions are as crucial for positive outcome of the critical care experience as any physiological intervention.

The Patient

Patients admitted to the intensive care unit (ICU) are faced with a multitude of stressors. Some obvious stressors related to the ICU environment include loss of privacy, artificial lighting on continuously for 24 hours, lack of windows in the unit, constant noise stemming from the various monitoring and life-support machines, and a lack of meaningful stimuli to the patient.

Ballard (1981) studied the stressors faced by ICU patients and found that the top three stressors were the feeling of being tied down by tubes, being in pain, and being thirsty. Patients viewed all of the various life-support and monitoring equipment attached to them as restricting movement. Being in pain and being thirsty are consequences of the injury or even the treatment of the critical care event. The nurse should be able to eliminate or at least decrease all three stressors by providing adequate pain medication and using comfort measures. However, even with intervention, the presence of these physical stressors can lead to psychological stress. It has been estimated that 30 to 70% of patients experience severe psychological stress (Reigel, 1989) with resulting feelings of powerlessness, anger, and the development of the ICU syndrome.

POWERLESSNESS

Powerlessness is a lack of power. Webster's (1986) dictionary defines powerlessness as being helpless and without authority. When the concept of powerlessness is defined in relation to the ICU environment, the definition changes slightly. Reigel (1989) defines powerlessness as the lack of personal control over events or situations. Another definition by Steinhart (1987) states powerlessness is the inability to make decisions and control the environment. It is not uncommon for the patients to feel powerless when placed in the ICU.

The environment of the ICU contributes to the patient's feeling of powerlessness. First, the patient with a critical illness may feel a lack of control over the disease process. The illness is of such magnitude that the patient was unable to control it at home and needed medical intervention. The illness has led to an ICU admission that has further decreased the patient's control of his/her environment and activities of daily living. Because of the illness, the patient may have lost control over normal bodily functions. A ventilator may be the means of breathing and a Foley catheter of emptying the bladder.

In the ICU, the patient also loses control of other activities of daily living. The nursing and medical staff control when, what, and how to eat. If the patient is allowed to eat, the nurses determine when and assist as needed. Restricted diets are often required and the patient may not be allowed to choose foods he/she enjoys. Frequently, the patient is unable to eat and receives nutrition via the intravenous route or through a nasogastric or gastric tube. Besides nutritional assistance, the patient must rely on the nursing staff for baths, turning, and other activities each of us takes for granted.

Other areas in which the patient loses control are the frequency of family visits and the timing of treatments. The visiting hours are restricted and the patient is unable to see significant others when or as often as desired. The patient frequently has no control as to when treatments such as breathing treatments, physical therapy, and occupational therapy will be done.

Finally, the patient has a lack of knowledge. Knowledge is frequently a source of power, since those who possess knowledge can often control a situation. The patient frequently does not have the knowledge to know that what he/she does affects the situation. The patient with inadequate knowledge about the disease and treatment may imagine the worst. Without adequate knowledge, the patient may think he/she is dying, or that the hardware related to external fixation of fractures is permanent.

When patients feel powerless, they may manifest certain behaviors in a variety of ways. A list of behaviors the patient experiencing powerlessness may exhibit is shown in Table 2–1.

Each patient may manifest different combinations of these behaviors. The powerless patient is often frightened and anxious, which often leads to frustration. Activities and decisions he/she was once capable of making are now being done and decided by others. This frustration can lead to anger, hostility, withdrawal, or depression. These consequences can often delay the recovery period.

Table 2–1. BEHAVIORS EXHIBITED BY PATIENTS EXPERIENCING POWERLESSNESS

Apathy
Withdrawal/Depression
Resignation
Fatalism
Malleability
Low knowledge of illness
Statements of low control
Anxiety
Restlessness
Sleeplessness
Wandering
Aimlessness
Lack of decision making
Aggression
Anger

Data from Roberts, S. L. Behavioral Concepts and the Critically Ill Patient. 2nd ed. East Norwalk, CT, Appleton & Lange, 1986.

There are several nursing interventions that may be helpful. First, recognition of the potential for the presence of feelings of powerlessness is essential. Although not all patients will experience the phenomenon to the same extent, they will all experience it. The nurse can help the patient decrease the feelings of powerlessness by restoring some control to the patient. If it is not harmful to the patient, the nurse can allow the patient to determine when treatments will be given. For example, the patient can decide to have physical therapy in the morning or afternoon, or decide when to get up out of bed to sit in the chair or bathe. Additionally, the nurse can allow the patient to decide where to place personal belongings such as pictures and get-well cards. As the patient's condition improves, more control can be given to the patient. The nurse must be vigilant in identifying situations in which the patient can exercise control.

ANGER

Anger is an emotional defense to protect the individual's integrity to a perceived threat and an agent of harm (Roberts, 1986). Frustration frequently produces anger when one is blocked from achieving a goal. Anger can also be viewed as a derivative of anxiety and powerlessness with both negative and positive effects. Anger that is turned inward, or internalized, can lead to depression, whereas anger that is turned outward, or externalized, can motivate the individual.

The critical care environment has many factors that can lead the patient to become angry. The two most prominent factors are powerlessness and a loss of some kind. Powerlessness with its resulting frustration and anger has already been discussed. The loss in this situation can be a loss of bodily function or of a limb or the perceived loss of one's former life owing to illness, disability, or disfigurement. Both powerlessness and loss can lead to anxiety and frustration.

The patient responds to the anxiety and frustration with anger. The loss or powerlessness is viewed as a threat to the individual, and the individual responds with anger. The behaviors that may be displayed in anger include the following (Roberts, 1986):

Clenching of the muscles or the fist
Turning away
Avoiding eye contact
Silence
Sarcasm
Insulting remarks
Verbal abuse
Argumentativeness
Demanding

Frequently, the nurses, doctors, and family members become the scapegoats as the patient ventilates anger. The patient may verbally lash out at them as a way of coping with the situation. In other cases, the patient may be afraid to show anger for fear of reprisals. Some patients find it frightening to be angry at the people who are delivering the care, since they are totally dependent on these people. If the patient is afraid of being angry at the staff, anger may be directed at the family.

If the patient is unable to externalize the anger, depression may occur. In this instance, the nurse must look for behaviors indicative of depression. Some of the obvious symptoms seen in a depressed patient are loss of interest in people, dissatisfaction, difficulty in making decisions, and crying. Or the depressed patient may express that he/she feels like a failure, is being punished, or has suicidal ideation.

The patient who externalizes the anger may be able to use it as the motivation for getting well. The anger can motivate the patient to change the situation that is the cause of the frustration. For example, if the patient has experienced a myocardial infarction that was partially prompted by a high-cholesterol diet, high blood pressure, and lack of exercise, the anger may motivate the patient to change his/her existing unhealthy behaviors. The nursing staff can utilize this anger to assist the patient in getting well. However, the nurse must first assist the patient in identifying the source of the anger. Additionally, the nurse must give the patient permission to be angry and assist him/her in identifying appropriate ways to express the anger. Above all, the nurses and family must realize that anger is a normal response and can be a healthy indication of coping.

ICU SYNDROME

The ICU syndrome was first studied by Egerton and Kay (1964). Their purpose was to study the psychosis experienced by postcardiotomy patients. Since then, multiple studies have examined the ICU syndrome. Some of the terms used to describe the ICU syndrome are *ICU psychosis, postcardiotomy delirium, postoperative psychosis, intensive care delirium,* and *impaired psychological response.*

The ICU syndrome is defined as a syndrome that occurs on the third to seventh day in the ICU. The common features of the syndrome are clouding of the consciousness, decreased attention span, disorientation, memory loss, and labile emotions. The syndrome occurs in 14% (Layne and Yudofsky, 1971) to 72% (Sadler, 1979) of adult patients admitted to the ICU. It clears within 48 hours after the patient is transferred out of the ICU. Egerton and Kay (1964) noted an absence of the syndrome in children.

The environmental factors that have been identified as causing the ICU syndrome are sleep deprivation, sensory deprivation, and sensory overload. The factors related to the patient are age, severity of illness, history of psychological problems, cardiopulmonary bypass, prolonged surgery and anesthesia time, metabolic abnormalities, and medications.

Sleep deprivation occurs in the ICU as a result of noise, pain, and frequent interruptions of the sleep cycle. Furthermore, the lights are on continuously for 24 hours and there is often a lack of windows to help orient the patient to night and day. Studies on experimental sleep deprivation have shown symptoms similar to patients with ICU syndrome after 2 to 5 days of sleep deprivation. The symptoms dissipated after the subjects had one night of recovery sleep. Likewise, patients with ICU syndrome have a resolution of the symptoms within 1 to 2 days after being transferred out of the ICU.

Besides sleep deprivation, patients in the ICU are also faced with sensory deprivation. Sensory deprivation is defined as a decrease in the amount and intensity of *meaningful* sensory input (Ballard, 1981). The constant noise, lights, technical language, and a lack of familiar faces all constitute sensory deprivation. Everything around the patient is unfamiliar and strange; the familiar environment of home and the family are missing.

Although the constant noise and lights constitute sensory deprivation, they also contribute to sensory overload. Not only is there a lack of meaningful input, but there is an overabundance of unfamiliar input. Sensory overload implies that two or more stimuli are confronting the patient at a greater level than normal. Sensory overload also implies that too many stimuli are confronting the patient at one time and thus causing confusion.

All of these factors lead to the ICU syndrome. The behavioral changes one might notice in these patients are similar to the symptoms related to sleep deprivation, sensory deprivation, and sensory overload. The symptoms commonly associated with the ICU syndrome are shown in Table 2–2.

A main nursing goal for patients with ICU psychosis is to reduce the sleep deprivation, sensory deprivation, and sensory overload confronting the patient. The patient should be reoriented frequently and addressed directly. The nursing staff should not talk about the patient or about another patient and should not have personal conversations within the patient's hearing range as this can increase the confusion. Activities can be planned to allow the patient to have uninterrupted sleep periods of 70 to 90 minutes. Additionally, the nurses can decrease the noise level by decreasing the volume on alarms and limiting or decreasing the volume of idle conversations. Lighting should be adjusted to simulate night and day, which will also help orient the patient and introduce some normal stimuli. The family should be encouraged to visit and bring personal items to place at the bedside. These interventions will help decrease the sleep deprivation, sensory deprivation, and sensory overload that lead to the ICU syndrome.

ALTERATION IN CIRCADIAN RHYTHMS

Circadian rhythms affect everything we do and are easily disrupted in the critically ill. Recognition of the cyclic patterns or rhythms present in all life forms is not new. Records from the fourth

Table 2–2. SYMPTOMS ASSOCIATED WITH THE ICU SYNDROME

Lassitude
Lethargy
Hallucinations/Sound distortions
Disorientation
Confusion
Restlessness
Irritability
Apathy
Poor judgment
Memory disturbance
Delusions
Paranoid ideation
Hostility
Disturbed sense of time
Feeling like one is floating in space
Psychotic behavior

Data from Roberts, S. L. Behavioral Concepts and the Critically Ill Patient. 2nd ed. East Norwalk, CT, Appleton & Lange, 1986.

century BC note that the activities of plants and animals corresponded to the day-night light variations. However, scientific experimentation to identify and closely examine these rhythms did not begin until the 1700s (Moore-Ede et al., 1982). The investigation of biological rhythms in relation to health care has only recently begun (Reinberg and Smolensky, 1983).

The term *circadian rhythm* was first used by Franz Halberg in 1959 to describe those biological rhythms that displayed cycles that were about (Latin *circa*) 24 hours, or one day (Latin *dies*). Research has also demonstrated the existence of rhythms less than 24 hours, termed *ultradian*, and rhythms greater than 24 hours, termed *infradian* (Minors and Waterhouse, 1981). Table 2–3 lists examples of circadian, ultradian, and infradian rhythms (Conroy and Mills, 1970; Moore-Ede et al., 1982).

The exact nature of circadian rhythms is a subject of continuing controversy. The debate centers around whether they are endogenous, that is, located within the organism itself, or exogenous, the result of external environmental cues or synchronizers. The primary synchronizer is thought to be the day-night cycle. Environmental temperature, humidity, noise, odors, food availability, and other factors are also thought to function as synchronizers (Reinberg and Smolensky, 1983). The term *desynchronization* refers to the disruption of the previous 24-hour pattern in a circadian rhythm. Research suggests that a combination of endogenous and exogenous factors are present in the circadian rhythms of most physiological variables (Minors and Waterhouse, 1981). A goal of the critical care nurse is to help the patient maintain circadian synchrony.

Table 2–3. EXAMPLES OF BIOLOGICAL RHYTHMS

- Circadian rhythms
  - Sleep-wakefulness
  - Body temperature
  - Blood pressure
  - Urine flow
- Ultradian rhythms
  - REM/NREM sleep
  - Sinoatrial node firing
  - Nerve action potential
- Infradian rhythms
  - Menstrual cycle
  - Hibernation
  - Aging

Circadian rhythms have been demonstrated in most human physiological processes (Conroy and Mills, 1970). Examples of the most prominent circadian rhythms with implications for critical care nursing are multiple.

Sleep-Wake Rhythms. The sleep-wake cycle of humans under normal conditions exhibits a relatively consistent pattern that is synchronized with the light-dark pattern of the solar day. Most adults sleep an average of 8 hours and are awake 16 hours of each day. Within the sleep period there are well-known sleep stages that follow an ultradian rhythm (Minors and Waterhouse 1981; Moore-Ede et al., 1982).

Thermoregulation Rhythms. Core body temperature is one of the most stable circadian rhythms. Although it is independent of the sleep-wake cycle, under most circumstances the two are closely aligned. In the healthy adult, core body temperature fluctuates 1.5°F during a 24-hour period. The lowest temperature, the trough, occurs in early morning (4 AM to 6 AM) and the highest temperature, the peak, occurs in late afternoon (4 PM to 6 PM) (Cole and Rogers, 1984; Minors and Waterhouse, 1981; Moore-Ede et al., 1982).

Cardiovascular Rhythms. Blood pressure and heart rate exhibit circadian rhythms that are strikingly similar. Both parameters peak in later afternoon and trough in the early morning hours. Both parameters also appear to parallel the sleep-wake cycle and endocrine rhythms. Although the influence of these synchronizers is substantial, research using recently developed monitoring techniques has demonstrated the existence of separate circadian rhythms in each (Cornelissen et al., 1987). Circadian variations have also been demonstrated in vascular tone, stroke volume, and cardiac output (Lemmer, 1987).

There is a discernible circadian pattern in the incidence of angina, myocardial infarctions (MIs), and sudden death. The peak incidence for these occurrences is between 6 AM to 12 noon. The trough lies between 12 midnight and 6 AM (Muller et al., 1985, 1987). Henderson (1982) noted that the mortality subsequent to MIs also demonstrates a circadian rhythm. The highest mortality rates in this study were between 4 PM and 8 PM. Conversely, the lowest mortality rates were between 4 AM and 8 AM.

Respiratory Rhythms. Circadian rhythms have been demonstrated in airway patency and bronchial responsiveness and are believed to play a major role in nocturnal asthma (Barnes, 1985; Smolensky and D'Alonzo, 1987).

Renal Rhythms. Urine volume and urinary excretion of sodium, potassium, chloride, and calcium show a circadian rhythm that peaks during late morning to early afternoon and troughs during the night. The peak and trough of urine volume will remain relatively constant despite large fluctuations in fluid intake (Moore-Ede et al., 1982).

Immunological Rhythms. Circadian rhythms within the immune system have been recorded and are currently being researched. However, the role of endocrine rhythms in the coordination of immune function is widely supported (Angeli and Carandante, 1987). Peak susceptibility to allergens is seen in the late evening and corresponds to the trough of corticosteroid production. Eosinophil production peaks at this time and is thought to be a protective mechanism in response to low corticosteroid levels (Cole and Rogers, 1984).

Cellular Rhythms. Research has also demonstrated the presence of circadian rhythms at the cellular level in humans, especially in cell reproduction. These rhythms appear to be responsible, at least in part, for variation found in tissue absorption and metabolism of drugs and tissue responsiveness to toxins (Mayerbach, 1983; Scheving et al., 1983).

Circadian Rhythms and Critical Care Nursing. The study of human circadian rhythms is growing rapidly. As new information becomes available, it will be essential that the critical care nurse modify nursing interventions to maximize patient outcomes. Table 2-4 outlines some of the ways current knowledge of circadian rhythms can be used to enhance nursing practice by providing nursing interventions to support circadian synchrony.

Table 2-4. NURSING INTERVENTIONS TO SUPPORT CIRCADIAN SYNCHRONY

1. Align nursing care interventions with the individual's usual patterns of activity-rest and sleep-wakefulness to prevent desynchronization.
2. Evaluate temperature elevations based on known circadian peaks and troughs.
3. Plan patient activities to coincide with times of peak cardiovascular responsiveness.
4. Closely monitor patients at risk for cardiovascular and pulmonary events during documented peak periods of morbidity and mortality.
5. Evaluate serum and urine electrolyte levels and urine volume levels based on known circadian fluctuations.
6. Coordinate medication administration to coincide with the circadian fluctuations of the physiological variables of systems they affect. For example, corticosteroid administration should be coordinated with endogenous corticosteroid peaks to prevent suppression of normal adrenal activity. Theophylline is most effective when given in a form that has maximum drug availability at night when airway patency is at its trough.
7. Administer new medications during the morning when histamine activity is at its lowest and corticosteroid levels are optimum to reduce the likelihood of an allergic reaction.
8. Maintain consistent day-night patterns by control of external lighting and temperature.

THE ELDERLY PATIENT

The demographic changes that have influenced the population of the United States have also influenced the population of patients within critical care units. Specifically, the number of elderly patients is increasing. The United States population is projected to increase by 9.2% between 1988 and 2000. The age groups growing the fastest during this period are likely to be the 45- to 59-year age group with a 45% increase, and the 75+ age group with a 98.3% increase between 1988 and 2025 (Spencer, 1984).

The elderly require an increase in the provision of inpatient care. Elderly people account for 30% of all hospital discharges, and 33% of health care expenditures despite the fact that they compose only 12% of the population (U.S. Senate, 1988).

These demographic changes will result in more and more patients over the age of 65 being cared for in critical care units. These patients present multiple challenges to the critical care nurse, since they not only experience a critical event, but most commonly have some chronic illness superimposed on the acute event.

Physiological Changes

Multiple physiological changes accompany the aging process. Every body system, including the processes of mentation and cognition, are affected. The reader is referred to other sources to review these physiological events (see Recommended Reading). In the following discussion, nursing care of the critically ill elderly is highlighted.

Psychosocial Changes

Alteration in Family Process. It is currently projected that 90% of people over the age of 65 do not live in institutions. Shamas (1979) found that 53% of a group of aged over 65 had seen one of their children within the preceding 24 hours. Therefore, critical care nurses can expect that the family will be an important part of the care of the critically ill elderly. Members of the elderly's family may include spouse, children, or grandchildren. Friends as well as pets may also be important members of the elder's "family."

Once recognizing the unique components of the elder's family situation, several nursing interventions may be helpful. Since the family serves as an anchor for the elder, assisting him/her to maintain a strong grasp on reality, it is important to allow adult family members to visit as often as possible. Under some circumstances, it may be necessary to consider special arrangements to allow the elder's grandchildren to visit. The goal of these interventions is to provide an environment for the elder that will support his/her orientation and normal routine as much as possible.

In developing plans to work with family members, it is also important to recall that the research on care of the families of the critically ill has not attended to the specific needs of families of the elderly. Until this database is developed, the critical care nurse can use some of the existing research in combination with experience to provide the best care.

Sensory-Perceptual Alteration. A normal consequence of the aging process is an increase in the threshold needed to produce a response. Therefore, older people need stimuli of greater intensity to respond. For example, older people need greater stimulation to respond to taste; therefore, they frequently prefer spicy to mild foods.

For the critically ill elderly, vision and hearing are the most important senses to consider. In the elderly, the size of the pupil decreases, making the pupil less responsive to light (Ebersole and Hess, 1985). The same change makes the elderly less able to focus on close objects. As the lens of the eye becomes cloudy, thicker, and less elastic, discrimination between colors becomes more difficult. With these changes, it is possible that the elderly may find the intense lights of the intensive care unit very painful. In addition to normal changes in vision, there is an increased incidence of many of the pathologies of the visual system with advancing age—cataracts, glaucoma, senile macular degeneration, and diabetic retinopathy.

Nursing interventions should be developed to reach two goals; limit damage from existing eye disorders and to minimize frustrations imposed by visual loss. To meet the first goal, approaches such as the use of prescribed medications and eye lubricants are important.

To meet the second goal, interventions include frequent assessment of visual ability and being always careful to introduce oneself and to explain procedures. If the patient wears glasses, the correct prescription should be available.

Hearing changes also accompany the aging process. Normally, there is a slowing of nerve transmission that will decrease hearing acuity (Ebersole and Hess, 1985). In addition, many elderly also experience "noise" or "ringing" in the ears that represents a potential normal degenerative process. Both of these phenomena make hearing more difficult.

Interventions to assist the hearing-impaired elder should begin by touching the patient before initiating conversation. While standing close to the patient, speak loudly and slowly. Generally, the use of short phrases and repeating phrases as necessary will improve the elder's ability to hear.

Knowledge Deficit. Aging leads to predictable changes in the cognitive process. One of the changes is difficulty in solving problems; thus, the elderly may easily feel overwhelmed by the changes imposed by the critical care experience. Recalling information and ignoring superfluous data are more difficult for the elderly, which may increase the feeling of being overwhelmed. They may have problems in remembering aspects they have been taught and may have difficulty focusing on important points of teaching or other types of information.

Memory also decreases with age. Studies show, however, that when a learner participates in determining what is to be remembered, they remember better. Frequently, long-term memory in the elderly is preserved, whereas short-term memory is greatly affected. The elderly also experience a slowed reaction time, causing them to need more time for input processing and response.

Alteration in Sleep Patterns. Overall, the elderly experience an increase in the total amount of sleep, which generally occurs as an increase in the number of daytime naps. Although sleep time may be increased, they also experience an increase in the number of nighttime awakenings. Many elderly also need more time to fall asleep.

Some changes in sleep cycles have been identified for the elderly. The total duration and number of shifts into stage 1 (nonrapid eye movement, NREM) sleep are increased (Eliopoulos, 1987). Although the duration of stage 2 sleep remains the same, awakening is more frequent. No changes are seen in stage 3. However, stage 4 appears to decrease with age, so that by age 50, it has decreased by about one half. Stage 4 is almost absent in old age. The amount of REM sleep in the elderly is also decreased.

One of the first steps in improving the elder's sleep pattern is allaying their fears and concerns. Dimming the lights at night, lowering noise, and limiting the number of interruptions while the patient sleeps are important. Napping is a normal sleep pattern for the elderly and should be supported in the critically ill when possible (Kartmann, 1985). Sedatives and hypnotics can be given, but only as a last resort.

The preceding nursing diagnoses represent some of the major ones encountered by critical care nurses caring for the elderly. Nursing care of the elderly is a specialty of its own. Currently, there is very little information available in the care of these individuals while they are critically ill. For that reason, the critical care nurse may wish to utilize gerontology clinical nurse specialists to assist in the development of age-specific nursing care plans for these patients.

The Family

While the experience of being critically ill most directly affects the individual, the family also experiences many changes. In caring for the critically ill, the nurse must recognize the influence of the family on the overall recovery of the individual. When one family member is ill, all family roles and functions are affected. Serious illness precipitates a crisis within the family that can throw a highly organized family into disequilibrium. In a very real sense, the illness or injury of one family member influences all members of the family. The AACN (1989) standards emphasize the importance of assessment of the family and the continual involvement of the family in the nursing care of the patient.

To begin to care successfully for the family, the nurse must identify the framework from which it operates. Thus, the nurse can approach the situation through recognition of the need to provide care for the family as a unit. The nursing role is to be sympathetic to what the family is experiencing, to understand the members, and to provide guidance throughout the experience.

FAMILY ASSESSMENT

Once the patient has been admitted to the critical care unit, an assessment of the family will provide valuable information for the preparation of the nursing care plan. Assessment of the family structure is the first step and is essential before specific interventions can be designed. An evaluation of communication patterns within the family will help to develop an understanding of the role relationships within the family. For example, this assessment can help to reveal the individuals who are involved in making decisions, and how conflicts are resolved within the family. Communication patterns may also illuminate role relationships within the family. As illness changes roles, the nurse begins to evaluate how these changes are implemented and whether or not they are actually acceptable to the individuals. For example, a wife who has been dependent upon her husband for most decisions may be very uncomfortable accepting a more dominant role in the face of her husband's illness. During this time, it is also important to seek an evaluation of the family's values, goals, and aspirations.

Family functioning is another important aspect for the critical care nurse to assess. Observation of the family will help to identify general aspects of interaction among members of the family. Answers to such questions as whether family members get along or if the atmosphere surrounding the family is one of support and nurturance or one of competition will provide important information about the family's ability to work together during a crisis. Other more external factors such as the availability of resources to support the family is another important consideration. For example, availability of child care or friends and neighbors to help with other aspects of daily life are very influential in assisting the family to cope during the crisis of a critical illness.

FAMILY NEEDS

Multiple studies have been completed to identify the needs of families of the critically ill (Bauman, 1984; Daley, 1984; Leske, 1986; Mathis, 1984; Molter, 1979; O'Neill-Norris and Grove, 1986; Rodgers, 1983; Spatt et al., 1986). Results of these studies suggest that information is the highest priority need for families. Throughout the stay within the critical care unit, the family needs a constant flow of information concerning their loved one's status and progress. Several studies have also identified that families seek consistent methods for the delivery of information about the hospital stay. Some facilities have utilized a daily telephone call to a family member or a consistent nurse to work with the family as techniques to meet this need. Families also report the need for updated information as the patient's status changes.

Another major area of needs for the family is related to reassurance. Several studies identified that families wanted to experience "hope." That is, the family members wanted to know that there was a possibility for recovery for their loved one. They report that they want to know that the staff cares about their relative and that the care delivered is the best possible. Some studies also suggest that family members want to feel accepted by the staff so that their needs and questions will be heeded. The reassurance also includes having the information needed in order to alleviate associated anxiety.

Families also report personal needs to be important during this period of time. Personal needs include convenient availability of bathroom facilities, cafeteria, and telephone. Families also report the need for areas in which they can be alone or for private consultation with physicians, counselors, or religious leaders.

INTERVENTIONS

There are specific interventions that the critical care nurse can use while working with the family. Several options are available to help meet the informational needs of the family. Hodovanic (1984) reported on a "telefamily" program in which a daily telephone call to one family member was made by a designated nurse. The purpose of this call was to provide continuous communication with the family. Another method recommended to both provide information and to lessen anxiety was the support group (Richmond et al., 1987).

Adequate education about the experience of being in a critical care unit may also help to meet the family's informational needs. A brochure describing the unit, the personnel caring for the patients, the usual activities, and other specifics is very helpful to the family. With the family's increased anxiety, having a brochure available that reinforces important information is very helpful. As specific questions arise, the family can refer back to the brochure and glean the necessary information.

Several additional strategies may also be beneficial in working with the family. Begin by personalizing communication; that is, call family members by their names. This will demonstrate your sincere interest in them and identify yourself as being responsible for the patient's care. Learn to recognize and respect the family members' usual role behaviors. For example, the wife who is used to close physical contact with her husband will appreciate opportunities to hold her husband's hand and participate in his care. This simple step is likely to greatly decrease her anxiety. The critical care nurse may also find it helpful to role model behavior for the family so they will know how to interact with their loved one.

When the patient's behavior is surprising to the family (confusion, for example), it is helpful to explain the reasons for the behavior to the family. Forewarning them before they enter the patient's room will also help them to keep the patient's behavior in perspective. Above all, the critical care nurse can help the family recognize the temporary nature of the behavior.

The Nurse

STRESSORS

The critical care unit can be a rewarding and satisfying area to work; however, it is not without its stressors. Although all areas of nursing are stressful, critical care is known for the stress it places on nurses. Critical care units are highly technological areas where nurses are required to make rapid life-sustaining and life-saving decisions.

Even very experienced critical care nurses experience the stressors found in the critical care unit. Major stressors reported by nurses are outlined in Table 2-5. Shift work is stressful, but rotating shifts is reported to be even more stressful. Rotating shifts causes a disruption in the nurse's circadian rhythm. Working weekends while other family members and friends are involved in activities can be a stressor. Even with every other weekend off, it never fails that the nurse receives a last-minute invitation from a friend on the scheduled work weekend. Many days are so busy that the nurse is unable to take a break or eat a meal. Constant interruptions

Table 2-5. STRESSORS FOR THE NURSE WORKING IN A CRITICAL CARE UNIT

Shift work
Working weekends
Missed breaks and meals
Constant interruptions
Death
Undignified deaths
Emergency situations
Long-term patients in the acute care setting
Exposure to infectious diseases
Cramped work area
Increased noise level
Burnout among other staff members
Performing non-nursing duties
Floating to other areas
Low salary
Conflict with other departments
Nonsupportive administration
Lack of input into decisions affecting nursing

Data from Randolph, G. L., Price, J. L., and Collins, J. R.: The effects of burnout prevention on burnout symptoms in nurses. Journal of Continuing Education in Nursing 17(2):43–49, 1986.

disrupt the organization of the nurse, thereby adding to the stress.

Another stressor identified by nurses is the death of patients. Although death occurs routinely in the intensive care unit, witnessing patients who die without dignity is particularly stressful. An example of an undignified death is a confused 80-year-old woman from a nursing home who had diabetes and multisystem organ failure. She had a below-the-knee amputation that was bubbling with an infection. Her other leg was pulseless and there were several infected areas on her toes, heel, and lower leg. The physicians continued aggressive therapy with talk of further amputation up to her hip. To add to the complexity of the situation, the family supported all aggressive treatment despite the seemingly hopeless picture. Caring for this patient was extremely stressful for the nurses. The family and the physicians made sporadic visits, but the nurses were with the patient around-the-clock. The physicians and the family did not see the constant pain and suffering of the patient but the nurses did. Sometimes critical care nurses have a difficult time putting this type of situation into perspective and out of their thoughts after they leave the unit.

Emergency situations require rapid decision-making skills that place additional stress on many nurses. However, some nurses report that caring for long-term patients in the acute care setting places more stress on them than emergency situations. Stress is very much an individualized phenomenon.

Other stressors in the work environment are exposure to infectious diseases, cramped work areas, and high noise levels. Other staff members displaying signs of burnout add stress to the critical care nurse. Nurses report that performing nonnursing duties, "floating" to other areas, low salary, and conflict with other departments are sources of stress. Administrators can cause stress when they are nonsupportive and do not seek nursing input into decisions that affect nursing practice. While these factors are stressful to critical care nurses, they are also stressful to nurses working in other areas of the hospital. Obviously, stress is an expected part of the nurse's work. However, if the stress becomes overwhelming, the nurse may experience burnout.

Burnout

DEFINITION

Webster's (1986) dictionary defines burnout as emotional exhaustion from mental stress. This definition, however, does not include the physiological and behavioral responses associated with burnout. The cause of burnout is failure to cope with job stressors. In addition, unrealistic goals, low self-esteem, self-criticism, and overcommitment are factors associated with burnout. Burnout has been attributed to the workaholic, Type A personality (Swogger, 1986). However, burnout is contagious and every nurse is at risk for burnout.

Symptoms

Burnout occurs gradually. Maslach (1976) describes four stages of burnout (Table 2–6). In the

Table 2–6. MASLACH'S FOUR STAGES OF BURNOUT

1. Emotional and physical exhaustion
2. Negativism, cynicism
3. Self-isolation
4. Terminal burnout

Data from Maslach, C.: Burnout. Human Behavior 5(9):18–20, 1976.

first stage, the nurse shows signs of emotional and physical exhaustion. Emotionally, the nurse has difficulty going to work. Physically, the nurse feels tired and is prone to headaches and colds. In the second stage, the nurse is cynical and negative toward coworkers and patients. As burnout progresses into the third stage, the nurse isolates herself/himself and performs as little work as necessary. The nurse only wants to perform the job and go home. The final stage is terminal burnout. This stage is manifested by total disgust for humanity in general. According to Maslach (1976), burnout may include physiological, behavioral, and emotional symptoms (Table 2–7).

Prevention

Burnout can be prevented by recognizing stress overload. Since critical care units are filled with stressful conditions, the nurse needs to learn stress-reduction methods. These methods can be as simple as taking a break and listening to a stress-reduction tape to practicing visual imagery (Table 2–8). A technique utilized by one nurse is to go to his car and read the newspaper on break. He says when he comes back into the hospital, he feels fresh, like he is coming in at the beginning of the shift. Nurses are encouraged to take breaks off the unit, take regular days off, and take extra time if signs of early burnout are observed.

As burnout is contagious, so is optimism. Nurses can work to surround themselves with optimistic coworkers. Focusing on the positive rather than the negative aspects of one's job and life may be helpful. Critical care nurses can also improve their odds against burnout by making time for themselves (e.g., read a favorite book, hobbies), attending assertiveness training and time-management courses, and developing problem-solving skills. Ceslowitz (1989) performed a study on burnout and coping among hospital staff nurses. The results showed lower burnout scores in nurses who used problem solving, used positive reappraisal, sought social support, and used self-controlled coping.

For the person with low self-esteem, Husted et al. (1989) recommend self-esteem enhancement to reduce the chances of burnout. Burnout can be prevented by recognizing the signs and symptoms. Awareness of the signs and symptoms of burnout is the first step in halting the process. Like an alcoholic who must first admit he/she is an alcoholic for successful therapy, so must a nurse experiencing burnout admit feelings of burnout.

Table 2–7. SYMPTOMS OF BURNOUT

Physiological	Behavioral	Emotional
Fatigue	Increased absenteeism	Withdrawal from work and family
Headaches	Impatience	Depression
Cold, clammy hands	Alcohol and drug addiction	Irritability
Nausea/Vomiting	Rigidity	Anger
Upset stomach	Accident prone	Indifference
Diarrhea	Low productivity	Detachment
Muscle tension	Overactivity	Hostility
Elevated blood pressure	Compulsive eating	Avoidance
Excessive urination	Inability to eat	Pessimism
Profuse sweating	Forgetfulness	Crying
Increased respirations	Restlessness	Anxiety
Increased pulse rate	Sleeplessness	Frustration
	Loss of interest	

Adapted from Maslach, C.: Burnout. Human Behavior 5(9):18–20, 1976.

Table 2–8. PREVENTION OF BURNOUT

- Recognize symptoms
- Learn stress-reduction methods
- Take breaks away from nursing unit
- Take time off
- Surround yourself with optimistic coworkers
- Make time for yourself
- Attend assertiveness training
- Attend time-management courses
- Develop problem-solving skills
- Do not set unrealistic goals
- Enhance your self-esteem

STRATEGIES FOR JOB SATISFACTION AND A SUCCESSFUL CAREER

A career is defined as one's progress through life and a profession. A nurse can move from one job to another and start at the bottom of the pay and benefits scale each time. A nurse can have many jobs but never have a career. A career includes additional responsibilities and salary. Any nurse can have a job, but in order for nursing to be a profession, nurses need careers.

A nurse who has been employed in the critical care unit for 1 year since graduation listed 5 tips for the new graduate in the critical care unit.

1. Ensure that a critical care course and a preceptor program will be provided.

2. Ensure that you feel comfortable with the preceptor. If not, do not worry about hurting someone's feelings. You need a good learning environment!

3. Attend some seminars on self-image, communication, and assertiveness. These will help you give a more professional image and you will feel more professional.

4. *Always* ask questions, no matter how stupid you feel they may sound. It is more stressful to pretend you know something than to admit you do not know and to learn it.

5. Do not work overtime for the first few months. This can be very stressful. Take time to rest and absorb what you have learned.

■ Continuing Education

Increased job satisfaction occurs when the nurse knows decisions were the best possible choices in the patient's care. Acquisition of knowledge through continuing education enables nurses to make these sound decisions. The increased level of competence helps reduce the stressors related to lack of knowledge. Many high-quality, low-cost seminars are available. A professional nurse must assume the responsibilities for educational seminars, including the cost of the seminar. The nonprofessional nurse assumes the employer is responsible for the cost of seminars and paid days off. Another alternative is to take advantage of seminars sponsored by an employer.

■ Summary

The experience of critical illness has a profound effect on the individual, family, and the nurse. This chapter has provided information concerning the response of these groups to the experience. By understanding the experience, it will become possible to develop strategies to lessen potential negative effects.

■ References

American Association of Critical-Care Nurses (1989): *Standards for Nursing Care of the Critically Ill.* 2nd ed. Norwalk, CT: Appleton & Lange.

Angeli, A., and Carandante, F. (1987): An update on clinical chronoendocrinology. In: W. T. J. M. Hekkens, G. A. Kerkhof, and W. J. Rietveld (eds.). *Advances in the Biosciences:* Vol. 73, *Trends in Chronobiology.* New York: Pergamon Press, pp. 319–334.

Ballard, K. S. (1981): Identification of environmental stressors for patients in a surgical intensive care unit. *Issues in Mental Health Nursing* 3:89–108.

Barnes, P. J. (1985): Circadian variation in airway function. *American Journal of Medicine* 79(6A):5–9.

Bauman, C. C. (1984): Identifying priority concerns of families of ill patients. *Dimensions of Critical Care Nursing* 3:313–319.

Ceslowitz, S. B. (1989): Burnout and coping strategies among hospital staff nurses. *Journal of Advanced Nursing* 14(7):553–557.

Cole, F. L., and Rogers, B. L. (1984): Biological rhythms: Implications for critical care. *Critical Care Nurse* 4(6):30–35.

Conroy, R. T., and Mills, J. N. (1970): *Human Circadian Rhythms.* London: Churchill.

Cornelissen, G., Scarpelli, P. T., Halberg, F., Halberg, J., Halberg, F., and Halberg, E. (1987): Cardiovascular rhythms: Their implications and applications in medical research and practice. In W. T. J. M. Hekkens, G. A. Kerkhof, and W. J. Rietveld (eds.). *Advances in the Biosciences:* Vol. 73, *Trends in Chronobiology.* New York: Pergamon Press, pp. 335–357.

Daley, L. (1984): The perceived immediate needs of families with relatives in the intensive care setting. *Heart and Lung* 13:231–237.

Ebersole, P., and Hess, P. (1985): *Toward Healthy Aging.* St. Louis, C. V. Mosby.

Egerton, N., and Kay, J. H. (1964): Psychological disturbances associated with open-heart surgery. *British Journal of Psychiatry* 110:1365–1370.

Eliopoulos, C. (1987): *Gerontological Nursing.* Philadelphia: J. B. Lippincott.

Hayter, J. (1983): Sleep behaviors of older persons. *Nursing Research* 32(4):242–246.

Henderson, V. V. (1982): Circadian rhythm and hours of postmyocardial infarction mortality. *Journal of Emergency Nursing* 8(2):63–66.

Hodovanic, B. H., Reardon, D., Reese, W., and Hedges, B. (1984): Family crisis intervention program in the medical intensive care unit. *Heart and Lung* 13(3):243–249.

Husted, G. L., Miller, M. C., and Wilczynski, E. M. (1989): Retention is the goal: Extinguish burnout with self-esteem enhancement. *Journal of Continuing Education in Nursing* 20(6):244–248.

Kartmann, J. L. (1985): Sleep and the elderly critical care patient. *Critical Care Nurse* 5(6):52–56.

Layne, O. L., and Yudofsky, S. C. (1971): Postoperative psychosis in cardiotomy patients. *New England Journal of Medicine* 273:287–292.

Lemmer, B. (1987): Chronopharmacology of cardiovascular medications. In W. T. J. M. Hekkens, G. A. Kerkhof, and W. J. Rietveld (eds.). *Advances in the Biosciences:* Vol. 73, *Trends in Chronobiology.* New York: Pergamon Press, pp. 219–243.

Leske, J. S. (1986): Needs of relatives of critically ill patients: A follow-up. *Heart and Lung* 15:189–193.

Maslach, C. (1976): Burnout. *Human Behavior* 5(9):18–20.

Mathis, M. (1984): Personal needs of family members of critically ill patients with and without acute brain injury. *Journal of Neurosurgical Nursing* 16:36–44.

Mayerbach, H. (1983): An overview of the chronobiology of cellular morphology. In A. Reinberg and M. H. Smolensky (eds.). *Biological Rhythms and Medicine: Cellular, Metabolic, Physiopathologic, and Pharmacologic Aspects.* New York: Springer-Verlag, pp. 47–78.

Minors, D. S., and Waterhouse, J. M. (1981): *Circadian Rhythms and the Human.* Boston: Wright.

Molter, N. C. (1979): Needs of relatives of critically ill patients: A descriptive study. *Heart and Lung* 8:332–339.

Moore-Ede, M. C., Sulzman, F. M., and Fuller, C. A. (1982): *The Clocks That Time Us: Physiology of the Circadian Timing System.* Cambridge, MA: Harvard University Press.

Muller, J. E., Stone, P. H., Turi, Z. G., Rutherford, J. D., Czeisler, C. A., Poole, W. K., Passamani, E., Roberts, R., and Robertson, T. et al. (1985). Circadian variation in the frequency of onset of acute myocardial infarction. *New England Journal of Medicine* 313(21):1315–1322.

Muller, J. E., Ludmer, P. L., Willich, S. N., Tofler, G. H., Aylmer, G., Klangos, I., and Stone, P. H. (1987): Circadian variation in the frequency of sudden cardiac death. *Circulation* 75:131–138.

O'Neill-Norris, L., and Grove, S. K. (1986). Investigation of selected psychosocial needs of family members of critically ill patients. *Heart and Lung* 15:194–199.

Randolph, G. L., Price, J. L., and Collins, J. R. (1986): The effects of burnout prevention training on burnout symptoms in nurses. *Journal of Continuing Education in Nursing* 17(2):43–49.

Reigel, B. (1989): Stressor of critically ill patients. In B. Reigel and D. Ehrenreich (eds.). *Psychological Aspects of Critical Care Nursing.* Rockville, MD: Aspen, pp. 17–29.

Reinberg, A., and Smolensky, M. H. (1983): *Biological Rhythms and Medicine: Cellular, Metabolic, Physiopathologic, and Pharmacologic Aspects.* New York: Springer-Verlag.

Richmond, T. S., Metcalf, J. A., and Winterhalter, J. (1987): Support group for families of acute neurological patients. *Journal of Neuroscience Nursing* 19(1):40–43.

Roberts, S. L. (1986): *Behavioral Concepts and the Critically Ill Patient.* 2nd ed. East Norwalk, CT: Appleton & Lange.

Rodgers, C. D. (1983): Needs of relatives of cardiac surgery patients during the critical care phase. *Focus on Critical Care* 10(5):50–55.

Sadler, P. D. (1979): Nursing assessment of postcardiotomy delirium. *Heart and Lung* 8:745–750.

Scheving, L. E., Pauly, J. E., Tsai, T. H., and Scheving, L. A. (1983): Chronobiology of cellular proliferation: Implications for cancer chemotherapy. In A. Reinberg and M. H. Smolensky (eds.). *Biological Rhythms and Medicine: Cellular, Metabolic, Physiopathologic, and Pharmacologic Aspects.* New York: Springer-Verlag, pp. 79–130.

Shamas, E. (1979): The family as support system in old age. *Gerontologist* 9:169–175.

Smolensky, M. H., and D'Alonzo, G. E. (1987): Nocturnal asthma: Circadian components and implications for chronotherapeutic strategies. In W. T. J. M. Hekkens, G. A. Kerkhof, and W. J. Rietveld (eds.). *Advances in the Biosciences:* Vol. 73, *Trends in Chronobiology.* New York: Pergamon Press, pp. 243–260.

Spatt, L., Ganas, E., Hying, S., Kirsch, E., and Koch, M. (1986): Informational needs of families of intensive care patients. *Quarterly Review Bulletin* 12:16–21.

Spencer, G. (1984). *Projections of the Population of the United States by Age, Sex and Race: 1983 to 2080.* Washington, D.C.: U.S. Department of Commerce, Bureau of the Census.

Steinhart, M. J. (1987): Psychosocial concerns of critically ill patients and their families. In I. A. Fein and M. A. Strosberg (eds.). *Managing the Critical Care Unit.* Rockville, MD: Aspen, pp. 325–337.

Swogger, G. (1986): The Type A personality, overwork, and career burnout. *Dental Clinics of North America* 30(4)(suppl.):537–544.

U.S. Senate Special Committee on Aging Report (1988).

Webster's Third New International Dictionary (1986). Springfield, MA: Merriam-Webster.

Recommended Reading

Baker, C. F. (1984): Sensory overload and noise in the ICU: Sources of environmental stress. *Critical Care Quarterly* 3:66–79.

Benner, Z. R. (1987): Nursing elderly cardiac clients. *Critical Care Nurse* 7(2):78–87.

Carnevali, D. L., and Patrick, M. (1986): Nursing management for the elderly. Philadelphia: J. B. Lippincott.

Helton, M. C., Gordon, S. H., and Nunnery, S. L. (1980): The correlation between sleep deprivation and the intensive care syndrome. *Heart and Lung* 9(3):464–468.

Matteson, M. A., and McConnell, E. S. (1988): *Gerontological Nursing.* Philadelphia: W. B. Saunders.

Morath, M. J., and Lynch, M. (1989): Intensive care psychosis. In M. S. Sommers (ed.). *Difficult Diagnosis in Critical Care Nursing.* Rockville, MD: Aspen, pp. 193–209.

Wallace-Barnhill, G. (1989): Psychological problems for patients, families and health professionals. In W. Shoemaker, S. Ayers, A. Grenvik, P. R. Holbrook, and W. L. Thompson (eds.). *Textbook of Critical Care.* 2nd ed. Philadelphia, W. B. Saunders, pp. 1414–1420.

Wilson, V. S. (1987): Identification of stressors related to patient's psychological responses to the surgical intensive care unit. *Heart and Lung* 16(3):267–273.

PART

II

Tools for the Critical Care Nurse

Chapter

3

Stephanie Woods, R.N., M.S.N., CCRN

Understanding Basic Electrocardiography and Interpreting Dysrhythmias

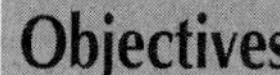

Objectives

At the completion of this chapter, the learner should be able to:

- Understand the basics of electrocardiography.
- Interpret the basic dysrhythmias of the sinoatrial node, atrioventricular node, atria, and ventricles.
- Treat the basic dysrhythmias based on the general therapeutic principles.
- Understand the basic concepts of cardiac pacing.

The ability to analyze and interpret dysrhythmias is a fundamental skill required of the critical care nurse. The objective for this chapter is to provide a basic understanding of electrocardiography for the purpose of analyzing and interpreting cardiac dysrhythmias. Electrocardiography is the process of creating a visual tracing of the electrical activity of the cells in the heart. This tracing is called the electrocardiogram (ECG).

The critical care nurse often deals with patients who are having their electrocardiograms monitored. Whether these patients are encountered in the acute setting of the critical care unit or on intermediate or step-down units, the expectation remains the same. The nurse must have a clear understanding of electrocardiography and be able to quickly assess and treat the patient's cardiac rhythm.

Basic Electrophysiology

AUTOMATICITY

The electrocardiographic tracing is our evidence that the cardiac muscle is generating electrical activity. The basis for this electrical activity is automaticity. Automaticity is what makes the heart muscle different from other forms of muscle in the human body. Automaticity simply means that the cardiac muscle can generate its own electrical activity, even during brief times when blood supply or nervous stimulation is absent.

Students demonstrate the concept of automaticity in basic biology courses. When the heart of a small animal is dissected out of the body it continues to beat, although blood and nervous supply have been removed. In the human body, special groups of cells generate automatic impulses for the purpose of exciting the remainder of the heart's muscle cells. While this process is facilitated by blood flow from the coronary arteries and stimulation from the sympathetic and parasympathetic nervous systems, the heart can continue to generate electrical activity for a brief time after blood and nervous supply have ceased.

The Cardiac Cycle

The cardiac cycle is composed of both the electrical activity due to automaticity and the mechanical, or muscular, response known as contraction. The electrical activity can be divided into two phases called depolarization and repolarization. The mechanical, or muscular, response is divided into diastole and systole. Depolarization is the active phase of electrical activity. Repolarization is the resting phase during which electrical activity is minimal. Both phases occur as a result of the movement of the electrolytes sodium and potassium across the cardiac cell membrane.

Both sodium and potassium are positively charged ions. This seems ironic, since the interior of the cardiac cell is normally in a negatively charged state. This negatively charged state is referred to as the cardiac cell's resting membrane potential (RMP). The normal resting membrane potential is −90 millivolts (mV) when the cell is in a repolarized state. Although the cardiac cell is normally in a negative state, it is the very presence of this negative state that stimulates the formation of an electrical impulse, or the beginning of depolarization.

Sodium is found outside and potassium inside the cardiac cell just before depolarization begins. The movement of the positively charged sodium ions into the cardiac cell begins the active electrical process known as depolarization. Depolarization is considered an active process because cellular energy in the form of adenosine triphosphate (ATP) is required. In response to the influx of sodium, the positively charged potassium ions begin to move to the outside of the cardiac cell. Potassium's movement leads to a slightly less positive or less negative state preferred by the cardiac cell.

Toward the end of depolarization, sodium will cease its movement into the cardiac cell and potassium will continue its movement to the outside of the cardiac cell. The net result will be a restoration of the normal RMP of −90 mV and the resting phase, or repolarization, will begin. Sodium and potassium are then returned to their proper places inside or outside the cell via the sodium-potassium pump. Again, it is this return to a resting, or repolarized state, that will stimulate the next depolarization.

Repolarization of the cardiac cell leads to a resting state for the muscle. *Diastole* is the term used when the muscle is in a resting, or uncontracted, state. It is during this resting state that the ventricles are filled with blood from the atria. A sufficient time of rest is necessary to adequately fill the ventricles before the next depolarization and subsequent systole.

RELATIONSHIP BETWEEN ELECTRICAL ACTIVITY AND MUSCULAR CONTRACTION

Under normal circumstances, depolarization is followed by contraction of a cardiac muscle fiber. The term *systole* refers to the contraction of the cardiac muscle.

It is important to understand that the electrocardiographic tracing, henceforth known as the ECG tracing, is evidence of electrical activity only. The presence of an ECG pattern does not necessarily ensure that the patient's heart is also contracting. To confirm that cardiac muscle contraction, or systole, is occurring, clinical signs such as a palpable pulse and the presence of an adequate blood pressure are sought.

Nurses may encounter situations in which a patient is pronounced dead despite the fact that there is an ECG tracing present. These patients are most often suffering from terminal disease processes for which no cure is possible, or they may be the victims of unsuccessful resuscitation efforts. A patient is pronounced dead when no pulse or blood pressure can be established. Despite the fact that the heart is no longer contracting and pumping blood to the coronary arteries and the nervous tissues, the patient's heart may continue to generate electrical impulses, thereby creating an electrocardiographic tracing.

In this scenario, automaticity continues despite lack of blood and nervous supply. The length of time that the heart can continue to create electrical impulses varies, but the electrical activity will usually cease within minutes. In this case, there is electrical activity without subsequent muscle contraction. This phenomenon is referred to as electromechanical dissociation, or EMD (American Heart Association, 1987).

NORMAL CARDIAC CONDUCTION PATHWAY

Theoretically, any cardiac cell can generate an electrical impulse. However, under normal conditions, only special groups of cardiac cells are responsible for impulse generation and conduction. These special cells make up the normal cardiac conduction pathway (Fig. 3-1). The cardiac cells are networked so that depolarization can spread easily from cell to cell. Depolarization normally begins in the sinoatrial (SA), or sinus, node, a special group of cardiac cells located high in the right atrium. The SA node is often referred to as the master, or dominant, pacemaker of the heart. This dominance is due to the SA node's anatomical position as well as its intrinsic ability to generate 60 to 100 beats per minute under normal circumstances. Once the impulse is formulated in the SA node, it is conducted through the atria via the internodal pathways. These pathways connect the SA and the atrioventricular (AV) nodes and are responsible for conducting the impulse throughout the right and left atria.

As stated in Chapter 8, the atria serve as reservoirs to collect blood returning from the head, body, and lungs. The right atrium receives deoxygenated blood from the head via the superior vena cava and from the body via the inferior vena cava. The left atrium receives oxygenated blood returning from the lungs.

Atrial depolarization precedes atrial contraction. The time during which atrial depolarization is occurring correlates with the time the atria are draining their blood into the ventricles. Most of this process will occur as a result of gravity flow. However, as depolarization ends, the atria will contract, sending any remaining blood down to the ventricles. Many sources refer to atrial systole as atrial kick. Contraction of the atria results in roughly a 30% increase in the blood sent to the ventricles, thereby dramatically affecting stroke volume and cardiac output for the next ventricular systole (Guzzetta and Dossey, 1984).

From the atria, depolarization proceeds to the AV node, which sits in the middle of the heart between the upper chambers (atria) and the lower chambers (ventricles). The AV node has two very important functions. First, the AV node delays entry of the electrical impulse into the

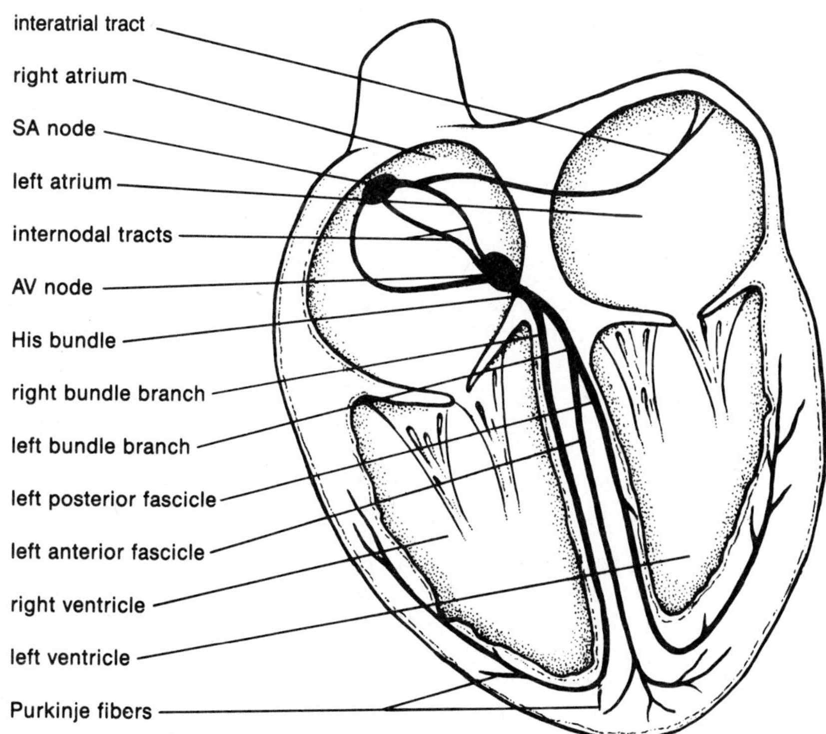

Figure 3-1. Normal cardiac conduction pathway. (From Patel, J., McGowan, S., and Moody, L.: Arrhythmias: Detection, Treatment, and Cardiac Drugs. Philadelphia, W. B. Saunders, 1989, Fig. 1, p. 2.)

ventricles. If the impulse immediately proceeds into the ventricle, contraction occurs before the ventricles have had the necessary time to fill with blood from the atria. The result would be a decreased stroke volume for the next systole, and therefore a decrease in cardiac output. This delay in impulse conduction is very short, only 0.02 second; however, it does allow for adequate ventricular filling.

A second important function of the AV node is to act as a back-up pacemaker for the heart should the SA node fail. When acting as the back-up pacemaker, the AV node generates 40 to 60 beats per minute under normal conditions. The AV node can emerge as the dominant pacemaker when the SA node's rate falls below 40 beats per minute, or when there is increased automaticity in the AV node.

Increased automaticity in the AV node can result in an increased heart rate. If the AV node is able to beat faster than the SA node, it can temporarily take over as the dominant pacemaker. Stress, caffeine, and nicotine are common causes of increased automaticity (Fenstermacher, 1989).

Once ventricular filling has been accomplished, the impulse leaves the AV node and moves down into the ventricles via the common bundle of His. The bundle of His is a thick cord of nerve fibers that runs down the first one-third of the ventricular septum. The common bundle then divides into the right and left bundle branches. The right bundle branch runs down the right side of the ventricular septum, and the left bundle branch runs down the left. The bundle branches have divisions known as fascicles. The right bundle branch has one division, or fascicle. The left bundle branch divides into two fascicles, the anterior-superior and the posterior-inferior. The large muscle mass of the left ventricle requires two fascicles for adequate depolarization, whereas the smaller right ventricle requires only one (see Fig. 3–1).

The impulse first enters the left ventricle via the left bundle branch, then moves across the septum for conduction down the right bundle branch. The impulse enters the left ventricle first so as to allow more time for its depolarization. However, despite this slight lead time, the overall effect is virtually simultaneous depolarization of both ventricles. From the bundle branches the electrical impulse is carried deep within the ventricular muscle by fine conductive fibers known as Purkinje fibers. The Purkinje fibers also act as a final back-up pacemaker for the heart. Should both the SA and AV nodes fail, the Purkinje fibers could generate an intrinsic rhythm of 15 to 40 beats per minute.

In summary, any change in the normal generation or conduction of impulses will lead to the development of dysrhythmias. Therefore, a thorough understanding of the normal conduction pathway and its intrinsic capabilities is prerequisite to understanding the genesis of dysrhythmias.

The 12-Lead ECG System

When monitoring electrical activity of the heart, the bedside practitioner has 12 leads at his/her disposal. There are three standard limb leads, three augmented limb leads, and six precordial leads.

STANDARD LIMB LEADS

The three limb leads are designated as leads I, II, and III. Limb leads are placed anywhere on the arms and legs. These leads are bipolar, meaning that a positive lead is placed on one limb and a negative lead is placed on another.

Electricity flows from negative to positive. Lead I records the flow of electricity from a negative lead on the right arm to a positive lead on the left arm. Lead II records activity between a negative lead on the right arm and a positive lead on the left arm. Lead III records activity between a negative lead on the left arm and a positive lead on the left leg (Fig. 3–2). The normal ECG waveforms are upright in the limb leads, with lead II producing the most upright waveforms.

AUGMENTED LIMB LEADS

The augmented limb leads are designated aVR, aVL, and aVF. These leads are unipolar, meaning that they record electrical flow in only one direction. A reference point is established in the center of the heart and electrical flow is recorded from that reference point toward the right arm (aVR), the left arm (aVL), and the feet (aVF) (Fig. 3–3). The "a" in these leads means augmented, and because these leads produce small ECG complexes, they must be augmented or enlarged for analysis. The ECG machine increases the size of these complexes 1.5 times. Normally, the ECG complexes will be upright or positive in lead aVF and downward or negative in aVR. Lead aVL usually produces an equiphasic QRS complex. This means that half of the complex

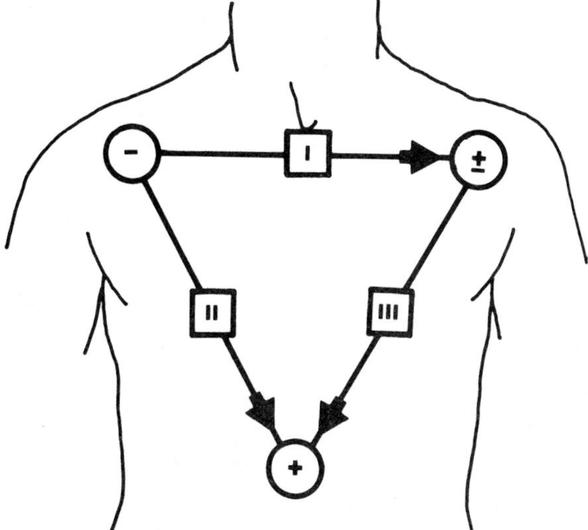

Figure 3-2. The bipolar limb leads. (From Abedin, Z., and Conner, R.: Twelve-Lead ECG Interpretation. Philadelphia, W. B. Saunders, 1989, Fig. 2-1, p. 15.)

rises above the baseline and half falls below the baseline (Fig. 3-4). The augmented leads are monitored using the limb leads already in place.

PRECORDIAL LEADS

The six precordial leads are positioned on the chest wall directly over the heart. The landmarks for placement of these leads are the intercostal spaces, sternum, and clavicular and axillary lines.

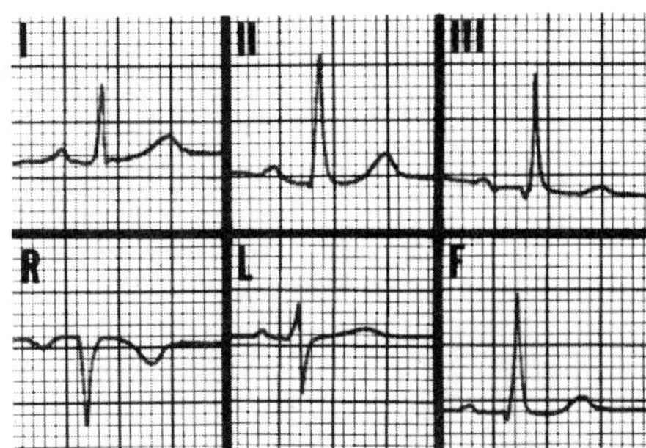

Figure 3-4. Note positive QRS complex in aVF and negative QRS complex in aVR. The QRS in aVL is equiphasic. Note that half of the QRS complex falls below the baseline and half rises above the baseline. (From Abedin, Z., and Conner, R.: Twelve-Lead Interpretation. Philadelphia, W. B. Saunders, 1989, Fig. 2-23, p. 32.)

Positions for these six leads are as follows (Fig. 3-5):

V_1 – Fourth intercostal space, right sternal border

V_2 – Fourth intercostal space, left sternal border

V_3 – Halfway between V_2 and V_4

V_4 – Fifth intercostal space, proximal anterior axillary line

V_5 – Fifth intercostal space, distal anterior axillary line

V_6 – Fifth intercostal space, midaxillary lines

The precordial leads are particularly useful in the localization of anterior and lateral myocardial

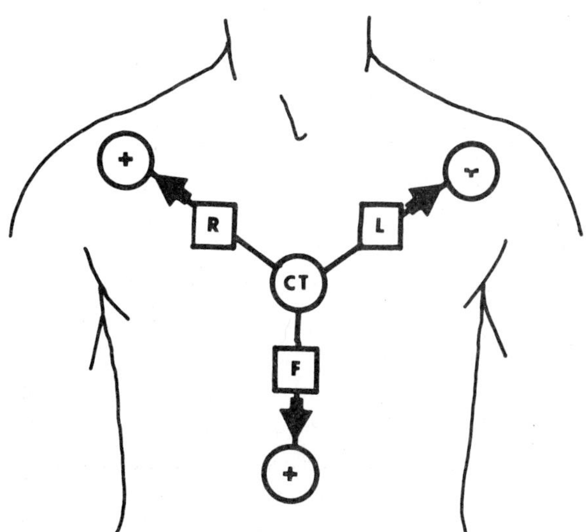

Figure 3-3. The unipolar limb leads. (From Abedin, Z., and Conner, R.: Twelve-Lead ECG Interpretation. Philadelphia, W. B. Saunders, 1989, Fig. 2-2, p. 15.)

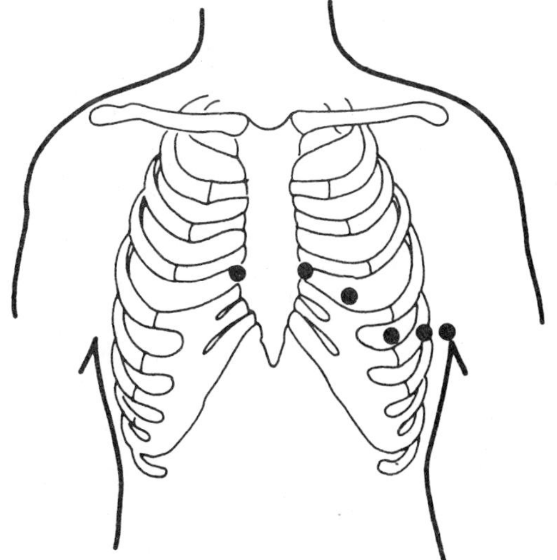

Figure 3-5. The precordial leads. (From Conover, M. B.: Understanding Electrocardiography: Arrhythmias and 12-Lead ECG. St. Louis, C. V. Mosby, 1988, Fig. 5-2.)

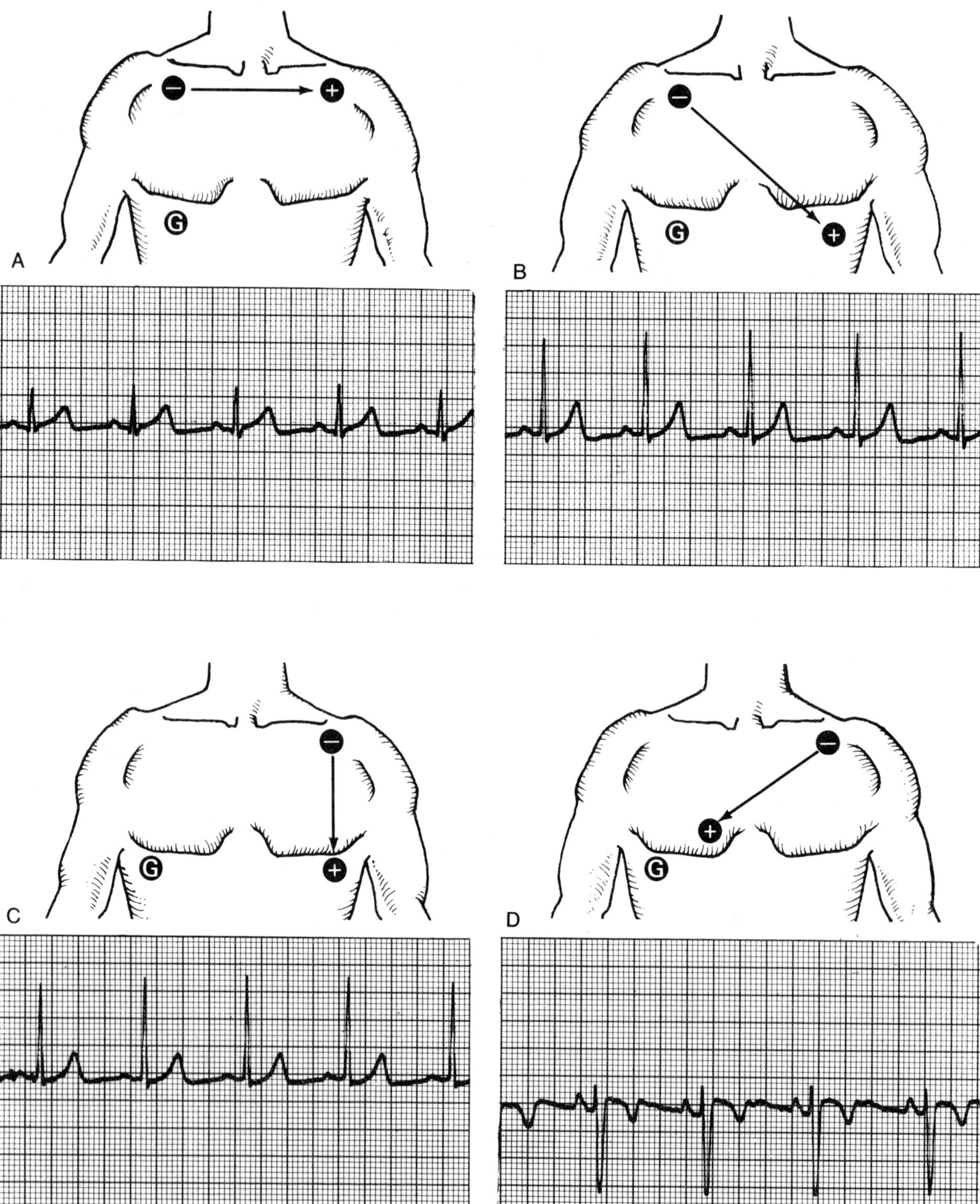

Figure 3–6. Limb leads and MCL1 electrode placement and their respective waveforms: (A) lead I, (B) lead II, (C) lead III, and (D) MCL1. (Reproduced with permission. Textbook of Advanced Cardiac Life Support. 1987, 1990. Copyright American Heart Association, Chap. 5, Fig. 8.)

ischemia, injury, and infarction. Since these leads lay directly over the surface of the heart, changes in the normal ECG can indicate which areas of the heart are experiencing difficulty. V_1 lies over the right ventricle, V_2 and V_3 lie over the ventricular septum, V_3 and V_4 lie over the anterior or frontal surface of the left ventricle, and V_5 and V_6 lie over the lateral, or side, surface of the left ventricle. None of the 12 leads discussed records activity directly over the posterior, or back side, of the heart.

In the clinical setting, the standard limb leads are most often used for monitoring. Lead II, in particular, is often preferred by novice practitioners, since it produces upright, or positive, waveforms. Another useful cardiac lead is the modified chest lead, or MCL1. This lead simulates the precordial lead V_1. A negative electrode is placed on the left, just below the midclavicle. The positive electrode is placed at the right sternal border and between the fourth and fifth intercostal spaces. This is the same position as for V_1 (Fig. 3-6).

The MCL1 allows for earlier detection of dysrhythmias, including changes associated with myocardial ischemia, and diagnosis of bundle branch blocks. It can also be helpful for differentiating whether abnormal beats are arising from the right versus the left ventricle. The MCL1 typically produces negative P, Q, R, S, and T waveforms (Alspach, 1991).

Many bedside monitors in critical care units have the capability of doing 12-lead ECGs. With the ability to monitor any of 12 leads, the practitioner can choose the lead that produces the clearest and most upright waveforms. Often two different leads can be displayed on the same patient simultaneously. A complete 12-lead ECG is usually done daily on patients with cardiac disease. A 12-lead ECG is also obtained when the patient experiences a change in cardiac status, particularly chest pain.

In most monitored settings, it is protocol to obtain and post a 6-second strip of the patient's rhythm every 4 hours. In addition to scheduled times, a rhythm strip should be obtained when the practitioner assumes care of a patient. Again, rhythm strips should also be obtained when a patient experiences any change in cardiac status.

The remainder of this chapter deals with analysis of rhythm strips rather than analysis of 12-lead ECGs.

Analyzing the Basic ECG Tracing

Prior to the discussion of the normal ECG tracing, it is helpful to discuss how waveforms and intervals are measured. ECG paper has standard measures, whether obtaining single-lead rhythm strips or 12 leads (Fig. 3-7). ECG paper is used to measure time of conduction and height of waveforms. When using ECG paper to measure time, the least unit of measure is the small box, which is equal to 0.04 second or 40.0 milliseconds. The next greater unit of measure is the large box, which contains five small boxes. One large box represents 0.20 second, or 200 milliseconds. Five large boxes represents 1 second, or 1000 milliseconds.

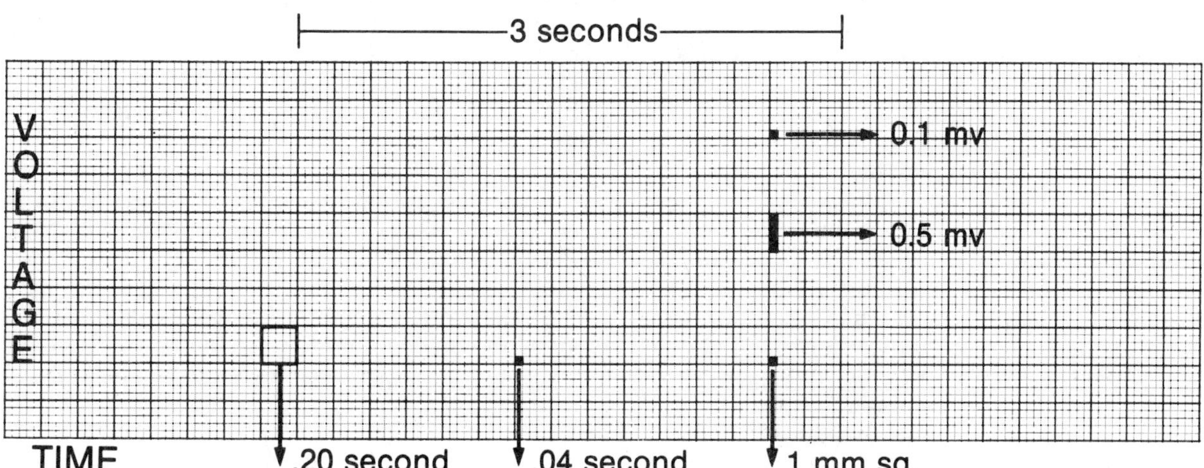

Figure 3-7. Standard ECG paper. (From Patel, J., McGowan, S., and Moody, L.: Arrhythmias: Detection, Treatment, and Cardiac Drugs. Philadelphia, W. B. Saunders, 1989, p. 10.)

The largest unit of measure is in seconds and is marked off at the top of the ECG paper by vertical hash marks (see Fig. 3–6). There may be 1, 2, or 3 seconds between two hash marks. Five large boxes between hash marks equals 1 second. Ten large boxes between hash marks equals 2 seconds. Fifteen large boxes between hash marks equals 3 seconds. In the clinical setting, it is standard to obtain 6-second rhythm strips for analysis and mounting in the patient's chart. To obtain a 6-second strip, count off the appropriate number of hash marks.

The value of measuring time on the ECG tracing is that speed of depolarization and repolarization in the atria and ventricles can be determined. In the next section, the normal intervals of conduction for each waveform are discussed.

Standardized ECG paper also allows the practitioner to measure the height, or amplitude, of waveforms. Amplitude is the height of each waveform, as measured by the number of small boxes (see Fig. 3–7). Amplitude is measured on the vertical axis of the ECG paper. Each small box is equal to 1 millimeter (mm) in amplitude or voltage. Waveform amplitude indicates the amount of electrical voltage being generated in the various areas of the heart. When waveforms are small, voltage is low. When waveforms are large, voltage is high. Low voltage and small waveforms are expected from the small muscle mass of the atria. High voltage and large waveforms are expected from the larger muscle mass of the ventricles.

WAVEFORMS AND INTERVALS

The normal ECG tracing is composed of a P, Q, R, S, and T wave (Fig. 3–8). These waveforms emerge from a flat baseline called the isoelectric line. Isoelectric means neither positive nor negative, i.e., a flat line. Any waveform that projects above the isoelectric line is considered positive, and any that projects below the line is considered negative.

P Wave. The P wave is an indication of atrial depolarization. Normally, it is an upright wave in leads I and II and has a rounded configuration. The amplitude of the P wave is measured at the center of the waveform and should not exceed three boxes, or 3 mm in height.

Normally, a P wave indicates that the SA node initiated the impulse that depolarized the atrium. However, as the various dysrhythmias are discussed, a change in the form of the P wave can indicate that the impulse did not come from the SA node, but rather from an abnormal pacemaking site, such as the atria or AV node.

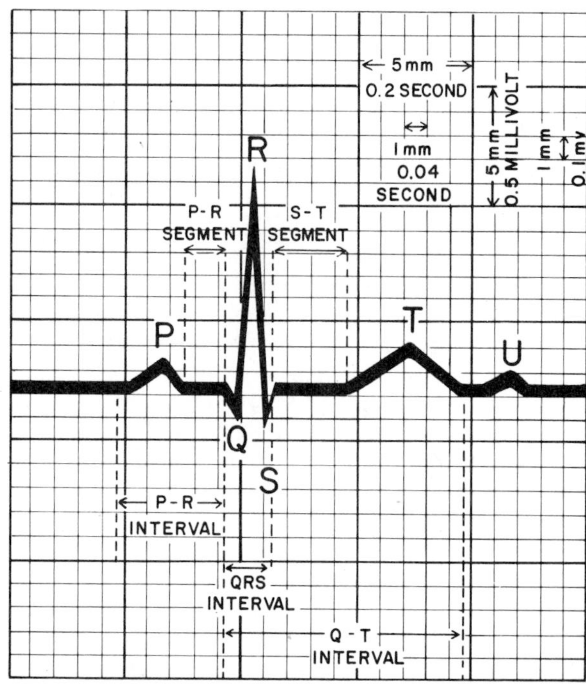

Figure 3–8. Normal ECG tracing: Waveforms and intervals. (From Sanderson, R., and Kurth, C.: The Cardiac Patient: A Comprehensive Approach. 2nd ed, Philadelphia, W. B. Saunders, 1983, p. 149.)

PR Interval. The P wave is connected to the next set of waveforms, the QRS complex, by the PR interval. The interval is measured from the beginning of the P wave, where the positive deflection of the P wave leaves the isoelectric line, to where the QRS complex begins. The PR interval measures the time it takes for the impulse to depolarize the atria, travel to the AV node, and then dwell there briefly before entering the bundle of His. These activities normally take less than 0.20 second. The normal PR interval is 0.12 to 0.20 second, which is three to five small boxes wide (see Fig. 3–8). When the PR interval is longer than normal, conduction of the impulse through the atria and down to the AV node is abnormally slow. When the PR interval is shorter than normal, conduction of the impulse is abnormally fast.

The word *dromotropy* is used to describe the speed of conduction. Many cardiac drugs increase the speed of conduction in the heart, and therefore are called positive dromotropic agents. Drugs that decrease the speed of conduction are called negative dromotropic agents. Both types of drugs are discussed further in the section on treatment of dysrhythmias.

QRS Complex. The QRS complex is a set of three distinct waveforms that are indicative of ventricular depolarization (see Fig. 3–8). The term *QRS complex* is an imprecise term. The QRS complex is a generic term for the waveforms that indicate ventricular depolarization. However, many people do not have all three distinct waveforms, Q, R, and S, in their QRS complex (Fig. 3–9).

The textbook normal QRS complex begins with a negative, or downward, deflection immediately following the P wave. This negative deflection is known as a Q wave (see Fig. 3–8). If the initial waveform following the P wave is positive, the patient does not have a Q wave. The absence of a Q wave is not abnormal. Q waves are normally small waveforms and are usually present in leads I, III, and aVL.

To determine if the Q wave is of normal size, it is compared to the next positive waveform, which is called an R wave. A Q wave should be no larger than one-fourth the size of the R wave. When Q waves exceed this normal size, they are referred to as pathological. Pathological Q waves are found on ECGs of patients who have had myocardial infarctions. The deep Q wave in these patients indicates that an area of myocardial tissue has died. The ECG machine reads no electrical activity in the area and this creates a deep, negative waveform (Fig. 3–10).

The first positive, or upright, waveform following the P wave is designated the R wave. Again, there may or may not be a Q wave prior to the R wave. The R wave is normally tall and positive in lead II (see Fig. 3–8). The amplitude of the R wave varies across leads. Leads V_4 to V_6 usually have the tallest R waves, since they measure electricity in the large muscle mass of the left ventricle. Some patients may have a second positive waveform in their QRS complex. If so, then that second positive waveform is called R prime (R′) (see Fig. 3–9).

The S wave is a negative waveform that follows the R wave. To have an S wave, the waveform must go below the isoelectric line (see Fig. 3–8). The amplitude of the S wave is measured from the point it leaves the isoelectric line to its deepest point.

QRS Interval. The QRS interval is measured from the beginning to the end of the QRS com-

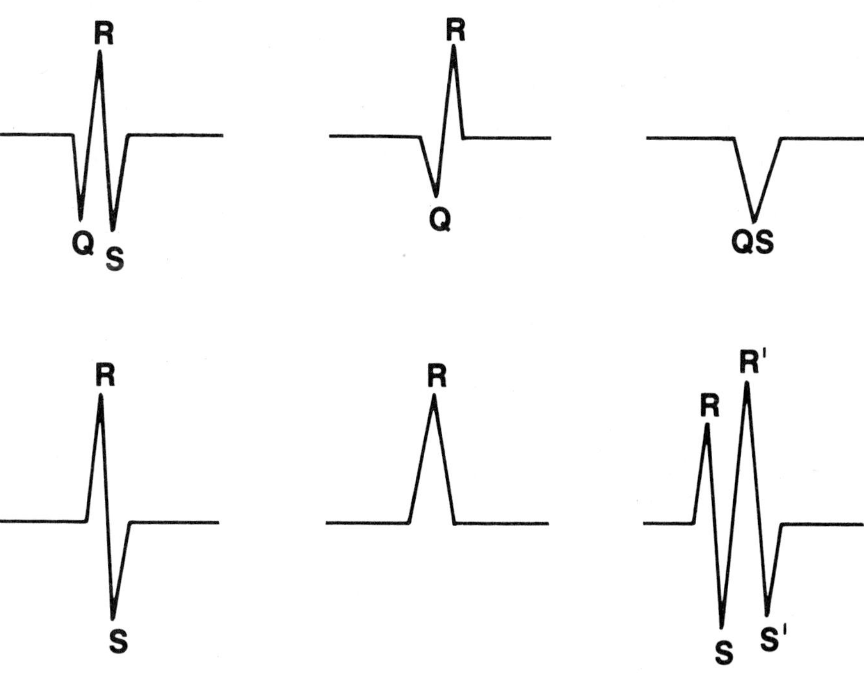

Figure 3–9. Different types of QRS complexes. (From Davis, D.: How to Quickly and Accurately Master ECG Interpretation. Philadelphia, J. B. Lippincott, 1985, p. 29.)

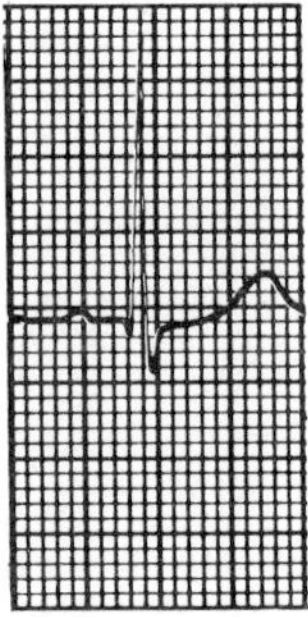

Normal Q wave

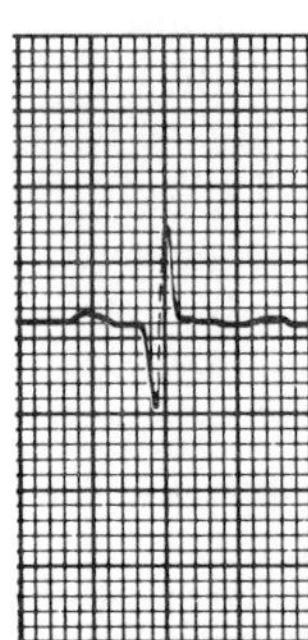

Pathological Q wave

Figure 3-10. Normal versus pathological Q wave. (From Davis, D.: How to Quickly and Accurately Master ECG Interpretation. Philadelphia, J. B. Lippincott, 1985, p. 175.)

plex (see Fig. 3-8). Whichever waveform begins the QRS complex, whether it is a Q or an R, marks the beginning of the interval. Therefore, you will be looking for the *first* deflection, either positive or negative, following the P wave. The QRS interval is measured from the point of first deflection up to where the *final* deflection returns to baseline. The final deflection may be an R or an S wave.

The normal width of the QRS complex is 0.06 to 0.10 second. This equates to one and a half to two and a half small boxes in length. When the QRS interval is longer than normal, conduction of the impulse through the ventricle is delayed.

When the QRS width is greater than 0.10 second, the patient is said to have a bundle branch block (BBB), or as is sometimes noted, an intraventricular conduction delay (ICD). The delay in conduction is most commonly caused by coronary artery disease. Either or both of the bundle branches can be blocked. A BBB causes a change in the normal conduction of impulses through the ventricles; hence, the prolonged interval. Bundle branch blocks also result in a change in the QRS complex morphology.

A right BBB produces a QRS with two distinct R waves in V_1 (Fig. 3-11). The second R wave occurs because conduction is delayed through the right ventricle. Normally, the QRS complex is evidence of biventricular depolarization. However, in right BBB, the first R wave is evidence of left ventricular depolarization and the second R wave is evidence of the delayed right ventricular depolarization.

A left BBB usually produces a wide, negative QRS complex in V_1. The widening of the QRS complex occurs as a result of the impulse being delayed in entry into the left ventricle (see Fig. 3-11).

T Wave. The T wave represents ventricular repolarization (see Fig. 3-8). You may notice that we did not describe a waveform indicating atrial repolarization. There is probably such a waveform, but it would be obscured by the large QRS complex.

Some beginning students of electrocardiography state that they have problems differentiating the P wave from the T wave. This should not be a problem, since the P wave immediately precedes the QRS, and the T wave immediately follows the QRS. Additionally, the T wave will usually be of greater size and amplitude than the P wave. This is because the atria are smaller muscle masses and therefore produce smaller waveforms than do the larger ventricles. T wave amplitude is measured at the center of the waveform and should be no greater than five small boxes, or 5 mm high. Changes in T wave amplitude can indicate electrical disturbances resulting from electrolyte imbalance or myocardial infarction (MI). For instance, hyperkalemia can cause an increase in T wave amplitude.

ST Segment. The ST segment connects the QRS complex to the T wave. Under normal conditions, the ST segment should be isoelectric, or flat. However, in some conditions such as myocardial ischemia, injury, and infarction, there may be depression, falling below baseline, or elevation, rising above baseline. The ST segment is not measured as a separate interval. However, its

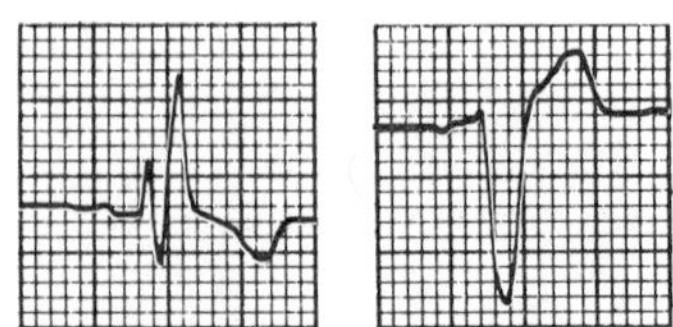

Figure 3-11. Right and left bundle branch blocks. (From Davis, D.: How to Quickly and Accurately Master ECG Interpretation. Philadelphia, J. B. Lippincott, 1985, pp. 152 and 154.)

measurement is encompassed in a larger interval known as the QT interval (see Fig. 3-8).

The QT interval is measured from the beginning of the QRS complex to the end of the T wave. This interval measures the time taken for ventricular depolarization and repolarization. There is no one standard QT interval. Normal QT intervals are those based on heart rate. The slower the heart rate, the longer the normal QT, and the faster the rate, the shorter the normal QT. QT intervals are normally longer in females. A QT chart is used to determine the outer limits for normal intervals (Table 3-1).

A final waveform that might be noted on the ECG is the U wave. The U wave is a small waveform of unknown origin. If present, it will immediately follow the T wave and will be of the same deflection (see Fig. 3-8). That is, if the T wave is positive, the U wave will also be positive. U waves may be seen in patients with electrolyte imbalance, particularly hypokalemia, and in myocardial infarction. However, the U wave is sometimes a normal finding, and therefore diagnosis of pathology should be dependent upon more specific indicators.

Systematic Interpretation of Dysrhythmias

The above discussion serves as a foundation of basic principles to be applied in the discussion of dysrhythmias. It is important to have a thorough understanding of the basic principles before continuing.

This section of the chapter proposes a systematic approach for the analysis and interpretation of dysrhythmias. Systematic analysis focuses attention on the following areas:

1. Assessment of rhythmicity, both atrial and ventricular
2. Assessment of rate, both atrial and ventricular
3. Assessment of waveform configuration and location
4. Assessment of intervals

Table 3-1. UPPER LIMITS OF THE QT INTERVAL, CORRECTED FOR HEART RATE

Rate (bpm)	QT Interval (sec)
40	0.49-0.50
50	0.45-0.46
60	0.42-0.43
70	0.39-0.40
80	0.37-0.38
90	0.35-0.36
100	0.33-0.34
110	0.32-0.33
120	0.31-0.32

(From Abedin, Z., and Conner, R.: Twelve-Lead ECG Interpretation. Philadelphia, W. B. Saunders, 1989.)

RHYTHMICITY

Rhythmicity refers to the regularity or pattern of the heart beats. P waves are used to establish atrial rhythmicity, and R waves establish ventricular rhythmicity. When an atrial rhythm is perfectly regular, each P wave is an equal distance from the next P wave. When a ventricular rhythm is perfectly regular, each R wave is an equal distance from the next R wave. An important part of the systematic interpretation of rhythms strips is looking at both atrial and ventricular rhythmicity.

Rhythmicity can be established through the use of calipers or paper and pencil. It is important to look at rhythmicity in both the atria and ventricle. To establish atrial rhythmicity, place one caliper point on one P wave and the other caliper point on the next consecutive P wave. Leaving the second point stationary, flip the calipers over. If the first caliper point lands exactly on the next P wave, the atrial rhythm is perfectly regular. If the point lands one small box or less away from the next P or R wave, the rhythm is essentially regular. If the point lands more than one small box away, the rhythm is considered irregular.

The same process is followed for assessing ventricular rhythmicity *except* you will place your caliper points on R waves. To establish ventricular rhythmicity, place one caliper point on one R wave and the other caliper point on the next consecutive R wave. Leaving the second point stationary, flip the calipers over. If the first caliper point lands exactly on the next R wave, the ventricular rhythm is perfectly regular (Fig. 3-12).

Rhythmicity can also be established by using paper and pencil. Slide a piece of blank paper over the rhythm strip and place the straight edge along the peak of the P wave to assess atrial rhythmicity, or along the peak of the R wave to assess ventricular rhythmicity. With the pencil, mark the peak of either the P or the R wave on

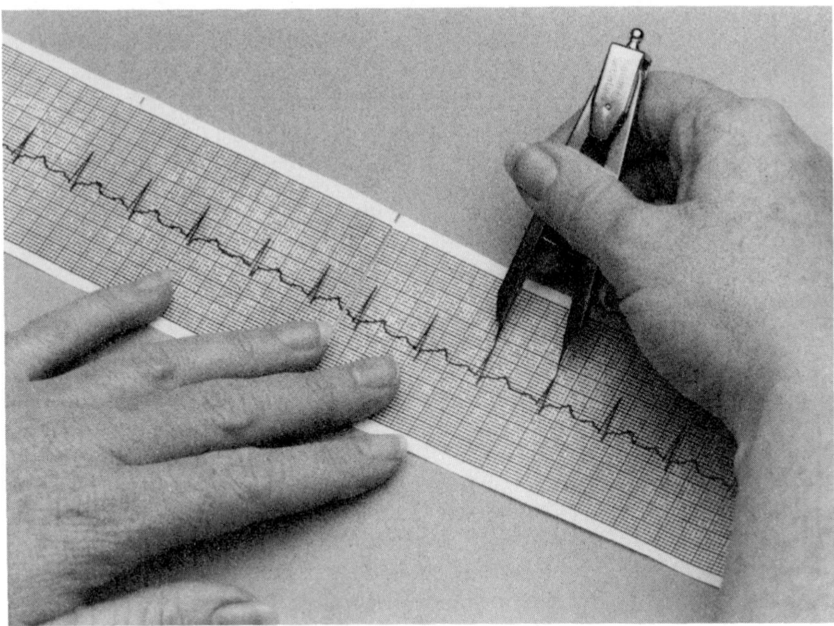

Figure 3-12. Establishing ventricular rhythmicity with calipers.

the paper. Without moving the paper, make another mark on the next P or R wave. Now slide the paper over to the next P or R waveform. If the pencil mark lands exactly on the next P or R wave, rhythm is perfectly regular. If the pencil mark is one small box or less away from the next P or R wave, the rhythm is essentially regular. If the pencil mark lands more than one small box away from the next P or R wave, the rhythm is irregular (Fig. 3-13).

Irregular rhythms can be regularly irregular or irregularly irregular. Regularly irregular rhythms have a pattern to them. In other words, the irregularity occurs in a predictable fashion,

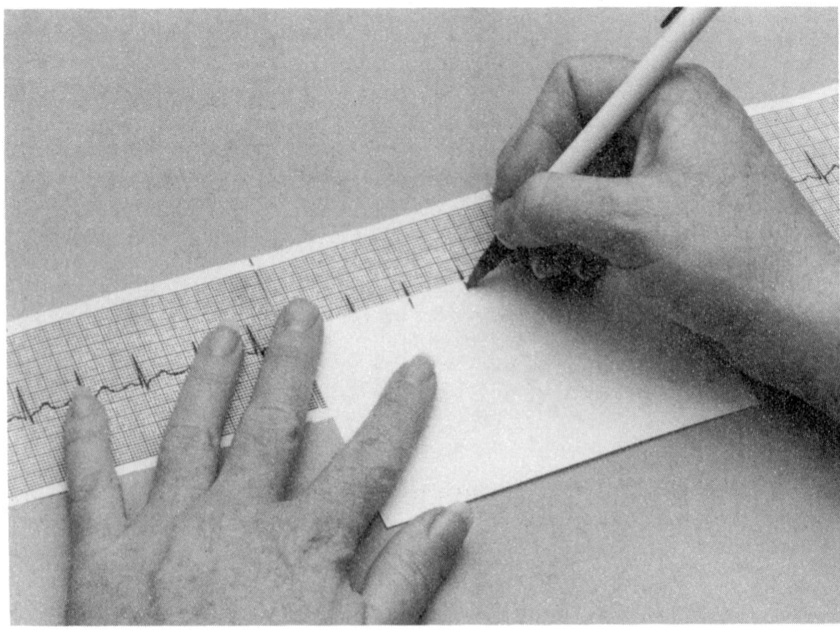

Figure 3-13. Establishing ventricular rhythmicity with paper and pencil.

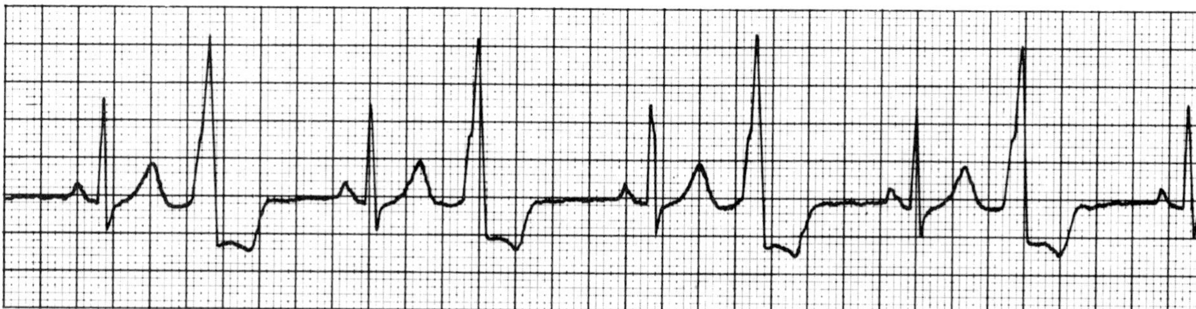

Figure 3-14. Note the irregularity in rhythm is predictable. The abnormal complexes occur every other beat. (From Patel, J., McGowan, S., and Moody, L.: Arrhythmias: Detection, Treatment, and Cardiac Drugs. Philadelphia, W. B. Saunders, 1989, p. 67.)

for instance, every second beat (Fig. 3-14). Irregularly irregular rhythms have no pattern and no predictability (Fig. 3-15).

RATE

Obviously, rate equates to how fast the heart is beating. Under normal conditions, the atria and the ventricles beat at the same rate. However, it is important to know that each can beat at a different rate. An important part of systematic analysis is calculation of both the atrial and ventricular rates. P waves are used to calculate the atrial rate, and R waves are used to calculate the ventricular.

Rate can be assessed in a variety of ways. This text will address two popular methods as follows:

1. The rule of 1500 is used to calculate the *exact* rate of a *regular* rhythm. To utilize the rule of 1500, locate two consecutive P or R waves. Use P waves if calculating the atrial rate, and R waves if calculating the ventricular rate. Locate the tallest point of either the P wave or the R wave. Count the number of small boxes between the highest points of two consecutive P or R waves. Divide that number of small boxes into 1500 to determine the exact heart rate in beats per minute. For example, if there are 20 small boxes between two consecutive R waves, divide 20 into 1500 for a rate of 75 ventricular beats per minute (Fig. 3-16).

Remember, this method is reserved for use with regular rhythms. If the rule of 1500 is used for irregular rhythms, the calculated rate will be accurate only between the two consecutive beats chosen. Charts are available based on the rule of 1500 to calculate heart rate.

2. The rule of 10 is a popular method for calculating the *approximate* rate. This method can be used for either regular or irregular rhythms. The rule of 10 is accomplished by counting the number of P or R waves in a 6-second strip and then multiplying that number by 10. This yields an approximate heart rate for 60 seconds, or 1 minute. For example, if there are

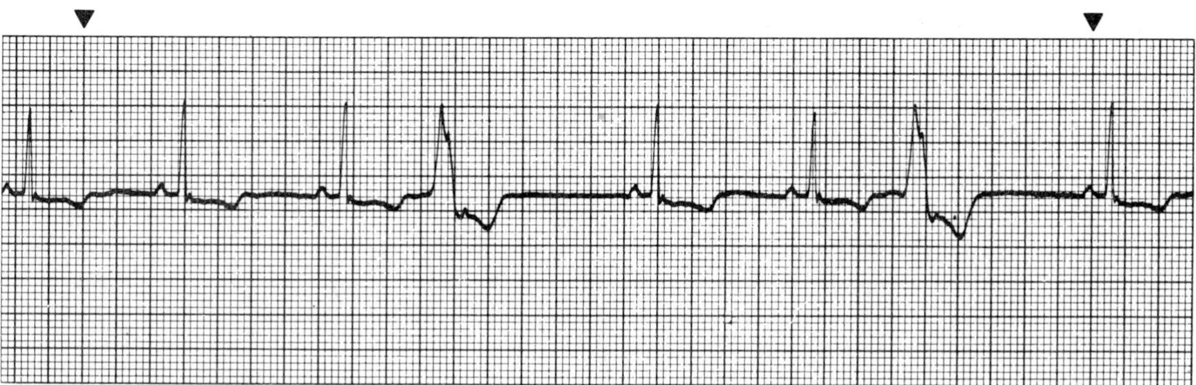

Figure 3-15. Note the irregularity in rhythm is unpredictable. The abnormal complexes occur randomly, without pattern. (From Huff, J., Doernbach, D., and White, R.: *ECG Workout: Exercises in Arrhythmia Interpretation.* Philadelphia, J. B. Lippincott, 1985, Fig. 4.41.)

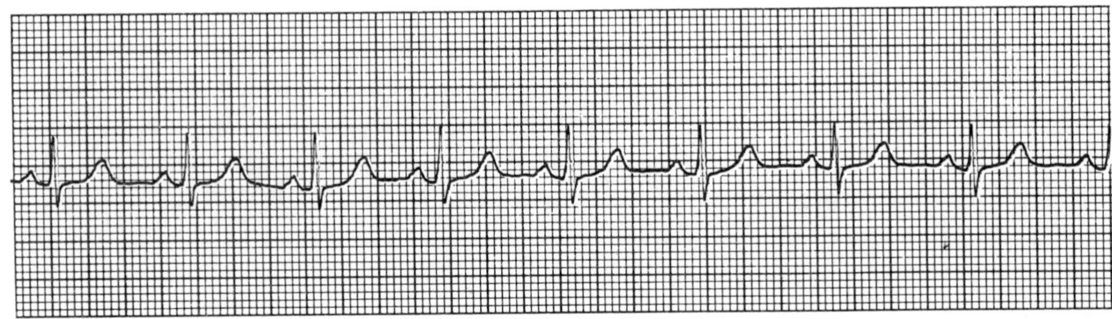

Figure 3-16. Calculating ventricular rate with the rule of 1500. Count the number of small boxes between two consecutive QRS complexes, then divide that number into 1500. In this rhythm strip there are 16 small boxes between QRS complexes. Sixteen boxes divided into 1500 gives a resultant rate of 94. (From Davis, D.: How to Quickly and Accurately Master Arrhythmia Interpretation. Philadelphia, J. B. Lippincott, 1989, p. 38, sinus rhythm.)

six R waves found on one 6-second strip, multiply those 6 complexes by 10 for an approximate rate of 60 ventricular beats per minute. This method is used when a quick assessment of rate is needed or when a patient is having an irregular rhythm.

Cardiac monitors display heart rates, usually in a digital form. However, these monitor-calculated rates may be inaccurate and should *always* be verified by one of the above-cited rate-calculation methods.

WAVEFORM CONFIGURATION AND LOCATION

The normal waveforms P, Q, R, S, and T have been previously discussed. When systematically analyzing ECG rhythms, configuration and location of these waveforms are very important.

Configuration. Each cardiac cell is capable of generating electrical impulses. This capability is referred to as automaticity. Each cardiac cell, once depolarized, creates a distinct waveform configuration that is manifest on the ECG rhythm strip. Various waveforms can be recognized as originating from certain areas of the heart by their shape and appearance. For instance, small slightly rounded waveforms known as P waves are associated with atrial depolarization, combinations of positive and negative waveforms known as QRS complexes with ventricular depolarization, and larger, rounded waveforms known as T waves with ventricular repolarization.

Under normal conditions, if all the P waves are originating from the SA node, then all P waves on a 6-second strip should look the same. If all impulses travel through the ventricle in the same way, then all QRS complexes in a 6-second strip should look the same. Also, if ventricular repolarization is always accomplished in the same way, all T waves in a 6-second strip should look the same. It also follows that if a waveform is coming from an abnormal place, that waveform will not look like the normal waveforms.

Configuration, or shape and appearance of a waveform, is often the first clue in the assessment of dysrhythmias. Once knowledgeable regarding normal waveform configuration, abnormal waveforms are readily apparent. No systematic analysis and interpretation is complete without carefully studying and comparing each waveform on the 6-second strip, looking for both normal and abnormal configuration.

Location. Location of waveforms is very important in a systematic analysis of dysrhythmias. The normal waveforms P, Q, R, S, and T should occur in their natural order. A P wave should precede each QRS. QRS complexes should be followed by T waves and T waves followed by P waves.

When analyzing rhythm strips, it is very important to note if waveforms are occurring in the natural order. If not, the location should be closely reviewed. In the later discussion of the basic dysrhythmias, several rhythms will be characterized by abnormal location or sequencing of waveforms (Fig. 3-17).

INTERVALS

A final important aspect of the systematic analysis of rhythm strips is the assessment of the intervals discussed previously in the section on analysis of the normal ECG tracing. No rhythm strip analysis is complete, and interpretation is impossible, without the assessment of the PR, QRS, and QT intervals.

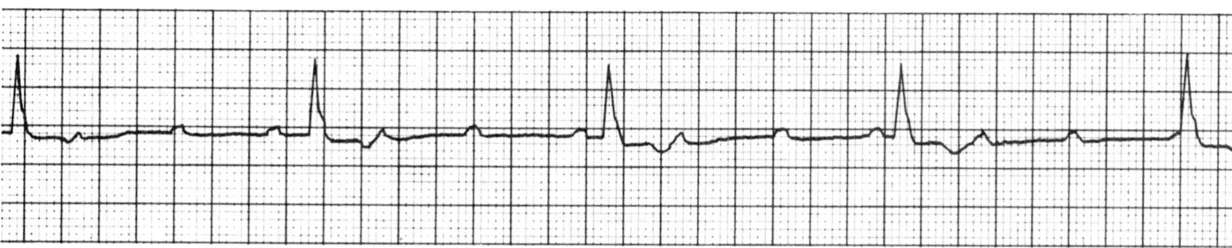

Figure 3-17. Note how P, Q, R, S, and T waves are out of normal sequence and location. (From Patel, J., McGowan, S., and Moody, L.: Arrhythmias: Detection, Treatment, and Cardiac Drugs. Philadelphia, W. B. Saunders, 1989, Fig. 107.)

The Basic Dysrhythmias

Review of the basic concepts of electrocardiography, and a systematic approach to analyzing ECG rhythm strips, are prerequisite to the discussion of the basic dysrhythmias. The word *dysrhythmia* means difficult or abnormal rhythm. In this case, dysrhythmia refers to abnormal cardiac rhythms. People also speak of cardiac arrhythmias. The word *arrhythmia* means no rhythm. Therefore, dysrhythmia is a more useful and descriptive term for the rhythms encountered in the clinical setting. The basic dysrhythmias can be grouped under the following anatomical areas:

Dysrhythmias of the SA node
Dysrhythmias of the AV node
Dysrhythmias of the atria
Dysrhythmias of the ventricles
Atrioventricular blocks

A section has been developed for each anatomical area and will include rhythm strip examples of common dysrhythmias associated with that anatomical area or structure. However, of more importance will be the description of characteristics that make each dysrhythmia unique and recognizable to the practitioner. These characteristics will be listed as the criteria for the diagnosis of that particular dysrhythmia. The most critical criteria for diagnosis are listed first and are designated with an asterisk.

It is these critical criteria that remove the shroud of mystery from dysrhythmia analysis and interpretation. Intuition or a sixth sense has no place here. Instead, the practitioner learns the criteria for each rhythm and then makes a diagnosis based on these criteria.

When beginning the study of basic electrocardiography, these critical criteria will need to be memorized or kept in a notebook for easy referencing. Initially, the task seems overwhelming. There is a great deal of information. Focusing on the critical criteria will help organize the information for easier analysis and interpretation of the dysrhythmias.

The criteria will become easier to use and remember as patients with the dysrhythmia are encountered. Dysrhythmia analysis and interpretation are truly skills that develop only through practice.

Each dysrhythmia discussed will have an impact on the body's ability to maintain a normal hemodynamic status. Normal hemodynamic status is defined as an adequate cardiac output, as evidenced by a normal arterial blood pressure. The hemodynamic effects of each dysrhythmia are discussed. The treatments for the dysrhythmias are discussed at the end of the chapter.

Dysrhythmias of the Sinoatrial Node

Before launching into a discussion of the dysrhythmias of the sinoatrial node, the most important rhythm of this chapter, normal sinus rhythm, must be covered. Normal sinus rhythm (NSR) is the rhythm against which all others are compared. Without a thorough understanding of what is normal, abnormal cannot be understood. Initial analysis of a rhythm strip should determine whether the rhythm is normal sinus or a dysrhythmia requiring further analysis.

NORMAL SINUS RHYTHM

The SA, sinus, node is the master pacemaker of the heart. Under normal circumstances, this special group of cardiac cells generates an electrical impulse that will be conducted down the normal conduction pathway depolarizing all cardiac cells (Fig. 3-18).

Critical Criteria for Diagnosis: Normal Sinus Rhythm

* 1. Upright, small, rounded P waves will be present in lead II.

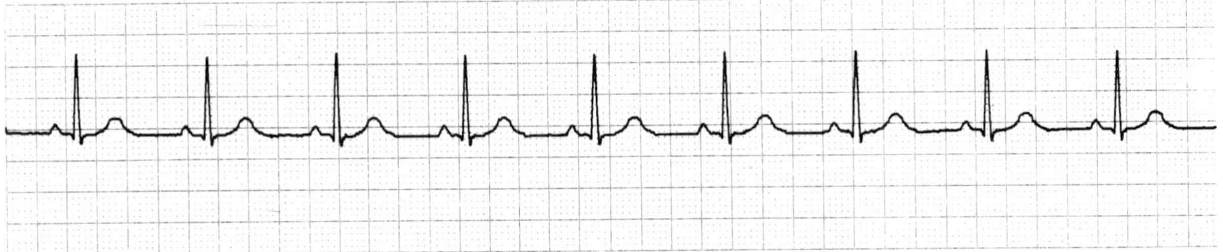

Figure 3–18. Normal sinus rhythm. Rhythm strip generated by the AA-700 Rhythm Simulator. (Reproduced with permission from Armstrong Medical Industries, Lincolnshire, Illinois, *DataSim*, Fig. 0.)

* 2. P waves will precede each QRS complex.
* 3. Both the atrial rate and the ventricular rate will be the same, and that rate will be between 60 and 100 beats per minute.
* 4. Rhythm will be regular or essentially regular.

5. The PR interval will be 0.12 to 0.20 second in duration.
6. The QRS interval will be 0.06 to 0.10 second in duration.

Hemodynamic Effects

The NSR is the optimal cardiac rhythm for maintaining an adequate cardiac output and blood pressure.

SINUS BRADYCARDIA

Bradycardia is defined as a slowed heart rate. Sinus bradycardia results when the SA node generates fewer than 60 beats per minute. Several processes can lead to sinus bradycardia:

Increased Vagal Stimulation. The parasympathetic nervous system exerts influence on heart rate via the vagus nerve. When the vagus nerve is stimulated, an impulse is sent to the heart and rate is decreased. The Valsalva maneuver, coughing, gagging, and vomiting all stimulate the vagus nerve and can cause sinus bradycardia.

Drug Effects. Many of the drugs administered to patients with cardiac disease decrease heart rate. This slowing in heart rate is often a desired result of treatment. When a patient's heart beats at a slower rate, oxygen demands are lessened. When bradycardia occurs as a side effect of a drug, the drug is said to have a negative chronotropic effect. Chronotropy means heart beats per minute. Negative chronotropic drugs decrease heart rate. Drugs with positive chronotropic effects increase heart rate.

Sinoatrial Node Ischemia. When the patient has myocardial ischemia, injury or infarction in the area surrounding the SA node, the node may become less able to generate impulses. Bradycardia can result.

Effects of Suctioning. Sinus bradycardia can occur during endotracheal suctioning. Bradycardia results as the SA node is robbed of oxygen.

Bradycardia as a Normal Finding. Athletes and others who are physically fit may have a slower than normal heart rate. Physical conditioning leads to increased strength of the cardiac muscle, and therefore increased effectiveness of the heart as a pump. An effective pump can deliver adequate amounts of blood to the body at a slower heart rate.

Increased Intracranial Pressure. Cushing's reflex is a hemodynamic response to increased intracranial pressure. Blood pressure increases and heart rate decreases and often becomes irregular. Respiratory patterns also change (Fig. 3–19) (Kenner et al., 1991).

Critical Criteria for Diagnosis: Sinus Bradycardia

* 1. Same criteria as for NSR *except* for a heart rate of <60 beats per minute.

Hemodynamic Effects

Patients demonstrate a variety of hemodynamic responses to sinus bradycardia. Many patients will continue to maintain an adequate cardiac output and blood pressure despite a lowered heart rate. This ability to compensate is better in patients with a healthy heart. Other patients will begin to decrease both their cardiac output and blood pressure as their pulse slows.

SINUS TACHYCARDIA

Tachycardia is defined as a rapid heart rate. Sinus tachycardia results when the SA node generates more than 100, but fewer than 150, beats per minute. Sinus tachycardia is a normal finding in children under the age of 6. Heart rate in children, as in adults, is also dependent upon oxygen consumption (Mott et al., 1985, p. 1171).

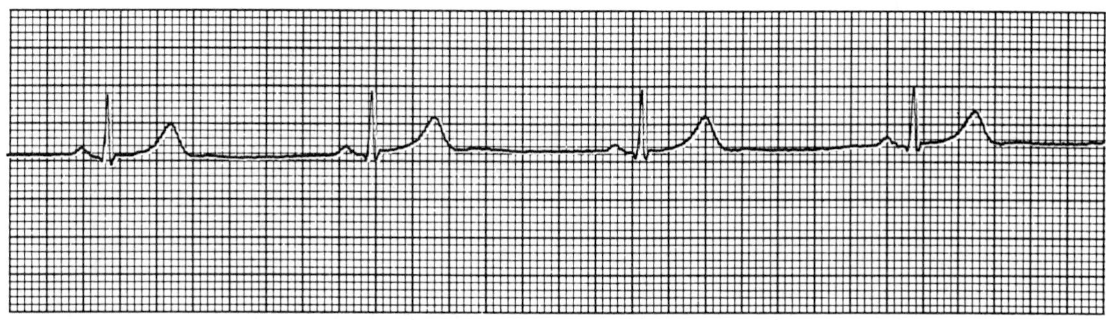

Figure 3-19. Sinus bradycardia. (From Davis, D.: ECG Workout: Exercises in Arrhythmia Interpretation. Philadelphia, J. B. Lippincott, 1985, p. 38, sinus bradycardia.)

Several other processes can also lead to sinus tachycardia:

Stimulants. There are many types of stimulants that can induce increased heart rate. Exercise is a natural stimulant to the heart. Heart rate increases as the body's oxygen demand and consumption increase. Commonly used and abused drugs like caffeine and nicotine both stimulate heart rate. Additionally, drugs such as decongestants and appetite suppressants can markedly increase heart rate. Stress and pain also stimulate the sympathetic nervous system, which stimulates the SA node to beat faster.

Increased Body Temperature. Elevation in body temperature can cause increases in heart rate (Kinney et al., 1988).

Alterations in Fluid Status. Both hypovolemia and hypervolemia can result in increased heart rate. When the circulating blood volume is low, such as in dehydration or after hemorrhage, the heart must beat faster to maintain an adequate cardiac output and blood pressure. When the circulating blood volume is increased, such as in fluid overload, again the heart must beat faster in order to compensate for the increased blood coming into the heart (Fig. 3-20).

Critical Criteria for Diagnosis: Sinus Tachycardia

* 1. Same criteria as for NSR *except* for heart rate of >100 beats per minute.

Hemodynamic Effects

Sinus tachycardia leads to a decrease in ventricular filling time. Decreased ventricular filling time leads to less blood volume in the ventricle for the next systole and consequently a lower cardiac output and arterial blood pressure. Another possibly severe consequence to sinus tachycardia is increased myocardial oxygen consumption. This is especially detrimental in the patient with inadequate coronary artery perfusion.

SINUS DYSRHYTHMIA

Sinus dysrhythmia is a cardiac rhythm disturbance that is associated with normal respiration. During inspiration air is brought into the lungs by a negative sucking pressure in the thorax. Since the heart lies within the thoracic cavity, this negative sucking pressure, associated with breathing, also causes more blood to be brought into the right atrium from the superior and inferior venae cavae. To compensate for this increased amount of blood coming to the heart, heart rate is increased.

With expiration, the pressure in the thoracic cavity is changed to positive and air is forced from the lungs. During expiration flow of blood

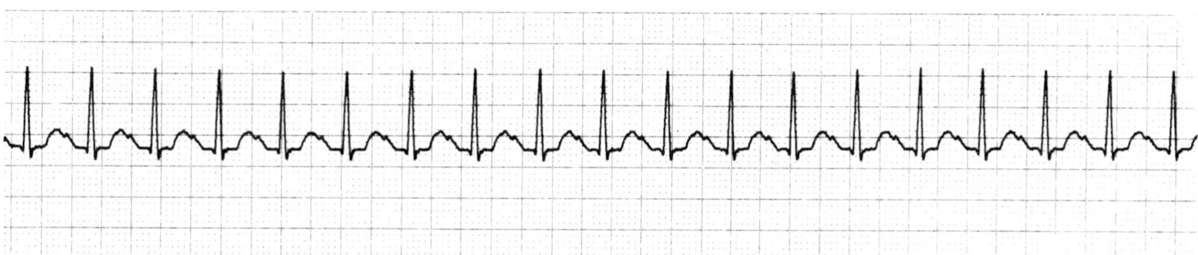

Figure 3-20. Sinus tachycardia. Rhythm strip generated by the AA-700 Rhythm Simulator. (Reproduced with permission from Armstrong Medical Industries, Lincolnshire, Illinois, *DataSim*, Fig. 1.)

into the heart returns to normal as does heart rate.

The ECG tracing will demonstrate an alternating pattern of faster heart rate, associated with inspiration, then slower heart rate, associated with expiration. This rhythm is considered a normal phenomenon; however, certain conditions can enhance the rhythm changes such as increased intracranial pressure, increased vagal tone, and myocardial ischemia, injury, and infarction.

Critical Criteria for Diagnosis: Sinus Dysrhythmia

* 1. Same criteria as for NSR *except* for a phasic increasing and decreasing of heart rate.
* 2. Changes in heart rate are associated with respiration.
* 3. Rhythm is usually regularly irregular (Fig. 3–21).

Hemodynamic Effects

It is rare to have significant changes in cardiac output and blood pressure with this rhythm. It is normally tolerated well unless the periods of slowed heart rate are fewer than 60 beats per minute or unless periods of faster heart rate are greater than 100 beats per minute.

SINUS ARREST/SINUS EXIT BLOCK

Instances can occur when the sinus node temporarily fails as the dominant pacemaker. This failure may be due to arrest, or an inability to generate an electrical impulse, or the impulse may be generated but blocked from exiting the SA node. This may happen for one or several beats. Since the impulse is either arrested in, or blocked from exiting, the SA node, no atrial or ventricular depolarization can occur.

When this occurs, there will be a complete absence of the normal cardiac waveforms. In other words, for one heart beat or more there will be no P, Q, R, S, and T waves.

This loss of the normal waveforms creates a pause of varying length on the ECG tracing. A pause is a long flat line between two beats that exceeds the normal amount of space found between other beats. If this pause is long enough to drop the heart rate to less than 60, then the AV node or the Purkinje fibers may come in as a back-up pacemaker and generate an escape beat or escape rhythm. The escape beat is so named because it allows the patient to escape the slowed heart rate, thus preventing further compromise.

Sinus arrest or sinus exit block may be caused by the following processes (Andreoli et al., 1987):

Enhanced Vagal Tone – The Valsalva maneuver, coughing, gagging, or vomiting may temporarily suppress impulse generation in, or conduction from, the SA node.

Coronary Artery Disease – Coronary artery disease (CAD) can lead to decreased perfusion of the SA node, resulting in impaired performance.

Effects of Drugs – Administration of various cardiac drugs that slow heart rate can lead to episodes of sinus arrest and exit block (Fig. 3–22).

Critical Criteria for Diagnosis: Sinus Arrest/Exit Block

* 1. Heart rate can be normal (60 to 100 beats per minute) or slower than normal.

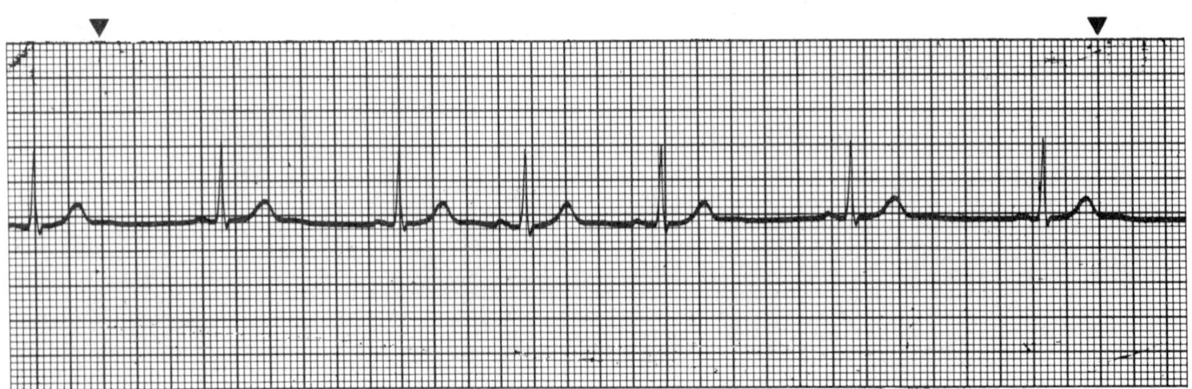

Figure 3–21. Sinus dysrhythmia. (From Huff, J., Doernbach, D., and White, R.: ECG Workout: Exercises in Arrhythmia Interpretation. Philadelphia, J. B. Lippincott, 1985, Fig. 1.57.)

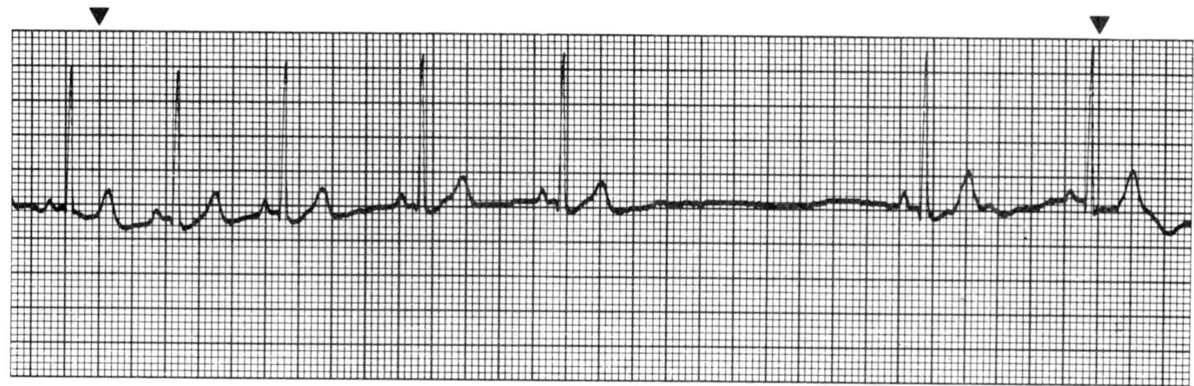

Figure 3-22. Sinus arrest/sinus exit block. (From Huff, J., Doernbach, D., and White, R.: ECG Workout: Exercises in Arrhythmia Interpretation. Philadelphia, J. B. Lippincott, 1985, Fig. 1.44.)

* 2. Pauses caused by missed beats will be noted on the ECG tracing.

* 3. Rhythm will be irregular on account of missed beats.

4. Pauses may be interrupted by an escape beat from the AV node or the Purkinje fibers.

Hemodynamic Effects

The hemodynamic effects of sinus arrest and/or exit block depend upon the number of sinus beats that are arrested or blocked, and the length of the resulting pause. When occasional beats are arrested or blocked, the hemodynamic effects are the same as for sinus bradycardia. Changes in cardiac output and blood pressure are dependent upon how low the heart rate falls.

When multiple beats are arrested or blocked, asystole results. The patient will cease to have any cardiac output and adequate blood pressure.

Dysrhythmias of the Atrioventricular Node

Dysrhythmias of the AV node are called junctional rhythms. However, in the literature and in clinical practice, the term *nodal rhythms* is also used. The AV node is located in the middle of the heart between the atria and the ventricles. The tissue immediately surrounding the AV node is referred to as junctional tissue. Both the AV node itself and the junctional tissue surrounding it are capable of generating cardiac rhythms. In this text, the terms *nodal* and *junctional* will be used interchangeably.

There are two primary causes of junctional or nodal rhythms, which are as follows:

1. Dysrhythmias can originate in the AV node or the junctional tissue surrounding it. When a singular beat, or ongoing rhythm, originates in an area other than the sinus node, that beat or rhythm is considered *ectopic.* Ectopic means out of the normal place.

Ectopic rhythms are usually due to increased automaticity. Increased automaticity is commonly due to stress, nicotine, or caffeine. However, it can also occur secondary to myocardial ischemia, injury, or infarction. Digitalis toxicity can also cause increased automaticity. Digitalis at toxic levels acts as a myocardial stimulant (Swonger and Matejski, 1988).

2. As mentioned earlier, escape rhythms can be generated from the AV node should the sinus node fail. The AV node is capable of generating 40 to 60 beats per minute as a back-up pacemaker.

There are ECG changes that are common to all the nodal dysrhythmias. These changes include P wave abnormalities and PR interval changes.

P Wave Changes. Because of the location of the AV node, in the center of the heart, impulses generated may be conducted either forward, backward, or both. Like a rock thrown into a pool of water, the impulse can radiate both forward and backward. With the potential of forward, backward, or bidirectional impulse conduction, three different P waveforms may be associated with nodal rhythms:

1. When forward conduction occurs, there will be an *absence of P waves.* This occurs because the atria do not receive the wave of depolarization. The atria also do not contract (Fig. 3-23).

2. When the impulse is conducted in a backward motion, an *inverted P wave* will be produced. Backward, or retrograde, conduction moves back toward the atria, allowing for at least partial depolarization of

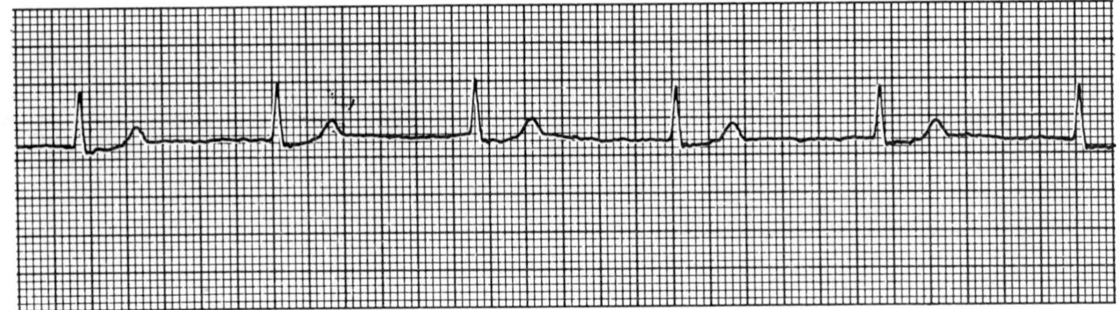

Figure 3–23. Nodal/junctional rhythm. Note absence of P waves. (From Davis, D.: How to Quickly and Accurately Master ECG Interpretation. Philadelphia, J. B. Lippincott, 1985, p. 288, junctional rhythm.)

the atria. When depolarization occurs in a backward fashion, an inverted P wave is created. Once the atria have been depolarized, the impulse then moves down the bundle of His and depolarizes both ventricles normally (Fig. 3–24).

3. When the impulse is conducted in both a forward and a backward fashion, *P waves may be present after the QRS*. In this type of conduction, the impulse first moves into the ventricles, depolarizing them and creating a QRS complex. Since the impulse is also conducted backward, some atrial depolarization occurs, and a late P wave is noted after the QRS complex (Fig. 3–25).

PR Interval Changes. The length of the PR interval in junctional rhythms depends upon where the impulse originates. When the impulse is generated high in the AV node or junctional tissue, near the atria, the PR interval will be normal or slightly shorter than normal. If the impulse is generated low in the AV node or junctional tissue, nearer the ventricle, then the PR interval will be shorter than normal. If the P wave is absent, the PR interval cannot be measured.

JUNCTIONAL/NODAL RHYTHM

See Figures 3–23, 3–24, and 3–25.

Critical Criteria for Diagnosis: Nodal/Junctional Rhythm

* 1. P waves may be absent, inverted, or follow the QRS complex.

* 2. The heart rate will be 40 to 60 beats per minute.

* 3. The PR interval will be at the low end of normal or shorter than normal.

4. The rhythm will usually be regular.

5. The QRS complex will be of normal width.

Hemodynamic Effects

In junctional, or nodal, rhythms, atrial depolarization is usually less effective, or in the case of forward conduction of the ectopic impulses, absent. With ineffective or absent depolarization of the atria, less than the normal amount of ventricular filling is accomplished. The net effect is diminished cardiac output and blood pressure. This effect may go unnoticed in some patients, whereas it may cause significant hypotension in others.

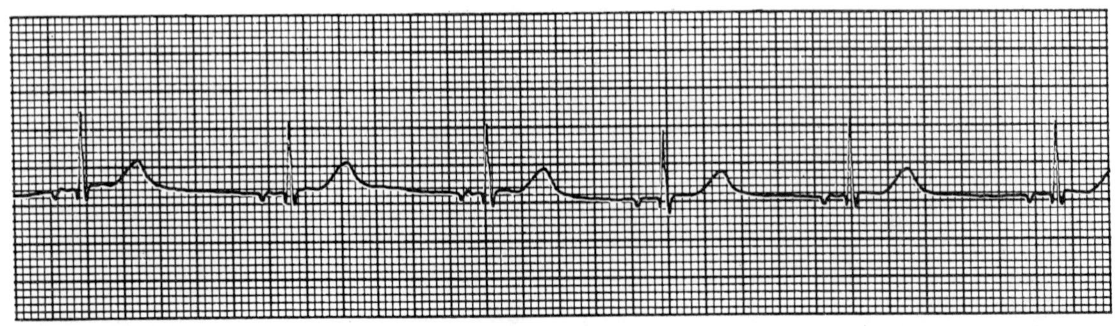

Figure 3–24. Nodal/junctional rhythm. Note inverted P waves prior to the QRS. (From Davis, D.: How to Quickly and Accurately Master ECG Interpretation. Philadelphia, J. B. Lippincott, 1985, p. 288, junctional escape rhythm.)

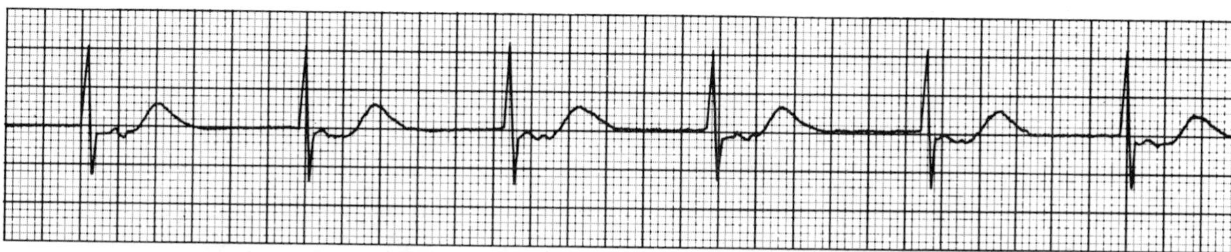

Figure 3-25. Nodal/junctional rhythm. Note P waves after the QRS. (From Patel, J., McGowan, S., and Moody, L.: Arrhythmias: Detection, Treatment, and Cardiac Drugs. Philadelphia, W. B. Saunders, 1989, Fig. 48.)

ACCELERATED NODAL RHYTHM (JUNCTIONAL TACHYCARDIA)

While the normal intrinsic rate for the AV node and junctional tissue is 40 to 60 beats per minute, rates can accelerate higher. Any rate higher than the normal upper limit of 60 beats per minute is considered junctional tachycardia. The upper rate capability for the AV node is considered to be 150 beats per minute (Fig. 3-26).

Critical Criteria for Diagnosis: Junctional/Nodal Tachycardia

* 1. Same as for junctional or nodal rhythm except for heart rate greater than 60 beats per minute.

Hemodynamic Effects

The hemodynamic effects of junctional tachycardia are the same as for a nodal rhythm. However, ventricular filling may be further compromised by the more rapid heart rate. On the other hand, the acceleration in heart rate may actually improve cardiac output. Cardiac output is affected by both the amount of blood available for pumping from the ventricles, and the heart rate. Improvement in cardiac output, secondary to increased heart rate, is dependent upon the health state of the heart.

PREMATURE NODAL (JUNCTIONAL) CONTRACTIONS (PNCs/PJCs)

Irritable areas in the AV node and junctional tissue can generate beats that are premature, or earlier than the next expected beat. These premature beats most often occur in the setting of normal sinus rhythm and temporarily upset the rhythmicity of the ECG tracing. The SA node response to premature beats is important in the analysis and interpretation of dysrhythmias. The SA node will either compensate for the one premature beat and continue the normal rhythm, or it will not compensate and the normal rhythm will be upset.

The closer the site of premature impulse generation to the sinus node, the less likely it is that the SA node will compensate. When a premature impulse fires close to the SA node, a wave of depolarization moves backward toward the sinus and excites the tissue of the SA node. After depolarization has occurred, the sinus requires time for repolarization before generating the next beat. This creates a pause on the ECG called a *noncompensatory pause* (Fig. 3-27).

To determine if a pause is compensatory or noncompensatory, a rhythm strip with a premature beat is analyzed. Calipers or paper and pencil will be needed. Two consecutive normal beats are located just prior to the premature beat, and the caliper points or pencil marks are placed on

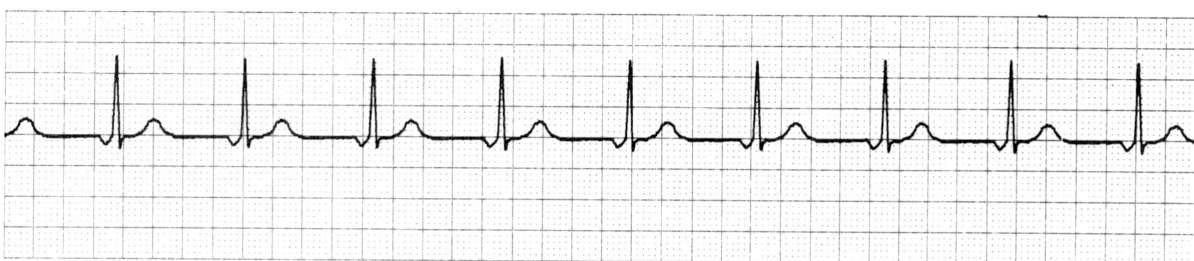

Figure 3-26. Accelerated nodal rhythm (junctional tachycardia). Rhythm generated by the AA-700 Rhythm Simulator. (Reproduced with permission from Armstrong Medical Industries, Lincolnshire, Illinois, *DataSim*, Fig. 22.)

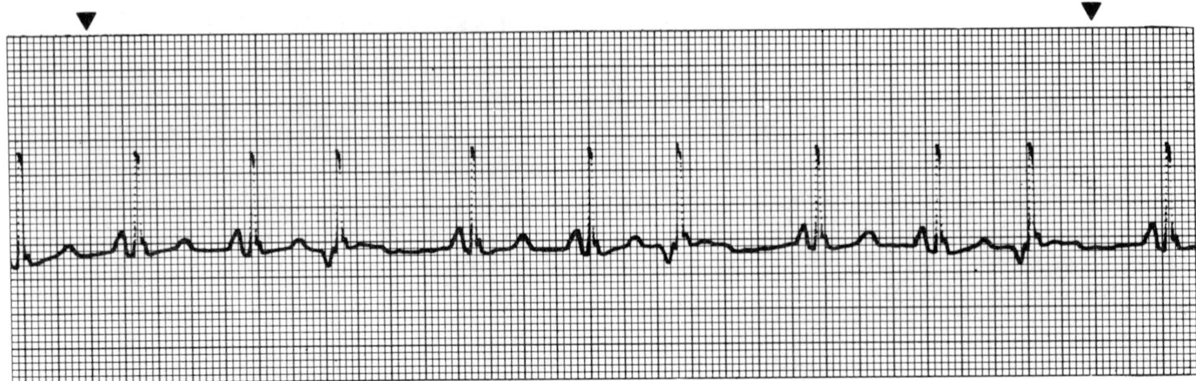

Figure 3-27. Premature nodal (junctional) contractions. Note noncompensatory pause. (From: Huff, J., Doernbach, D., and White, R.: ECG Workout: Exercises in Arrhythmia Interpretation. Philadelphia, J. B. Lippincott, 1985, Fig. 3.58.)

the R wave of each normal beat. Now flip the calipers over, or slide the paper over, to where the next normal beat should have occurred. The premature beat will come in early.

Now, being careful not to lose placement, flip the calipers or slide the paper over one more time. If the point of the calipers or the mark on the paper lands exactly on the next normal beat's R wave, the sinus node *compensated* for the one premature beat and kept its normal rhythm (Fig. 3-28). If the caliper point or pencil mark does not land on the next normal beat's R wave, then the sinus did *not compensate* and had to establish a new rhythm.

Critical Criteria for Diagnosis: Premature Nodal (Junctional) Contractions (PNCs/PJCs)

* 1. The ectopic beats are premature.

* 2. If a P wave is present, before the QRS, the PR interval will usually be shorter than normal.

* 3. PJCs are *usually* followed by a noncompensatory pause.

* 4. P waves may be absent, inverted, or occur after the QRS complex.

Hemodynamic Effects

Premature nodal contractions do not usually alter the cardiac output or blood pressure in a significant way. However, many patients do report palpitations. Be aware that increasing numbers of PJCs may herald the development of nodal tachycardia.

Dysrhythmias of the Atria

Increased automaticity in either the right, left, or both atria can result in abnormal cardiac rhythms. These dysrhythmias are most often due to increased automaticity. Increased automaticity can result from a wide variety of processes (Guzzetta and Dossey, 1984) as follows:

Stress. The stress response causes the liberation of norepinephrine. This can cause increased automaticity in the atria. Drugs that stimulate the sympathetic nervous system, such as amphetamines, cocaine, and decongestants, can also cause atrial dysrhythmias (American Heart Association, 1987).

Electrolyte Imbalances. Electrolyte imbalances, particularly hypokalemia, can result in increased automaticity in the atria.

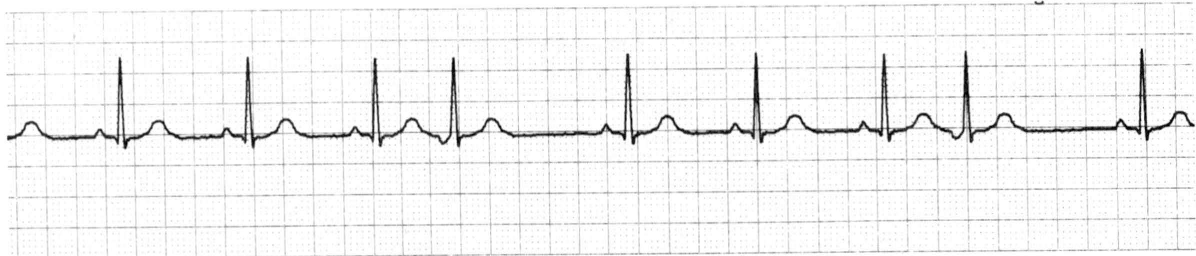

Figure 3-28. Premature nodal (junctional) contraction with a compensatory pause. Rhythm generated by the AA-700 Rhythm Simulator. (Reproduced with permission from Armstrong Medical Industries, Lincolnshire, Illinois, *DataSim*, Fig. 24.)

Hypoxia. The atria become very irritable when deprived of oxygen. Patients with chronic obstructive pulmonary disease are at high risk for atrial dysrhythmias.

Injury to the Atria. When the atria are injured, such as with trauma related to cardiac surgery, they are more prone to generating ectopic beats.

Digitalis Toxicity. Digitalis in toxic doses is very stimulating to the myocardium, and in particular to the atria.

Hypothermia. Lowered body temperature predisposes a patient to atrial dysrhythmias. For this reason it is important to maintain a patient's temperature near normal. The hypothermic patient should be warmed back to normal body temperature as rapidly as possible through the use of warming blankets, inhalation of warmed, humidified mist, and radiant warmers.

Hyperthyroidism. Hyperthyroidism places a patient in a metabolic state very similar to the stress response. The hormones produced by the thyroid gland are very similar to norepinephrine and have a stimulating effect on the heart.

Alcohol Intoxication. Alcohol is a cardiac stimulant and has an irritating effect on the heart.

Pericarditis. When the pericardial lining surrounding the heart is inflamed or infected, the atria become more irritable. Indeed, atrial dysrhythmias may be one of the first signs of pericarditis.

WANDERING ATRIAL PACEMAKER

A wandering atrial pacemaker (WAP) is a rhythm most often seen in a patient with chronic obstructive pulmonary disease (COPD) and is secondary to hypoxia (Fenstermacher, 1989). This dysrhythmia is characterized by a wandering of pacemaking activity throughout the atria. To meet the criteria for this rhythm, at least three sites of atrial pacemaking must be documented.

When impulses are generated from different pacemaking sites, different waveforms will be manifest. Therefore, if at least three different atrial cell groups are generating impulses, then at least three different P wave morphologies will be present on the ECG. Varying waveform morphology is another way of saying that the P waves look different in shape, slope, or orientation. P waves in wandering atrial pacemaker can be upright, inverted, flat, pointed, notched, and/or slanted in different directions.

The PR interval will vary, since the impulses are originating from different locations within the atria. The length of the PR interval will depend upon how far the impulse is generated from the ventricle (Fig. 3–29).

Critical Criteria for Diagnosis: Wandering Atrial Pacemaker

* 1. Must see *at least* three different-looking P waves.

* 2. The heart rate must not be greater than 100 beats per minute.

* 3. The PR intervals will vary.

* 4. The rhythm is usually irregular.

Hemodynamic Effects

Like in the nodal rhythms, atrial depolarization may be less effective in WAP. Therefore, ventricular filling may be affected with consequent decrease in cardiac output and blood pressure.

MULTIFOCAL ATRIAL TACHYCARDIA

Multifocal atrial tachycardia (MAT) is essentially the same as wandering atrial pacemaker except that the rate exceeds 100 beats per minute. It is almost exclusively found in the COPD patient population. The cause of the dysrhythmia is thought to be right atrial dilation secondary to increased pulmonary pressures (Guzzetta and Dossey, 1984) (Fig. 3–30).

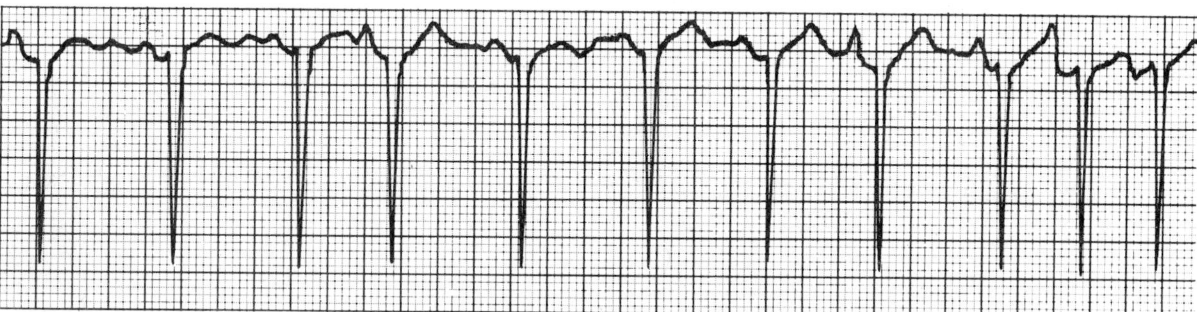

Figure 3–29. Wandering atrial pacemaker. Note the varying P wave morphologies. (From Patel, J., McGowan, S., and Moody, L.: Arrhythmias: Detection, Treatment, and Cardiac Drugs. Philadelphia, W. B. Saunders, 1989, Fig. 41.)

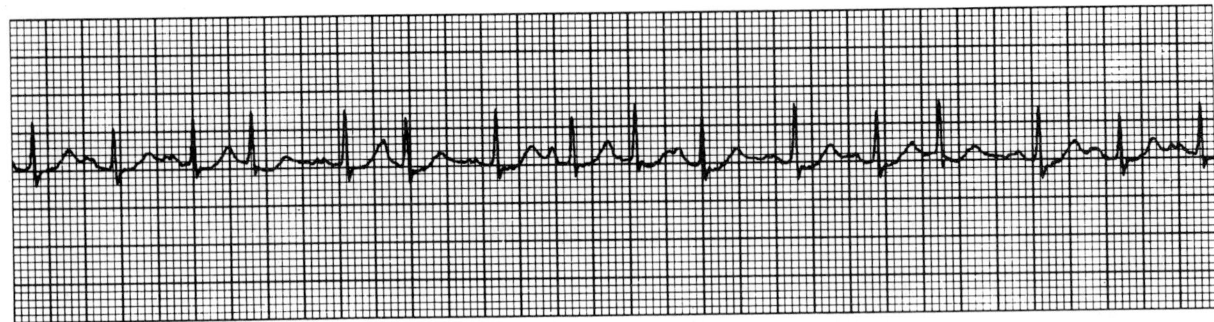

Figure 3-30. Multifocal atrial tachycardia. (From Patel, J., McGowan, S., and Moody, L.: Arrhythmias: Detection, Treatment, and Cardiac Drugs. Philadelphia, W. B. Saunders, 1989, Fig. 42.)

Critical Criteria for Diagnosis: Multifocal Atrial Tachycardia

* 1. Same as for wandering atrial pacemaker except for a rate greater than 100 beats per minute.

Hemodynamic Effects

The hemodynamic effects of MAT are the same as those for WAP. The faster the rate, the more pronounced the hemodynamic effects, primarily lowered cardiac output and blood pressure.

PREMATURE ATRIAL CONTRACTIONS

Premature atrial contractions (PACs) are a common dysrhythmia and are usually seen in the setting of normal sinus rhythm. Like the PJCs/PNCs discussed earlier, they are generated very near the SA node. This frequently leads to depolarization of the tissue surrounding the SA node, and causes a pause on the ECG. Again, this pause is usually noncompensatory (Fig. 3-31).

Critical Criteria for Diagnosis: Premature Atrial Contractions

* 1. The ectopic beats are premature.

* 2. The PR interval is usually normal or slightly shorter than normal.

* 3. PACs are *usually* followed by a noncompensatory pause.

* 4. P wave of the premature beat may be found in the T wave just prior to the premature beat (see rhythm below, Fig. 3-31). When this occurs, the T wave of the preceding beat will be distorted. Compare the T wave of the beat preceding the premature beat with other normal T waves on the ECG strip.

Occasionally, a premature atrial contraction is generated and conducted down to the AV node just after a normal impulse has been conducted. The PAC arrives at the AV node when the bundle of His and its branches are refractory to, or unable to conduct, the premature impulse. The impulse is blocked and not allowed to enter the ventricle. This blocked PAC can be detected as a

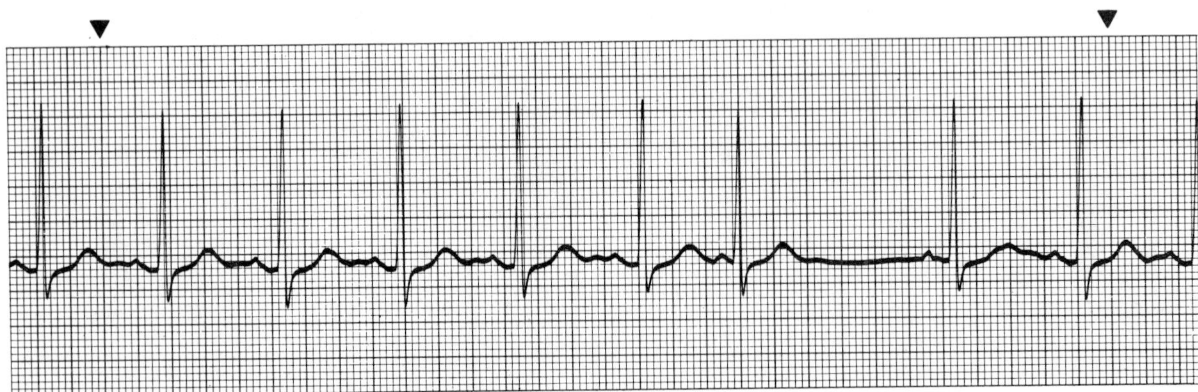

Figure 3-31. Premature atrial contraction. Note noncompensatory pause. (From Huff, J., Doernbach, D., and White, R.: ECG Workout: Exercises in Arrhythmia Interpretation. Philadelphia, J. B. Lippincott, 1985, Fig. 2.5.)

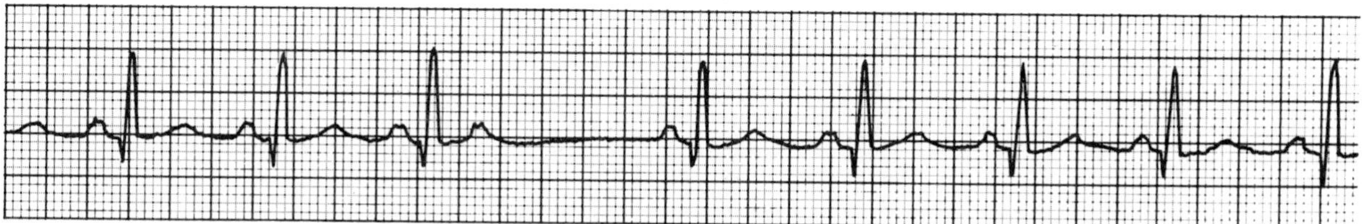

Figure 3-32. Blocked premature atrial contraction. Note unusual looking T wave following the PAC. (From Patel, J., McGowan, S., and Moody, L.: Arrhythmias: Detection, Treatment, and Cardiac Drugs. Philadelphia, W. B. Saunders, 1989, Fig. 26.)

pause on the ECG. Prior to the pause, a different-looking T wave can usually be noted. The unusual T wave is caused by the PAC's premature P wave imposed on the normal T wave (Fig. 3-32).

Critical Criteria for Diagnosis: Blocked Premature Atrial Contraction

* 1. A pause will be noted on the ECG tracing.

* 2. A premature P wave, which differs from the normal P wave, will be found in the T wave, or just after the T wave, of the last normal beat before the pause.

Hemodynamic Effects

Premature atrial contractions do not usually alter the cardiac output or blood pressure in a significant way. However, many patients do report palpitations. Be aware that increasing numbers of PACs may herald the development of atrial fibrillation or flutter.

PAROXYSMAL ATRIAL TACHYCARDIA

Paroxysmal atrial tachycardia (PAT) is a rapid rhythm that arises from the atria without warning. Because of the fast rate, PAT can be a life-threatening dysrhythmia. It is usually seen in patients with cardiac disease; however, it may also occur in healthy patients. In some instances, increased numbers of PACs precede the onset of PAT.

When the atria generate impulses more rapidly than the AV node can conduct, varying degrees of block may result. Blocking of impulses by the AV node will be noted by P waves that are not followed by QRS complexes. P waves may merge with T waves. Sometimes the AV node will block impulses in a set pattern, such as every third or fourth beat. When the AV node conducts every third atrial impulse, a three to one block exists. In other words, for every three atrial impulses, or every three P waves, there is only one conducted QRS (Fig. 3-33).

When the AV node randomly decides which atrial impulses it will conduct and there is no pattern, varying degrees of block are said to exist (Fig. 3-34).

Critical Criteria for Diagnosis: Paroxysmal Atrial Tachycardia

* 1. Occurs suddenly, usually without warning.

* 2. Heart rate is usually 150 to 250 beats per minute.

* 3. Rhythm is absolutely regular.

4. P waves, if present, will usually merge with the preceding T waves, altering the appearance of the T wave.

5. Existence of AV block. May be a fixed or varying degree of block.

6. Width of QRS is usually normal.

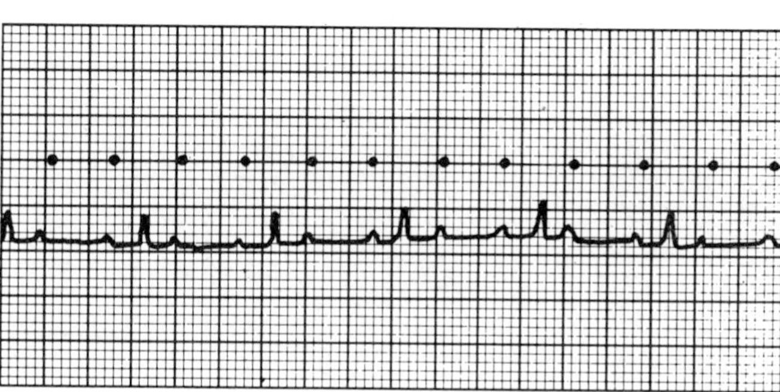

Figure 3-33. Paroxysmal atrial tachycardia with fixed degree of block. Note every second P wave is conducted. (Reproduced with permission. Textbook of Advanced Cardiac Life Support. American Heart Association, 1987, 1990, Chap. 5, Fig. 33.)

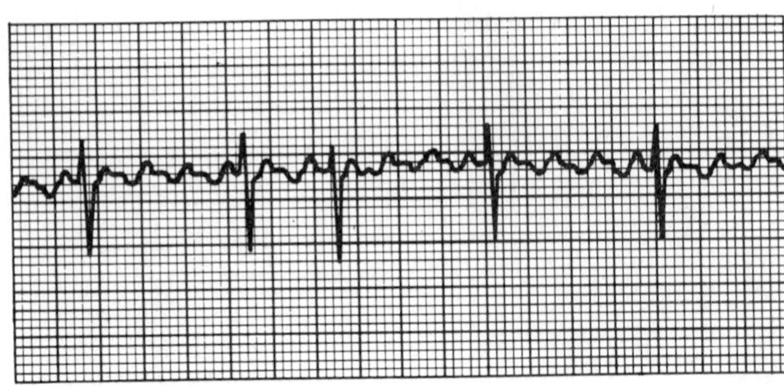

Figure 3-34. Paroxysmal atrial tachycardia with varying degrees of block. (Reproduced with permission. Textbook of Advanced Cardiac Life Support. American Heart Association, 1987, 1990, Chap. 5, Fig. 36.)

Hemodynamic Effects

The hemodynamic effects of PAT can vary from palpitations to shock. The faster the rate, the less time there is for ventricular filling. At faster rates, cardiac output and blood pressure can be severely compromised.

ATRIAL FLUTTER

Atrial flutter is a dysrhythmia that arises from a single irritable focus in the atria. Atrial flutter is most commonly seen in patients with heart disease. Patients who have valvular disease seem particularly susceptible to its development (Andreoli et al., 1987).

The waveforms associated with atrial flutter are flutter, or "F," waves. Flutter waves have a sawtooth configuration and are best seen in leads II, III, and aVF. They are usually inverted or negative (Fig. 3-35).

It is important to understand that flutter waves are occurring incessantly and with perfect regularity. The irritable focus in the atria never stops firing. This means that the flutter waves continue throughout the ECG strip, often altering the appearance of the QRS complex and the T wave (see Fig. 3-35).

Flutter waves are usually generated at a rate of 250 to 350 beats per minute. However, the AV node is physiologically unable to conduct all of these impulses. Therefore, as in PAT, the AV node selectively conducts a given number of flutter waves down to the ventricle. If, for example, the atrial focus is generating 300 beats per minute, the AV node might be able to conduct every fourth beat. This would be a 3:1 ratio of conduction and the resultant ventricular rate would be 100 beats per minute (300 divided by 3 equals 100). In Figure 3-36, there is such an example.

Like PAT, the degree of block may be fixed and predictable, 2:1, 3:1, 4:1, or unpredictable and varied (Fig. 3-37).

Critical Criteria for Diagnosis: Atrial Flutter

* 1. Presence of negative flutter waves in leads II, III, and aVF.

* 2. Atrial rate is usually 250 to 350 beats per minute. Ventricular rate varies with the degree of AV block.

3. Onset is usually rapid.

Hemodynamic Effects

The hemodynamic effects of atrial flutter are completely dependent upon the ventricular rate, sometimes called the ventricular response. In patients who are conducting high numbers of atrial impulses through the AV node, compromise of

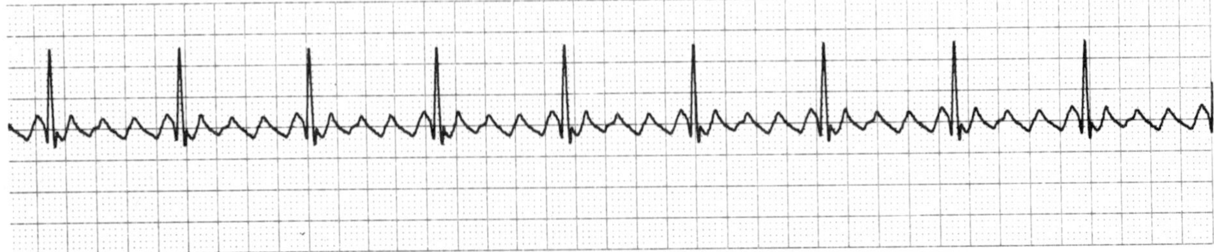

Figure 3-35. Atrial flutter. Note sawtooth configuration and negative orientation of the flutter waves. Rhythm generated by the AA-700 Rhythm Simulator. (Reproduced with permission from Armstrong Medical Industries, Lincolnshire, Illinois, *DataSim*, Fig. 4.)

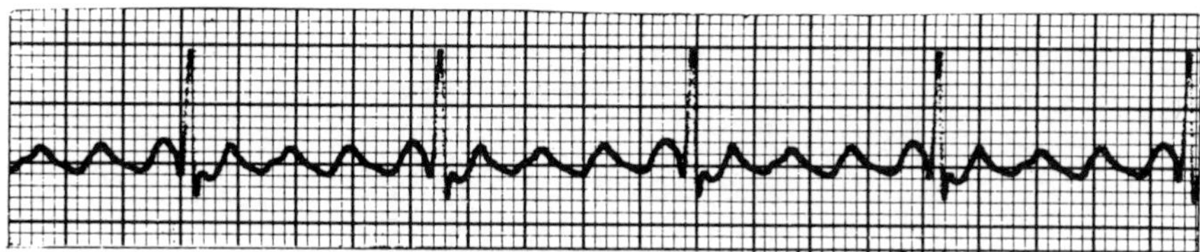

Figure 3-36. Atrial flutter with fixed degree of block (3:1). Atrial rate is 300 bpm and ventricular is 100 bpm. Note a QRS occurs only after every third flutter wave. (From Fenstermacher, K.: Dysrhythmia Recognition and Management. Philadelphia, W. B. Saunders, 1989, p. 32, atrial flutter, lead II.)

the cardiac output and blood pressure is more likely.

Patients whose AV nodes are blocking greater numbers of the atrial impulses tend to maintain a more normal cardiac output and blood pressure.

ATRIAL FIBRILLATION

Atrial fibrillation is a dysrhythmia characterized by erratic impulse formation throughout the atria. Widespread irritability and increased automaticity lead to a chaotic state of impulse formation.

Atrial fibrillation produces a wavy baseline with no discernible P waves. As the AV node is bombarded with rapidly fired atrial impulses, it conducts impulses to the ventricles in an unpredictable fashion. This erratic conduction results in an irregularly irregular ventricular rhythm.

As the AV node attempts to regulate the movement of impulses into the ventricle, it may allow an impulse through before the bundle and the branches are able to conduct. Premature impulses are more likely to be conducted successfully down the left bundle branch. However, the right bundle branch is often found to be refractory, or unable to conduct. When an impulse is unable to be conducted via the right bundle branch, it must cross the ventricular septum and move down the left bundle branch first and then cross back over the septum and depolarize the right ventricle. When this occurs, the impulse is said to be aberrantly conducted.

Aberrant conduction refers to the abnormal, or roundabout, way in which the impulse travels through the ventricles. When an impulse takes an aberrant pathway, depolarization takes longer. This results in a widened time interval for the QRS complex. In atrial fibrillation, aberrantly conducted beats are referred to as Ashman's beats. Aberrantly conducted Ashman's beats are more likely to occur when an atrial impulse arrives at the AV node just shortly after a previously conducted impulse (Fig. 3-38) (Kenner et al., 1991).

Fibrillation results in an ineffective quivering of the atria. The atria are never fully depolarized and therefore do not contract. This loss of atrial systole, or kick, diminishes the effectiveness of ventricular filling.

Additionally, the blood that collects in the atria is agitated by fibrillation atria, and normal clotting is accelerated. Small thrombi begin to form along the walls of the atria. Should the patient convert back to a normal sinus rhythm and the atria begin to contract normally, these clots could be dislodged and sent out to the lungs and the body.

For this reason, if a patient has been in atrial

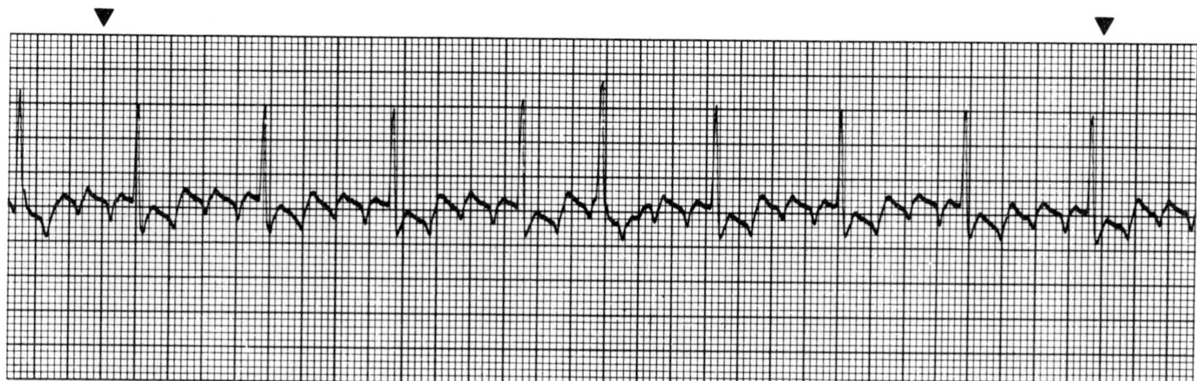

Figure 3-37. Atrial flutter with varying degree of block. There are varying ratios of flutter waves to QRS complexes. (From Huff, J., Doernbach, D., and White, R.: ECG Workout: Exercises in Arrhythmia Interpretation. Philadelphia, J. B. Lippincott, 1985, Fig. 2.60.)

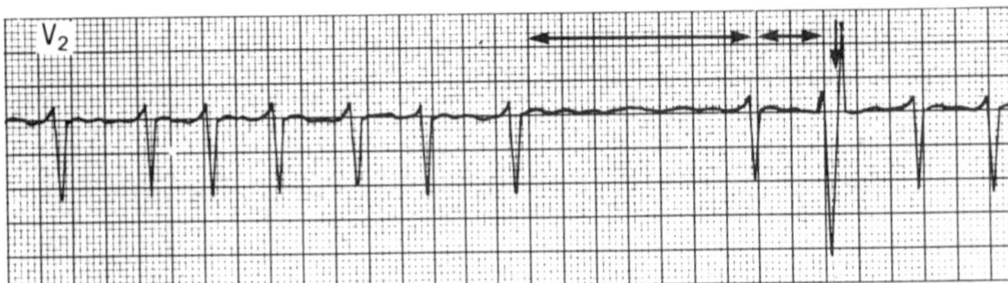

Figure 3-38. Atrial fibrillation. Note Ashman's beat, following a long, short cycle. (From Laver, J.: Electrical activity of the heart and dysrhythmias. In: Guzzetta, C., and Dossey, B. [eds.]: Cardiovascular Nursing: Bodymind Tapestry. St. Louis, C. V. Mosby, 1984, Fig. 7-25.)

fibrillation for an unknown amount of time, and if there is a stable blood pressure, the patient should be anticoagulated before any attempt is made to convert his/her atrial fibrillation to NSR. Heparin is the drug of choice for anticoagulation.

For patients who suffer from chronic atrial fibrillation, long-term coumadin therapy is usually prescribed to diminish the risk of thromboembolism (Fig. 3-39) (Swonger and Matejski, 1988).

Critical Criteria for Diagnosis: Atrial Fibrillation

* 1. Wavy baseline with no discernible P waves.

* 2. Irregularly irregular ventricular rhythm.

3. QRS width may vary between normal and slightly widened.

4. Presence of Ashman's beats.

Hemodynamic Effects

The hemodynamic effects of atrial fibrillation relate to the rate at which atrial impulses are conducted down through the ventricles. Patients who conduct 60 to 100 atrial impulses per minute tend to better tolerate the rhythm. Those who conduct at markedly slower or faster rates are more likely to experience a decrease in cardiac output and blood pressure.

Dysrhythmias of the Ventricle

Ventricular dysrhythmias originate in the ventricles. Since impulses for ventricular dysrhythmias are generated in the lower portion of the heart, depolarization occurs in an abnormal way. Depending upon where the impulse originates, it must travel in a backward or sideways fashion to depolarize the ventricles. This abnormal or aberrant flow of electricity lengthens the normal time interval for depolarization of the ventricles. The result is a widened QRS complex. The QRS interval extends beyond the normal of 0.06 to 0.10 second.

Depolarization, following an abnormal ventricular beat, rarely moves as far backward as the atria. Therefore, most ventricular dysrhythmias have no evident P waves. However, if a P wave is evident, it will usually be seen in the T wave of the prior beat. There are two types of ventricular dysrhythmias, ectopic and escape:

1. The ectopic rhythms are abnormal and disturb or override the normal sinus rhythm. These ectopic rhythms are capable of firing at fast rates and may be life threatening.

2. The Purkinje fibers, deep in the ventricles, can act as a site for back-up pacemaking should the SA and AV nodes fail. The Purkinje fibers can generate an escape rhythm of 15 to 40 beats

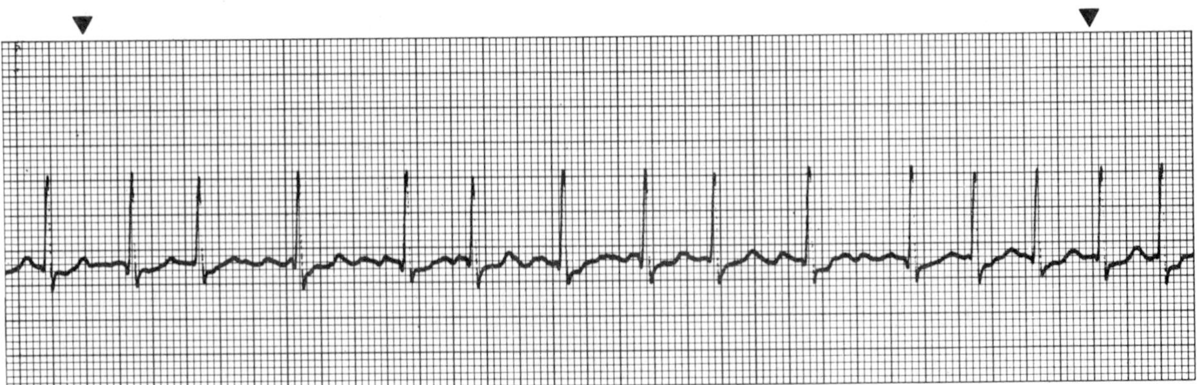

Figure 3-39. Atrial fibrillation. (From Huff, J., Doernbach, D., and White, R.: ECG Workout: Exercises in Arrhythmia Interpretation. Philadelphia, J. B. Lippincott, 1985, Fig. 2.50.)

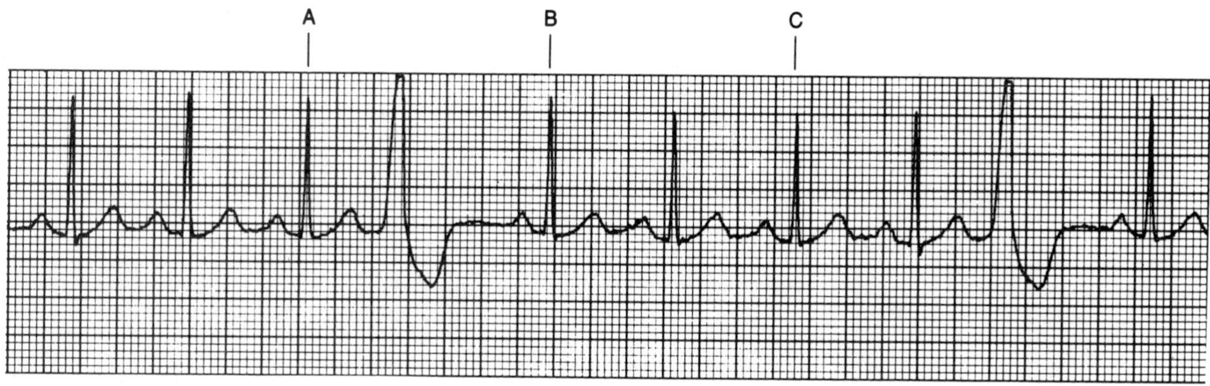

Figure 3-40. Unifocal premature ventricular contractions. (From Patel, J., McGowan, S., and Moody, L.: Arrhythmias: Detection, Treatment, and Cardiac Drugs. Philadelphia, W. B. Saunders, 1989, Fig. 56.)

per minute under normal circumstances. While this is a very slow intrinsic rate, some patients are able to maintain a near adequate cardiac output and blood pressure with rates closer to 40 beats per minute. However, most patients will be compromised.

Generation of ventricular dysrhythmias can be secondary to (Patel et al., 1989):

Myocardial Ischemia, Injury, and Infarct. When blood supply is decreased to an area of the ventricle, the blood-deprived area becomes irritable and will be more likely to have increased automaticity. Prolonged ischemia can lead to permanent injury to the area, creating an even greater potential for ectopic impulse formation. Ultimately, the area deprived of blood supply will infarct or die. Once cellular death has occurred, *no* electrical activity will be generated.

Hypokalemia. Low serum potassium can facilitate the development of ventricular dysrhythmias. As discussed earlier, potassium plays an important role in the normal depolarization/repolarization process.

Hypoxia. Inadequate amounts of oxygen are irritating to the ventricles and often stimulate ectopic beats and/or rhythm formation.

Acid-Base Imbalances. Both alkalosis and acidosis can stimulate ventricular ectopy.

PREMATURE VENTRICULAR CONTRACTIONS

Premature ventricular contractions (PVCs) are a common ventricular dysrhythmia. The beats can be generated anywhere in the ventricles. When there is only one focus of ventricular irritability, all of the ectopic beats will appear the same. Ventricular beats coming from one area are called unifocal, meaning having one focus (Fig. 3-40).

There can also be multiple areas, or foci, of ventricular irritability. When multiple areas are generating abnormal impulses, waveform configuration will vary. Ventricular beats coming from more than one area are called multifocal ectopy (Fig. 3-41).

Since PVCs are generated in the ventricles, a considerable distance from the SA node, the SA node is usually able to compensate for the premature beat. This compensation is noted on the

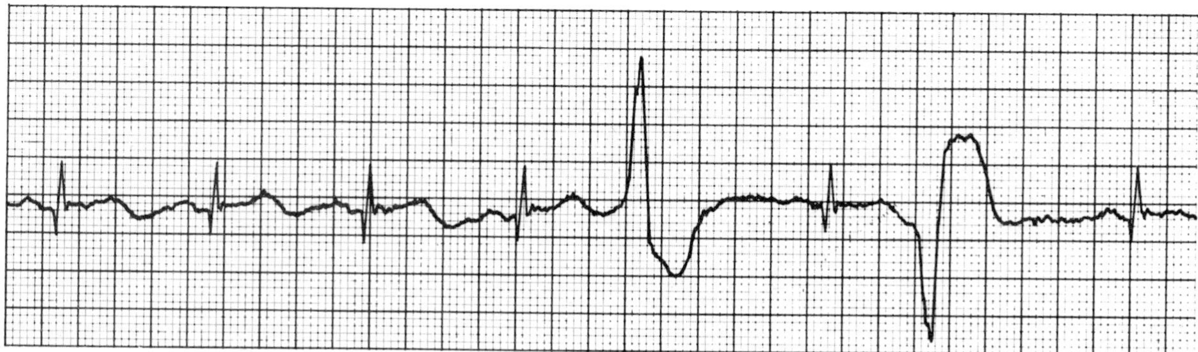

Figure 3-41. Multifocal premature ventricular contractions. (From Patel, J., McGowan, S., and Moody, L.: Arrhythmias: Detection, Treatment, and Cardiac Drugs. Philadelphia, W. B. Saunders, 1989, Fig. 63.)

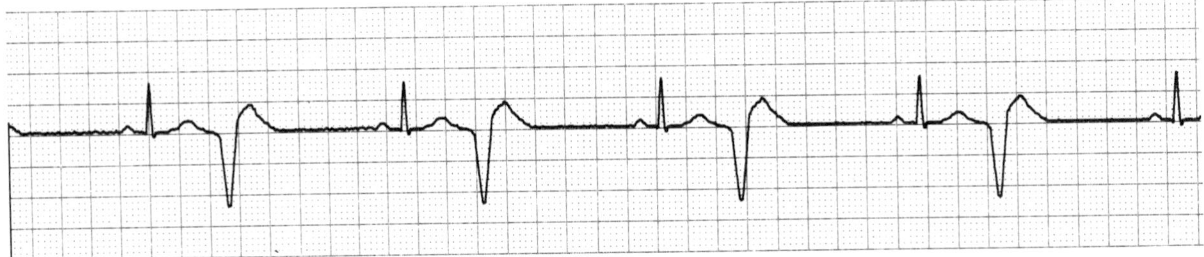

Figure 3–42. Premature ventricular contractions in a bigeminal pattern. Rhythm strip generated by the AA-700 Rhythm Simulator. (Reproduced with permission from Armstrong Medical Industries, Lincolnshire, Illinois, *DataSim,* Fig. 27.)

ECG tracing as a long pause following the PVC (see Fig. 3–41).

To determine if a pause is compensatory, place the points of the calipers, or mark a piece of paper, at the peak of the R waves of two consecutive normal beats *prior* to the PVC. Now flip the calipers over, or slide the paper over, one beat. The PVC will come in earlier than expected. Now flip the calipers, or move the paper over, to where the next normal sinus beat should come in. If the caliper point or pencil mark lands exactly on the next sinus beat, the sinus node has compensated for the one irregular beat and continued with the same rhythm. Therefore, the pause is compensatory.

Premature ventricular contractions may also occur in a predictable pattern. For example, PVCs may occur every other beat, every third, or every fourth beat. When PVCs occur every other beat, the pattern is referred to as bigeminy (Fig. 3–42). When the PVCs occur every third beat, the pattern is called trigeminy, and every fourth beat, quadrigeminy.

Premature ventricular contractions can also occur sequentially. Two PVCs in a row are termed a couplet (Fig. 3–43). Three PVCs in a row are termed a triplet, or salvo (Fig. 3–44).

Critical Criteria for Diagnosis: Premature Ventricular Contractions

* 1. Ectopic beat occurs prematurely, before the next anticipated sinus beat.
* 2. The QRS complex of the premature beat will be wider than 0.10 second.
* 3. The rhythm will be irregular due to the premature beats. However, the irregular beats may occur in a regular pattern.
* 4. The premature beat will usually be followed with a compensatory pause.
* 5. The ST segment of the PVC will slope away from, or be in the opposite direction from, the QRS of the PVC. In other words, if the QRS complex of the PVC is upright, or positive, then the ST segment will be downward, or negative (see Fig. 3–44).

6. P waves are usually absent prior to the ectopic beat.

7. PVCs may be unifocal or multifocal.

Hemodynamic Effects

The hemodynamic effects associated with PVCs are varied. Some patients may be asymptomatic, whereas others will report palpitations and lightheadedness. Symptoms usually worsen with an

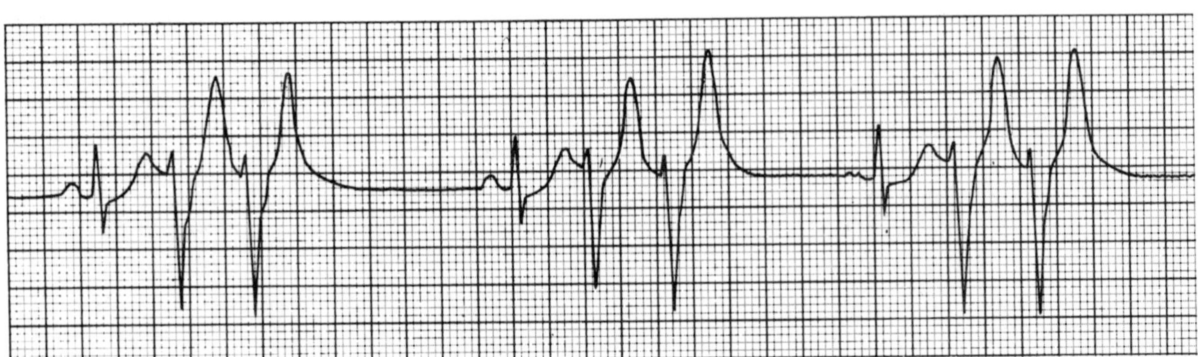

Figure 3–43. Two premature ventricular contractions in a row (couplet). (From Patel, J., McGowan, S., and Moody, L.: Arrhythmias: Detection, Treatment, and Cardiac Drugs. Philadelphia, W. B. Saunders, 1989, Fig. 61.)

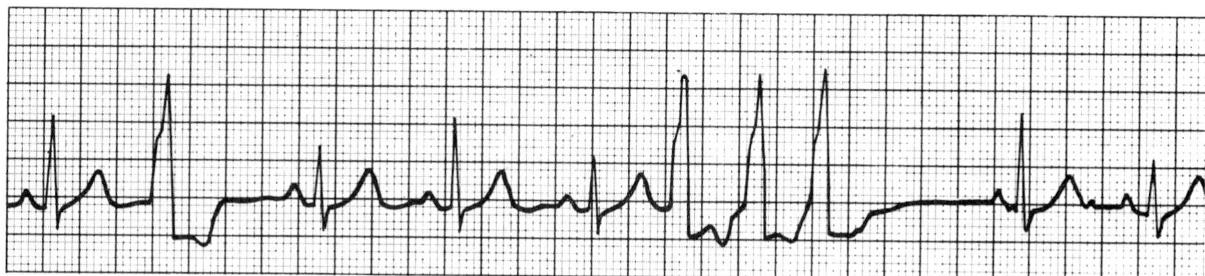

Figure 3-44. Three premature ventricular contractions in a row (triplet). (From Patel, J., McGowan, S., and Moody, L.: Arrhythmias: Detection, Treatment, and Cardiac Drugs. Philadelphia, W. B. Saunders, 1989, Fig. 72.)

increase in the number of ectopic beats. An increasing number of PVCs may serve as a warning for the potential development of ventricular tachycardia.

VENTRICULAR TACHYCARDIA

Ventricular tachycardia is a rapid rhythm that originates in the ventricles. Ventricular tachycardia is characterized by at least three premature ventricular complexes in a row. Ventricular tachycardia occurs at a rate greater than 100. This is a life-threatening dysrhythmia. The site of irritability in the ventricle is unifocal; therefore, all waveforms produced appear the same. Since ventricular tachycardia is considered an ectopic rhythm, depolarization of the ventricles occurs in an abnormal way. Abnormal or aberrant depolarization of the ventricles produces a widened QRS.

The wave of depolarization associated with ventricular tachycardia rarely reaches the atria. Therefore, P waves are not usually evident on the ECG. However, if P waves are present, they will usually be embedded in the T wave of the prior beat (Fig. 3-45).

Critical Criteria for Diagnosis: Ventricular Tachycardia

* 1. Greater than three PVCs in a row is considered ventricular tachycardia.

* 2. Heart rate is greater than 100 beats per minute.

* 3. QRS complex width is greater than 0.10 second.

4. P waves may or may not be visible. If visible, P waves will probably be embedded in the T wave of the preceding beat.

Hemodynamic Effects

Hemodynamic effects associated with ventricular tachycardia may vary. Most patients will have a significant loss of cardiac output with a resultant low blood pressure. Many patients will become pulseless with no obtainable blood pressure.

However, in rare instances, some patients will maintain a pulse and a blood pressure with ventricular tachycardia. Treatment of the dysrhythmia is dependent upon the presence or absence of a pulse and a blood pressure (American Heart Association, 1987).

VENTRICULAR FIBRILLATION

Ventricular fibrillation is a chaotic rhythm characterized by a quivering of the ventricles that results in a total loss of cardiac output. Patients experiencing ventricular fibrillation are in a state of clinical death. Clinical death means that the patient's heart has stopped contracting; therefore,

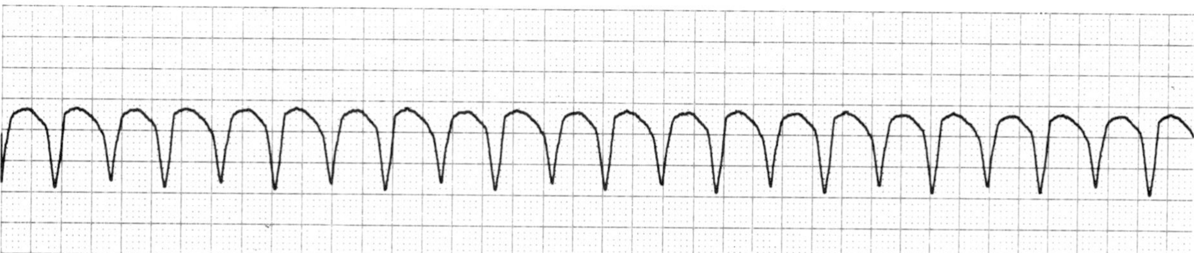

Figure 3-45. Ventricular tachycardia. Rhythm strip generated by the AA-700 Rhythm Simulator. (Reproduced with permission from Armstrong Medical Industries, Lincolnshire, Illinois, *DataSim*, Fig. 13.)

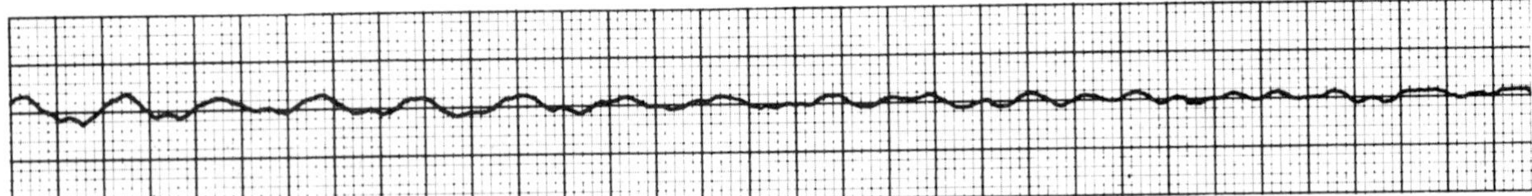

Figure 3-46. Fine ventricular fibrillation. (From Patel, J., McGowan, S., and Moody, L.: Arrhythmias: Detection, Treatment, and Cardiac Drugs. Philadelphia, W. B. Saunders, 1989, Fig. 86.)

there is no blood flow to the vital organs, including the brain, heart, lungs, and kidneys.

Ventricular fibrillation can occur without a known cause. When a patient fibrillates without the presence of cardiac disease, it is considered primary ventricular fibrillation. More commonly, however, patients fibrillate secondary to the processes listed under the discussion of PVCs.

The electrical energy created by ventricular fibrillation varies in amplitude. When voltage is low in the fibrillating ventricle, the result is a small-amplitude waveform. This form of ventricular fibrillation is referred to as fine (Fig. 3-46).

When voltage is greater in the fibrillating ventricle, the result is a larger-amplitude waveform. This form of ventricular fibrillation is referred to as coarse (Fig. 3-47). Coarse ventricular fibrillation responds better to defibrillation than does fine ventricular fibrillation (American Heart Association, 1987).

Critical Criteria for Diagnosis: Ventricular Fibrillation

* 1. Fluctuating, jagged baseline. No discernible P, Q, R, S, and T waves.
 2. Ventricular fibrillation may be coarse or fine.

Hemodynamic Effects

Hemodynamic effects are profound in ventricular fibrillation. All atrial and ventricular contractions cease, leading to total loss of cardiac output. There will be no palpable pulse or obtainable blood pressure. Brain death will occur within 4 to 6 minutes if life support is not instituted (American Heart Association, 1987).

IDIOVENTRICULAR RHYTHM

Idioventricular rhythm is an escape rhythm generated by the Purkinje fibers. This rhythm should emerge only when the SA and AV nodes have failed. The Purkinje fibers are capable of an intrinsic rate of 15 to 40 beats per minute. Since this rhythm originates in the deepest portion of the ventricles, normal depolarization is impossible. Aberrant conduction results. Therefore, the QRS of the idioventricular rhythm will be wider than normal. Because of the distance of the impulse formation from the atria, it is doubtful that atrial depolarization will occur. There is usually no evidence of P waves on the ECG strip.

Some patients with cardiac disease may experience idioventricular rhythm while sleeping. During deep sleep the metabolic demands of the body are diminished. The number of sinus depolarizations per minute, or heart rate, normally decreases with the decrease in metabolic demands. Should the patient be in a sinus bradycardia to begin with, this further slowing can encourage competition between the SA node and the Purkinje fibers.

The group of cardiac cells capable of beating the fastest will pace the heart. For example, if the sinus rate falls to 39 beats per minute and the Purkinje fibers can beat at 40 beats per minute, an idioventricular rhythm may emerge. This occurrence is more common in patients with severe

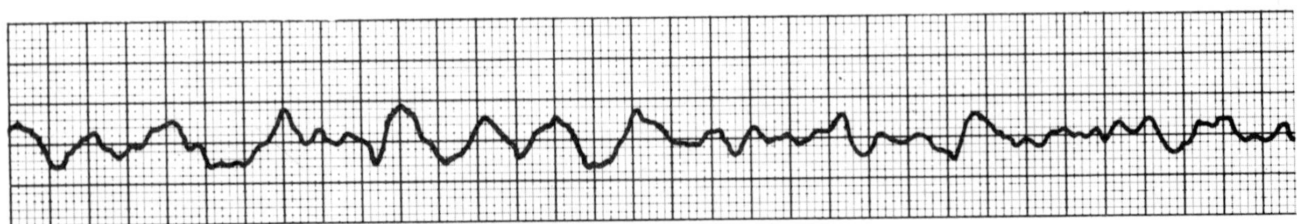

Figure 3-47. Coarse ventricular fibrillation. (From Patel, J., McGowan, S., and Moody, L.: Arrhythmias: Detection, Treatment, and Cardiac Drugs. Philadelphia, W. B. Saunders, 1989, Fig. 84.)

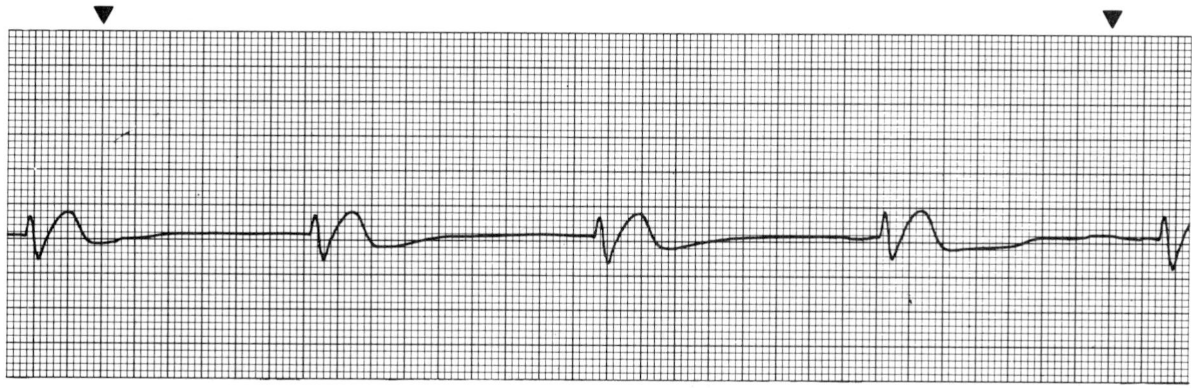

Figure 3-48. Idioventricular rhythm. (From Huff, J., Doernbach, D., and White, R.: ECG Workout: Exercises in Arrhythmia Interpretation. Philadelphia, J. B. Lippincott, 1985, Fig. 4.23.)

coronary artery disease and those whose SA and AV nodes are suppressed by drugs (Fig. 3-48).

Critical Criteria for Diagnosis: Idioventricular Rhythm

* 1. Heart rate is 15 to 40 beats per minute and regular.

* 2. Widened QRS interval, usually 0.12 second or greater.

3. P waves are not usually visible.

Hemodynamic Effects

Hemodynamic effects vary with idioventricular rhythm. Some patients will be able to maintain an adequate cardiac output and blood pressure, whereas others will become hypotensive.

When the rhythm occurs during sleep, it is often difficult to impossible to obtain the blood pressure while the rhythm is present. Since the patient is usually awakened suddenly for the taking of vital signs, his or her sympathetic nervous system will be stimulated. This liberates norepinephrine into the blood stream and stimulates the SA node to increase its rate and regain pacemaking function.

ACCELERATED IDIOVENTRICULAR RHYTHM

This rhythm is the same as that discussed for idioventricular rhythm except that the rate exceeds 40 beats per minute. The faster rate is due to increased automaticity in the Purkinje fibers. This is most often due to myocardial ischemia, injury, and infarction but it can also occur as a result of hypokalemia, digitalis toxicity, or various forms of heart disease (Fig. 3-49) (Patel et al., 1989).

Critical Criteria for Diagnosis: Accelerated Idioventricular Rhythm

* 1. Same as for idioventricular rhythm except that heart rate is greater than 40 beats per minute but less than 100 beats per minute.

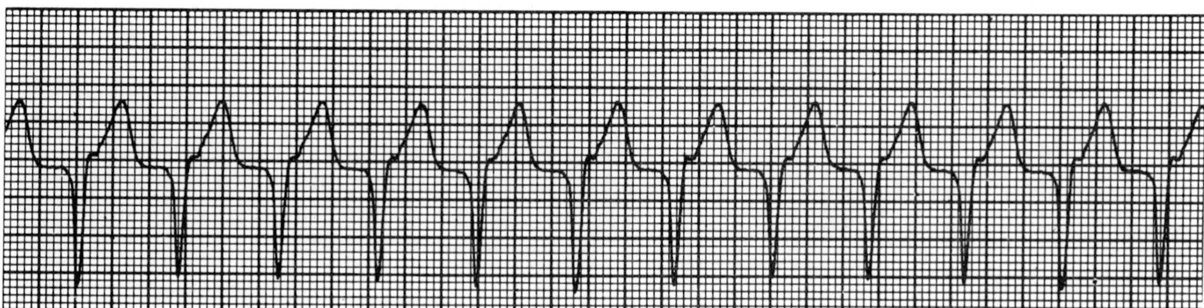

Figure 3-49. Accelerated idioventricular rhythm. (From Patel, J., McGowan, S., and Moody, L.: Arrhythmias: Detection, Treatment, and Cardiac Drugs. Philadelphia, W. B. Saunders, 1989, Fig. 80.)

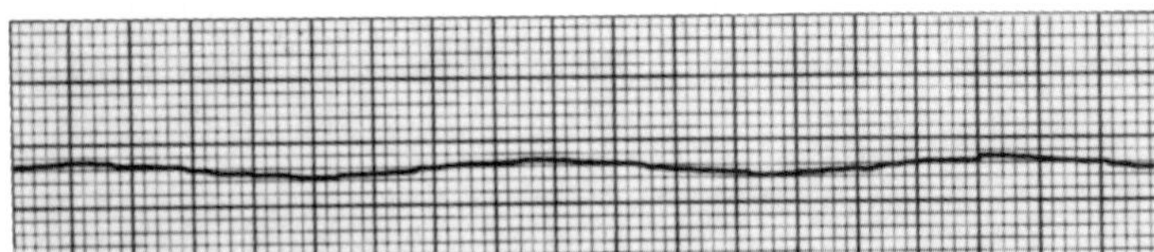

Figure 3–50. Ventricular standstill or asystole. (From Fenstermacher, K.: Dysrhythmia Recognition and Management. Philadelphia, W. B. Saunders, 1989, p. 54, asystole.)

Hemodynamic Effects

Hemodynamic effects of accelerated idioventricular rhythm correspond to the rate. Patients with rates less than 60 seem to tolerate this rhythm best. Patients with rates of 100 or greater will suffer the same effects as those for ventricular tachycardia.

VENTRICULAR STANDSTILL (ASYSTOLE)

Ventricular standstill is characterized by complete cessation of all electrical activity. A flat baseline is seen without any evidence of P, Q, R, S, or T waveforms. Ventricular standstill is also called asystole, since all contraction of the heart muscle stops. Ventricular standstill, or asystole, is the one arrhythmia discussed in this chapter.

Be aware that asystole may occur as the end result of a severe bradycardia, or sinus arrest. When questioning asystole, *always* remember to check to see that the patient's electrodes and ECG monitor patches are intact. If an electrode or patch is loose, the ECG pattern may be lost, creating a flat line that appears to be asystole (Fig. 3–50).

Critical Criteria for Diagnosis: Ventricular Standstill (Asystole)

* 1. Flat baseline observed with no evidence of P, Q, R, S, or T waveforms.

Hemodynamic Effects

The hemodynamic effects are the same as for ventricular fibrillation. The patient will lose all perfusion to the major organs and death will occur.

■ Atrioventricular Blocks

AV block refers to an impairment in the conduction of impulses from the atria to the ventricles. This impairment may cause slowed conduction of impulses, or it may lead to complete blockage of impulse conduction from the atria to the ventricles.

The most common processes related to impairment of impulse conduction are as follows (Guzzetta and Dossey, 1984):

Coronary Artery Disease (CAD). Both acute and chronic CAD can lead to impairment of impulse conduction. Coronary artery disease robs the conduction pathway of its normal blood supply, impairing impulse generation and conduction.

Infectious/Inflammatory Processes. Infectious and inflammatory processes can damage the conduction pathway, leading to impairment or blockage of impulses. These processes include systemic lupus erythematosus (SLE) and myocarditis.

Enhanced Vagal Tone. When the vagus nerve is stimulated, heart rate decreases and a transient impairment in impulse conduction may occur. The vagus nerve is stimulated by pressure on the carotid arteries, gagging, vomiting, coughing, and the Valsalva maneuver. Once the effect of the vagus nerve is removed, the impairment usually resolves.

Effects of Drugs. Many cardiac drugs have a negative dromotropic effect, or slowing down of conduction of impulses from the atria to the ventricles. This is a desired effect, in that a slower heart rate decreases the myocardial oxygen demand. In patients with a bradycardic rhythm, this effect may cause compromise.

There are four types of atrioventricular blocks, each categorized in terms of degree. The four types are first-degree, second-degree type I, second-degree type II, and third-degree block. The higher the degree of block, the more severe the consequences. First-degree block has minimal consequences, whereas third-degree block may have life-threatening consequences.

Each form of AV block is distinctly different from the others. However, the critical criteria for diagnosis for each type of block relate to some abnormality in the PR interval. Remember, the PR interval measures the amount of time it takes for an impulse to be generated in the atria, travel down to the AV node, and then be delayed there before entering the ventricles. When the impulse is delayed for longer than usual, the PR interval will lengthen.

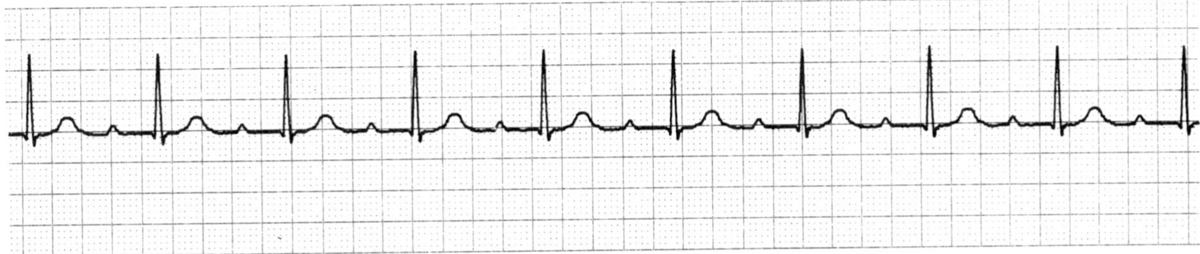

Figure 3-51. First-degree block. Rhythm strip generated by the AA-700 Rhythm Simulator. (Reproduced with permission from Armstrong Medical Industries, Lincolnshire, Illinois, *DataSim*, Fig. 19.)

FIRST-DEGREE BLOCK

First-degree block is a common dysrhythmia in the elderly and in patients with cardiac disease. As the normal conduction pathway ages and/or becomes diseased, impulse conduction becomes slower than normal. First-degree block often occurs in the setting of normal sinus rhythm or sinus bradycardia (Fig. 3-51).

Critical Criteria for Diagnosis: First-Degree Block

* 1. Underlying rhythm is usually normal sinus rhythm.
* 2. The PR interval is longer than the normal 0.12 to 0.20 second.
* 3. The PR interval of each beat is the same.

4. Often accompanied by sinus bradycardia.

Hemodynamic Effects

There are usually no hemodynamic changes associated with first-degree block. Changes in blood pressure are more likely if first-degree block is associated with bradycardia.

SECOND-DEGREE BLOCK

There are two types of second-degree block. Both types are characterized by distinctive criteria for diagnosis.

Second-Degree Block Type I: Mobitz I (Wenckebach's Phenomenon)

Second-degree AV block type I usually occurs at the level of the AV node and is characterized by progressive delay of impulse conduction.

The normal conduction tissue becomes progressively unable to conduct impulses from the atria to the ventricles. This progressive inability is demonstrated by a steadily lengthening PR interval, beat to beat.

The conduction tissue finally becomes unable to conduct the next sinus beat. Therefore, a P wave will be seen on the ECG tracing that is not followed by a QRS complex. By not conducting this one beat, the AV node is able to recover and then conduct the next atrial impulse (Fig. 3-52).

Critical Criteria for Diagnosis: Second-Degree Block Type I

* 1. PR interval progressively lengthens on a beat-by-beat basis until a P wave is not conducted. The lengthening of the PR may occur over three to four beats, or it may occur over less.
* 2. Pauses will be noted on the ECG following the unconducted P waves.

3. It will appear that there is a patterning or grouping of beats prior to each missed beat.

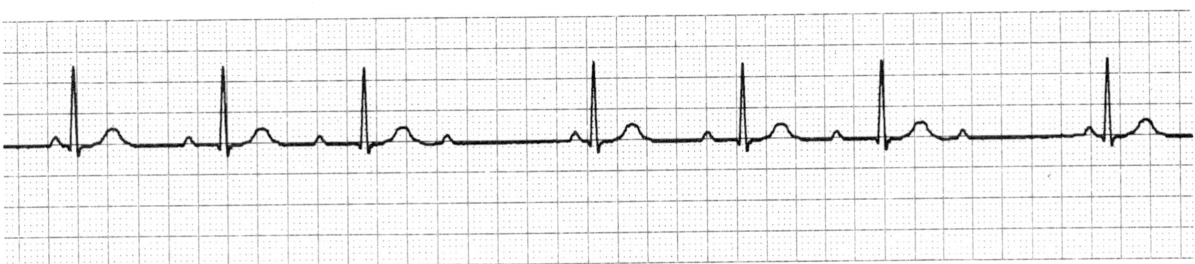

Figure 3-52. Second-degree block, Mobitz type I, or Wenckebach. Note steadily lengthening PR interval. Rhythm strip generated by the AA-700 Rhythm Simulator. (Reproduced with permission from Armstrong Medical Industries, Lincolnshire, Illinois, *DataSim*, Fig. 6.)

4. P to P intervals will usually be regular. This interval is measured with calipers or pencil and paper. Place the caliper points, or make a pencil mark on paper, at the peak of two consecutive P waves. Now flip the calipers over or slide the paper over. If the caliper point or pencil mark lands exactly on the next P wave's peak, the P to P interval is regular.

5. R to R intervals will usually be irregular. R to R intervals are measured using the technique described for P to P intervals. However, the peak of two consecutive R waves will be used instead.

6. QRS width is usually normal.

Hemodynamic Effects

Second-degree block type II is considered a self-limiting rhythm. In other words, it rarely progresses to a higher or more severe degree of block (American Heart Association, 1987). If the patient experiences any hemodynamic effects, they relate to the pauses seen on the ECG. If the patient is already bradycardic, these pauses will cause a further decrease in heart rate and a more pronounced effect on the cardiac output and the patient's blood pressure.

SECOND-DEGREE BLOCK TYPE II: MOBITZ II

Second-degree block type II is a more severe form of AV block. Like in type I, there are atrial impulses that are blocked from entering the ventricle. Unlike type I, however, these blocked beats are not preceded by a steadily lengthening PR interval. Instead, the PR interval remains the same, or is fixed, beat to beat. Despite the fact that the PR remains unchanged, a P wave occasionally, and without warning, will not be conducted down to the ventricles.

In some instances, the unconducted beats occur in a pattern, such as every other beat or every third beat. At other times, the unconducted beats will occur randomly, without pattern (Fig. 3-53).

Critical Criteria for Diagnosis: Second-Degree Block Type II

* 1. Occasional P waves are not followed by a QRS complex. These unconducted P waves may occur in a regular pattern such as every other beat or randomly without pattern.

* 2. The PR interval of conducted beats is consistently the same or fixed.

* 3. The P to P interval is regular.

Hemodynamic Effects

The hemodynamic effects of second-degree block type II correspond to the decrease in rate caused by the unconducted beats. Essentially, missed beats create a bradycardia. The greater the number of unconducted beats, the greater the impact on the cardiac output and blood pressure.

THIRD-DEGREE BLOCK (COMPLETE HEART BLOCK)

Third-degree block is often called complete heart block because no atrial impulses are conducted down to the ventricles. The block in conduction can occur at the level of the AV node, the bundle of His, or the bundle branches (Patel et al., 1989).

When a complete block exists between the atria and the ventricles, the rhythm of the heart beat becomes uncoordinated. The atria beat at one rate and the ventricles beat at a different rate. There is no communication between the two. This is why third-degree block is sometimes called AV dissociation.

In third-degree block, the atria are paced by the SA node, usually at a rate of 60 to 100. However, the atrial impulses are blocked from

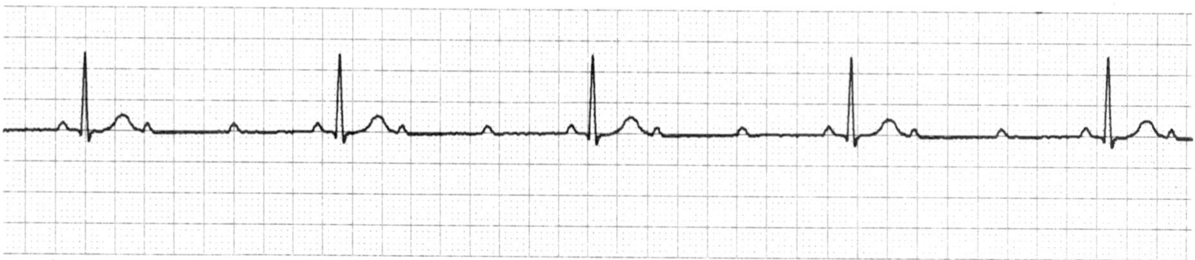

Figure 3-53. Second-degree block, Mobitz type II. Note fixed PR interval. Rhythm strip generated by the AA-700 Rhythm Simulator. (Reproduced with permission from Armstrong Medical Industries, Lincolnshire, Illinois, *DataSim*, Fig. 7.)

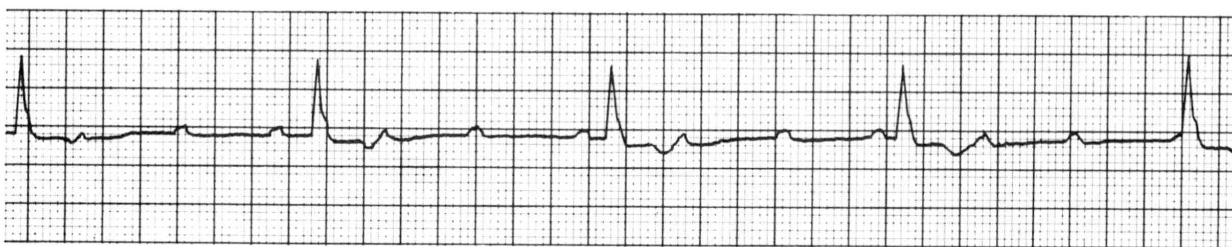

Figure 3-54. Third-degree block with nodal escape. (From Patel, J., McGowan, S., and Moody, L.: Arrhythmias: Detection, Treatment, and Cardiac Drugs. Philadelphia, W. B. Saunders, 1989, Fig. 107.)

entering the ventricles. When the ventricles do not receive an impulse from the atria, either the AV node or the Purkinje fibers can generate an escape rhythm. If the AV node acts as the back-up pacemaker, the rate will be 40 to 60 (Fig. 3-54). Since AV impulses are formed above the level of the ventricle, they proceed down the normal ventricular conduction pathway. This produces a QRS complex of normal width. If the Purkinje fibers act as the back-up pacemaker, the rate will be 15 to 40 (Fig. 3-55). Impulses generated in the ventricles must depolarize the heart in an abnormal way, resulting in a widened QRS complex.

In third-degree block, the ECG waveforms do not occur in normal sequence. Since the atrial rate is usually faster than the ventricular rate, there will be more P waves than R waves noted on the ECG. This produces a very unusual looking ECG. The P waves are regularly spaced throughout the strip. The R waves are also regularly spaced, but occur at a slower rate.

Even if P waves appear before QRS complexes, the P waves are not related to the QRS complex. They cannot be related, since there is a block in conduction between the atria and the ventricles. This lack of communication between the P waves and the QRS complexes can be further demonstrated by the widely varying PR interval. This variation in PR interval is totally unpredictable, unlike the progressive lengthening in second-degree block type I or the fixed interval in second-degree block type II (see Fig. 3-55).

Critical Criteria for Diagnosis: Third-Degree Block (Complete Heart Block)

* 1. There will be a difference in the atrial and ventricular heart rates. The atrial rate is usually greater than the ventricular rate.
* 2. The P to P intervals are regular.
* 3. The R to R intervals are regular.
* 4. The PR interval will vary constantly from beat to beat.
* 5. Waveforms occur in an abnormal sequence and appear to be dissociated from one another.
* 6. The QRS interval will be narrow, and the ventricular rate 40 to 60 beats per minute if the AV node is acting as the back-up pacemaker (see Fig. 3-54). If the Purkinje fibers act as the back-up pacemaker, the QRS complex will be wider than normal, and the ventricular rate will be 15 to 40 beats per minute (see Fig. 3-55).

Hemodynamic Effects

The hemodynamic effects of third-degree block depend upon the adequacy of the ventricular rate in maintaining cardiac output and blood pressure. Cardiac output and blood pressure are usu-

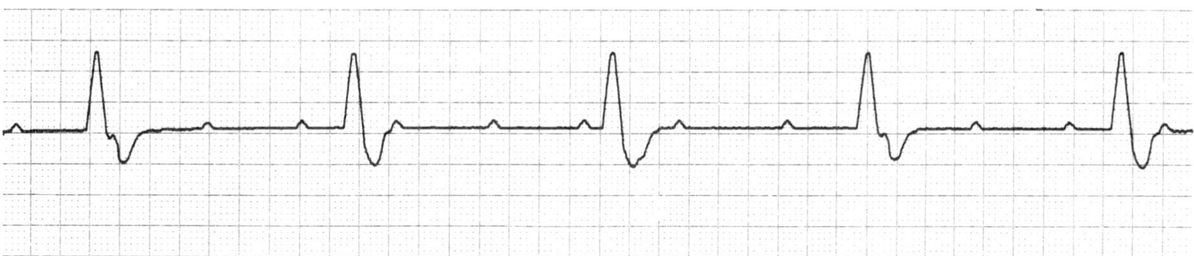

Figure 3-55. Third-degree block with ventricular escape. Rhythm strip generated by the AA-700 Rhythm Simulator. (Reproduced with permission from Armstrong Medical Industries, Lincolnshire, Illinois, *DataSim,* Fig. 8.)

ally improved with nodal escape rhythms owing to the faster rate.

Intervening with Patients Experiencing Dysrhythmias

Dysrhythmia interpretation is a required skill for the nurse working in the critical care unit. However, interpreting a rhythm correctly is only part of an important task. The nurse must be able to respond appropriately to, and intervene with, patients experiencing cardiac dysrhythmias.

Learning the criteria for each rhythm is a difficult enough challenge, and attempting to learn the treatment for each dysrhythmia may seem overwhelming. To simplify this process, the treatments for dysrhythmias discussed in this chapter are organized into the four following categories:

Intervening with patients experiencing rapid heart rates

Intervening with patients experiencing slow heart rates

Intervening with patients experiencing unpredictable rhythms

Intervening with patients experiencing life-threatening rhythms

Treatments discussed under each category are based upon recommendations presented in the second edition of the *Textbook of Advanced Cardiac Life Support,* published by the American Heart Association in 1987. Advanced cardiac life support (ACLS) combines basic life support (BLS) and dysrhythmia recognition with the more aggressive techniques, including entubation, drugs, and pacemaking.

The ACLS textbook details the standards commonly accepted by health care professionals for the care of patients requiring advanced life-saving techniques and interventions. These standards are presented, in an abbreviated form, in a decision tree known as an algorithm. These algorithms are reproduced in Chapter 6: Code Management. This discussion of treatments is an elaboration of the ACLS algorithms.

Intervening with Patients Experiencing Rapid Heart Rates

Of the dysrhythmias covered in this chapter, several are characterized by rapid rates: sinus tachycardia; atrial tachycardia, fibrillation, and flutter; and nodal tachycardia.

All of these dysrhythmias listed originate above the level of the ventricles. Therefore, tachycardias originating in the SA node, atria, or AV node are often referred to as supraventricular tachycardias (SVTs). Supraventricular tachycardia is a generic and nonspecific term that clarifies that the tachycardic rhythm is *not* from the ventricles, and therefore will not require or respond to many of the treatments used for ventricular tachycardia.

Ventricular tachycardia is the only rapid rhythm that is not covered in this section. Ventricular tachycardia will be discussed under the life-threatening rhythms.

Treatment of rapid-rate dysrhythmias, or SVTs, may include the following:

1. Mediating the effects of the parasympathetic and sympathetic nervous systems
2. Intervening with appropriate cardiac drugs
3. Utilizing electrical energy to convert the rapid rhythm to a slower, more normal rhythm

Successful treatment of these dysrhythmias may include one or all of these approaches. Severity of the patient's symptoms will also dictate treatment choice and timing. When a patient has a stable blood pressure, less aggressive means of treatment, such as those discussed under mediation of the nervous system effects, can be employed. When a patient is experiencing hypotension, intervention is more aggressive and includes either cardiac drugs, electrical energy, or both.

MEDIATING THE EFFECTS OF THE NERVOUS SYSTEM

When the sympathetic nervous system (SNS) is stimulated by pain or anxiety, it releases norepinephrine. Norepinephrine increases SA node automaticity, and thereby causes sinus tachycardia. If there are other areas of the heart that are irritable, such as the atria or the AV node, norepinephrine will also enhance their automaticity. Atrial fibrillation, flutter, or nodal tachycardia can develop.

If a patient is hemodynamically stable while experiencing one of the rapid-rate dysrhythmias, a noninvasive maneuver can be used to decrease the stimulating effect of norepinephrine. Noninvasive maneuvers are those that do not require alteration of the skin's integrity or insertion of any device into the body. These maneuvers include relaxation techniques, pain and anxiety relief, and vagal maneuvers.

Relaxation Techniques. Relaxation techniques are used to diminish the stress response. Guided imagery, biofeedback, and audiotapes may be useful for some patients who experience rapid-rate dysrhythmias that are stress related (Guzzetta and Dossey, 1984). Often, patients have recurrent episodes of these dysrhythmias. The patient can be taught various relaxation techniques to slow the heart rate as well as to prevent recurrences.

Pain and Anxiety Relief. Pain and anxiety relief should be a nursing goal for any patient who has, or is at risk for, dysrhythmias. Anxiety is a commonly expressed patient response to hospitalization, particularly in the critical care unit. In addition to providing the cited relaxation therapies, the nurse must remember to keep the patient and family informed of all procedures. Knowledge deficit can lead to increased anxiety, which may be manifest in the form of dysrhythmias. Therefore, patient education is an important part of the patient care plan.

Additionally, the use of mild sedatives may be indicated in some patients. Drugs such as diazepam (Valium) and alprazolam (Xanax) may be ordered on schedule or as required for patients at high risk for anxiety-related dysrhythmias. Valium is often the drug of choice, since it can be given both orally and intravenously.

Pain relief should also be a primary goal included in the patient care plan. Any source of pain, whether acute or chronic, can lead to stimulation of the SNS and increase the heart rate. Consequently, alteration in comfort should be continually assessed and treated appropriately. While chest pain is of ultimate concern to the nurse caring for the patient with cardiac disease, other sources of pain should not be ignored or remain untreated.

Appropriate drugs should be ordered to treat both acute and chronic pain. Morphine sulfate is often the drug of choice for acute pain. It is administered intravenously in 1- to 2-mg increments. Meperidine hydrochloride (Demerol) may also be used in patients who are allergic to morphine. Any medication that the patient has been taking for chronic pain prior to hospitalization should also be administered to the patient during hospitalization.

Vagal Maneuvers. Vagal maneuvers are used to stimulate the vagus nerve of the parasympathetic nervous system (PNS). The vagus nerve slows the heart rate when it is stimulated. Therefore, the PNS acts as a counterbalance for the sympathetic nervous system. The vagus nerve is usually stimulated in one of two following ways:

1. When a patient is in a rapid-rate dysrhythmia, carotid massage can be used to stimulate the vagus nerve. Gentle, downward pressure on *one* carotid artery, just beneath the mandible, can lead to increased vagal tone with resultant slowing of the heart rate. This effect is caused by suppression of automaticity in the SA node as well as decreased conduction through the AV node.

   This maneuver is usually performed by the physician. The patient must be closely observed for changes in mental status as the carotid is massaged. If a patient has poor blood flow through the carotids, this maneuver may lead to inadequate cerebral perfusion.

2. The Valsalva maneuver will also elicit strong vagal tone. Ask the patient to tense his/her abdominal muscles briefly. This bearing down causes increased vagal stimulation. This maneuver should not be used in patients with increased intracranial pressure (Kenner et al., 1991).

As vagal maneuvers are performed, the bedside ECG is closely monitored. If the maneuver is successful, the heart rate will begin to return to normal. If the patient is in paroxysmal atrial tachycardia (PAT), fibrillation, or flutter, you may notice that fewer of the rapid atrial impulses are being conducted to the ventricles.

INTERVENING WITH CARDIAC DRUGS

Many classes of cardiac drugs are used to control or decrease heart rate. These include the beta-blockers, calcium channel blockers, cardiac glycosides, and antidysrhythmics.

Beta-Blockers. The SNS exerts two types of effects, alpha and beta. The alpha effects of the SNS primarily relate to vasoconstriction and the resultant increase of blood pressure. The beta effects of the SNS are increased heart rate, increased strength of cardiac contraction, and bronchodilation. Beta-blocking drugs block or diminish the beta effects of the sympathetic nervous system (Swonger and Matejski, 1988).

In the setting of myocardial infarction, beta-blockers are particularly useful for preventing and treating tachycardic rhythms. In addition to suppressing automaticity in the SA node, beta-blockers also effectively suppress automaticity in irritable areas surrounding the infarct area. The beta-blockers are particularly useful in slowing down the rate of sinus tachycardia, atrial tachycardia, fibrillation, and flutter. A secondary benefit in the use of beta-blockade in myocardial infarction is the decreased oxygen consumption associated with decreasing heart rate (Andreoli et al., 1987).

Propranolol (Inderal) and labetalol (Normodyne) are two beta-blocking drugs that can be given intravenously or orally. These drugs suppress SA node depolarization and AV conduction. These are desired effects in patients experiencing rapid-rate dysrhythmias. There may also be an associated alpha-blocking effect of lowered blood pressure.

In addition to monitoring the effects of slowed heart rate, the nurse must also watch for other potential effects, decreased strength of contractility, and bronchoconstriction. Blocking of the beta effect of increased strength of contractility can lead to a less effective cardiac contraction. This can result in decreased cardiac output and lowered blood pressure. Patients who are known to have a history of congestive heart failure or myocardial infarction should be monitored closely for signs of decreased contractility while on beta-blockers (Swonger and Matejski, 1988).

Calcium Channel Blockers. The calcium channel blocking drugs are very useful in the slowing of rapid heart rates. Calcium is the third electrolyte involved in the cardiac cycle. Calcium moves across the cardiac cell membrane during depolarization. By blocking some of calcium's movement, the rate of depolarization can be slowed. When depolarizations are slowed, heart rate and oxygen consumption are decreased.

The calcium channel blocker verapamil (Isoptin) is frequently used in patients with paroxysmal atrial tachycardia (PAT), fibrillation, and flutter. It is the only calcium channel blocker that is available in intravenous form. Five to ten milligrams is injected intravenously, slowly over 2 minutes. The ECG is closely monitored during and following the injection. Effects will be seen within 5 to 15 minutes. If effective, the heart rate will slow and then convert back to a sinus rhythm. If the tachycardic rhythm persists, the same dose can be repeated in 30 minutes.

Cardiac Glycosides. The drugs digitalis (Lanoxin) and digitoxin (Crystodigin) are cardiac glycosides, or cardiotonics. They are known for their ability to increase the strength of contraction; however, they are also very useful in suppressing sinus depolarization and atrial irritability and slowing conduction through the AV node. Available in oral and intravenous forms, these drugs can be used for sinus and nodal tachycardia and acute or chronic atrial dysrhythmias (Swonger and Matejski, 1988).

To ensure adequate drug levels and effectiveness, the patient must be "digitalized" over a period of time. Intravenous digitalization is accomplished by giving 0.5 mg in divided doses over 24 hours. This can also be accomplished by oral doses. For oral digitalization, up to 1 mg is given as a loading dose and is then followed by 0.125 to 0.5 mg daily.

When a patient's hemodynamic status becomes compromised secondary to a rapid atrial dysrhythmia, intravenous dosing is the route of choice. The ECG is monitored closely as the initial dose is given. Effects may not occur until 30 minutes to 2 hours following the initial dose (Skidmore-Roth, 1991).

One sign of digitalis or digitoxin toxicity is the development of dysrhythmias. The toxic patient may present with the same dysrhythmias that he/she was taking the cardiotonic to treat. In addition to atrial dysrhythmias, the patient may also develop bradycardia or AV block. To determine if the patient is toxic, a serum digoxin level is drawn.

Antidysrhythmics. Multiple agents may be used for the treatment of dysrhythmias. These are discussed in Chapters 6 and 8.

UTILIZING ELECTRICAL ENERGY

When patients with rapid-rate dysrhythmias are hypotensive but have a pulse, it often becomes necessary to utilize electrical energy to convert the rapid rate to a more normal one.

Synchronized cardioversion involves using varying amounts of electrical energy, 10 to 360 joules (J), applied to the chest wall to convert undesirable rhythms into more normal ones. Rhythms such as atrial flutter usually require low initial doses of electricity (25 J), and no more than 200 J total. Atrial and nodal tachycardia usually require 75 to 100 J and atrial fibrillation usually requires 100 J initially. Up to 360 J may be used in atrial and nodal tachycardia and atrial fibrillation (American Heart Association, 1987). Care of the patient before, during, and after cardioversion is outlined in detail in Chapter 6 on code management.

The defibrillator is used for synchronized cardioversion; however, the machine is first placed into the synchronized mode. The electrical energy is delivered directly on top of one of the patient's R waves. In other words, it is synchronized with the patient's QRS complex. By synchronizing the electricity with the patient's own ventricular depolarization, there is a better chance of halting the rapid-rate dysrhythmia.

It is hoped that when the shock is delivered directly on the QRS, the irritable area creating the dysrhythmia will be depolarized (Andreoli et al., 1987). Repolarization always follows depolarization. During this resting phase the SA node has the opportunity to emerge as the dominant pacemaker. It sometimes takes multiple shocks to convert the abnormal rhythm to NSR. The amount of electricity is increased with each sequential shock until the rapid-rate dysrhythmia is converted.

If the patient's ECG does not demonstrate a clear R wave, delivery of a synchronized dose of electricity on the R wave will be inaccurate, if not impossible. Particularly in the very rapid rhythms, the ECG machine may not be able to distinguish between the various waveforms. In this case, defibrillation may be required. If a patient with rapid-rate dysrhythmia is pulseless, defibrillation is also required (American Heart Association, 1987).

Intervening with Patients Experiencing Slow Heart Rates

Many of the dysrhythmias discussed in this chapter have the overall effect of slowing the heart rate. Slowing of the heart rate whether due to decreased automaticity, blocking of impulses, or the emergence of a lower-rate pacemaker creates the same hemodynamic response and requires the same basic treatment. These slow-rate dysrhythmias include sinus bradycardia, dysrhythmia, and arrest/exit block; nodal rhythm; atrioventricular blocks; and idioventricular rhythm.

Treatment of slow heart rates may include the following:

1. Suppression of the parasympathetic nervous system effects
2. Utilization of appropriate cardiac drugs
3. Utilization of electrical energy to increase heart rate

It is most important to realize that treatment of the slow dysrhythmias should be based upon the patient's blood pressure *not* the heart rate itself. An arbitrary heart rate, for instance, fewer than 60 beats per minute, cannot be established as a magical point at which a patient should be treated. When a patient with bradycardia becomes hypotensive, the heart rate is too low and should be treated (Guzzetta and Dossey, 1984).

SUPPRESSION OF THE PARASYMPATHETIC NERVOUS SYSTEM

Stimulation of the PNS via the vagus nerve results in a slowing of heart rate. It is important that the nurse be aware of processes that can increase vagal tone, such as vomiting, gagging, carotid massage, and performing the Valsalva maneuver.

Nausea and vomiting should be controlled with antiemetics or nasogastric suctioning if necessary. Palpation of the carotid arteries should be done cautiously and avoided if possible. Prevention of constipation through the administration of stool softeners and laxatives will keep the patient from straining at stool (i.e., performing the Valsalva maneuver).

Hypoxia can also lead to slowing of the heart rate. In the critical care setting, endotracheal suctioning is a common cause of hypoxia and often results in bradycardia. Endotracheal suctioning should be based upon breath sounds and not performed on an arbitrary schedule. Suctioning should be accomplished within 15 seconds if possible, and the bedside monitor should be watched as you suction.

To further ensure the patient's safety, hyperoxygenation is recommended prior to and following endotracheal suctioning. Hyperoxygenation is accomplished by Ambu bagging the patient with 100% oxygen for several breaths (Moorhouse et al., 1987). Closed-system suction equipment is also helpful in decreasing suction-related hypoxia.

Utilization of Appropriate Cardiac Drugs

The drugs atropine and isoproterenol are commonly used to increase heart rate in the hypotensive patient. Both are positive dromotropic agents.

Atropine is classified as a vagolytic drug because it blocks the effect of the vagus nerve and increases heart rate. Atropine is given in 0.05- to 1.0-mg doses, intravenous push. This dose may be repeated *up to* a total dose of 2 mg.

Isoproterenol (Isuprel) has a chemical composition similar to norepinephrine. It causes an increase in heart rate via stimulation of the beta effects of the sympathetic nervous system. Isoproterenol is given in an intravenous drip. Four milligrams of isoproterenol is mixed in a 250-ml bag of 5% dextrose in water and then titrated until heart rate and blood pressure begin to increase.

Both atropine and isoproterenol must be used cautiously and appropriately. Increased heart rate results in increased myocardial oxygen consumption. In the patient with cardiac disease, this increased rate and oxygen consumption may lead to ischemia, injury, and ultimately infarction (American Heart Association, 1987). Therefore, these drugs should be reserved for use *only* when bradycardia is accompanied by hypotension.

Utilization of Electrical Energy

In severe cases of bradycardia, utilization of electrical energy will be necessary to pace the heart. This energy will be delivered in the form of a temporary cardiac pacemaker. A pacemaker is required when the SA node fails and when the AV node and the Purkinje fibers prove inadequate or fail to act as back-up pacemakers (Guzzetta and Dossey, 1984).

Cardiac pacemakers can deliver varying amounts of electrical energy at varying rates. The pacemaker is set at a rate and electrical output that will maintain an adequate cardiac output and blood pressure. Second-degree type II block and third-degree block often require the use of a pacemaker. The need for the pacemaker may be temporary or permanent.

Temporary Pacemakers

There are three types of temporary pacemakers used for slow heart rates in the clinical setting. They will be discussed in the order in which they appear in the ACLS algorithm for bradycardia: external, transvenous, and transthoracic (American Heart Association, 1987).

External Pacemaking. The external pacemaker, also called the external noninvasive pacemaker, may be a free-standing piece of equipment or a part of the defibrillator (see Fig. 6–21).

The external pacemaker delivers electrical current directly to the skin via two electrodes. External pacing is accomplished by positioning two large monitor patches. One patch is placed on the anterior chest, over the heart. The other patch is placed on the patient's back, over the posterior surface of the heart. An electrode is attached to each monitor patch and then connected to the external pacemaker. Electricity conducts through the skin, the skeletal muscle, and then through the heart muscle, causing depolarization.

The external pacemaker has two modes: demand and asynchronous. The demand mode paces the heart based on need. A heart rate is set, for instance, 60 beats per minute, and if the patient's heart rate falls below 60, the pacemaker will generate an impulse to pace the heart. The asynchronous mode paces the heart at a set rate independent of any activity the patient's heart generates. The demand mode is safer for the patient, and is therefore the mode of choice.

Once the mode is set, the electrical output is adjusted until the patient is 100% paced. Heart rate is then adjusted until an adequate blood pressure is obtained (Kinkade and Lohrman, 1990). A more thorough discussion will follow under the discussion of transvenous pacemaking.

External pacemaking can be instituted within seconds. It does not require a physician and can be initiated by a nurse. However, this means of pacing is truly *temporary*. The direct application of electrical current to the skin is uncomfortable. If the patient's situation requires ongoing support for pacemaking, a transvenous pacemaker should be inserted as soon as possible.

Transvenous Pacemaking. Transvenous pacemaking is employed by introducing a large-bore catheter into a large vein, such as the subclavian, brachial, femoral, or jugular, using sterile technique. A special pacing catheter can then be threaded via the introducer into the appropriate chamber for pacing. The atria, the ventricles, or both can be paced. If atrial pacing is needed, the flexible catheter is threaded via the introducer through the superior or inferior vena cava and into the right atrium. If ventricular pacing is needed, the catheter is threaded into the right ventricle. An ideal position is achieved when the catheter tip touches the wall of the heart and stabilizes in the folds of the endocardium (Kinkade and Lohrman, 1990).

Most pacing catheters utilize a bipolar lead. Bipolar means that there are two electrodes encased within the pacing catheter. One electrode terminates at the end of the pacing catheter, and as such is designated the distal electrode. The second electrode terminates above the level of the distal electrode, and as such is designated the proximal electrode (Fig. 3–56). Electrical energy flows between these two electrodes and causes depolarization.

Temporary pacing catheters are available for atrial, ventricular, and AV pacing. There are straight tips, J-shaped tips, and balloon-tipped catheters in a range of sizes from 3 to 7 French.

Once the pacemaking catheter is in contact with the wall of the heart, a pacemaking generator is attached to the ends of the pacemaking wire left outside of the patient's body. There are generators for accomplishing AV pacing and for simpler ventricular pacing.

Pacemaking generators have five basic controls:

1. On/off switch.
2. Rate control—usually varies between 30 and 180 beats per minute.

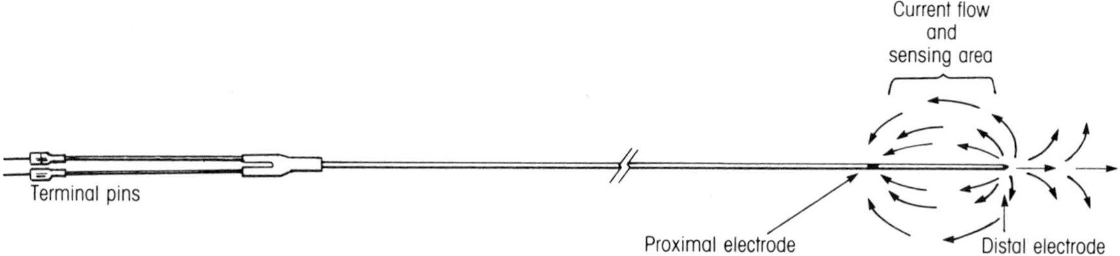

Figure 3-56. A bipolar pacing catheter. (From Sager, D.: The person requiring cardiac pacing. In: Guzzetta, C., and Dossey, B. [eds.]: Cardiovascular Nursing: Bodymind Tapestry. St. Louis, C. V. Mosby, 1992, Fig. 13-6.)

3. Electrical output—registered in milliamperes (mA). Electrical output can be varied between 0.1 and 20 mA.

4. Sensitivity control—registered in milliamperes. Sensitivity can be varied between 0.5 and 20 mA.

5. Mode—The pacemaker can function in either a demand or asynchronous mode.

When the atria alone or both the atria and ventricles require pacing, an AV sequential pacemaking generator is usually used. The generator has dual controls for setting electrical output and heart rate for both the atria and the ventricles. To begin temporary pacing, the generator is turned on. Generators are battery powered. If the unit fails to come on, the battery may be dead. Most pacemakers have a safety lock for the on/off switch that prevents the generator from being accidentally turned off.

Once the generator is turned on, the rate control is usually set at 60 to 70 beats per minute. Now the electrical output is turned up until the patient's heart is 100% paced by the pacemaker. When the patient's heart is being paced, the ECG strip will demonstrate an electrical artifact called the pacer spike. If the atria are being paced, the spike will appear before the P wave (Fig. 3-57). If the ventricles are being paced, the spike will appear before the QRS (Fig. 3-58). If both the atria and the ventricles are being paced, spikes will appear before the P wave and the QRS (Fig. 3-59).

This thin, vertical spike will typically be followed by a larger than normal P wave or wider QRS complex. Since the heart is being paced in an artificial, or abnormal, fashion the path of depolarization is altered and consequently waveforms and intervals are altered.

Depolarization of the atria or ventricle, as evidenced by a pacer spike and the enlarged P wave or widened QRS complex, is called capture. The minimum amount of electrical energy required to achieve capture is called threshold. It usually takes less than 1 mA to achieve capture (American Heart Association, 1987). To maintain capture, the electrical output is set at two to three times threshold.

Once capture has been assured, the heart rate can be set so that an adequate blood pressure results. The lowest heart rate possible is used so as to diminish myocardial oxygen demands and consumption.

The generator has an asynchronous mode and a demand mode. Again, asynchronous means that the pacer does not synchronize its pacemaking with the patient's own intrinsic pacemaking. Demand mode means that the pacemaker generates an impulse only when the patient is unable to generate his/her own. Like in external pacemaking, demand is the mode of choice.

The final control to be set on the generator

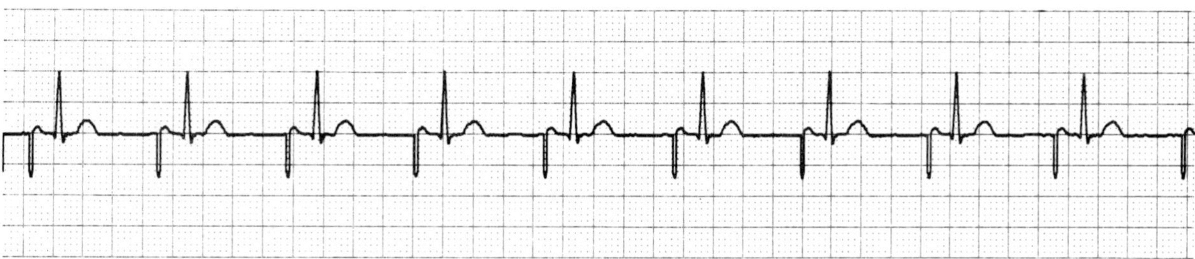

Figure 3-57. Paced rhythm: Atrial. Note spike in front of the P wave. Rhythm strip generated by the AA-700 Rhythm Simulator. (Reproduced with permission from Armstrong Medical Industries, Lincolnshire, Illinois, *DataSim*, Fig. 32.)

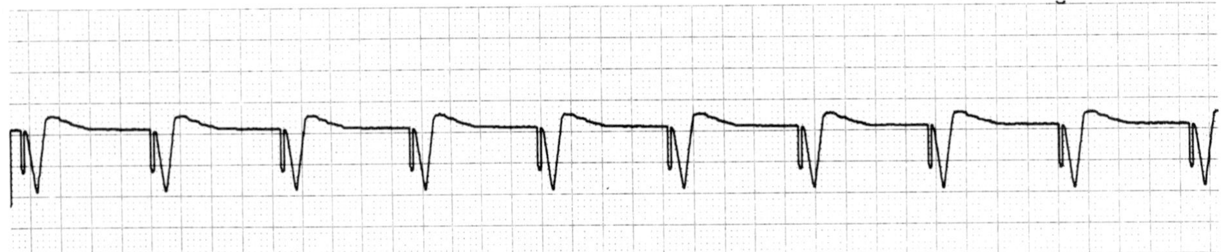

Figure 3-58. Paced rhythm: Ventricular. Note spike in front of the QRS. Rhythm strip generated by the AA-700 Rhythm Simulator. (Reproduced with permission from Armstrong Medical Industries, Lincolnshire, Illinois, *DataSim,* Fig. 36.)

is sensitivity. Sensitivity relates to the generator's ability to "sense" that the patient is having his/her own heart beat. There is a sense/pace indicator light or needle at the top of every generator. When the generator delivers a paced beat, the pace light will come on or the needle will indicate paced. If the patient generates his/her own beat, the sense indicator should register. Sensitivity is adjusted until the indicator registers all patient beats.

After all controls have been set, the pacemaker generator should be secured. In addition, precautions should be taken to protect the patient from microshock. For safety, the generator should be secured with a cloth-fastening strap to the patient's chest or arm for a subclavian, jugular, or brachial insertion and to the thigh for a femoral insertion. The generator should *never* be secured to the patient's gown, bed, or IV pole (Guzzetta and Dossey, 1984). The patient should be taught how to turn and move in bed so as not to dislodge pacing wire placement.

In the older generators, the connection between the pacing wire and the generator is exposed. These generators should be covered by a rubber glove. By insulating the generator with the rubber glove, the patient and the nurse will be protected from any leakage of electricity. Newer generators conceal the terminal connections within the generator. However, for safety, the nurse should still wear rubber gloves when working with the generator.

Other electrical safety precautions include limiting the use of line-powered electrical devices, such as volume infusion pumps, lamps, and ECG machines. There is a potential for electrical interference from these machines with the pacemaker. If these devices are used, avoid allowing them to touch the metal bed frame. The patient should not use an electrical razor.

Troubleshooting the Transvenous Pacemaker. In addition to the usual risks of bleeding and infection associated with invasive techniques, there are two primary problems that can occur with a temporary pacemaker. The first is failure to capture and the second is failure to sense.

FAILURE TO CAPTURE. When the pacemaker generates an electrical impulse and there is no cardiac muscular response, there is failure to capture. On the ECG, a pacer spike will occur with no evidence of depolarization. If an atrial pacer fails to capture, the atrial pacer spike will not be followed by a P wave. If a ventricular pacer fails to capture, the ventricular pacer spike will not be followed by a QRS (Fig. 3-60). Failure to capture can occur secondary to pacing wire displacement or fracture and to battery failure. If the battery is not the problem, the pacing wire can be repositioned to assure that it is in close contact with the wall of the heart.

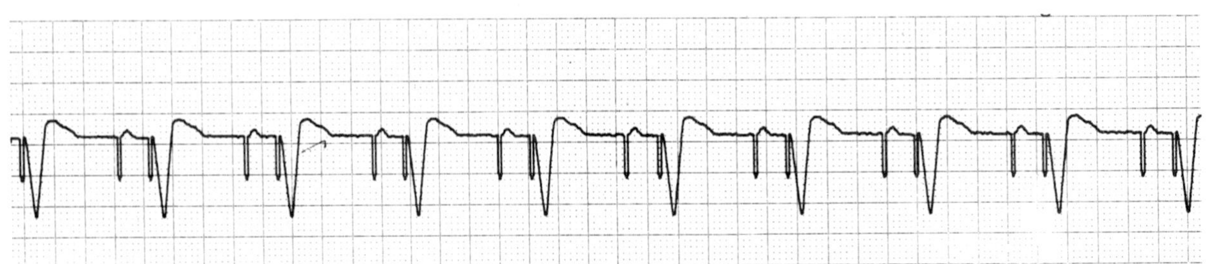

Figure 3-59. Paced rhythm: Atrioventricular sequential. Note spikes prior to the P wave and the QRS. Rhythm strip generated by the AA-700 Rhythm Simulator. (Reproduced with permission from Armstrong Medical Industries, Lincolnshire, Illinois, *DataSim,* Fig. 33.)

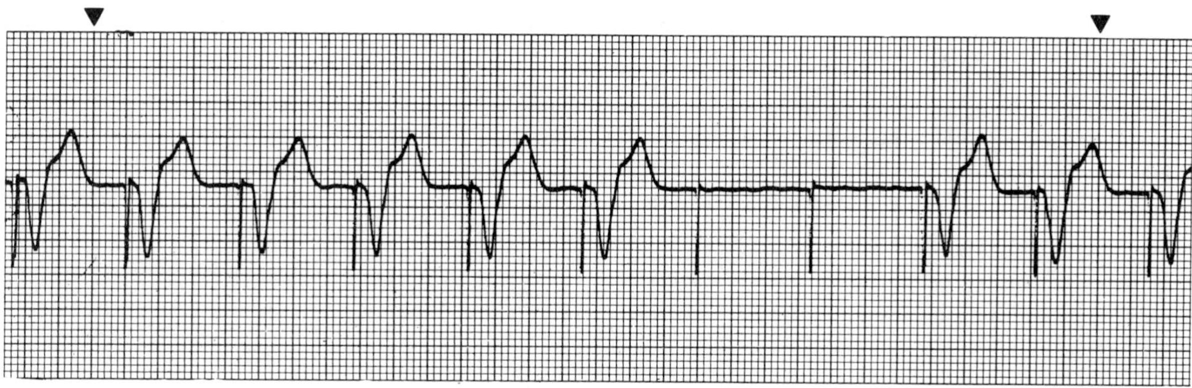

Figure 3-60. Paced rhythm with failure to capture. (From Huff, J., Doernbach, D., and White, R.: ECG Workout: Exercises in Arrhythmia Interpretation. Philadelphia, J. B. Lippincott, 1985, Fig. 5.26.)

If there is still failure to capture, a chest x-ray should be ordered to check for lead fracture. The pacing catheter is radiopaque, and therefore interruption in the wire can sometimes be seen on x-ray. If lead fracture has occurred and the patient continues to need pacing, a new pacing catheter must be inserted.

If all of the above are ruled out and there is still failure to capture, the electrical output (mA) can be increased. If the pacing catheter has drifted into an area of muscular injury or infarct, higher milliamperes may be required to obtain capture.

FAILURE TO SENSE. It is imperative that the pacemaker generator be able to sense when the patient's heart is generating an intrinsic beat. Otherwise, the pacemaker generator could deliver an electrical impulse on top of the patient's own heart beat. When a pacemaker impulse falls on the T wave, there is a possibility of stimulating a life-threatening dysrhythmia, such as ventricular fibrillation (Andreoli et al., 1987).

Failure to sense is manifest as inappropriate pacer spikes on the ECG tracing; inappropriate in that the spikes fall on or near the patient's own beats (Fig. 3-61). Again, this problem can occur when the catheter has become dislodged or fractured. The physician can attempt repositioning the pacing catheter, and can obtain a chest x-ray to check for dislodgement or fracture.

If the inappropriate pacer spikes are falling on the patient's T wave, or if ectopic beats are being generated, the nurse can turn the pacemaker off. If the pacemaker is turned off, the patient must be closely monitored. If the patient does have an irregular rhythm, the ECG and blood pressure should be monitored closely. The situation can then be evaluated and either pacing discontinued or a new pacing wire inserted. If the patient is unable to generate a heart rate, or if

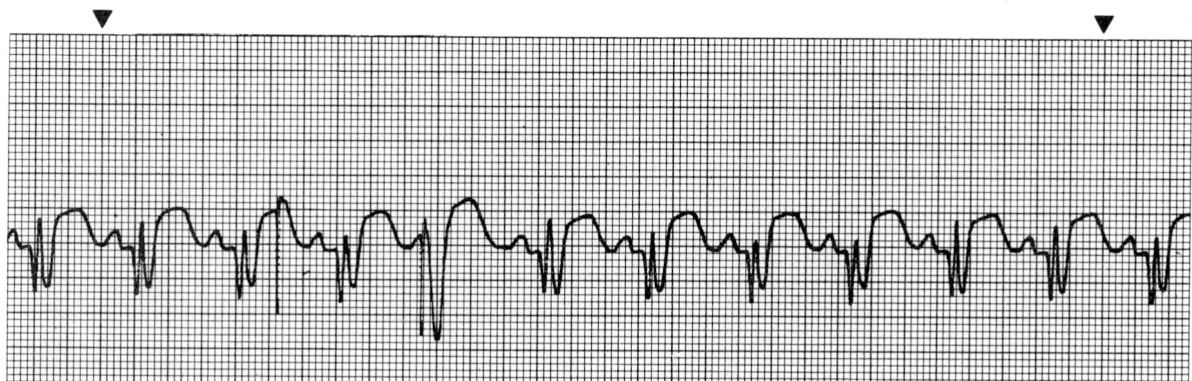

Figure 3-61. Paced rhythm with failure to sense. Note spike without a QRS to follow. (From Huff, J., Doernbach, D., and White, R.: ECG Workout: Exercises in Arrhythmia Interpretation. Philadelphia, J. B. Lippincott, 1985, Fig. 5.28.)

that heart rate is inadequate to sustain a normal blood pressure, external pacing may be required.

Insertion of a transvenous pacemaker can be time consuming, and requires an adept physician. When time is limited, the patient is compromised, and/or there is no physician available to place the transvenous pacemaking catheter, external temporary pacing should be employed.

Transthoracic Pacing. In emergency situations when all other pacing methods have failed, a pacing catheter can be inserted directly *into* the heart through the chest wall. Special pacing stylets are kept on the crash cart for this purpose. A pacing stylet is a needle with an inner trocar. This stylet is inserted, using a subxiphoid approach, into the heart (Fig. 3–62). Once inside the heart, as evidenced by the ability to aspirate blood through the needle, the inner trocar is removed and the pacing stylet is inserted.

The needle is removed and the pacing stylet is left in place in the heart. The pacing stylet is attached to the generator with an adapter. The patient's heart can then be paced as described in the discussion of transvenous pacemaking.

INTERVENING WITH PATIENTS EXPERIENCING UNPREDICTABLE RHYTHMS

Three rhythms presented in this chapter deal with unpredicted or premature beats. Premature atrial, nodal, and ventricular contractions can occur without warning and may herald the development of more severe dysrhythmias. These premature beats are caused by increased irritability or automaticity in the atria, AV node, or ventricles.

Treatment of these premature beats is based upon patient symptoms and the risk of further dysrhythmia development. If the patient is asymptomatic and not at high risk for further dysrhythmia development, no treatment is necessary. However, if the patient reports palpitations, light-headedness, or syncope, treatment may be required. Premature beats in the setting of myocardial infarction will usually be treated.

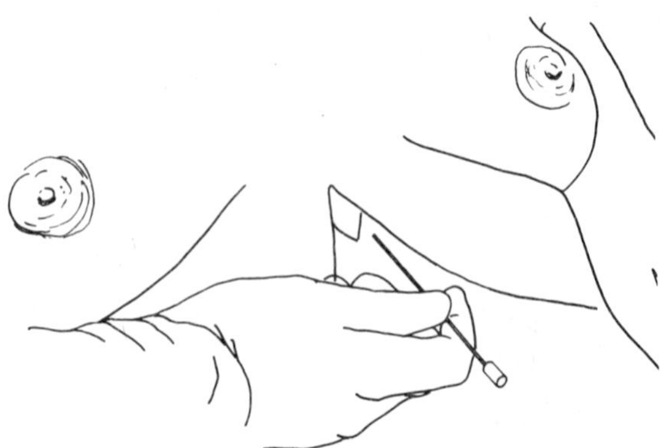

Figure 3–62. Subxiphoid approach for insertion of transmyocardial pacing stylet. (Reproduced with permission. Textbook of Advanced Cardiac Life Support. American Heart Association, 1987, 1990, Chap. 13, Fig. 2.)

If treatment is required, it will usually include modification of known risk factors and the utilization of appropriate cardiac drugs.

Modification of Known Risk Factors. Patients experiencing premature beats often have known risk factors for dysrhythmia development. Reduction of stress, withdrawal from caffeine and nicotine, and correction of hypoxia may be sufficient to control or suppress the irritable areas producing the premature beats.

Utilization of Appropriate Cardiac Drugs. The drugs cited in the previous discussion of intervening with patients experiencing rapid heart rates will again be applicable for the atrial and nodal premature beats.

Premature ventricular beats will not be suppressed by the drugs used for atrial and nodal premature beats. For PVCs, lidocaine is the drug of choice. Lidocaine suppresses irritability in the ventricle by stabilizing the cardiac membrane. If the patient is allergic to lidocaine, the drugs procainamide and bretylium may be used. There is a more detailed discussion of these antidysrhythmic drugs in Chapter 6.

INTERVENING WITH PATIENTS EXPERIENCING LIFE-THREATENING RHYTHMS

There are three remaining dysrhythmias that create life-threatening situations. These rhythms are ventricular fibrillation, ventricular tachycardia, and asystole. Treatment of each of these dysrhythmias will be discussed separately, again following ACLS guidelines.

Ventricular Fibrillation. Ventricular fibrillation is a life-threatening dysrhythmia. Survival is dependent upon rapid detection and immediate intervention. The rhythm must be correctly assessed.

The amplitude of ventricular fibrillation can be very low, producing a fine, wavy baseline. Because of this, asystole can be diagnosed in error. Coarse ventricular fibrillation can be mistaken for ventricular tachycardia. For these reasons, at least two leads should be reviewed before diagnosing ventricular fibrillation.

The primary treatment for ventricular fibrillation is defibrillation. If a defibrillator is not immediately available, cardiopulmonary resuscitation (CPR) is initiated in the interim. As soon as a defibrillator is accessible, immediate defibrillation should be accomplished.

The ACLS guidelines state that the initial defibrillation should be accomplished with 200 J. If the rhythm does not convert, defibrillation is repeated at 300 J. If the patient continues in fibrillation, 360 J is used. After this initial series of 200, 300, and 360, CPR is continued. Intravenous access is established and drugs including epinephrine, lidocaine, and bretylium are used. Concurrent with these activities, the patient is intubated and respirations supported.

Throughout the rest of the arrest, defibrillation at 360 J follows administration of the various drugs. A sequence of drugs then defibrillation will be repeated until the patient is successfully resuscitated or the code is terminated. A thorough discussion of the drugs used to treat ventricular fibrillation is included in Chapter 6.

Ventricular Tachycardia. The treatment of ventricular tachycardia (VT) is dependent upon whether the patient has a pulse or not. The patient experiencing VT with a pulse usually requires less aggressive therapy, such as drugs. The patient experiencing VT without a pulse requires the use of electricity to convert the rhythm.

In VT with a pulse, an IV access is established and the patient is bolused with 1 mg/kg of lidocaine. The usual bolus is between 50 and 100 mg intravenous push (IVP). Lidocaine can be repeated at half the original dose every 8 minutes until the rhythm converts, or until a total dose of 3 mg/kg has been given.

It is important to note here that lidocaine comes in a variety of packaging. Prefilled syringes containing 100 mg, 1 g, and 2 g are available. It is imperative that the nurse select and administer the correct dosage. The 100-mg syringe is appropriate for IV boluses. Erroneous administration of the 1- or 2-g syringe can result in patient death. The nurse must *always* check and double check that the correct syringe is in hand prior to administration.

If a patient is allergic to lidocaine, Pronestyl or bretylium can be used instead. These drugs are covered in greater detail in Chapter 6. If after utilizing the various drugs VT persists, then cardioversion should be attempted. A series of 50, 100, 200, and 360 J can be used.

In the patient without a pulse, treatment should proceed directly to cardioversion. Again, a series of 50, 100, 200, and up to 360 J can be used. If there is time, the patient can be sedated prior to delivering the electrical shocks. If the VT recurs, the drugs described above can be used. Should there be any delay in delivering the electrical shocks, CPR should be performed to support the patient.

Asystole. Asystole carries a grave prognosis. Asystole is usually the result of end-stage cardiac disease. However, it can also be the end result of severe sinus bradycardia or sinus arrest/exit.

In the patient experiencing asystole, CPR should be the initial supporting treatment. Epinephrine, 1:10,000, 0.5 to 1.0 mg IVP, can be used to stimulate automaticity. Atropine, 1 mg, should also be used in case the asystole is the end result of bradycardia. Pacing should be considered if the drugs prove ineffective. Sodium bicarbonate may also be considered if the patient is acidotic.

It should also be remembered that what is thought to be asystole may indeed be fine ventricular fibrillation (VF). If there is some doubt as to the rhythm, defibrillation should be attempted following the algorithm for VF.

Summary

The intention of this chapter is to demystify the analysis and interpretation of the basic dysrhythmias. ECG interpretation is a basic skill that develops only through practice. For the beginning student, the critical criteria for diagnosis provide the structure by which rhythms are analyzed. Initial effort should be toward the memorization of these criteria.

It is hoped that this chapter will prove to be a valuable reference in the delivery of quality care to patients with cardiac dysrhythmias and to their families.

References

Abedin, Z., and Conner, R. (1989): *Twelve-Lead ECG Interpretation.* Philadelphia: W. B. Saunders.

Alspach, J. G. (1991): *Core Curriculum for Critical Care Nurses.* Philadelphia: W. B. Saunders.

American Heart Association (1987): *Textbook of Advanced Cardiac Life Support.* Dallas: American Heart Association.

Andreoli, K., Zipes, D., Wallace, A., Kinney, M., and Fowkes, V. (1987): *Comprehensive Cardiac Care.* St. Louis: C. V. Mosby.

Conover, M. B. (1988): *Understanding Electrocardiography: Arrhythmias and the 12-Lead ECG.* St. Louis: C. V. Mosby.

Fenstermacher, K. (1989): *Dysrhythmia Recognition and Management.* Philadelphia: W. B. Saunders.

Guzzetta, C., and Dossey, B. (eds.) (1984). *Cardiovascular Nursing: Bodymind Tapestry.* St. Louis: C. V. Mosby.

Kenner, C., Guzzetta, C., and Dossey, B. (1991): *Critical-Care Nursing: Body-Mind-Spirit.* Boston: Little, Brown.

Kinkade, S., and Lohrman, J. (1990): *Critical Care Nursing Procedures: A Team Approach.* St. Louis: C. V. Mosby.

Kinney, M., Packa, D., and Dunbar, S. (1988): *AACN's Reference for Critical-Care Nursing.* St. Louis: C. V. Mosby.

Moorhouse, M., Geissler, A., and Doenges, M. (1987): *Critical Care Plans: Guidelines for Patient Care.* Philadelphia: F.A. Davis.

Mott, S., Fazekas, N., and James, S. (1985): *Nursing Care of Children and Families: A Holistic Approach.* Reading, MA: Addison-Wesley.

Patel, J., McGowan, S., and Moody, L. (1989): *Arrhythmias: Detection, Treatment, and Cardiac Drugs.* Philadelphia: W. B. Saunders.

Skidmore-Roth, L. (1991): *Mosby's 1991 Nursing Drug Reference.* St. Louis: C. V. Mosby.

Swonger, A., and Matejski, M. (1988): *Nursing Pharmacology.* Boston: Scott, Foresman.

Recommended Reading

Davis, D. (1985): *How to Quickly and Accurately Master ECG Interpretation.* Philadelphia: J. B. Lippincott.

Davis, D. (1989): *How to Quickly and Accurately Master Arrhythmia Interpretation.* Philadelphia: J. B. Lippincott.

Kelly, S. J. (ed.) (1988): Pediatric cardiac dysrhythmias. In: *Pediatric Emergency Nursing.* Norwalk: Appleton & Lange.

Kinney, M., Zipes, D., Andreoli, K., and Packa, D. (1991): *Comprehensive Cardiac Care.* St. Louis: C. V. Mosby.

Thelan, L., Davie, J., and Urden, L. (1990): *Textbook of Critical Care Nursing.* St. Louis: C. V. Mosby.

Chapter 4

Joan M. Vitello-Cicciu, R.N., M.S.N., CCRN, C.S.
Cynthia Kline O'Sullivan, R.N., M.S.N.

Introduction to Hemodynamics

Objectives

- Identify the physiologic basis for hemodynamic monitoring in critically ill patients.
- Describe indications, measurement, complications, and nursing implications associated with monitoring of central venous pressure, left atrial pressure, pulmonary artery pressure, and intra-arterial pressure.
- Identify normal values of the above pressures.
- Analyze conditions which alter hemodynamic values.
- Explain clinical relevance and methods for measuring cardiac output.
- Discuss rationale and methods for continuous monitoring of mixed venous oxygen saturation.

A person's initial exposure to the critical care environment may be a rather mystifying experience. Comprehending the complicated equipment such as digital readouts, waveforms, alarms, and the tangle of wires, tubings, and cables may at first seem an impossible feat. However, even when the technical equipment and data obtained are well understood, it is important to know that this technology only serves to augment patient care and should not detract from a holistic perspective. Furthermore, viewing the patient as a person first, and utilizing the equipment as merely an adjunct, should be the focus in critical care no matter how much our clinical practice is influenced by technology.

A considerable portion of the equipment utilized in the critical care setting is for the purpose of hemodynamic monitoring. The term *hemodynamics* refers to the interrelationship of the various physical forces that affect the blood's circulation through the body. Developing a working knowledge of the concepts known as pressure, flow, and resistance will provide the foundation for this understanding. Insight into the factors affecting the heart's ability to pump effectively is also essential. Thus, this chapter discusses the basic principles of hemodynamics, the heart as a pump, and hemodynamic monitoring. Essential nursing considerations for patients being hemodynamically monitored are also introduced.

The Basics: Pressure, Flow, and Resistance

One of the basic laws of physics can be explained by the following equation:

$$\text{Pressure} = \text{Flow} \times \text{Resistance}$$

Illustrating this principle with a water pipe (Fig. 4-1), we know that by altering either the

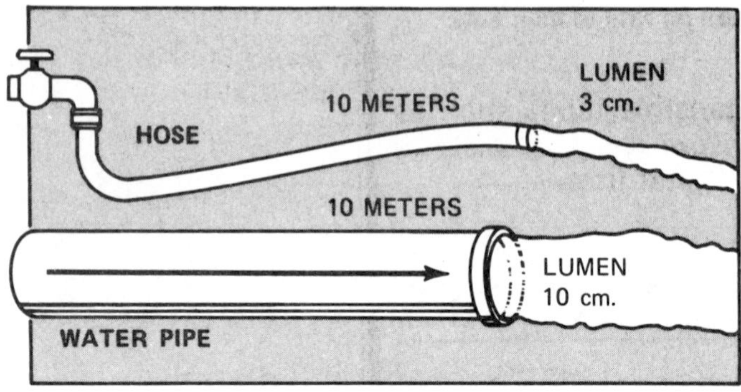

Figure 4-1. Schematic drawing illustrating the flow of fluid through a garden hose and a water pipe. Blood flow is decreased through the narrower lumen (hose) as compared to the wider lumen (pipe). (From Jackle, M., and Halligan, M.: *Cardiovascular Problems: A Critical Care Nursing Focus,* Bowie, MD, Robert J. Brady, 1980.)

flow or the resistance of the pipe, the water pressure inside it will be affected. For example, turning the faucet will increase the flow of water through the pipe, thereby increasing the pressure. Similarly, by partially occluding the pipe with sand or leaves, and narrowing the opening, the flow of water is met with increased resistance, and pressure builds up within the pipe.

Another law of physics is that there is a natural tendency for liquids to flow from an area of higher pressure to an area of lower pressure. This phenomenon occurs frequently in the body, and is exemplified by the movement of blood through the cardiac chambers.

Clinically, these concepts may be better understood when the above equation is applied to blood pressure, such that

Blood Pressure = Cardiac Output (Flow) × Peripheral (Systemic) Vascular Resistance

In this equation, we see that blood pressure is affected by both cardiac output and peripheral (systemic) vascular resistance. You may recall that cardiac output is defined as the volume of blood that circulates through the body per minute, and therefore represents flow. Peripheral (systemic) vascular resistance is the opposition to blood flow exerted by the blood vessels, and is affected by blood viscosity, vascular tone, and the friction that is imposed by the inner lining of the blood vessels. In the clinical setting, you may observe that your patient's blood pressure has dropped from 136/70 mm Hg to 80/50 mm Hg. The fall in blood pressure has occurred because either the flow (cardiac output) has been reduced or the resistance has decreased. Conversely, if this patient's blood pressure should increase to 190/90 mm Hg, either the cardiac output or resistance has increased.

First, consider the peripheral (systemic) vascular resistance. A major factor that influences this resistance is the lumen size (diameter) of the vessel. For example, if the lumen size narrows, the resistance will increase and vice versa. In the critical care setting, vasoactive drugs are often used to alter the lumen size of the peripheral vessels (predominantly the arterioles) with the aim of either lowering or elevating the blood pressure.

Next, consider the patient's cardiac output. There are a number of factors that can influence the cardiac output, which may be illustrated by the following equation:

Cardiac Output = Heart Rate × Stroke Volume

Stroke volume may be defined as the volume of blood ejected by the heart per contraction. Therefore, a change in either the stroke volume or heart rate will affect the cardiac output. This concept is expanded on later in this chapter.

It will be helpful to refer back to these concepts as physiological principles relative to hemodynamics are introduced in the following sections.

The Blood and Circulatory System

The complex network of veins, arteries, and the heart that drives circulation is in many ways analogous to the water pipe illustration. However, the human circulatory system is unique for many reasons. Blood itself possesses characteristics that make it unlike any other bodily substance, in that it is a viscous liquid with both cellular and fluid components. The cells of the blood vary in shape, size, structure, and function. For example, neutrophils, monocytes, macrophages, and eosinophils are collectively known as white blood cells, or leukocytes. Leukocytes are found in relatively small numbers within the circulating blood, and perform a variety of immunological functions. Conversely, the red blood cells, or erythrocytes, comprise a much larger portion, contributing to approximately 99% of the total number of cells. The major function of erythrocytes is to transport oxygen, in the form of hemoglobin, from the lungs to the tissues. Because the majority of the blood's cellular component is made up of erythrocytes, they provide the blood with many of its physical properties.

Typically, approximately 40% of the total blood volume is cellular, whereas the remainder is plasma. Environmental factors, certain disease states, and the sex of the patient all affect the actual number of circulating blood cells. An increase in blood cells causes the blood to become more viscous. This increased viscosity results in greater friction, and therefore makes the flow of blood through small vessels more difficult. However, blood is able to flow freely through the tiny capillaries by the alignment of erythrocytes within these vessels. Thus, blood moves through the capillaries as a "plug" of erythrocytes rather than randomly, as occurs in the larger vessels. This is an important feature, since tissue oxygenation occurs at the capillary level, and it is the erythrocytes that provide this valuable function.

The human circulatory system is actually one continuous circuit (Fig. 4–2). Under normal conditions, the system contains a volume of blood that remains relatively constant. Therefore, when the body's metabolic demands increase, blood needs to be circulated more quickly through the circuit to meet those demands. Likewise, when the body is at rest and its demands are reduced, some of the blood volume is essentially "stored" (in veins) within the circulatory system itself.

The body utilizes several mechanisms to regulate the flow of blood through the blood vessels in order to meet metabolic demands (Fig. 4–3). The first mechanism involves the ability of blood vessels to change their diameter or lumen size (discussed above). Unlike the water pipe, the walls of the vessels, particularly the veins, have the ability to constrict or dilate according to need. For example, in response to increased demands, the veins constrict. As a result, more blood is forced back to the heart. It then passes through the lungs, where it is reoxygenated, and it is returned to the heart to be pumped out to the tissues. Likewise, when the body is at rest and demands are reduced, the veins become dilated.

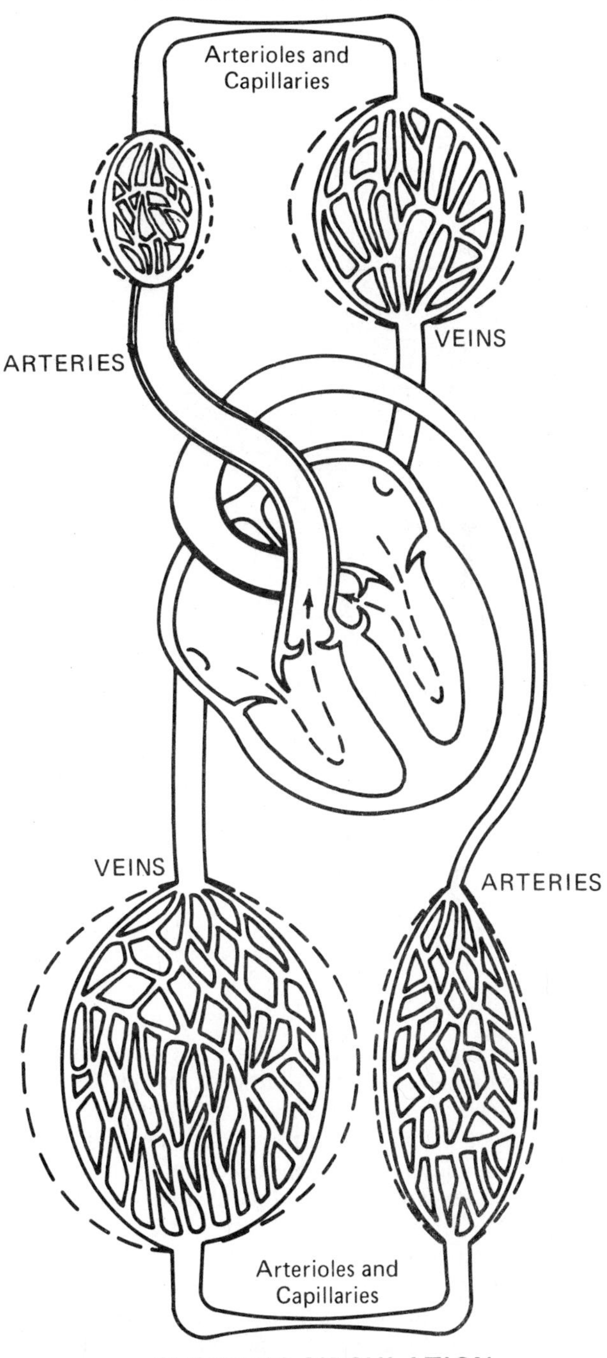

Figure 4–2. Illustration depicting the closed circuit which is composed of the systemic and the pulmonary circulation. (From Jackle, M., and Halligan, M.: *Cardiovascular Problems: A Critical Care Nursing Focus,* Bowie, MD, Robert J. Brady, 1980.)

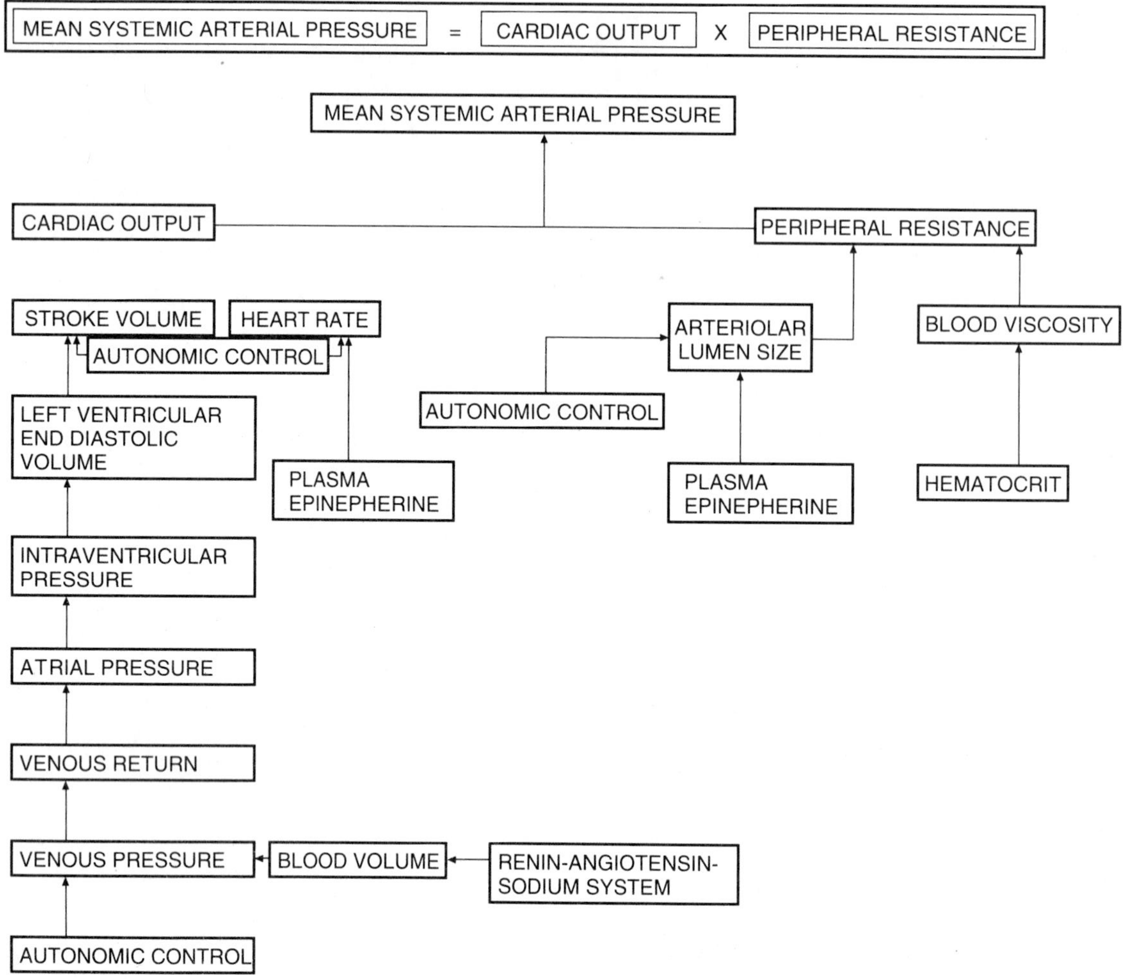

Figure 4-3. Mechanisms that regulate systemic arterial pressure. (From Vander, A., Sherman, J. H., and Luciano, D. S.: Human Physiology. 3rd ed. New York, McGraw-Hill, 1980. Reproduced with the permission of McGraw-Hill, Fig. 11-56, pp. 304-305.)

As their diameter increases, the veins are able to accommodate a larger volume of blood. In this way, they serve as a reservoir, so that a smaller volume of blood is returned to the heart. Circulation is therefore accomplished efficiently, reducing the cardiac workload, since only the amount of blood required to meet the demand is being pumped by the heart.

Two other mechanisms that control blood flow involve the heart's ability to control its heart rate and strength of contraction (contractility). These are regulated by a complex interaction between the autonomic and central nervous systems in conjunction with input from the circulatory and endocrine systems. The kidneys also play a role in regulating circulation through mechanisms that adjust blood pressure and blood volume via the renin-angiotensin system.

The Cardiac Cycle

In order to fully understand hemodynamics, a knowledge of the cardiac cycle is necessary. The cardiac cycle occurs in two phases: diastole, when the left and right ventricles receive blood from the atria, and systole, when the ventricles contract, thereby squeezing blood out of the heart through the aorta and the pulmonary artery. It is important to note that diastole occurs simultaneously between the left and right sides of the heart, as does systole. In order to illustrate the flow of blood through the circulatory system, the entire sequence will now be described, from the right side of the heart to the left side.

After supplying oxygen to the tissues, deoxygenated blood is collected by the systemic veins. Venous blood from the peripheral circulation enters the right atrium of the heart via the superior and inferior venae cavae. During diastole, as the right atrium begins to fill with blood, the tricuspid valve is closed (Fig. 4-4). As the right atrium fills more completely, right atrial pressure becomes higher than right ventricular pressure. This pressure difference forces the tricuspid valve to open. Blood then rushes from the right atrium into the right ventricle.

As the right ventricle fills with blood from the right atrium, pressure within the atrium drops, whereas it rises within the ventricle. Simultaneously, the right atrium contracts, ejecting enough blood into the right ventricle to fill it completely (Fig. 4-5). As this occurs, right ventricular pressure surpasses right atrial pressure, causing the tricuspid valve to snap closed, thereby preventing blood from entering the right ventricle.

During systole, the right ventricle begins to contract, increasing intraventricular pressure (Fig. 4-6). When the pressure rises sufficiently to overcome the pressure exerted on the pulmonic valve, the valve then opens. Blood is therefore ejected out of the right atrium into the pulmonary artery. In turn, blood travels through the pulmonary circulation and is oxygenated at the level of the capillaries and alveoli. Oxygenated blood is then transported back to the heart via the pulmonary vein.

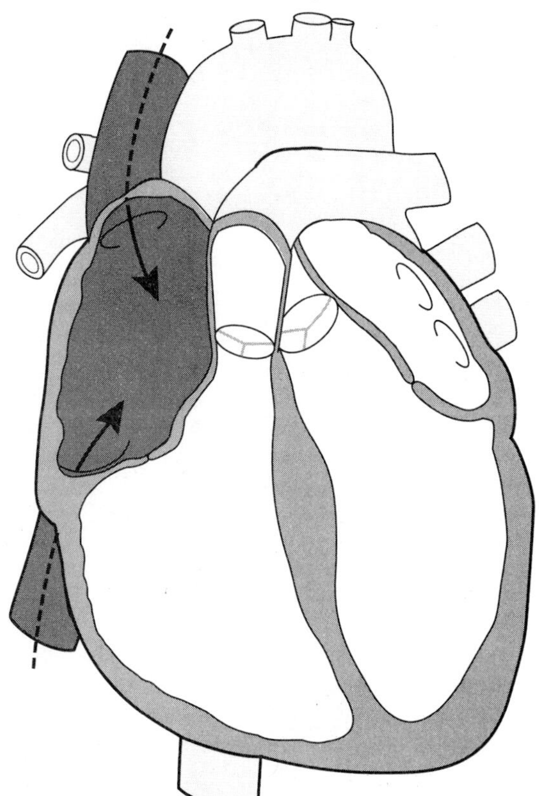

Figure 4-4. Illustration depicting blood flow into the right atrium during diastole.

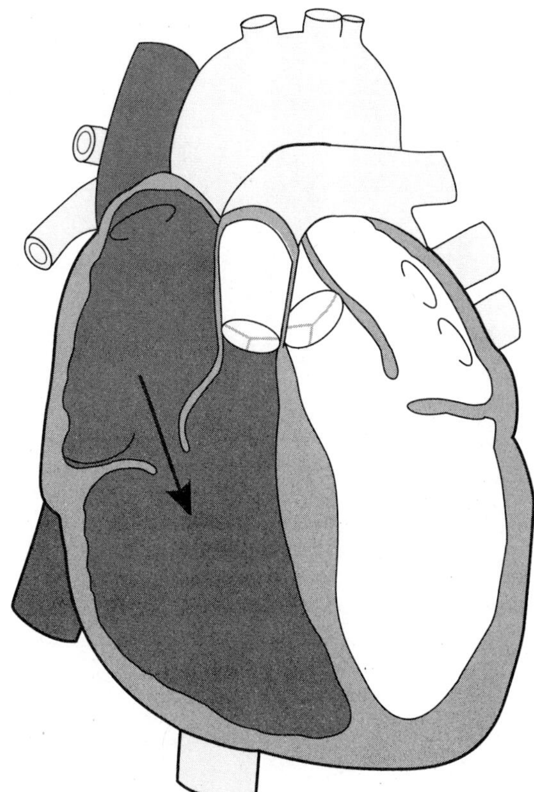

Figure 4-5. As blood continues to flow into the right atrium, the resulting pressure causes the tricuspid valve to open. Blood is then able to enter the right ventricle.

Oxygenated blood from the pulmonary circulation enters the left atrium during diastole. At this time, the mitral valve is closed. As the left atrium fills, left atrial pressure exceeds left ventricular pressure. The pressure difference forces the mitral valve to open, and blood then rushes into the left ventricle. As the left ventricle fills, the left atrium contracts, ejecting enough blood to fill the left ventricle (Fig. 4-7).

Left ventricular pressure now transcends left atrial pressure, causing the mitral valve to snap closed, and preventing additional blood from entering the left ventricle. The amount of blood in the left ventricle at this phase in the cardiac cycle is known as the left ventricular end-diastolic volume (LVEDV). This volume is significant because it determines the amount of blood that will be ejected into the systemic circulation. The LVEDV is commonly referred to as preload, and will be described in further detail in a later section.

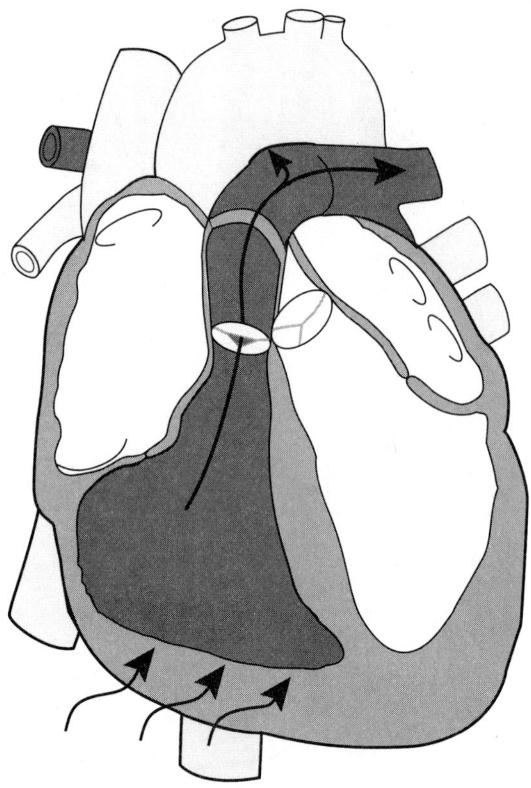

Figure 4-6. During systole the right ventricle contracts, squeezing its contents through the pulmonic valve and into the pulmonary circulation.

During systole, the left ventricle contracts, elevating the left ventricular pressure to such a degree that it overcomes the pressure exerted on the aortic valve from the systemic circulation (Fig. 4-8). Oxygenated blood is then ejected from the left ventricle through the aorta into the systemic circulation, where it ultimately supplies the tissues with oxygen.

As previously stated, the volume of blood that is ejected out during systole is referred to as the stroke volume. The volume that remains in the left ventricle at the end of systole is the left ventricular end-systolic volume (LVESV). The left ventricle never ejects its entire end-diastolic volume. It merely ejects a fraction of this volume, known as the ejection fraction, which is normally 60 to 70%.

■ Cardiac Output/Stroke Volume

The cardiac output (CO) is the amount of blood ejected from the heart per minute, and is essentially equal to the amount of venous blood that is returned to the right atrium from the peripheral circulation. Physiologically, cardiac output is equal to the stroke volume times the heart rate. Therefore, anything that can affect either the heart rate, or the stroke volume, or both will affect the cardiac output. Moreover, stroke volume is influenced by three variables: (1) preload, (2) afterload, and (3) contractility (Fig. 4-9).

Preload may be defined as the amount of muscle fiber stretch prior to the next contraction. This muscle fiber stretch (also known as the presystolic fiber length) is directly affected by the end-diastolic volume in the ventricles. It is the end-diastolic volume that actually stretches the muscle fibers before contraction (during diastole). Thus, preload can also be defined clinically as either the ventricular end-diastolic volume (EDV) or pressure (EDP). Another important factor is that within physiological limits, ventricular contraction will be stronger as the muscle fiber

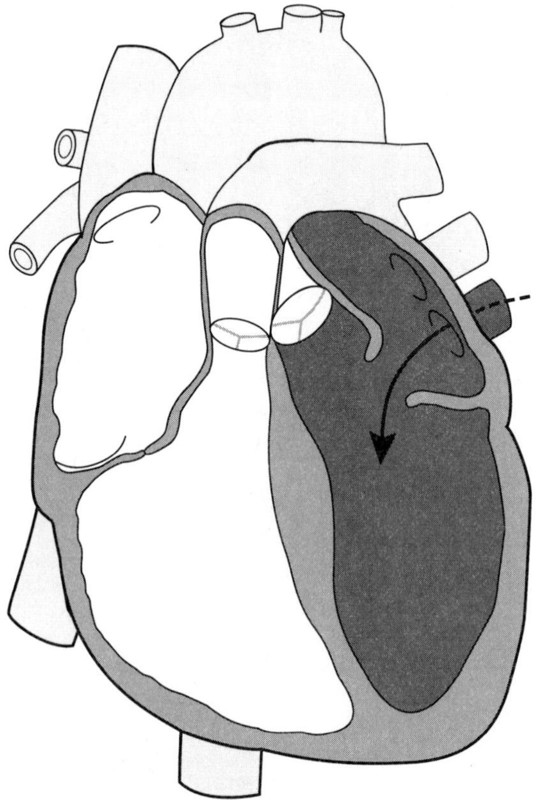

Figure 4-7. Oxygenated blood from the lungs now enters the left atrium. As atrial pressure builds, the mitral valve will be forced open so that blood may pass into the left ventricle (not shown).

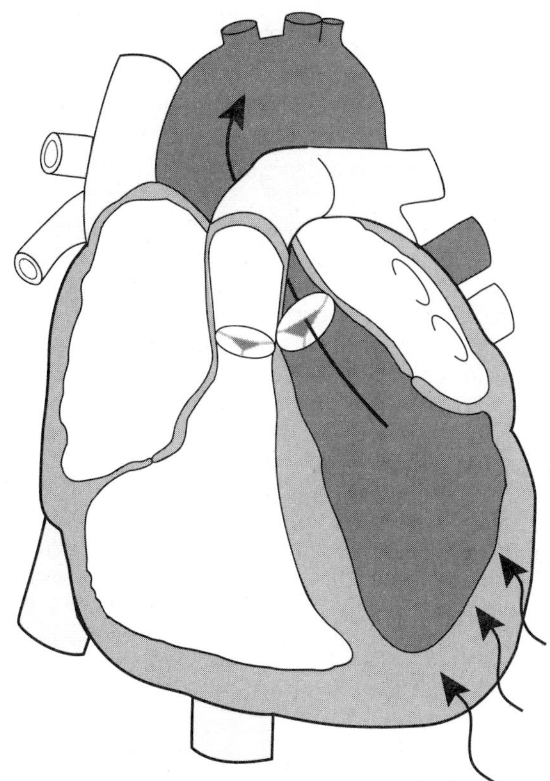

Figure 4-8. During systole, the left ventricle contracts, squeezing its contents through the aortic valve and into the systemic circulation to oxygenate the tissues.

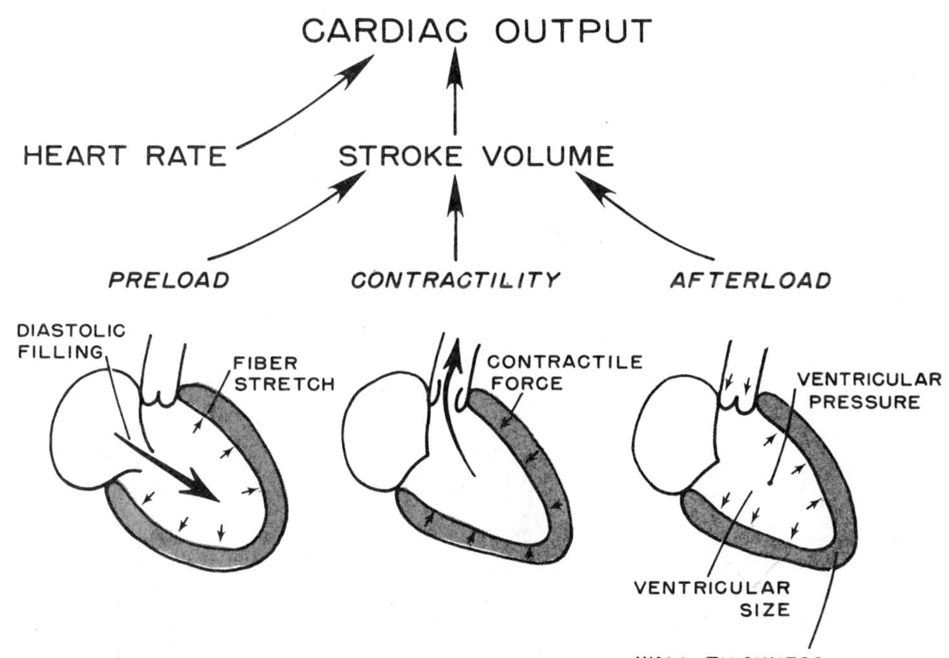

Figure 4-9. Factors affecting cardiac output (Reproduced by permission from: Price, S., and Wilson, L.: *Pathophysiology: Clinical Concepts of Disease Processes.* 3rd ed. New York, 1986, McGraw-Hill Book Co.; copyrighted by The C. V. Mosby Co., St. Louis, Fig. 25-11, p. 351.)

stretch (preload) increases. This is often referred to as the Frank-Starling principle in so far as cardiac output or stroke volume is related to the presystolic fiber length. Clinically, this means that a decrease in preload (↓ in EDV) for a patient will often result in a decrease in force of contraction.

Afterload is defined as the pressure or resistance to blood flow out of the ventricle. This pressure or resistance must be overcome in order for the ventricle to eject its stroke volume. The principal factor that offers resistance to this blood flow out of the ventricles is the arterial blood pressure. Thus, if the arterial blood pressure is high, the left ventricle must exert more force to effectively pump blood out of its chamber. Moreover, additional energy will be required to generate enough pressure or force to eject this blood; the oxygen requirements of the heart will increase in order to generate sufficient energy to accomplish this. Clinically, an increase in afterload may cause a decrease in stroke volume, especially if the left ventricle is unable to generate enough force to overcome this resistance.

Contractility, the third variable affecting stroke volume, is defined as a measure of how forcefully the ventricle contracts to eject its stroke volume. This is the intrinsic ability of the muscle fibers to shorten. How much (extent) and how fast (velocity) these fibers shorten will also affect stroke volume. For example, if the ventricular fibers can shorten effectively and rapidly, the rate of pressure rise in the ventricle during systole will be able to exceed the arterial blood pressure, resulting in a rapid forceful ejection of stroke volume. Conversely, if the ventricular fibers lose their strength of contraction, the stroke volume will decrease. Thus, contractility directly affects stroke volume, as do preload and afterload, as previously discussed.

■ Essential Components of Hemodynamic Monitoring

All hemodynamic monitoring equipment contains the following basic components: (1) transducer, (2) amplifier, (3) display instrument, (4)

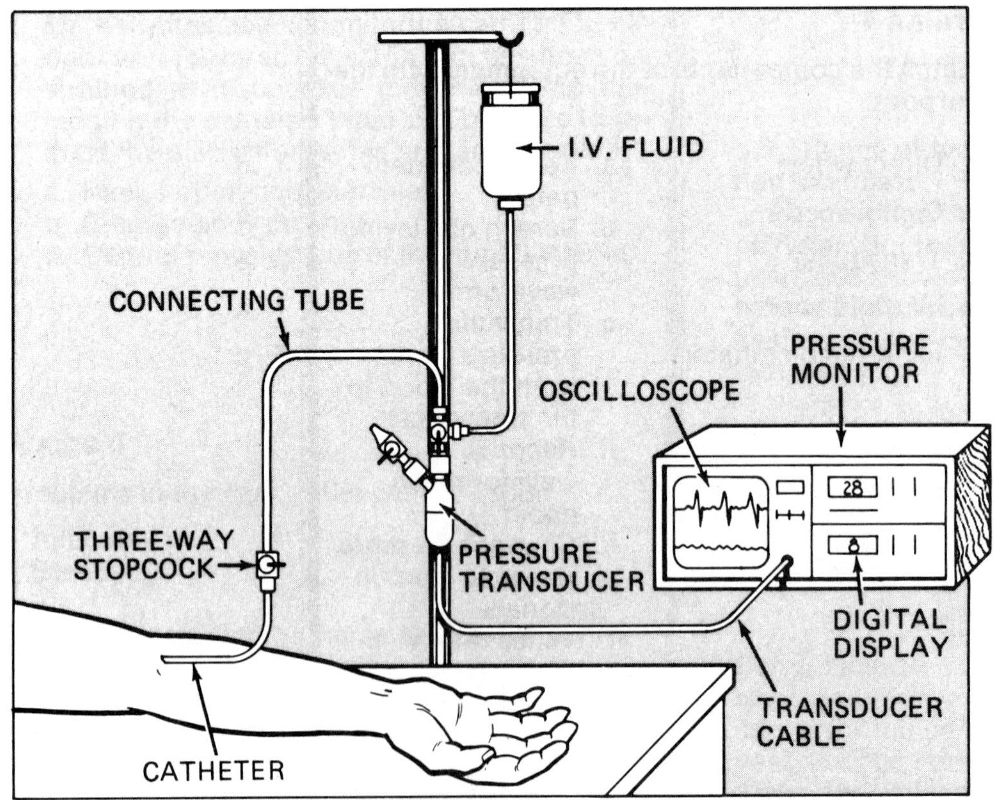

Figure 4-10. Essential components for invasive monitoring, using the brachial approach. (From Jackle, M., and Halligan, M.: *Cardiovascular Problems: A Critical Care Nursing Focus.* Bowie, MD, Robert J. Brady, 1980.)

fluid-filled catheter/tubing/flush system (Fig. 4–10).

The transducer is an instrument that is used to sense physiological events and transform them into electrical signals. Some of the physiological events commonly measured by a transducer include (1) pressure, (2) flow, (3) temperature, (4) light intensity, and (5) sound.

Housed within the pressure monitor are the amplifier and the display instrument. The amplifier connects to the transducer by an electrical cable. It functions by picking up the electrical event from the transducer, and amplifying it while also filtering out interference signals. The improved signal is then transmitted to an instrument where it can be displayed.

Display instruments may be used to record, or in some manner provide, a quantifiable display of the original signal. The signal may be seen as a waveform, digital readout, or a fluctuation on a meter. The method generally used to monitor hemodynamic pressures is to display a pressure waveform on an oscilloscope (a screen) and a digital reading of the pressure values on the pressure monitor.

The fourth component necessary to perform any hemodynamic monitoring is the catheter/tubing/flush system. This system comprises a blood-compatible catheter that may be inserted into either an artery, vein, or heart chamber depending on the type of hemodynamic monitoring required to care for a critically ill patient. The catheter is then attached to rigid, noncompliant tubing that is attached to some type of flush device that can control flow of solution through the tubing. In order to keep the tubing and catheter patent and free of blood clots, a flush solution (e.g., Ringer's lactate, normal saline) often containing heparin is used. The use of heparin to discourage clot formation and to promote catheter patency is currently under scientific investigation. To date, it is not known if the addition of heparin to a flush solution is necessary for the maintenance of patency in arterial lines. Therefore, the American Association of Critical-Care Nurses is sponsoring the Thunder Project, a national multicentered nursing research study designed to evaluate the effect of heparinized and nonheparinized flush solutions on the patency of arterial pressure lines. This project is designed to help us base our practice on research. Heparin is delivered from a compressible bag that is pressurized by either a pressure bag or an inflatable cuff. The pressure bag is required in order to provide enough pressure to the flush solution to drive the continuous flow of fluid through the tubing and catheter.

In order to obtain reliable measurements prior to initiating any type of hemodynamic monitoring, the equipment must first be standardized. To accomplish this, the transducers used for monitoring hemodynamic pressures must be leveled, balanced, and calibrated.

To level a transducer, you simply need to position the air-fluid interface of the stopcock at approximately the level of the patient's right atrium. This area is known as the phlebostatic axis, and is located at the fourth intercostal space, midway between the anterior and posterior aspects of the chest (often referred to as "mid-axillary" position; Fig. 4–11). The transducer may be placed directly on the patient's chest, or it may be attached to an IV pole positioned near the patient. A leveling instrument may be used to ensure the proper height of the transducer when mounting it on a pole rather than directly on the patient's body.

Balancing, or "zero referencing," is an operation performed to eliminate the influence of at-

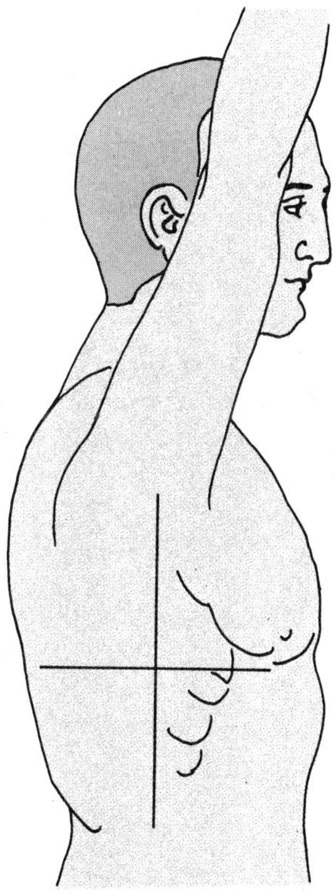

Figure 4–11. Locating the phlebostatic axis. (From Taylor, T.: Monitoring left atrial pressure in the open-heart surgical patient. *Critical Care Nurse* 6(2):64, 1986, Fig. 2.)

mospheric pressure on the monitoring system. In order to control for this, the stopcock on the flush system is turned so that the patient's pressure is no longer being displayed, and only environmental pressures are sensed by the equipment. The straight line that appears on the display screen and the corresponding digital readouts are then adjusted to read "zero." In this manner, atmospheric pressure is negated, even though it actually measures about 760 mm Hg at sea level.

Calibration is performed to ensure numerical accuracy within the electrical system. Most monitors are designed with a specific mechanism to accomplish this, such that a specific pressure reading will be displayed when pushing a button. By comparing the value indicated on the display screen, the digital readout, and the monitor's specific calibration factor, the accuracy of the system may be assessed.

Central Venous Pressure Monitoring

MEASUREMENT

The central venous pressure (CVP), or right atrial pressure, is a direct measurement of the pressure of the right atrium, but it may also be measured from the superior and inferior venae cavae. Since there are no valves between the right atrium and the venae cavae, the pressures within these areas are essentially equal. However, the clinical importance of CVP measurement lies in its ability to also reflect right ventricular pressure. During diastole, the heart's tricuspid valve is open, allowing a clear passage for blood to flow from the right atrium to the right ventricle. Because of this, the CVP measurement is a reliable reflection of right ventricular preload or right ventricular end-diastolic pressure (RVEDP).

The CVP measurement is particularly valuable in helping to reflect right ventricular pressure and right ventricular end-diastolic pressure. Generally, these factors are those situations that affect either circulatory volume status or right ventricular function. For example, a patient with a low CVP measurement may be hypovolemic, vasodilated, or experiencing any other condition that reduces venous return to the heart. On the other hand, a high CVP measurement may be indicative of any condition that reduces the right ventricle's ability to eject blood, thereby increasing right ventricular pressure, and hence right atrial pressure. These conditions include hypervolemia, vasoconstriction, right-sided heart failure, and pulmonary hypertension.

METHODS OF MEASURING CVP

Catheters used for CVP measurement are generally stiff and radiopaque. They may vary in length and diameter depending on the vein that is used: Shorter catheters are generally used for the subclavian insertion, and longer catheters for upper extremity veins.

There are several acceptable sites that may be used for CVP line insertion. The internal jugular site is often preferable because it allows the patient a high degree of mobility, and the risks of infection and thrombophlebitis are relatively low. The subclavian is another commonly used site, but subjects the patient to an additional risk of potential pneumothorax during insertion. Other veins that may be suitable include the cephalic, femoral, antecubital, and occasionally the basilic and saphenous veins.

The insertion procedure for central lines is analagous to the pulmonary artery insertion. However, the design of the CVP catheter is different in that it contains only a single lumen. Please refer to the section on pulmonary artery catheters for a description of this procedure.

Central venous pressure may be measured by

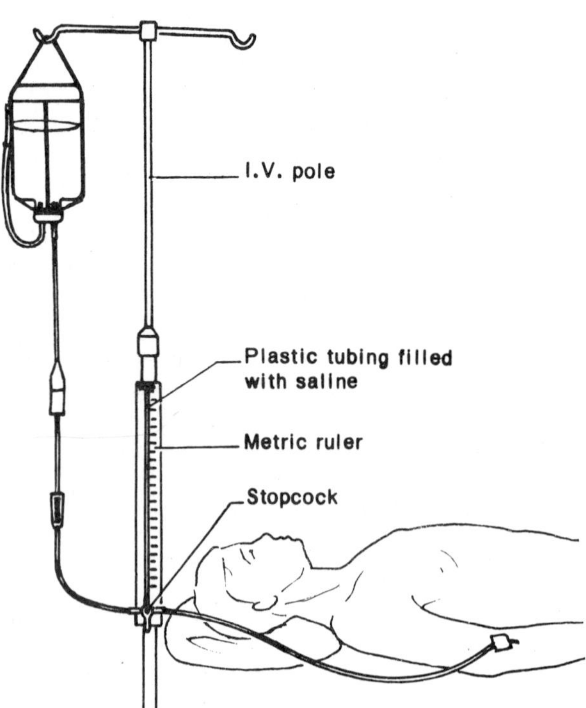

Figure 4-12. Measuring central venous pressure using a water manometer. (From Cyginski, J., and Tardieu, B.: *The Essentials in Pressure Monitoring—Blood and Other Body Fluids. An Illustrated Guide.* The Hague, Netherlands: Martinus-Nijhoff, 1980, Fig. 17, p. 85.)

using either a conventional pressure transducer system or a device called a water manometer (Fig. 4–12). The latter is a quick, simple method that requires little equipment to use. It essentially functions by the principle that fluids will move from an area of higher pressure to an area of lower pressure. A fluid-filled tube called a manometer is the measuring device that actually relays the patient's pressure reading without the use of electrical equipment. The manometer is connected to the patient's intravenous infusion system that in turn connects to the central venous catheter. When the stopcock is turned so that the infusion is turned off, fluid from the manometer flows into the patient's vein, and levels off when the patient's central venous pressure and the pressure exerted by the fluid in the manometer equalize. After the measurement is recorded, the stopcock may again be turned so that the infusion may resume. Measurements taken from a water manometer are recorded in centimeters of water. (cm H_2O).

Measuring CVP using a pressure transducer is analogous to most other types of pressure monitoring. It requires all the standard equipment as illustrated in Figure 4–11. Measurements taken from a pressure transducer are recorded in millimeters of mercury (mm Hg).

The typical CVP tracing consists of three upwardly deflected waves that correspond to various phases in the cardiac cycle. The "a" wave is produced by atrial contraction and the "c" wave is produced when the tricuspid valve closes. The "V" wave depicts the cumulative effect that occurs when the right ventricle contracts as the right atrium fills with blood, causing the tricuspid valve to bulge upward into the right atrium. Figure 4–13 illustrates a typical CVP tracing.

Figure 4–14 denotes normal pressures and oxygen saturation in the various locations in the heart.

The normal value for CVP measurement is 0–8 mm Hg, or 3–8 cm H_2O (using a water manometer). To convert a reading from one form to another, the following equation may be utilized, since the two measurements are not interchangeable:

$$\frac{\text{CVP in cm H}_2\text{O}}{1.36} = \text{CVP in mm Hg}$$

Abnormalities in CVP measurement, as discussed earlier, are generally caused by any condition that alters venous tone, blood volume, or right ventricular contractility. Because the right ventricle does not generate significant pressure during atrial contractions, the atrial pressure is recorded as a mean (average) pressure rather than as a systolic and diastolic pressure. Mean pressures may be obtained directly from the monitor display with most conventional systems.

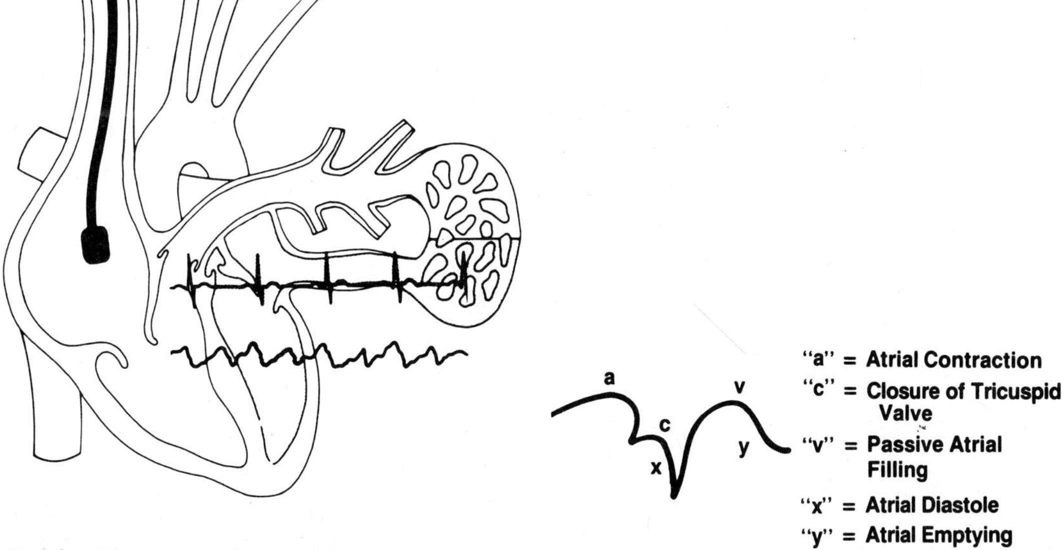

Figure 4–13. Right atrial pressure waveform correlating with ECG. (Courtesy of Baxter Healthcare Corporation, Baxter Edwards Critical-Care Division, Irvine, California.)

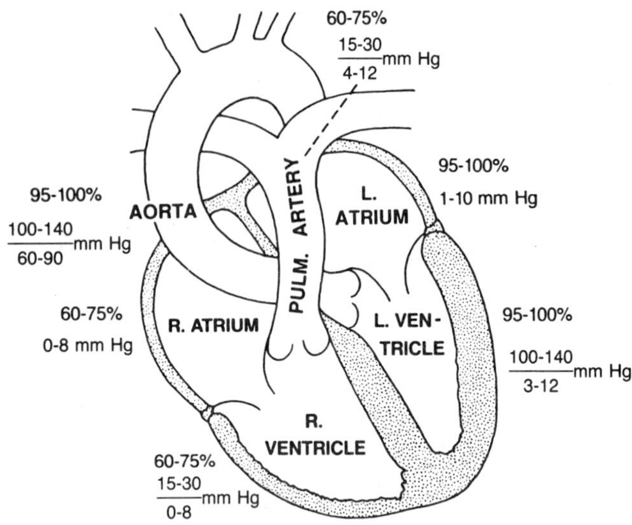

Figure 4–14. Schematic illustration of heart model depicting the pressure and oxygen saturation measurements in the various chambers of the heart. (From Gardner, P. E., and Woods, S. L.: Hemodynamic monitoring. *In*: Underhill, S. L., et al.: *Cardiac Nursing*. 2nd ed. Philadelphia, Lippincott, 1989, Fig. 34–1, p. 452.)

COMPLICATIONS OF CVP INSERTION AND MONITORING

Because insertion of a CVP catheter involves a disruption of skin integrity, the risk of infection is introduced. However, this risk is greatly reduced if attention to sterile technique during insertion and site care is observed.

Other complications may occur during the insertion itself. These include carotid puncture, pneumothorax, hemothorax, perforation of the right atrium or ventricle, and disturbances in cardiac rhythm, generally either atrial or ventricular dysrhythmias.

NURSING IMPLICATIONS FOR MONITORING CENTRAL VENOUS PRESSURE

In order to obtain accurate CVP measurements, it is important for the air-fluid interface of the transducer to be properly placed at the phlebostatic axis (described previously). Measurements are taken when the patient is in the supine position, either flat, or with the head of the bed slightly elevated (less than 30°). Changes in body position may be corrected for by adjusting the level of the transducer. These adjustments are also described in the next section.

Another method of recording central venous pressure is obtained by analysis of the CVP waveform from a strip/chart recorder which has been calibrated to the oscilloscope. This method is more precise than the numerical display or the waveform from the oscilloscope, both of which may be misleading owing to respiratory variation. These strip/chart recordings need to be examined whenever serious alterations in values occur. These recordings permit the clinician to take into account the influence of the respiratory cycle. All hemodynamic waveforms can be obtained using a strip/chart recorder.

Respiratory variation is a second consideration that must be addressed when monitoring CVP. Any situation that alters intrathoracic pressure, such as spontaneous inspiration and mechanical ventilation, will affect the CVP waveform. For this reason, the CVP measurement should be read at the end of expiration for the most accurate information.

Another important nursing consideration in the care of patients with CVP monitoring is close observation for any complications. The complications that may occur will be discussed in further detail in the section on pulmonary artery catheters. Infection, though uncommon, is a potentially dangerous situation for any patient, particularly one who is critically ill. Therefore, daily observation of the insertion site is of utmost importance. Signs of infection include an elevated body temperature and pain, warmth, redness, and purulent drainage at the insertion site. The manifestation of any of these signs should be reported to the patient's physician immediately.

Finally, one nursing consideration that is paramount in utilizing this method of monitoring is for accurate interpretation of the data obtained. Measurements of CVP are most valuable when comparing trends in the context of other physiological parameters rather than individual numbers. Furthermore, a careful physical assessment is no substitute for recording hemodynamic values, and it can help to identify false readings if they occur. Finally, a comparison of several hemodynamic values in conjunction with a thorough physical assessment will generally provide the most accurate interpretation of the patient's condition. The next section will focus on another useful hemodynamic index: the left atrial pressure.

Left Atrial Pressure

MEASUREMENT

The left atrial pressure (LAP) is a measurement of the pressure of the blood as it returns to the left side of the heart. The LAP is considered to be a reflection of the left ventricular preload. As you recall, preload is defined as the volume or pressure in the ventricle at the end of diastole (left ventricular end-diastolic volume [LVEDV] or pressure [LVEDP]). On the left side of the heart during diastole, the mitral valve is opened allowing for communication between the left atrium and the left ventricle. Thus, at the end of diastolic filling under normal circumstances, the LAP is nearly identical to the LVEDP. The normal LAP is in the range of 1 to 10 mm Hg (Fig. 4–14). Because the left atrium does not generate significant pressure during atrial contraction, the atrial pressure is recorded as an average (mean) pressure rather than as a systolic or diastolic pressure measurement.

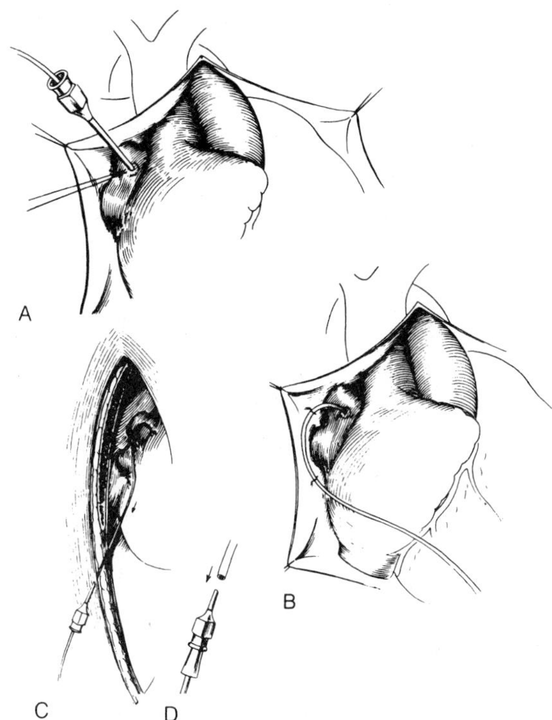

Figure 4–15. Left atrial line placement. Method of inserting left atrial pressure monitoring line. *(A)* A Teflon catheter is inserted through purse-string suture into right upper pulmonary vein through large needle. *(B)* It is then secured to pericardium to prevent accidental dislodgement. *(C)* Catheter is passed through chest wall with large needle. *(D)* Blunt needle adapter is used to connect catheter to extension tubing for measurement of pressure. (From Behrendt, D. M., and Austen, G.: *Patient Care in Cardiac Surgery.* Boston, Little, Brown, 1985, Fig. 2–13, p. 50.)

INSERTION

The left atrial catheter is inserted during cardiac surgery. The catheter itself is composed of a polyvinyl material and is approximately 6 in in length. The surgeon may insert this catheter in one of two ways. The most common technique is through a needle puncture of the right superior pulmonary vein that empties into the left atrium followed by insertion of the catheter into the left atrium (Taylor, 1986).

The second method is through direct insertion via a needle puncture into the intra-atrial groove into the left atrium just above the mitral valve (Fig. 4–15) (Taylor, 1986).

The catheter is then sutured into place and brought out through a stab wound into the chest wall, usually toward the right inferior end of the patient's sternal incision. Then the catheter is connected to a pressurized tubing system as previously described. The left atrial pressure waveform is then displayed on the oscilloscope. A sterile dressing is usually placed over the insertion site of the catheter and is changed daily. The LAP catheter is normally used for 24–72 hours and then is removed by a physician or other designated person depending on the policies of the institution.

NURSING IMPLICATIONS

In order to obtain accurate left atrial pressure recordings, the air-fluid interface of the transducer must be positioned at the phlebostatic axis (previously described) when the patient is in the supine position (see Fig. 4–11). If the patient assumes the lateral position facing the transducer, the air-filled interface of the transducer must be leveled as shown in Figure 4–16: An imaginary line is drawn at the fourth intercostal space along the chest wall and another line is drawn at the mid-sternum, and the point where the lines intersect is the approximate position of the left atrium and where the air-fluid interface of the transducer should be leveled.

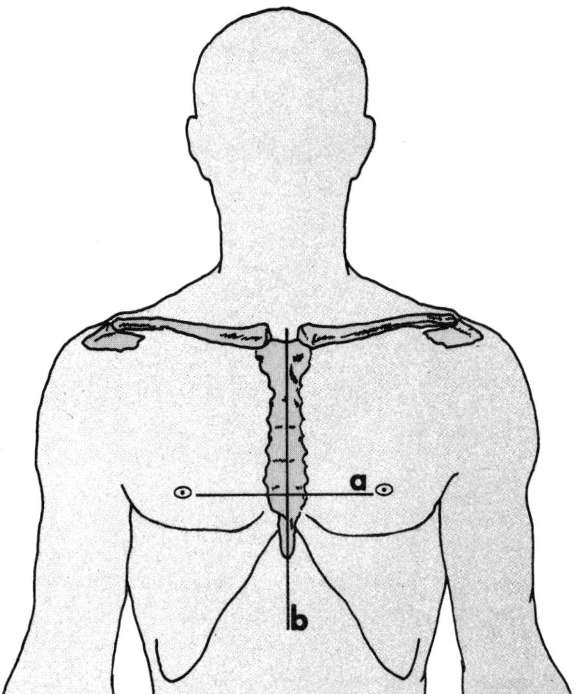

Figure 4-16. Site for leveling the transducer in the anterior lateral position. (From Taylor, T.: Monitoring left atrial pressures in the open-heart surgical patient. *Critical Care Nurse* 6(2):65, 1986, Fig. 3A.)

If the patient's back is facing the transducer, then another reference point to level the air-fluid interface of the transducer is necessary (Fig. 4-17). This is obtained by drawing an imaginary line along the fourth intercostal space at approximately the T4-T6 level and by drawing a second line along the midline of the spinal column. The transducer is then leveled at this point of intersection of both lines.

Another consideration for obtaining accurate LAP readings is the effect of the respiratory cycle. Again, LAP should be ideally obtained at the end of expiration, regardless of whether or not a patient is being mechanically ventilated. The rationale for this is that the end-expiratory pleural pressure usually remains at a relatively constant level and allows for a stable pressure waveform that facilitates accurate measurements.

A third consideration in obtaining accurate LAP measurements is for the patient on positive end-expiratory pressure (PEEP). The patient may be put on PEEP to correct hypoxemia (low Po_2). In this case, the LAP reading should be obtained while the patient is being mechanically ventilated on PEEP regardless of the level of PEEP because removing the PEEP to obtain any parameter has been found to be detrimental to the patient's oxygen level and may actually cause hypoxia. It is important to note that the strip/chart recordings as previously discussed in the CVP section can be used to ascertain the LAP.

COMPLICATIONS OF LAP MONITORING

The danger of introducing air or debris into the LAP catheter system is of paramount importance because of the peril of causing an embolism into the coronary or cerebral circulation. The nurse must ensure that all connections are tightly fitted and that all stopcocks have been capped. Medications or fluids should not be routinely administered through this catheter to again avoid the danger of introducing any air into the system.

Another complication of the LAP catheter is clot formation. Small clots can pose the same danger as air bubbles. If a clot is suspected, the nurse should manually try to aspirate the clot back into the syringe. However, if unsuccessful, the physician should be notified and the catheter should then be removed.

The third potential complication is infection. Prevention in this case is warranted. Remember

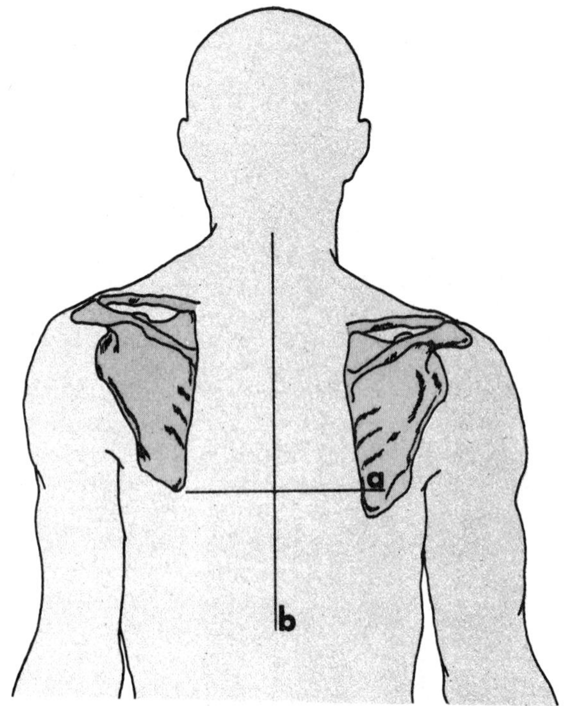

Figure 4-17. Site for leveling the transducer in the posterior lateral position. (From Taylor, T.: Monitoring left atrial pressures in the open-heart surgical patient. *Critical Care Nurse* 6(2):65, 1986, Fig. 3B.)

that this is a direct line into the heart and any microorganism that invades the cardiac tissue may directly affect the heart's performance. Thus, constant surveillance of the insertion site is mandatory and adherence to dressing changes per hospital policy should be maintained.

VARIABLES INFLUENCING LAP

The LAP can be either lowered or elevated depending on the clinical condition of the patient. A lowering of the normal LAP will be found in the following conditions: hypovolemia, massive vasodilation, and excessive PEEP (10 cm H_2O). Elevations in LAP may be found in the following conditions: hypervolemia, massive vasoconstriction, pulmonary congestion, mitral stenosis, mitral regurgitation, cardiac tamponade, constrictive pericarditis, and depressed contractile states such as in myocardial infarction, cardiomyopathy, or hypothermia.

It is important to remember that a series of LAP readings depicting trends is more informative than one single reading that deviates from the normal baseline range. Like any other hemodynamic parameter, the LAP should be correlated with other assessment data before any changes in therapy are instituted.

Pulmonary Artery Catheter

The introduction of the pulmonary artery catheter in 1970 by Swan and Ganz represented a major breakthrough in hemodynamic monitoring. Prior to this time, the central venous catheter was the only parameter that was available for monitoring cardiac function. No matter how important the CVP is in monitoring right-sided parameters, it is of little help in detecting left-sided problems.

The pulmonary artery catheter allows the clinician to indirectly monitor valuable information regarding left ventricular function. As was discussed earlier, through the contraction of the left ventricle, blood is ejected systemically to the tissues, where oxygen and nutrients are then made available to the cells. Any alterations in left ventricular function can severely compromise blood flow to the tissues. Since left ventricular stroke volume is influenced by the blood volume and contractility of the left ventricle during systole, the pulmonary artery catheter (PA catheter) is helpful in identifying conditions that contribute to abnormalities in both of these indices.

TYPES OF CATHETERS

The PA catheter is a long, hollow, pliable catheter that is radiopaque and is constructed with a variable number of lumens, or sections, that extend to several points (centimeters) along the length of the catheter. Distal and proximal lumens are for pressure monitoring, and these are filled with fluid. Medications or fluids should not be routinely administered through the distal lumen of the PA catheter. A thermistor lumen is used during cardiac output monitoring, and houses temperature-sensitive wires; and the balloon inflation lumen is equipped with a valve that enables a tiny balloon on the tip of the catheter to be inflated with a syringe. This balloon is inflated during insertion of the catheter to allow the catheter tip to flow through the various cardiac structures without causing damage to the cardiac tissue.

There are several types of PA catheters currently available. Catheters can either have two, three, four, or five lumens. Two-lumen PA catheters are the simplest type, which are currently rarely used (Fig. 4–18). They contain one lumen for pulmonary artery pressure monitoring, and a second lumen for inflation of the balloon during insertion.

Three-lumen catheters contain one PA lumen, one balloon-inflation lumen, and a third

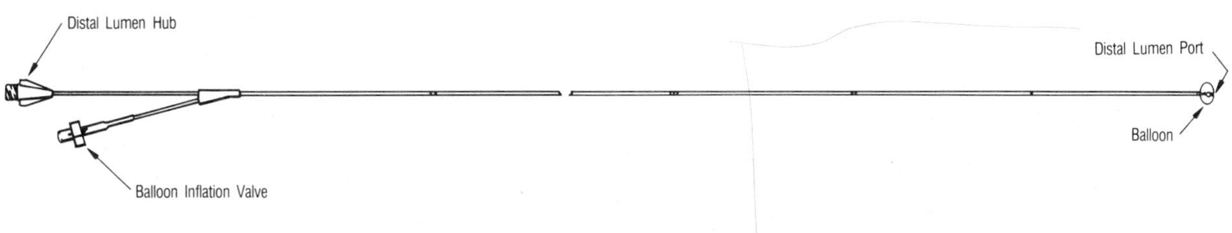

Double Lumen Catheter

Figure 4–18. Two-lumen pulmonary artery catheter which has the balloon inflation valve (to obtain wedge pressure) and distal lumen hub (to obtain PA pressure). (Courtesy of Baxter Healthcare Corporation, Baxter Edwards Critical-Care Division, Irvine, California.)

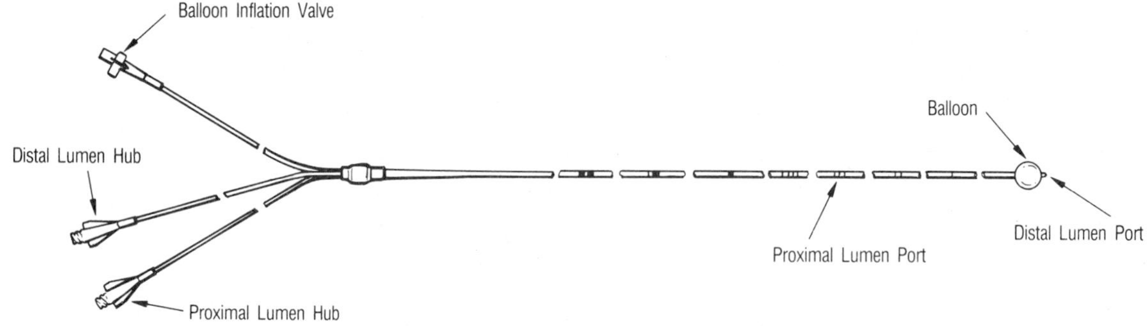

Figure 4–19. Triple lumen pulmonary artery catheter with balloon inflation valve, proximal injection hub (to obtain RA pressure) and distal injection hub. (Courtesy of Baxter Healthcare Corporation, Baxter Edwards Critical-Care Division, Irvine, California.)

lumen with a thermistor for cardiac output monitoring (Fig. 4–19).

Four-lumen catheters contain, in addition to a thermistor port and a balloon-inflation port, one port for positioning in the right atrium, often identified as the proximal port, and a fourth lumen, with a distal port for the positioning in the pulmonary artery (Fig. 4–20). The right atrial (proximal) lumen functions identically to the CVP, or right atrial catheter, discussed previously. The proximal port may therefore be used for monitoring purposes as well as for intravenous infusions.

Five-lumen catheters (Fig. 4–21) contain, in addition to the four ports described above, a fifth port situated high in the right atrium, which is used solely for infusion purposes. This fifth port is sometimes referred to as the venous infusion port (VIP). Five-lumen catheters have several advantages over the four-lumen type. First of all, they provide a mechanism for continuous monitoring of CVP pressure without interruption of the intravenous infusion. Second, because blood flows through the right atrium at a high velocity, two medications can be infused simultaneously, one through the right atrial lumen and another through the fifth lumen without fear of drug incompatibility.

Some pulmonary artery catheters are also designed for the purpose of transvenous pacing. This technique involves the insertion of pacemaker electrodes through the PA catheter in order to provide temporary ventricular pacing capabilities when other methods are not readily available. This modality is used in situations when the patient's own natural pacemaker is functioning ineffectively and dysrhythmias or absence of cardiac rhythm (asystole) result. Figure 4–22 illustrates a typical transvenous pacemaker system, which is inserted into a specially designed

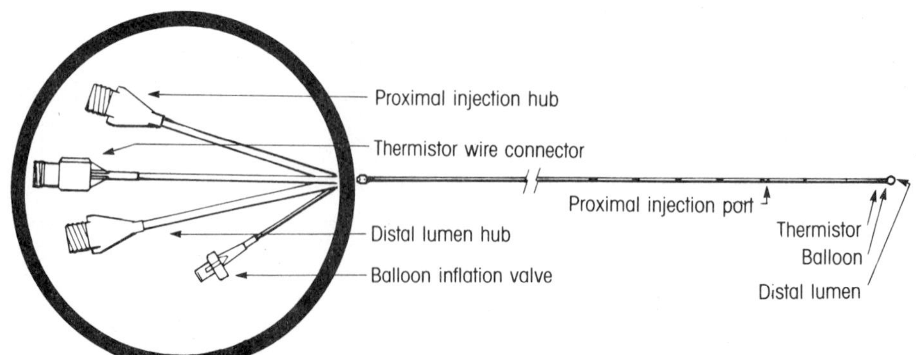

Figure 4–20. Quadruple-lumen pulmonary artery catheter containing the balloon inflation valve, proximal and distal injection hubs, and a thermistor lumen for obtaining cardiac output measurements. (From Davis, S. G., and Silverman, B.: Hemodynamic monitoring. *In*: Guzetta, C. G., and Dossey, B. M. (eds.). *Cardiovascular Nursing: Bodymind Tapestry*. St. Louis: C. V. Mosby, 1984, Fig. 10–3, p. 260.)

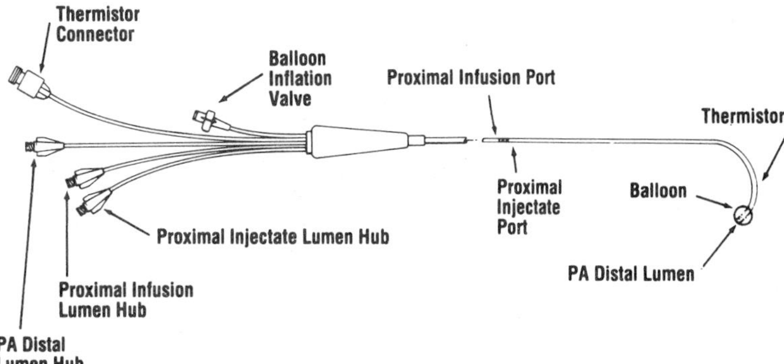

Figure 4-21. Five-lumen pulmonary artery catheter containing the quadruple lumen components in addition to a second proximal lumen for infusion of fluid or medications. (Courtesy of Baxter Healthcare Corporation, Baxter Edwards Critical-Care Division, Irvine, California.)

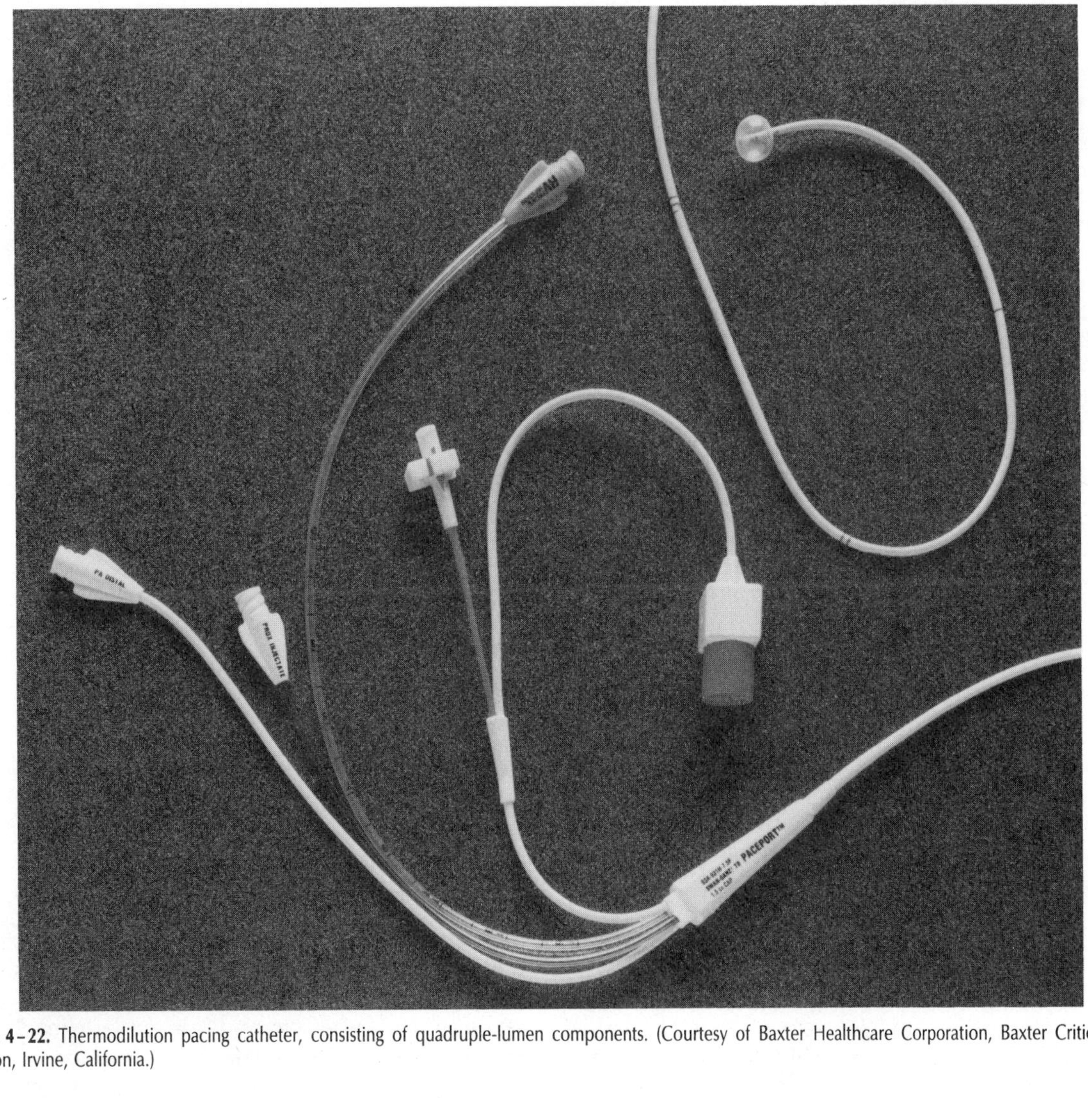

Figure 4-22. Thermodilution pacing catheter, consisting of quadruple-lumen components. (Courtesy of Baxter Healthcare Corporation, Baxter Critical-Care Division, Irvine, California.)

pulmonary artery catheter. An external generator is used to "fire" the pacing impulse. For more information regarding pacemakers, see Chapter 3.

A rather recent development in pulmonary artery technology has been in the area of fiberoptic catheters. Specially designed catheters are now available to continuously monitor mixed venous oxygen saturation (SvO_2), through a fiberoptic network housed inside a conventional PA catheter. To measure SvO_2, a tiny beam of light is transmitted through the catheter and into the patient's pulmonary artery circulation. Blood flowing through the pulmonary artery will be illuminated by this light. The patient's cardiac function and oxygenation will determine how much the blood reflects the light, and a tiny microchip located within the catheter quantifies this amount. These results are ultimately converted to a numerical value, which is displayed on a monitoring screen for continuous assessment. The concept of SvO_2 will be further discussed in a later section.

NURSING RESPONSIBILITIES PRIOR TO INSERTION

Despite the varying types of PA catheters currently available, the nursing responsibilities prior to inserting one remain relatively similar. Differences would depend on the patient's individual condition as well as personal preference of the physician and the brand of equipment used.

Of primary importance is the need for patient teaching prior to insertion. Patients are often anxious and uncertain about this procedure, and can benefit from simple, straightforward explanations. The following is a sample of the information that should be presented to the patient when the decision has been made to insert a PA catheter. The physician will provide additional information regarding the risks and benefits of the procedure, but the critical care nurse must be able to reinforce necessary information while providing emotional support.

> Hello, Mrs. Smith. The doctor has discussed the pulmonary artery catheter with you. I can help to clarify some points with you if you like.
>
> The PA catheter will give us valuable information about how your heart is working, and will help us to decide the best possible treatment.
>
> The procedure will probably take about 30 minutes. It won't be too painful, but it will involve the insertion of a small catheter through your skin and up into your heart. The skin will be numbed with a local anesthetic. It will be important for you to remain still while the catheter is being passed, but I'll be with you during the entire procedure to make sure you'll be as comfortable as possible.

As the physician continues the procedure, additional reinforcement should be provided to help decrease the patient's anxiety.

EQUIPMENT

The equipment required for pulmonary artery monitoring is similar to the pressure transducer system discussed in the section on CVP monitoring, using a transducer, amplifier, and display instrument with a tubing system for continuous flushing of the line. Variations from this method are possible when catheters contain both a right atrial (proximal port) and PA port (distal port). Rather than one set of tubing, two sections are needed to continuously flush both ports of the catheter. In order to simultaneously monitor both the right atrial and PA pressure, two transducers are necessary.

Because of certain risks involved with this procedure, it is necessary to have emergency medications and equipment readily available. Complications include hemothorax, pneumothorax, perforation of the vein or cardiac chamber, and cardiac rhythm disturbances. The pulmonary artery catheter passes through the right ventricle prior to coming to the pulmonary artery. As it does so, it can irritate the ventricle, causing ventricular rhythm disturbances, such as premature ventricular contraction and ventricular tachycardia (see above). For this reason, it is necessary to keep a prefilled syringe of 50 to 100 mg of intravenous lidocaine available to be infused emergently should these rhythm disturbances become hemodynamically significant.

INSERTION METHOD

Brachial Site

The site is cleaned and draped. A tourniquet is applied to the upper arm. A local anesthetic may be injected into the skin. The vein is needle punctured and placement in the vein is confirmed by a free flow of blood into the catheter. After the tourniquet is removed, the catheter is advanced.

Subclavian, Internal Jugular, or External Jugular Site

The patient's bed is placed in the Trendelenburg position to promote venous filling in the upper body for easier insertion of the catheter. This position can also prevent air embolism during insertion. If the Trendelenburg position is contraindicated such as in a patient with pulmonary edema, a blanket roll can be placed between the shoulder blades to facilitate insertion. The skin is cleaned and draped, and the skin is injected with a local anesthetic. A needled syringe is used to puncture the vessel and confirm placement by backward flow of blood into the syringe. The syringe is removed, and a guide wire is threaded through the needle into the vessel. The needle is then removed so that a hollow tube called an introducer may be passed over the guide wire. The wire is then removed and the pulmonary artery catheter passed freely into the vessel through the hollow introducer. It should be noted that there are several variations in this method of insertion, and physicians may have their own individual preferences as well. Technique may also vary according to the brand of equipment and patient anatomy.

Surgical Cutdown

Occasionally, it may be necessary to insert a pulmonary artery catheter using a surgical cutdown approach owing to the lack of suitable veins for the above method. In this method, the skin and surrounding muscle are surgically excised in order to expose the underlying vein. Once this is accomplished, the catheter may be placed similarly to the method described above.

NURSING RESPONSIBILITIES DURING INSERTION

As the catheter is passed through the cardiac chambers, the nurse must pay particular attention to heart rate, rhythm, and blood pressure. Therefore, vital signs should be recorded frequently. Any dysrhythmias that occur during the procedure should be documented, and the usual emergency equipment and medications made available.

As the tip of the catheter passes through each chamber, the waveform will change, and pressures displayed will need to be recorded. These waveforms will appear as follows: right atrial, right ventricular, pulmonary artery systolic and diastolic, pulmonary artery wedge pressure (Figs. 4–23 and 4–24). The last waveform signals the end of insertion, at which time the physician then

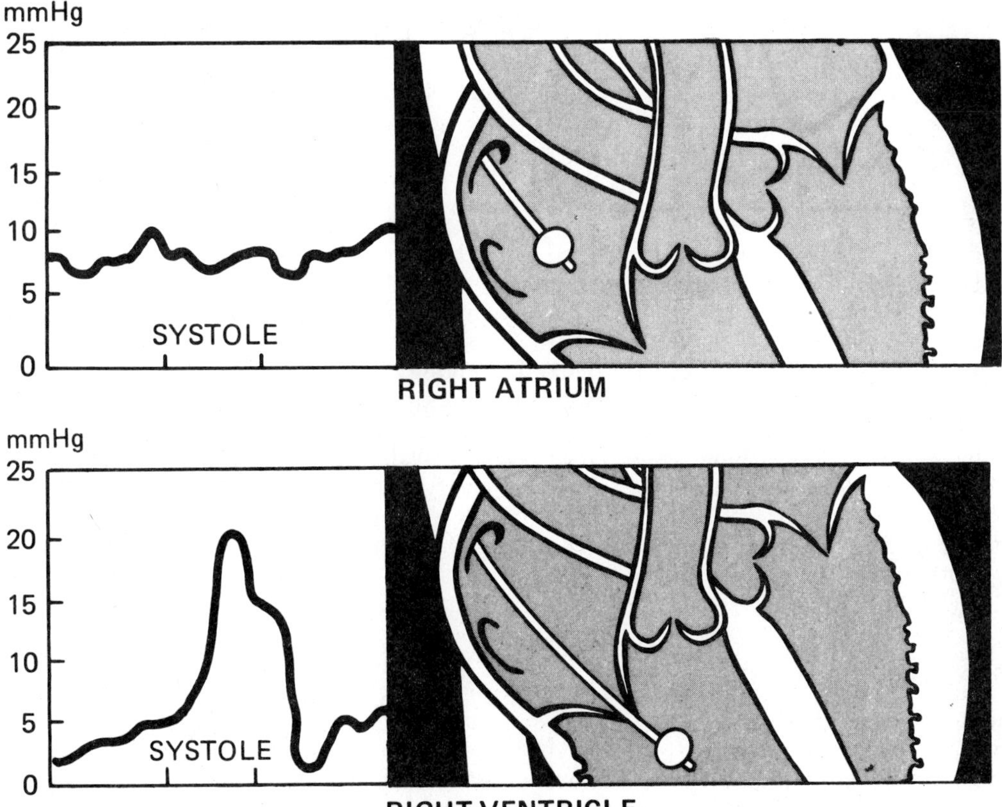

Figure 4–23. *(Top)* Pulmonary artery catheter as it floats into the right atrium, crossing the tricuspid valve, and then passing into the right ventricle *(bottom)*. (From Jackle, M., and Halligan, M.: *Cardiovascular Problems: A Critical Care Nursing Focus.* Bowie, MD, Robert J. Brady, 1980.)

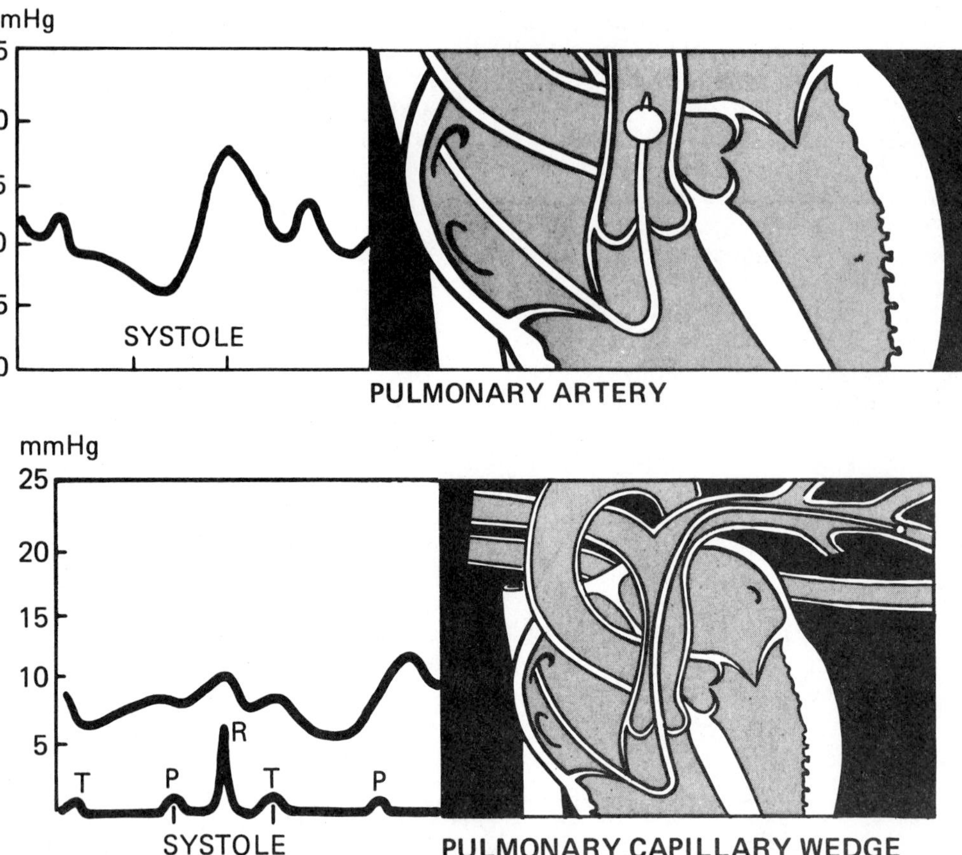

Figure 4-24. Pulmonary artery catheter being advanced through the pulmonic valve from the right ventricle to the pulmonary artery *(top).* Catheter is then floated into a smaller pulmonary arteriole in order to obtain the wedge pressure *(bottom).* (From Jackle, M., and Halligan, M.: *Cardiovascular Problems: A Critical Care Nursing Focus.* Bowie, MD, Robert J. Brady, 1980.)

deflates the balloon. Once the balloon is deflated, the tip of the catheter falls back in position in the pulmonary artery.

The nurse will reinflate the balloon to monitor pulmonary artery wedge pressures as ordered or according to unit protocol. The balloon should not be inflated for more than a few seconds to avoid causing ischemia to the lung tissue by obstructing blood flow. After the PA catheter is inserted, the centimeters (cm) should be noted to provide the clinician with an assessment clue should the catheter be accidentally pulled out or advanced.

CLINICAL SIGNIFICANCE OF PA CATHETER VALUES

The pulmonary artery pressure consists of a systolic, diastolic, and mean pressure (Fig. 4-25). The systolic pressure is the peak pressure attained as the right ventricle ejects out its stroke volume. The diastolic pressure is the lowest pressure on the waveform reflective of the movement of blood from the pulmonary artery out into the lung capillaries. The third parameter, the mean pressure, is the average pressure exerted on the pulmonary vasculature. The normal PAP is approximately 25/10 mm Hg, with a mean pressure of 15 mm Hg (see Fig. 4-14).

The fourth parameter, known as the pulmonary artery wedge pressure (PAWP) (Fig. 4-26), is a mean pressure with a normal value of 6 to 12 mm Hg (see Fig. 4-14). When the balloon is inflated, the PAWP actually reflects the pressure ahead of the catheter, which is both the left atrial pressure and left ventricular end-diastolic pressure. Thus, the PAWP is a good measurement of LV function. In the absence of valvular disease and pulmonary vascular congestion, the pulmonary artery diastolic pressure (PADP) also closely approximates the pressure in the left atrium and left ventricle just prior to contraction (end diastole) as well as the mean pressure in the pulmo-

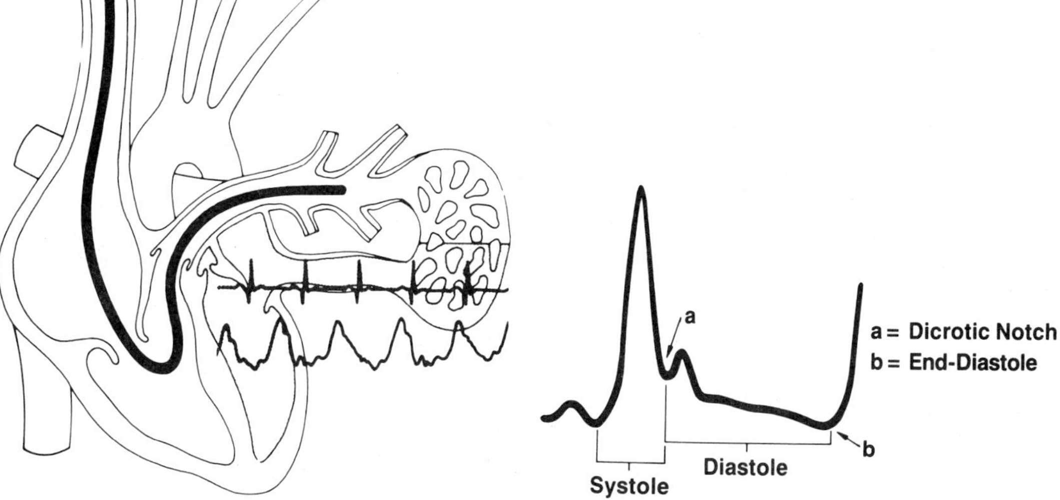

Figure 4-25. Pulmonary artery waveform corresponding to PA catheter position and patient's ECG. (Courtesy of Baxter Healthcare Corporation, Baxter Edwards Critical-Care Division, Irvine, California.)

nary capillaries (pulmonary wedge pressure). These pressures are equal because the mitral valve is open during end diastole, therefore providing an open circuit for the free movement of blood from the pulmonary artery to the lungs and back to the left atrium and left ventricle.

An understanding of the PADP and its relationship to LV end-diastolic pressure is of much value as a guide to therapy. In patients with normal left ventricles, an increase in LVEDP (and hence, PADP) indicates a rise in left ventricular blood volume that will be ejected with the next systole. Likewise, a drop in LVEDP (and a subsequently low PADP) signals a reduction in left ventricular blood volume available for the next contraction. Patients with elevated PADPs may include those who have been overhydrated with intravenous fluid as well as those patients with renal disease who cannot produce adequate urine output. Conditions causing low PADPs include dehydration, excessive diuretic therapy, and hemorrhage.

A rise in PADP can also provide the clinician with early information about impending left ventricular failure, as may be seen with myocardial infarction. An elevated PADP may be the

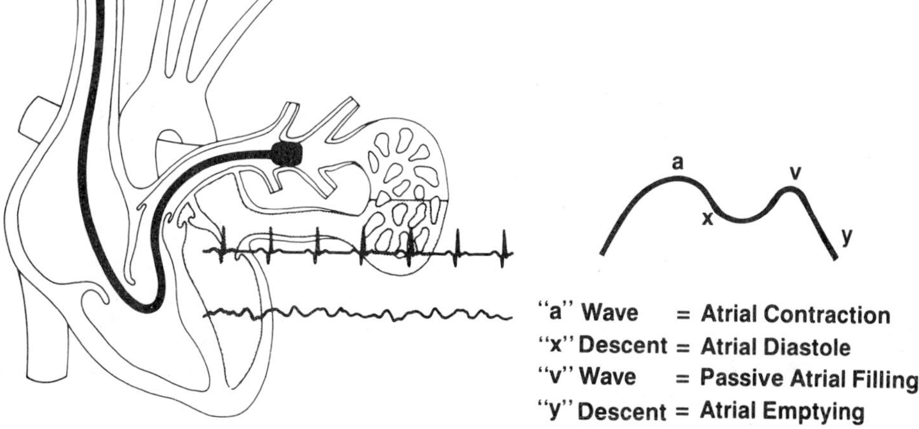

Figure 4-26. The pulmonary artery catheter in pulmonary artery wedge position measures left heart pressure. During diastole, the mitral valve is open, creating an open column of blood from the pulmonary arteries to the left atrium and left ventricle. When the balloon is inflated, blood flow from behind the catheter is obstructed so that the catheter tip reflects the pressure in front of the catheter (left heart pressure). (Courtesy of Baxter Healthcare Corporation, Baxter Edwards Critical-Care Division, Irvine, California.)

first observable change in the patient's condition before any other physical signs are apparent. By monitoring changes and tracking trends, the PADP can be invaluable in determining the most appropriate therapy to be administered as well as the effectiveness of that therapy.

The PAWP, being comparable to the PADP for the majority of patients, can also be used (mentioned previously) as a physiological indicator of LV failure and blood volume alterations. However, because the balloon of the catheter cannot be inflated for more than a few seconds at

Table 4–1. COMPLICATIONS OF PULMONARY ARTERY CATHETERS

Complication	Cause	Clinical Presentation	Nursing Implications
Infection	Violation of aseptic technique	Redness, pain, irritation, warmth, purulent drainage at insertion site; elevated body temperature	Daily observation for clinical signs of infection
	Catheter not secured to the surrounding skin	As above; the nonsterile section of the catheter can slip forward into the vessel	Adherence to aseptic technique during dressing changes
Dysrhythmias	Irritation to the endocardium caused when the balloon is deflated at the catheter tip. It can also occur when the catheter tip migrates back into the right ventricle	Premature ventricular contractions, ventricular tachycardia visible on monitor. Reduced perfusion with ventricular dysrhythmias may cause hypotension, mental status changes, decreased cardiac output, and other problems	Have lidocaine available to treat lethal dysrhythmias. Never advance the catheter without inflating the balloon. Continuous ECG monitoring
Air embolization	Balloon rupture. Poor technique during insertion. Disconnected infusion line	Signs of shock (drop in BP, rise in heart rate). Patient may appear to have had a CVA (change in level of consciousness, possibly seizures, motor weakness)	If embolization occurs, position the patient with head down (20°) and on left side. During catheter insertion, the patient needs to be positioned head down (Trendelenburg position). Notify physician immediately—this is an emergency situation
Pulmonary thromboembolism (PTE)	Thrombus formation on the catheter due to inadequate flushing, using nonheparinized flush solution	Sudden onset of dyspnea, chest pain, tachycardia, may lead to pulmonary infarction (see below)	Notify physician immediately of suspected PTE. Maintain anticoagulant therapy (heparin infusion) as ordered. Monitor partial thromboplastin time (PTT) while on heparin. Optimize ventilation. Administer inotropic medications as indicated. Preventive measures: use heparinized flush solution, ensure adequate flushing of lines, be alert for PA lines left in over 72 hr
Pulmonary artery rupture	Overinflation of the balloon. Deflated balloon tip passed during insertion of the catheter causing perforation. Frequent inflation of balloon	Signs of hemorrhage—↓BP, ↓CO, ↑HR. Decreased pulmonary blood flow	Use no more than 1.5 cc of air to inflate balloon. Never flush catheter when in the wedge position. If the waveform appears dampened, never force flush the line; instead, aspirate the clot
Pulmonary infarction	Catheter movement into the wedged position. Balloon left inflated. Thrombus formation around the catheter causing occlusion	Cough, hemoptysis (bloody sputum), pleuritic pain, high fever, bronchial breathing, and pleural friction rub. Hypoxemia, hypocardia, and respiratory alkalosis	Inflate the balloon with no more than 1.5 cc of air, and deflate it immediately after wedge tracing appears on monitor. If tracing appears to be wedged, and balloon is deflated, notify physician. A chest x-ray may be necessary to confirm position

Data compiled from Woods, S. L., and Grose, B. L.: Hemodynamic monitoring in patients with acute myocardial infarction. In: Underhill, S. L., Woods, S. L., Sivarajan-Froelicher, E. S., Halpenny, C. J.: *Cardiac Nursing*. Philadelphia, J. B. Lippincott, 1989, pp. 293–294.

a time, the PAWP cannot be used for continuous monitoring. Furthermore, frequent inflation of the balloon should be avoided to prevent the possibility of the balloon rupturing and causing air embolization (see below). However, periodic comparison of the PADP and PAWP is helpful in assessing the accuracy of the PADP measurement, especially in patients experiencing acute hemodynamic changes.

COMPLICATIONS OF PULMONARY ARTERY CATHETERS

Complications that may occur with PA monitoring are uncommon. Table 4–1 lists the most common complications as well as implications for the nurse in these situations.

NURSING IMPLICATIONS FOR PATIENT POSITIONING

It has been assumed that the patient must be flat and supine in order to obtain reproductive measurements. However, several studies have determined the effects of varying backrest positions, up to 60 degrees on PA, PA wedge, and LA pressures, and have found little effect on these hemodynamic measurements, provided the phlebostatic axis and proper leveling to the air-fluid interface of the stopcock are used as the zero reference level (Chulay and Miller 1984; Laulive, 1982; Retailliau et al., 1985).

One study looking at the effect of the side-lying position has found that reliable PA and PA wedge pressures can be obtained when the patient is in the 90-degree lateral decubitus position, provided the fourth intercostal space and midsternum are used as the reference level (Kennedy et al., 1984). The zero reference level for various degrees of lateral positioning are unknown; thus, PA and PA wedge pressures may not be reliable if obtained in other lateral positions less than 90 degrees (Whitman et al., 1982; Wild, 1984). Moreover, Kennedy et al. (1984) recommend that baseline measurements be performed and compared in the supine, right lateral, and left lateral decubitus positions before relying only on measurements in either of the lateral positions.

■ Cardiac Output Monitoring

As was previously discussed, cardiac output (CO) is the amount of blood that has been pumped out of each ventricle (stroke volume) each minute. Cardiac output can be calculated by multiplying the stroke volume (SV) (amount of blood pumped out of each ventricle during each contraction) by the heart rate (HR) (the number of ventricular contractions per minute). Thus, the formula is $CO = SV \times HR$.

In the critical care setting, cardiac output is an important hemodynamic parameter. It is used to assess if the heart is pumping enough blood to supply oxygen to all of the body tissues. Employing the thermodilution method, cardiac output can be measured at the bedside of a critically ill patient. This method involves injecting a known amount of solution at a known temperature (iced or room temperature) via the proximal port (CVP or right atrial) of a quadruple-lumen PA catheter and then measuring the resultant drop in temperature downstream (using the thermistor of the PA catheter) (Fig. 4–27). The cardiac output for the right side of the heart is calculated via a computer. It is important to note that although this cardiac output is a reflection of right ventricular blood flow, the cardiac output of the left ventricle closely equals the right side under normal conditions.

EQUIPMENT

The equipment needed to perform cardiac output includes (1) four- or five-lumen PA catheter with thermistor, (2) injectate (3, 5, or 10 ml of 5% dextrose in water or saline solutions), (3) cardiac output computer. There are two methods of injecting the solution into the CVP proximal port. The first method is referred to as the open injectate delivery system. This method involves preparing prefilled syringes (usually 10 ml of dex-

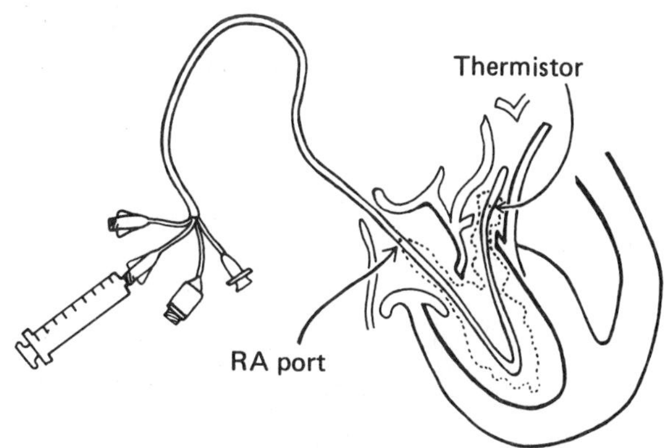

Figure 4–27. Illustration depicting injection into right atrium for cardiac output measurement. (From Gardner, P. E., and Woods, S. L.: Hemodynamic monitoring. *In:* Underhill, S. L. et al.: *Cardiac Nursing.* 2nd ed. Philadelphia, Lippincott, 1989, Fig. 34–13, p. 464.)

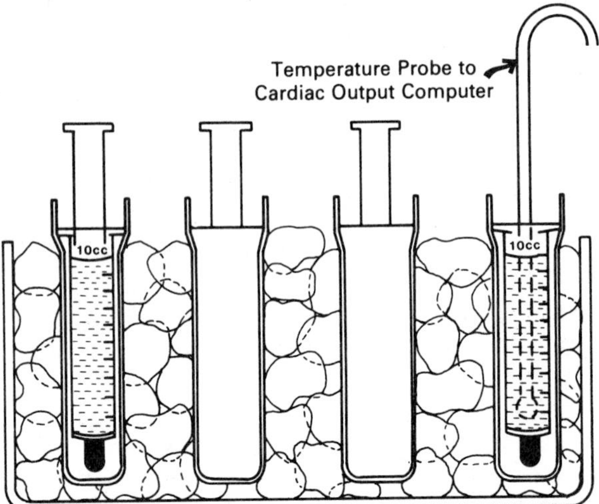

Figure 4-28. Illustration depicting iced injectate preparation. Preloaded syringes are placed in plastic or metal tubes, or in resealable bags that are suspended in an ice bath. (From Gardner, P. E., and Woods, S. L.: Hemodynamic monitoring. *In*: Underhill, S. L. et al.: *Cardiac Nursing*. 2nd ed. Philadelphia, Lippincott, 1989, Fig. 34-15, p. 465.)

trose or saline solutions), and then putting these syringes in a sterile bath of ice chips and water (Fig. 4-28). (Prefilled syringes are available from certain manufacturers.) Maintaining the sterility of the ice bath is a major concern. One nursing study that investigated the ice bath encasing the syringes found bacterial growth after 8 to 24 hours (Grose et al., 1981). It is, therefore, recommended that this ice bath be changed every 8 hours. Another consideration is that these syringes need to be chilled to the range of 0° to 5°C. In addition, it takes approximately 12 to 60 minutes to reach this temperature before these syringes can be used (Grose et al., 1981). Erroneous variations in cardiac output can occur if these syringes are not properly chilled.

The second method is known as the closed injectate delivery system. This method involves using a completely closed set-up of a sterile injectate solution, tubing coils, and a syringe attached near the proximal injectate port to instill the predetermined amount of solution (Fig. 4-29). The advantages of this method include eliminating the need to prepare prefilled syringes, reducing nursing preparation time, and reducing the risk of infections by avoiding multiple entries into a sterile system.

METHOD OF OBTAINING CARDIAC OUTPUT

Care must be exercised in obtaining accurate cardiac outputs. Table 4-2 depicts causes of faulty

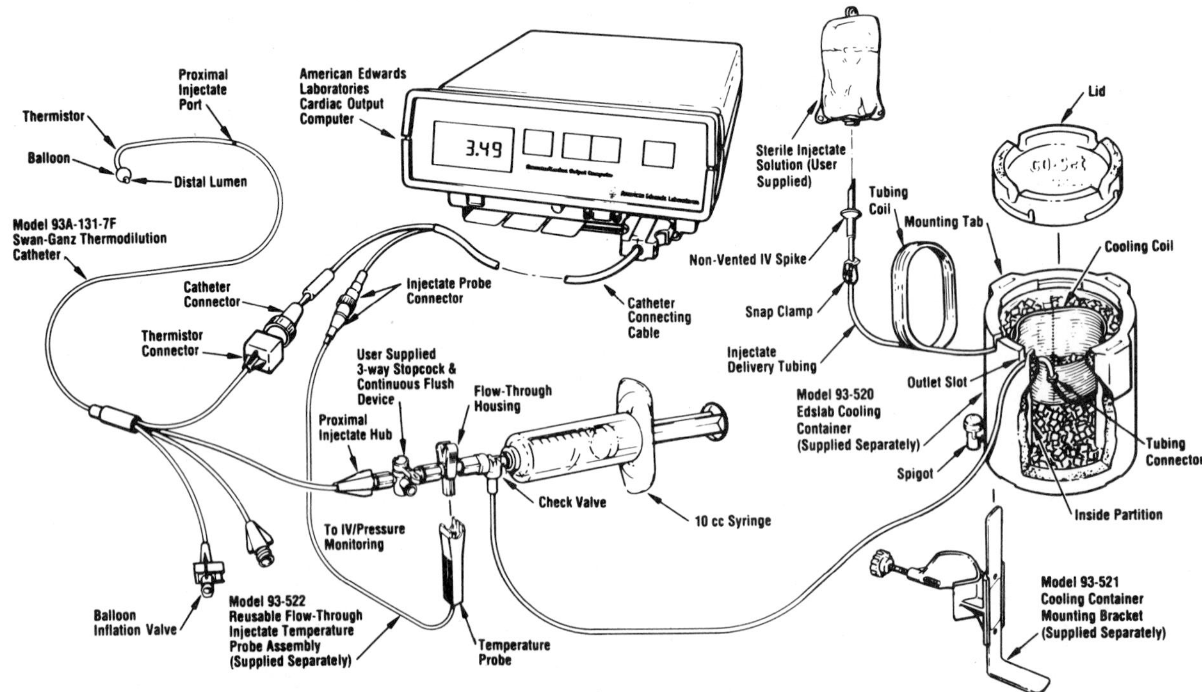

Figure 4-29. Schematic illustration of the closed injectate delivery system for use with iced injectate. A cooling container is not used for room-temperature injectate. (Courtesy of Baxter Healthcare Corporation, Baxter Edwards Critical Care Division, Irvine, California.)

cardiac outputs. The following points are important to bear in mind to ensure accuracy:

1. The correct position of the PA catheter should be verified by the waveform because malposition of the catheter will cause erroneous CO values.

2. The appropriate computation or calibration constant (per manufacturer's instruction) must be displayed on the computer. This constant is used to correct the computer for the gain of heat from the tubing and thermistor.

3. When chilled prefilled syringes are used, they should have been placed in the ice bath solution for at least 12 to 60 minutes. The temperature of syringes should not exceed 5°C when using the iced-injectate method (Levett and Replogle, 1979; Runciman et al., 1981).

4. Avoid handling the barrel of the syringe because heat gain during handling will cause an incorrect value.

5. When using the prefilled syringe, inject within 30 seconds of removal from ice bath (Gardner and Woods, 1989). When using either the prefilled or manual closed-injectate (5 or 10 ml) syringe, the manner of injection should be smooth and rapid (within 4 seconds) (Ganz and Swan, 1972), preferably at the end of expiration (Gardner, 1989).

6. The proximal port should be assessed for the patency and type of intravenous fluid infusing through this line during CO injectates. Vasoactive drugs should not be routinely administered through this line because harmful effects could result from rapid CO instillations.

7. The patient should ideally be positioned in the supine position in a backrest elevation of 0 to 20 degrees (Doering and Dracup, 1988).

8. It is recommended that three CO measurements be obtained and an average CO be calculated. The first CO may be erroneous, especially if the catheter is filled with room temperature fluid and ice injectate is used. If there is a 10% difference in this reading, then discard this value and do not use it to average the cardiac output.

High correlation has been found when COs using iced temperature and room temperature injectates have been compared. In some pathophysiological conditions resulting in high- or low-output states, investigators have recommended using 10 ml of iced injectate to allow for a more reliable reading (Gardner and Woods, 1989).

Table 4–2. CAUSES OF ERRORS IN CARDIAC OUTPUT

Faulty technique
Slow injection (>4 sec)
Injectate too warm (when using iced injectate method)
Incorrect computation constant set on computer
Incorrect position of PA catheter
Faulty thermistor
Catheter not properly connected to computer
Patient changes in position or movement
Dysrhythmias
Ventilators with positive end-expiratory pressure
Intracardiac shunts (atrial/ventricular septal defect)

CLINICAL RELEVANCE

In the critically ill patient, the thermodilution method has gained widespread acceptance because of accuracy, ease of use, safety, and ability to obtain repeated cardiac outputs. The normal cardiac output value is in the range of 4 to 8 liters per minute (L/min). It has been noted that the cardiac output varies with body size. Because of this variation, the cardiac index (CI) is used because this parameter takes into account the body size of a patient and is considered to be a more precise measurement of cardiac output. The normal CI is 2.5 to 4.0 liters/minute/square meter (L/min/m^2). The formula is as follows:

$$\text{Cardiac Index} = \frac{\text{Cardiac output in L/min}}{\text{Body Surface Area}}$$

The body surface area (BSA) in square meters can be calculated based on the patient's height and weight. The DuBois Body Surface Chart enables quick calculation of a patient's BSA (Fig. 4–30). Many cardiac output computers will automatically calculate the BSA based on the height and weight of the patient that has been entered and can also automatically calculate the CI.

The ability to obtain the CI enables health care personnel to assess patients' responses to pharmacological agents or fluid administration, since changes in cardiac output may occur soon after therapy has begun. Another use for the CI is to assess the ventricular pump performance. For example, if the left ventricle of a patient should begin to fail, one would expect to see a gradual decline in the CI. This decline in turn has implications regarding the patient's prognosis (Table 4–3).

Alterations in the CI result from variations in stroke volume or heart rate. Moreover, re-

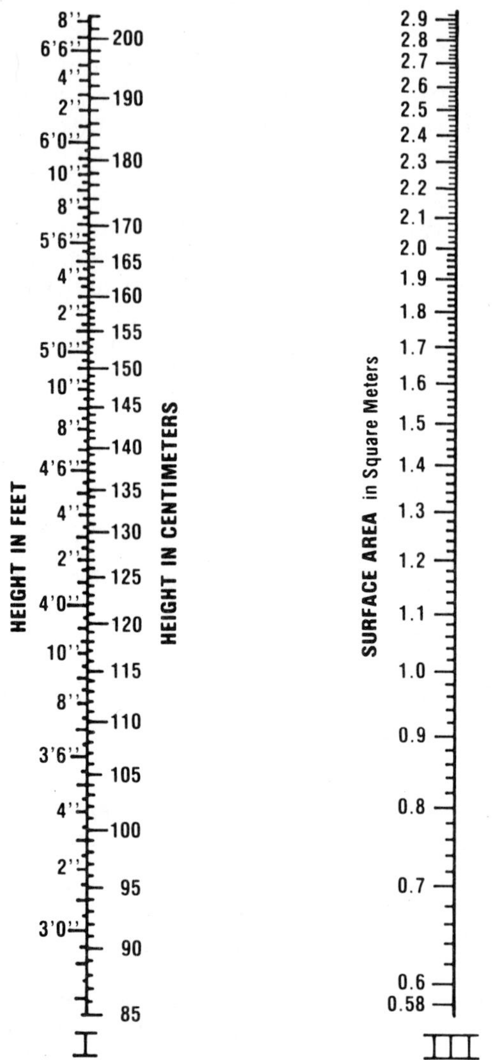

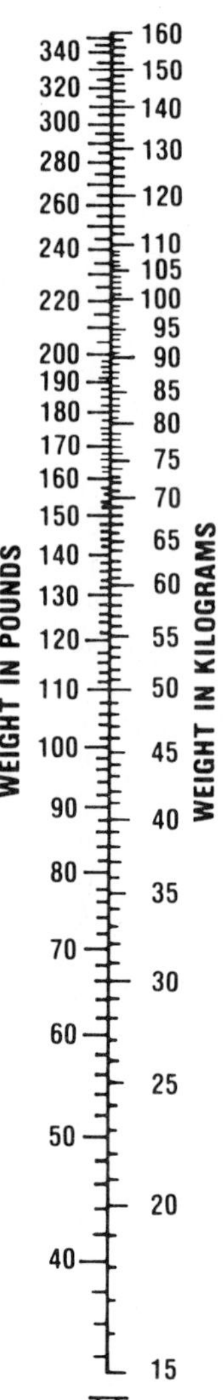

Figure 4-30. DuBois body surface chart. To find body surface of a patient, locate the height in inches (or centimeters) on scale I and the weight in pounds (or kilograms) on scale II and place a straight edge (ruler) between these two points, which will intersect scale III at the patient's surface area. (From DuBois, E. F.: *Basal Metabolism in Health and Disease*. Philadelphia, Lea & Febiger, 1936.)

member that three factors affect stroke volume; i.e. preload, afterload, and contractility (see above for a more detailed discussion).

Causes of low cardiac index may include the following:

Table 4-3. CLINICAL STATES OF DECREASED CARDIAC INDEX

CI	Clinical States
2.0–2.2 L/min/m²	Onset of cardiac failure
1.5–2.0 L/min/m²	Cardiogenic shock
Under 1.5 L/min/m²	Irreversible stage of shock

1. Abnormally fast or slow heart rate that will cause poor filling of the left ventricle
2. Low stroke volume due to a decrease in preload as a result of:
   a. Diuresis
   b. Dehydration
   c. Third space shift
   d. Hypovolemia
   e. Vasodilation (septic shock)
3. Low stroke volume due to an increase in afterload as a result of:
   a. Vasoconstriction due to hypothermia or low-flow states
   b. LV failure
   c. Increased blood viscosity
4. Low stroke volume due to a decrease in con-

tractility (decreased cardiac function) as a result of:

a. Myocardial ischemia/infarction
b. Cardiomyopathies
c. Cardiogenic shock
d. Cardiac tamponade

5. Valvular disorders such as stenosis or regurgitation (insufficiency)

Cause of high cardiac index can occur as a result of the following:

1. Increased physical activity (exercise)
2. Increased anxiety
3. Pulmonary edema
4. Increased metabolic states (e.g., hyperthyroid, fever, tachycardia, adrenal disorders)
5. Anemia
6. Sepsis (initial stages)
7. Mild hypertension with a wide pulse pressure

Treatment of low cardiac index in the critical care patient is often aimed at correcting the underlying problem. Thus, given the list of causes of low cardiac index, the following therapies may be instituted:

1. Correct the abnormal heart rate employing a pacemaker, pharmacological agents (beta-blockers, calcium channel blockers, antidysrhythmic drugs) or elective cardioversion.

2. Increase stroke volume by increasing preload via fluid administration (either crystalloid or colloid solutions) and avoiding diuretics.

3. Increase stroke volume by decreasing afterload through the use of diuretics or afterload-reducing drugs such as sodium nitroprusside (Nipride) or nitroglycerin (NTG).

4. Increase stroke volume by increasing contractility through the use of a positive inotropic agent; e.g., digitalis preparations, dobutamine, dopamine, epinephrine, isoproterenol (Isuprel).

5. Replace a severely diseased cardiac valve causing the problem.

Mixed Venous Oxygen Saturation

SvO_2 MONITORING SYSTEM

Mixed venous oxygen saturation (SVo_2) is another hemodynamic parameter that can be monitored on a continuous basis or obtained intermittently via blood sampling. The advent of the fiberoptic pulmonary artery catheter (discussed above) has enabled clinicians to obtain continuous SvO_2 measurements. Intermittent measurements can be obtained by drawing blood from the pulmonary artery distal port.

This blood is known as mixed venous blood because blood returns to the pulmonary artery from various organs having different oxygen needs. This venous blood is then "mixed" in the PA, and therefore reflects an overall picture of oxygen use by the various organs and tissues.

After the mixed venous sample is drawn, it is sent to the laboratory for blood gas analysis. The lab analysis will include an SvO_2 measurement as well as other mixed venous blood gas parameters.

The fiberoptic pulmonary artery catheter (Fig. 4–31) is inserted in the same manner as previously described in the section on PA catheters. However, there are three distinct components to enable continuous SvO_2 monitoring. These include (1) the fiberoptic catheter, which transmits and receives light waves; (2) the optical module, which sends/receives light to the end of the catheter via a fiberoptic channel; (3) a microprocessor, which interprets SvO_2 values by changing the light signal into an electrical signal that is then displayed as a digital numerical display (Fig. 4–32).

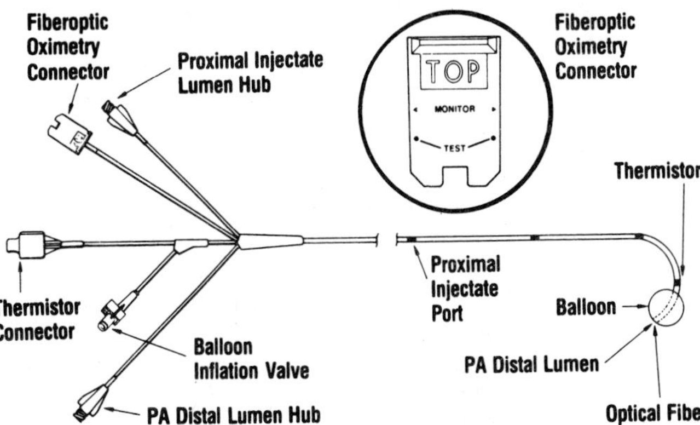

Figure 4–31. SvO_2 fiberoptic pulmonary artery catheter. (Courtesy of Baxter Healthcare Corporation, Baxter Edwards Critical Care Division, Irvine, California.)

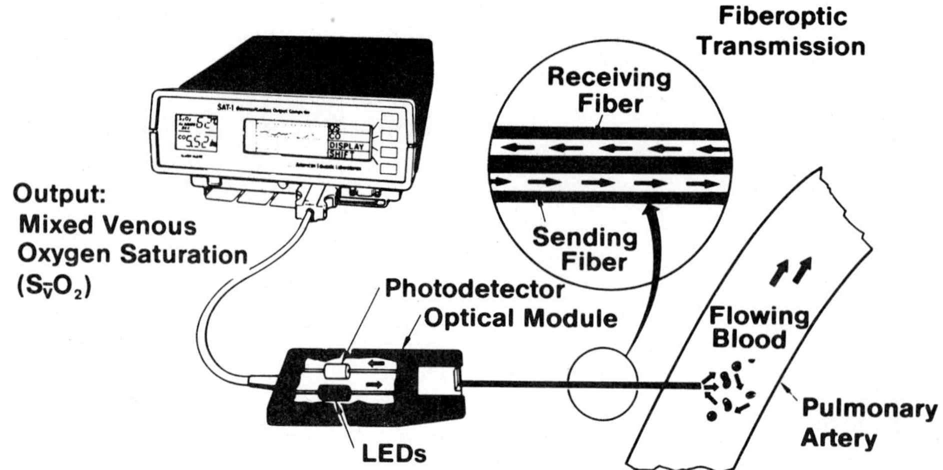

Figure 4-32. Illustration depicting the SAT-1 fiberoptic oximetry system from American Edwards Laboratories. (Courtesy of Baxter Health Care Corporation, Baxter Edwards Critical-Care Division, Irvine, California.)

SvO_2 MEASUREMENT

The SvO_2 is a measurement that reflects the degree to which the tissues of the body are using oxygen (demand) as well as the adequacy of the oxygen supply at the tissue level. In other words, it helps evaluate whether or not the oxygen supply can meet the oxygen demands of the tissues of the body. Oxygen supply is determined by several variables such as the content of oxygen in the arterial blood (assessed by the hemoglobin), the PaO_2 (partial pressure of arterial oxygen), the arterial oxygen saturation (SAO_2), and the delivery of this oxygen-rich blood to the tissues of the body (assessed by the cardiac output). Oxygen demand is determined by the patient's condition. Factors that increase the oxygen demand include shivering, exercise, fever, pain, anxiety, increased work of breathing, bathing, vasoactive drugs, and endotracheal suctioning. Therefore, if the oxygen supply cannot meet the increase in the oxygen demand, this will be reflected in the SvO_2 measurement.

The normal SvO_2 measurement is in the range of 60 to 80%, whereby 75% is often recorded as the average SvO_2. Whenever the oxygen supply fails to meet the oxygen demand, the SvO_2 will decrease to less than 60%, alerting the

Table 4-4. ALTERATIONS IN SvO_2

Alteration	Cause	Possible Causative Factor
Low SvO_2 (<60%)	$\downarrow O_2$ supply	Hypoxia or hemorrhage, anemic states, hypovolemia, cardiogenic shock, dysrhythmias, myocardial infarction, congestive heart failure, cardiac tamponade, massive transfusions of stored blood, restrictive lung disease, ventilation/perfusion abnormalities
	$\uparrow O_2$ demand	Strenuous exercise, hyperthermia, pain, anxiety or stress, hormonal imbalances, increased work of breathing, bathing, pheochromocytoma, thiamine/vitamin deficiency, septic shock, seizures, shivering
High SvO_2 (>80%)	$\uparrow O_2$ supply	Increase in FIO_2, hyperoxia
	$\downarrow O_2$ demand	Hypothermia, anesthesia, hypothyroidism, pharmacological paralysis (pancuronium bromide or vecuronium bromide), early stages of sepsis, cirrhosis
High SvO_2 (>80%)	Technical error	PA catheter in wedged position, fibrin clot at end of catheter, noncalibrated monitor

Data compiled from Halfman-Franey, M.: Current trends in hemodynamic monitoring of patients in shock. *Critical Care Nursing Quarterly* 11:9–18, 1988; and Briones, T. L.: SvO_2 monitoring. Part 1. Clinical Case Presentation *Dimensions of Critical Care Nursing* 7:70–78, 1988, Abbott Laboratories.

nurse that either the oxygen supply is too low or the oxygen demand is too high. Interventions are then aimed at either increasing the oxygen supply (increasing cardiac output or increasing oxygen saturation via blood transfusion) or by decreasing the oxygen demand (determining the factor that is increasing the demand and then alleviating or decreasing it).

Increases in SvO_2 may occur when the oxygen delivery (supply) exceeds the oxygen demand or when there is a decrease in demand. This may occur with the following conditions: hypothermia, anesthesia, early stages of septic shock, wedged PA catheter, or deposits of fibrin on the tip of the catheter. Table 4–4 summarizes many of the causative factors that increase or decrease the SvO_2.

Intra-Arterial Monitoring

Intra-arterial monitoring is an invasive technique of monitoring arterial blood pressure. This method, as opposed to the noninvasive cuff technique, allows for continuous and accurate measurement of arterial pressure.

Although the sphygmomanometer method of determining arterial pressure is simple and accessible, for the critically ill patient, it is not always the most accurate. As the patient's stroke volume falls, the Korotkoff sounds become more difficult to auscultate. This is why the intra-arterial method is preferred in unstable patients.

The noninvasive method of measuring blood pressure is most commonly by sphygmomanometry. With this method, an inflatable cuff attached to a mercury manometer is placed over an artery, generally at the brachial site. The cuff is then inflated with air until the artery is compressed against the underlying bones of the extremity. The pressure produced ultimately occludes the artery completely as the cuff pressure exceeds the systolic pressure of the extremity. A stethoscope is then placed below the cuff over the superficial artery. As the cuff is slowly deflated, blood is once again allowed to flow freely through the artery. As the first jets of blood pass through the artery, the sound produced is detected by the stethoscope. The corresponding pressure observed on the mercury manometer is recorded as systolic pressure, or the pressure generated by contraction of the ventricles. As the cuff continues to deflate, more blood is allowed to flow through the artery. When these sounds disappear, the corresponding measurement on the mercury manometer is recorded as diastolic pressure. Diastolic pressure is the pressure exerted on the arteries between cardiac contractions. The characteristic sounds auscultated with sphygmomanometry are called Korotkoff's sounds.

EQUIPMENT

In order to monitor the intra-arterial pressure, the following components are required:

1. A catheter is placed into a radial, brachial, or femoral artery either percutaneously or via surgical cutdown. If the catheter is placed into the radial artery an Allen test should be performed to assess patency of the radial and ulnar arteries (Fig. 4–33). In patients whose radial ulnar arch is not patent, a radial line should not be placed as any thrombosis could result in circulatory compromise to the hand, leading to possible limb loss.
2. A pressurized heparinized fluid source is attached to the arterial catheter to keep the catheter patent. The intravenous fluid should be pressurized to 300 mm Hg by using an inflatable bag to prevent backflow of arterial blood into the tubing-catheter system. Remember that enough pressure needs to be exerted so as to force the heparinized solution to flow against the patient's systolic pressure.
3. The transducer is attached to the hub of the catheter (see Fig. 4–10) via the connecting tubing. Once the transducer is attached to the monitor, it should be balanced, zeroed, and calibrated (see previous section on essential components of hemodynamic monitoring).
4. The bedside monitor amplifies the signal from the transducer and displays the arterial waveform on an oscilloscope. This arterial waveform is displayed continuously along with numerical values.

WAVEFORM/MEASUREMENTS

The normal arterial waveform consists of a steep ascent during systole followed by a gradual descent during diastole. As the left ventricle contracts, the systolic pressure wave is transmitted to the transducer and then depicted as a sharp rising wave. The systolic pressure is then measured at the peak of the waveform (Fig. 4–34). This pressure is considered to reflect the function of the left ventricle. Thus, if the left ventricle should contract poorly, the systolic pressure would become lower to reflect this decrease in function.

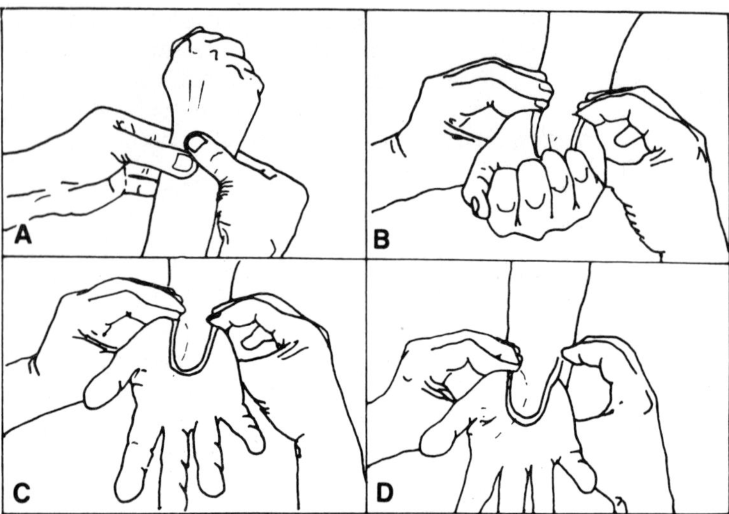

Figure 4-33. Modified Allen test. When the patient's hand is held above the head with the fist clenched, both the radial and ulnar arteries are compressed *(A)*. The hand is lowered *(B)* and opened *(C)*. Pressure is then released over the ulnar artery *(D)*. Color should return to the hand within 6 sec, indicating a patent ulnar artery and an intact superficial palmar arch. (From Kaye, W. Invasive monitoring techniques: Arterial cannulation, bedside pulmonary artery catheterization, and arterial puncture. *Heart Lung* 12(4):395-427, p. 400.)

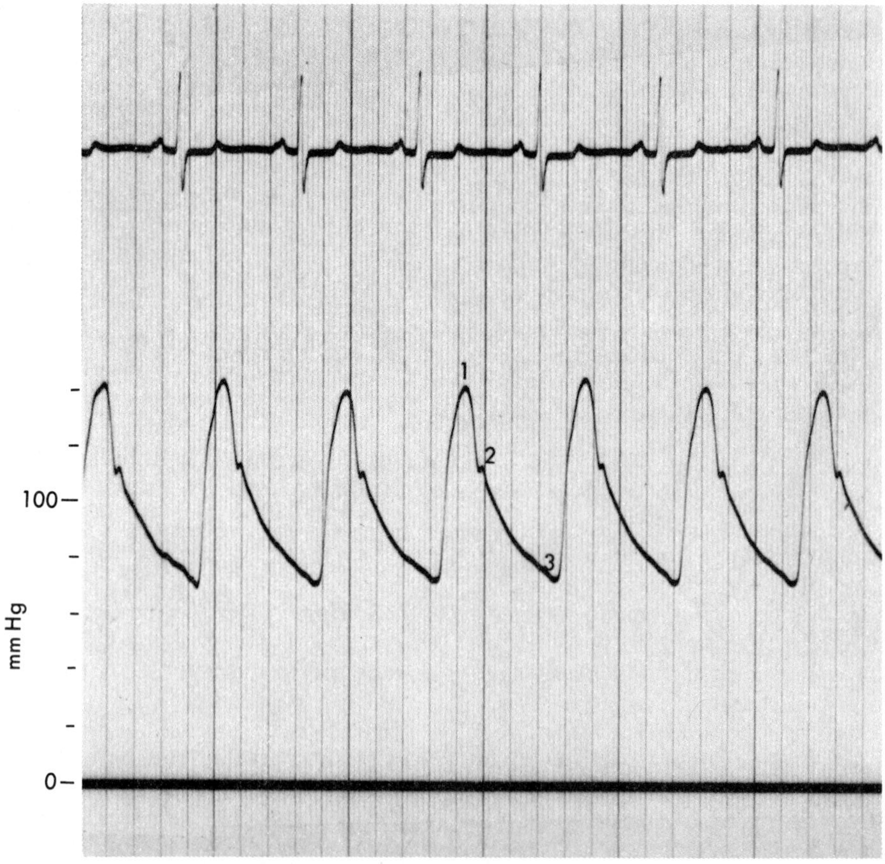

Figure 4-34. Normal arterial pressure tracing: (1) Systole; (2) Dicrotic notch; and (3) Diastole. (Reproduced with permission from: Daily, E. and Schroeder, J. S.: *Hemodynamic Waveforms.* 2nd ed. St. Louis, 1990, The C. V. Mosby Co., Fig. 5-1, p. 95.)

The normal value of the systolic pressure is 90 to 140 mm Hg.

The diastolic pressure is shown as the lowest point on the arterial waveform (see Fig. 4–34). This pressure is a reflection of peripheral resistance. Therefore, if the resistance should increase, the diastolic pressure would also increase. The normal diastolic pressure is 60 to 80 mm Hg.

The dicrotic notch is a small notch on the downstroke of the waveform (see Fig. 4–34). It occurs as a result of the closure of the aortic valve. Closure of the aortic valve (dicrotic notch) is commonly considered the reference point between the systolic and diastolic phases of the cardiac cycle.

The mean arterial pressure is a calculated pressure that closely estimates the perfusion pressure in the aorta and its major branches. It represents the average pressure in the peripheral arterial system during the entire cardiac cycle. However, it is not the average of the systolic and diastolic pressure but more closely approximates the diastolic pressure as opposed to the systolic pressure. It can be calculated via a computer encased in the monitor or arithmetically. The arithmetic formula is as follows:

$$\text{Mean Arterial Pressure} = \frac{\text{Systolic BP} + 2\ \text{Diastolic BP}}{3}$$

The normal MAP is 70 to 100 mm Hg. It is important to maintain a MAP greater than 60 mm Hg in order to perfuse the vital organs of the body.

The pulse pressure is defined as the arithmetic difference between the systolic and diastolic pressure.

Systolic pressure = 140 mm Hg
Diastolic pressure = 70 mm Hg
Pulse pressure = 70 mm Hg

The pulse pressure widens when the systolic and diastolic pressures get farther apart. As these pressures become closer, the pulse pressure narrows.

INDICATIONS FOR INTRA-ARTERIAL MONITORING

Intra-arterial pressure monitoring is indicated for critically ill patients in whom continuous arterial pressure monitoring is essential. Ideally, any patient who is receiving continuous intravenous vasoactive drugs should have intra-arterial monitoring in order to evaluate response to therapy. Other indications include the following:

1. Patients in whom frequent arterial blood sampling is necessary
2. Patients in whom the rapid removal of blood (phlebotomy) is vital
3. Patients in low-flow states (shock) or who have hypotension
4. Patients who are severely hypertensive
5. Patients who are critically vasodilated or vasoconstricted

COMPLICATIONS

The major complications of arterial pressure monitoring include (1) thrombosis, (2) embolism, (3) blood loss, and (4) infection. Thrombosis (blood clot) may occur if a continuous flush solution with heparin is not used. Also, a greater incidence of thrombosis has been reported when the catheter used is very long (Kaye, 1983). In addition, radial artery catheters left in place longer than 48 hours increase the risk of thrombosis (Kaye, 1983).

Embolism may occur as a result of small clot formation around the tip of the catheter. In addition, air embolism may result from air being allowed to enter the closed tubing system especially during intermittent flushing by hand.

Blood loss is usually a result of sudden dislodgement of the catheter from the artery in which it has been placed or from disconnection of the tubing. Rapid blood loss may occur (remember this is in an artery not a vein) if either of these occurrences are not promptly recognized.

Infection is usually the result of a catheter left in place for a prolonged period of time. Most infections occur when catheters are in for more than 72 hours (Band and Maki, 1979). The incidence of infection is also increased when a catheter has been inserted via a surgical cutdown approach (Mandel and Dauchot, 1977).

CLINICAL CONSIDERATIONS OF ARTERIAL MONITORING

The invasive method of obtaining blood pressure is considered to be more accurate because it actually gives beat by beat information as opposed to the noninvasive method that measures vibrations (Korotkoff's sounds) of the arterial wall over several beats (see previous discussion). In patients who are hypotensive, there may be a serious discrepancy between the invasive and noninvasive blood pressure, whereby the cuff pressure may be significantly lower, leading to dangerous mistakes in treating such a patient. Under normal circumstances, a difference of 5 to 20 mm Hg between invasive and noninvasive blood pressure is expected, whereby the invasive blood pressure should be greater than the noninvasive value (Kaye, 1983).

When a difference between the invasive and noninvasive BP is such that the noninvasive value is higher than the invasive number, one must become suspicious of equipment malfunction or a technical error (Kaye, 1983). Table 4–5 lists the possible causes. One sign of a possible problem is when the waveform appears to decrease in amplitude, lose the dicrotic notch on the downslope (Fig. 4–35), and depict low systolic pressure. This is referred to as a damped waveform. This phenomenon is indicative of interference with the transmission of the pulse through the fluid-filled catheter to the transducer. A damped waveform could result from the catheters becoming lodged against the arterial wall, a clot at the catheter tip or in the stopcock, air in the transducer, or kinks in the tubing system. In order to make sure that this damped waveform is not reflective of the patient becoming acutely hypotensive, the nurse should take a cuff pressure immediately and compare that value to the intra-arterial value. If the noninvasive value is indeed higher, the nurse is then alerted to a possible technical problem and should troubleshoot the system for one of the previously mentioned causes of damping. Damping due to catheter obstruction may be corrected by aspirating any visible clots or by carefully repositioning the catheter if it seems to be lodged against the arterial wall.

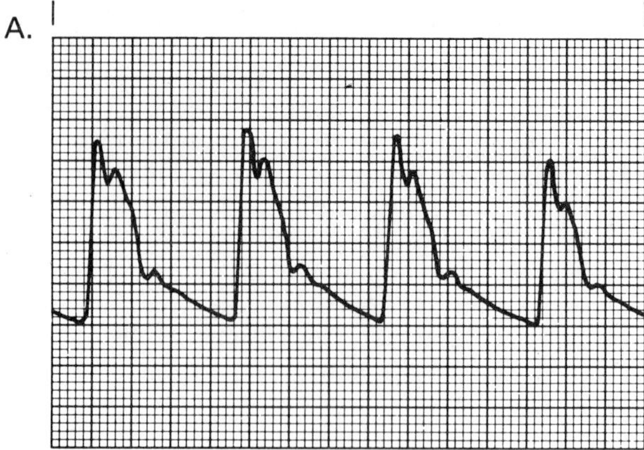

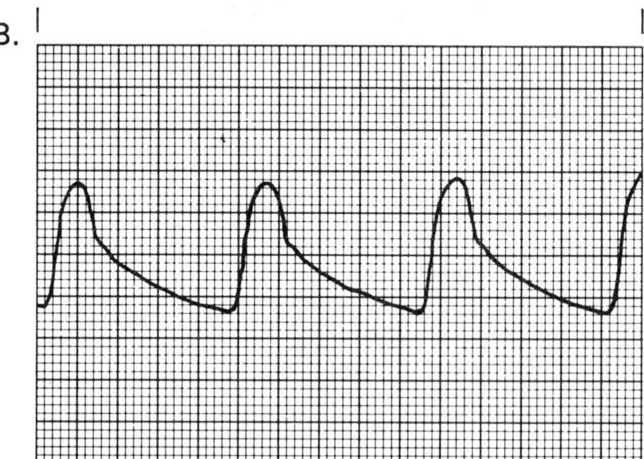

Figure 4–35. *(A)* Normal arterial waveform depicting sharp upstroke and clear dicrotic notch. *(B)* Damped waveform depicting slow upstroke, lower systolic pressure, and poor dicrotic notch. (From Jackle, M., and Halligan, M.: *Cardiovascular Problems: A Critical Care Nursing Focus.* Bowie, MD, Robert J. Brady, 1980.)

Table 4–5. CAUSES OF HIGHER NONINVASIVE VS INVASIVE BP

Air bubbles
Improper cuff size
Improper cuff placement
Incorrect calibration of sphygmomanometer
Improper calibration of transducer
Failure to zero the transducer
Blood in catheter system
Blood clot at catheter tip
Kinking of the tubing system
Loose or open connections
Dislodgement of catheter tip against arterial wall
Soft compliant tubing
Long tubing (greater than 4 ft)
Too many stopcocks (more than 3)

Data compiled from Kaye, W.: Invasive monitoring techniques: Arterial cannulation, bedside pulmonary artery catheterization, and arterial puncture. *Heart and Lung* 12:395–427, 1983; and Gardner, P. E., and Woods, S. L.: Hemodynamic monitoring. In: Underhill, S. L., Woods, S. L., Sivarajan-Froelicher, E. S., and Halpenny, C. J.: Cardiac Nursing. Philadelphia: J. B. Lippincott, 1989, pp. 451–481.

NURSING IMPLICATIONS

Any nurse caring for a patient with an arterial line should ideally try to prevent or reduce the incidence of complications. Thus, in order to prevent thrombosis, embolism, blood loss, or infection, the nurse's responsibilities include the following:

1. Maintain a continuous heparinized flush solution through the catheter to prevent clot formation.

2. Document insertion date of the catheter and keep physician aware of placement time (re-

member the longer the catheter is in place, the greater the risk of clot formation).

3. Keep tubing free of kinks.

4. Maintain a pressure of 300 mm Hg on the flush solution.

5. Avoid intermittent flushing by hand to minimize the problem of embolism.

6. Check extremity frequently for color, temperature, sensation, and capillary refill.

7. Keep wrist in a neutral position and place on an armboard.

8. Check for a damped waveform, and if noted, reposition catheter or aspirate for air or clots.

9. Tighten all connections and make sure that these connections remain tight so as to minimize possible blood loss.

10. Restrain an agitated patient to prevent sudden dislodgement of catheter or disconnection of tubing.

11. Set high and low alarms.

12. Ensure that adequate pressure is applied to the site of insertion for 10 minutes when the catheter is discontinued and withdrawn.

13. Keep sterile caps over the openings of stopcocks.

14. Change dressing using aseptic technique according to the Centers for Disease Control's recommendations.

Summary

This chapter was designed as an introduction to the basic principles of hemodynamics and the technological aspects of hemodynamic monitoring. Discussion focused on the various types of hemodynamic monitoring currently used in the critical care setting such as central venous pressure, left atrial pressure, pulmonary artery and wedge pressure, cardiac output, SvO_2, and arterial pressure monitoring. In addition, nursing considerations in caring for a patient undergoing each of these modalities was highlighted.

Hemodynamic monitoring is an important physiological assessment tool in caring for critically ill patients. Data obtained from this modality should serve as a guide to the health care team in determining and evaluating interventions for such patients.

References

Band, J. D., and Maki, D. C. (1979): Infections caused by indwelling arterial catheters for hemodynamic monitoring. *American Journal of Medicine* 67(5):735–741.

Chulay, M., and Miller, T. (1984): The effect of backrest elevation on pulmonary artery and pulmonary capillary wedge pressures in patients after cardiac surgery. *Heart and Lung* 13(2):138–140.

Doering, L., and Dracup, K. (1988): Comparisons of cardiac output in supine and lateral positions. *Nursing Research* 37(2):114–118.

Ganz, W., and Swan, W. J. C. (1972): Measurement of blood flow by thermodilution. *American Journal of Cardiology* 29:241–245.

Gardner, P. E. (1989): Cardiac output: Theory, technique and troubleshooting. *Critical Care Nursing Clinics of North America* 1(3):577–587.

Gardner, P. E., and Woods, S. L. (1989): Hemodynamic monitoring. In: S. L. Underhill, S. L. Woods, E. S. Sivarajan-Froelicher, and C. J. Halpenny, eds. *Cardiac Nursing.* 2nd ed. Philadelphia: J. B. Lippincott, pp. 451–481.

Grose, B. L., Adair, M., and Riem, M. (1981): Incidence of contamination of thermodilution cardiac output bath. *Circulation* 64(Suppl. IV):179.

Kaye, W. (1982): Catheter and infusion-related sepsis: The nature of the problem and its prevention. *Heart and Lung* 11(3):221–228.

Kaye, W. (1983): Invasive monitoring techniques: Arterial cannulation, bedside pulmonary artery catheterization, and arterial puncture. *Heart and Lung* 12(4):395–427.

Kennedy, G. T., Bryant, A., and Crawford, M. H. (1984): The effects of lateral body positioning on measurements of pulmonary artery and pulmonary wedge pressures. *Heart and Lung* 13(2):155–158.

Laulive, J. (1982): Pulmonary artery pressures and position changes in the critically ill adult. *Dimensions of Critical Care Nursing* 1(1):28–34.

Levett, J. M., and Replogle, R. L. (1979): Thermodilution cardiac output: A critical analysis and review of the literature. *Journal of Surgical Research* 27(6):392–404.

Mandel, M. A., and Dauchot, P. J. (1977): Radial artery cannulation in 1,000 patients: precautions and complications. *Journal of Hand Surgery* 2(6):482–485.

Retailliau, M. A., Leding, M. M., and Woods, S. L. (1985): The effect of backrest position on the measurement of left atrial pressure in patients who have had cardiac surgery. *Heart and Lung* 14(5):477–483.

Runciman, W. B., Ilsley, A. H., and Robert, J. G. (1981): Thermodilution cardiac output—A systematic error. *Anesthesiology Intensive Care* 9(2):135–139.

Taylor, T. (1986): Monitoring left atrial pressures in the open heart surgical patient. *Critical Care Nurse* 6:62–68.

Whitman, G. R., Howaniak, D. L., and Verga, T. S. (1982): Comparison of pulmonary artery catheter measurements in 20° supine and 20° right and left lateral recumbent positions. *Heart and Lung* 11(3):256–257.

Wild, L. R. (1984): Effect of lateral recumbent positions on the measurement of pulmonary artery and pulmonary artery wedge pressures in critically ill adults. *Heart and Lung* 13(3):305.

Recommended Reading

Briones, T. L. (1988): SvO_2 Monitoring: Part 1. Clinical Care Application. *Dimensions of Critical Care Nursing* 7(2):70–72.

Cross, F. A., and Vargo, R. L. (1988): Cardiac output: Iced versus room temperature solution. *Dimensions of Critical Care Nursing* 7(3):146–149.

Daily, E. K., and Schroeder, J. S. (1989): *Techniques in Bed-*

side Hemodynamic Monitoring. 4th ed; St. Louis: C. V. Mosby, Chapters 1–8.

Davis, S. G., and Silverman, B. (1984): Hemodynamic monitoring. In: C. E. Guzzetta and B. M. Dossey, eds. *Cardiovascular Nursing: Bodymind & Tapestry.* St. Louis: C. V. Mosby, pp. 253–275.

Enger, E. L. (1989): Pulmonary artery wedge pressure: When it's valid, when it's not. *Critical Care Nursing Clinics of North America* 1(3):603–618.

Erwin, G. W., and Long, S. (1984): *Memory Bank for Hemodynamic Monitoring.* Pacific Palisades, CA: Nurseco, pp. 1–200.

Gardner, P. (1989): Cardiac output: Theory, technique, and troubleshooting. *Critical Care Nursing Clinics of North America* 1(3):577–587.

Gardner, P. E., and Laurent-Bopp, M. (1987): Continuous SvO_2 monitoring: Clinical application in critical care nursing. *Progress in Cardiovascular Nursing* 2(1):9–18.

Gardner, P. E., and Woods, S. L. (1989): Hemodynamic monitoring. In: S. L. Underhill, S. L. Woods, E. Sivarajan-Froelicher, and C. J. Halpenny, eds. *Cardiac Nursing.* Philadelphia: J. B. Lippincott, pp. 451–481.

Halfman-Franey, M. (1988): Current trends in hemodynamic monitoring. *Critical Care Nursing Quarterly* 11(1):9–18.

Hardy, G. R. (1988): SvO_2 continuous monitoring techniques. *Dimensions of Critical Care Nursing* 7:(1)8–17.

Hurst, F. M. (1984): Invasive hemodynamic monitoring: An overview. *Journal of Emergency Nursing* 10:11–22.

Jackle, M., and Halligan, M. (1980): *Cardiovascular Problems: A Critical Care Nursing Focus.* Bowie, MD: Robert J. Brady, pp. 211–271.

Kadota, L. (1985): Theory and application of thermodilution cardiac output measurement: A review. *Heart and Lung* 14(6):605–612.

Kadota, L. T. (1986): Reproducibility of thermodilution cardiac output measurements. *Heart and Lung* 15(6):618–622.

Kaye, W. (1983): Invasive monitoring techniques: Arterial cannulation, bedside pulmonary artery catheterization, and arterial puncture. *Heart and Lung* 12(4):395–427.

Laulive, F. (1981): Nursing management of left atrial pressure monitoring. *Critical Care Quarterly* 4(2):75–82.

Loveys, B. J., and Woods, S. L. (1986): Current recommendations for thermodilution cardiac output measurements. *Progress in Cardiovascular Nursing* 1(2):24–28.

Norsen, L. H., and Fox, G. B. (1985). Understanding cardiac output and the drugs that affect it. *Nursing '85* 15(4):31–42.

Taylor, T. (1986): Monitoring left atrial pressures in the open heart surgical patient. *Critical Care Nurse* 6(2):62–66.

Urban, N. (1986): Integrating hemodynamic parameters with clinical decision making. *Critical Care Nurse* 6(2):48–61.

Vitello-Cicciu, J. M., and Eagan, J. S. (1988): Data acquisition from the cardiovascular system. In: M. R. Kinney, D. R. Packa, and S. B. Dunbar, eds. *AACN's Clinical Reference for Critical Care Nursing.* New York: McGraw-Hill, pp. 556–563.

Chapter

5

Mary Lou Noll, Ph.D., R.N., CCRN

Ventilatory Assistance

Objectives

- Review anatomy and physiology of the respiratory system.
- Describe methods for assessing the respiratory system, including physical assessment, interpretation of arterial blood gases, and noninvasive techniques.
- Compare commonly used oxygen delivery devices.
- Discuss methods for maintaining an open airway.
- Identify indications for initiating mechanical ventilation.
- Describe types and modes of mechanical ventilation.
- Relate complications associated with mechanical ventilation.
- Explain methods for weaning patients from mechanical ventilation.
- Formulate a plan of care for the mechanically ventilated patient.

Maintaining an adequate airway and ensuring adequate breathing, or ventilation, are nursing interventions essential to all patients. These nursing interventions provide the framework for this chapter. Respiratory anatomy and physiology are reviewed in order to provide a basis for discussing ventilatory assistance. Assessment of the respiratory system is discussed, including physical assessment, assessment of arterial blood gases, and noninvasive methods for assessing gas exchange. Airway management and mechanical ventilation are also discussed in this chapter.

Review of Respiratory Anatomy and Physiology

The primary function of the respiratory system is gas exchange. Oxygen (O_2) and carbon dioxide (CO_2) are exchanged via the respiratory system in order to provide adequate oxygen to the cell. The respiratory system can be divided into (1) the upper airway, (2) the lower airway, and (3) the lungs. The upper airway provides gas exchange to and from the lower airway, whereas the lower airway provides gas exchange to the alveoli. The anatomical structure of the respiratory system is shown in Figure 5–1.

UPPER AIRWAY

The upper airway consists of the nasal cavity and pharynx. The bony structure of the nasal cavity is referred to as the nasal conchae. The nasal cavity conducts air, filters large foreign particles, and warms and humidifies air. The nasal cavity also is responsible for voice resonance, smell, and sneeze reflexes. The throat, or pharynx, trans-

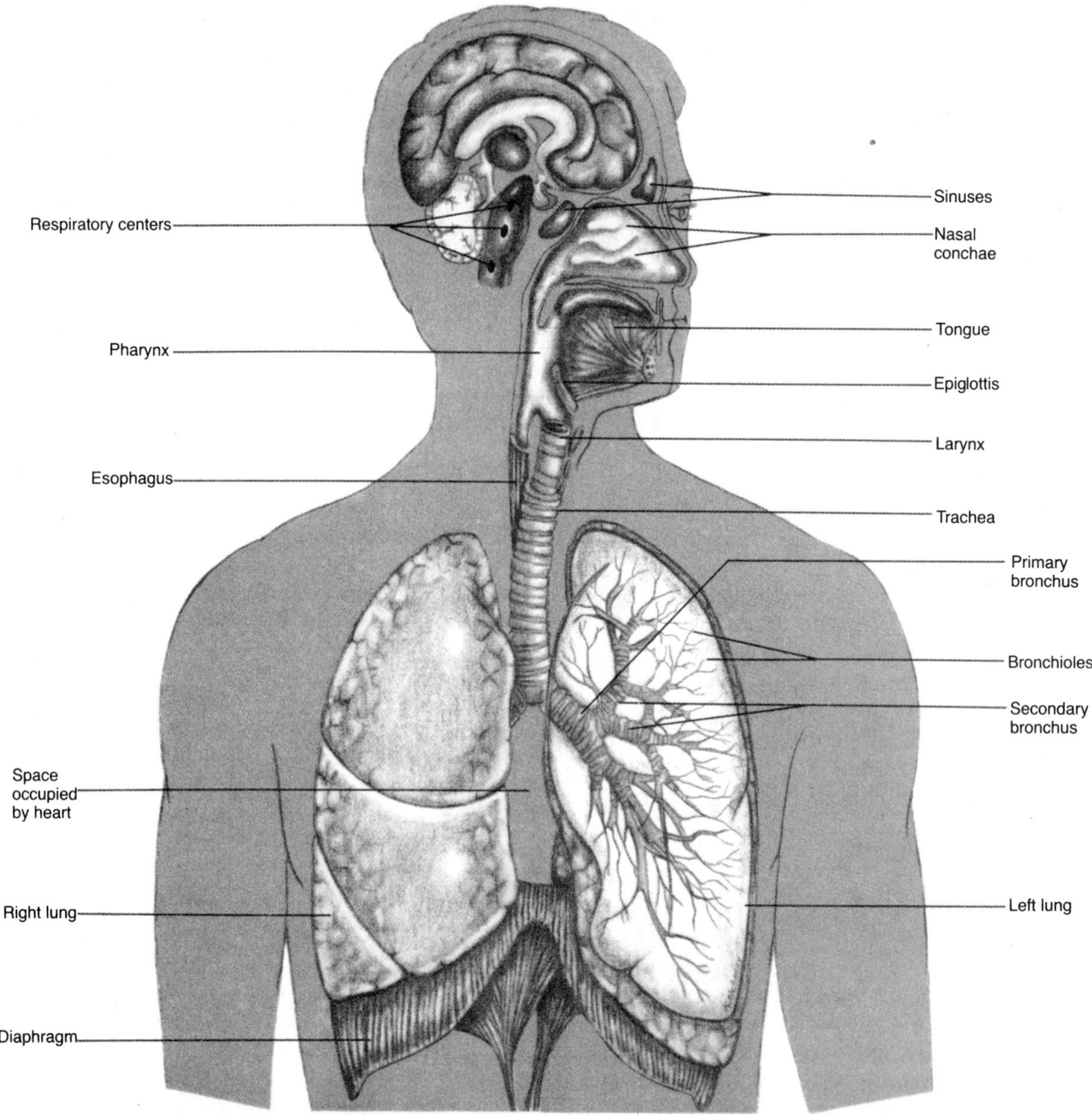

Figure 5-1. Anatomy of the respiratory system. The lungs are located in the thoracic cavity. The diaphragm forms the floor of the thoracic cavity, and separates it from the abdominal cavity. The internal view of one lung shows air passages. (From Solomon, E. P., and Phillips, G. A.: Understanding Human Anatomy and Physiology. Philadelphia, W. B. Saunders, 1987, Fig. 15-1, p. 262.)

ports both air and food. Air enters the superior part of the pharynx, the nasopharynx, and then passes behind the mouth through the oropharynx.

LOWER AIRWAY

The lower airway consists of the larynx, trachea, right and left mainstem bronchi, bronchioles, and alveoli. The larynx is the narrowest part of the conducting airways in adults. Also referred to as the voice box, the larynx contains the vocal cords. The larynx is partly covered by the epiglottis, which prevents aspiration during swallowing. The passage through the vocal cords is called the glottis.

The windpipe, or trachea, warms, humidifies, and filters air. Cilia in the trachea propel mucus and foreign material upward through the airway.

At about the level of the fifth thoracic vertebra, the trachea branches into the bronchi. This bifurcation is referred to as the carina.

The right and left mainstem bronchi conduct air to the respective lungs. The right mainstem bronchus is shorter, wider, and straighter than the left. Mucosal cells in the bronchi trap foreign materials. The bronchi branch into the bronchioles, which in turn branch into the alveoli.

The alveoli are the distal airway structures and are responsible for gas exchange at the capillary level. Over 300 million of these tiny air sacs are present in the lungs. The alveoli consist of a single layer of epithelial cells and fibers to permit expansion and contraction. The alveoli are covered by a network of capillaries. Gas exchange occurs between the alveoli and these capillaries. The alveoli are coated with surfactant, which prevents them from collapsing. The structure of the alveolus is shown in Figure 5-2.

LUNGS

The lungs consist of lobes. The left lung has two lobes, whereas the right lung has three lobes. Each lobe consists of lobules that are supplied by one bronchiole. The lungs are covered by the pleura, which consists of two layers. The parietal pleura is the inner layer that covers the lungs. The outer layer is referred to as the visceral pleura. The pleural space is the area in between the parietal and visceral pleurae. The pressure in the pleural space, intrapleural pressure, is always negative (less than atmospheric) to facilitate lung expansion on inspiration.

Table 5-1. CHANGES IN INTRAPLEURAL AND INTRAALVEOLAR PRESSURES DURING INSPIRATION AND EXPIRATION

Pressures	At Rest (mm Hg)	Inspiration	Expiration
Atmospheric	760	760	760
Intrapleural	756	750	756
Intra-alveolar	760	757	763

PHYSIOLOGY OF BREATHING

Changes in intrapleural pressure and intra-alveolar pressure (the pressure in the lungs) cause the act of breathing (Table 5-1; Fig. 5-3). At rest, intrapleural pressure is less than atmospheric (negative), whereas the intra-alveolar pressure equals atmospheric pressure. During inspiration, the diaphragm lowers and flattens and the intercostal muscles contract, increasing the size of the chest cavity (Fig. 5-4). Subsequently, the intrapleural pressure becomes even more negative and

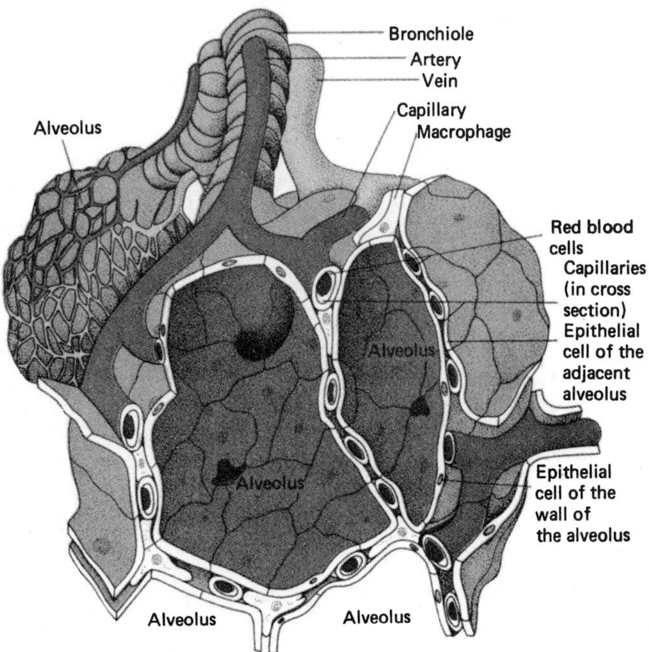

Figure 5-2. Structure and function of the alveolus. (From Solomon, E. P., and Phillips, G. A.: Understanding Human Anatomy and Physiology. Philadelphia, W. B. Saunders, 1987, Fig. 15-2, p. 265.)

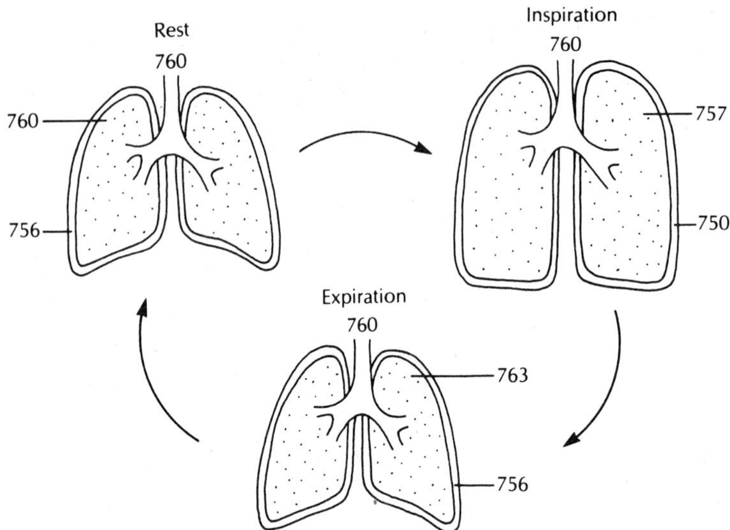

Figure 5-3. Changes in intra-alveolar and intrapleural pressures during inspiration and expiration. (From Harvey, M. A.: Study Guide to the Core Curriculum for Critical Care Nursing. Philadelphia, W. B. Saunders, 1986, Fig. 1-7, p. 3.)

the intra-alveolar pressure becomes negative. Since atmospheric pressure is greater than both intra-alveolar and intrapleural pressure, air flows into the lungs. Expiration is considered a passive phenomenon. When intrapulmonary pressure in the lungs exceeds atmospheric pressure, expiration occurs; the diaphragm and intercostal muscles relax and the lungs recoil (see Fig. 5-4). This recoil generates positive alveolar pressure.

GAS EXCHANGE

The process of gas exchange (Fig. 5-5) consists of four steps: (1) ventilation, (2) diffusion at pulmonary capillaries, (3) perfusion (transportation), and (4) diffusion to the cells.

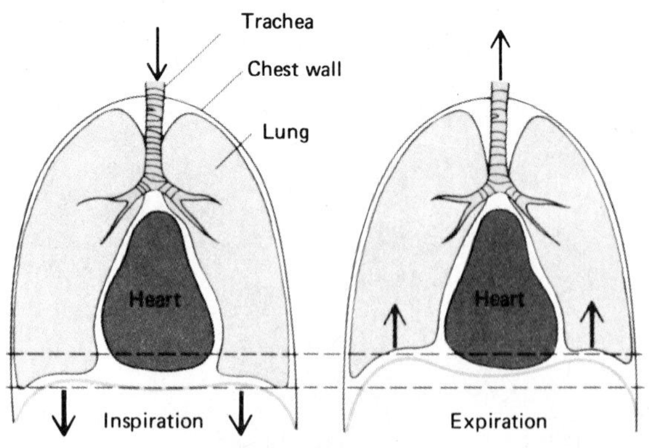

Figure 5-4. Changes in position of diaphragm during inspiration and expiration. (From Solomon, E. P., and Phillips, G. A.: Understanding Human Anatomy and Physiology. Philadelphia, W. B. Saunders, 1987, Fig. 15-3, p. 265.)

1. Ventilation is the transport of air in and out of the alveoli.
2. Diffusion of oxygen and carbon dioxide occurs at the pulmonary capillary level. The alveoli contain higher levels of oxygen than exist in the capillaries, causing oxygen to diffuse from the alveoli into the capillaries. Carbon dioxide (CO_2) levels are higher in the capillaries, causing CO_2 to diffuse into the alveoli for elimination through the lungs.
3. The oxygenated blood in the pulmonary capillary is transported via the pulmonary vein to the left side of the heart. The oxygenated blood is perfused or transported to the tissues. A good cardiac output is necessary for this process.
4. Diffusion of O_2 and CO_2 occurs at the cellular level.

REGULATION OF RESPIRATION

The rate, depth, and rhythm of respirations are controlled by respiratory centers in the medulla and pons. When the CO_2 level is high or the O_2 level is low, receptors in the carotid arteries and the aorta send messages to the medulla to regulate respiration. In individuals with normal lung function, respirations are stimulated by high levels of CO_2. Patients with long-term chronic obstructive pulmonary disease (COPD) normally have high levels of CO_2. In these individuals, the stimulus to breathe is low levels of oxygen. These patients with chronically high levels of CO_2 are not usually given high levels of supplemental oxygen because it would depress their respiratory drive.

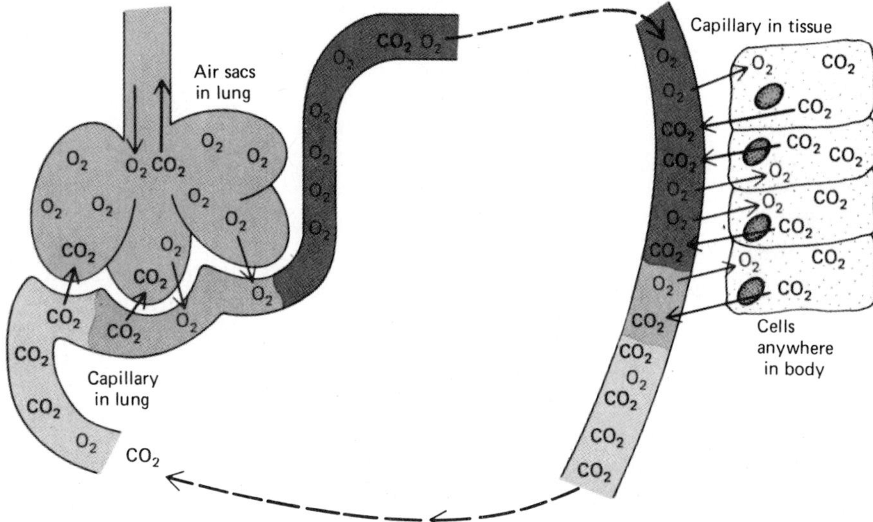

Figure 5-5. Diffusion of oxygen (O_2) and carbon dioxide (CO_2) (a) between alveoli and pulmonary capillaries, and (b) at the cellular level. (From Solomon, E. P., and Phillips, G. A.: Understanding Human Anatomy and Physiology. Philadelphia, W. B. Saunders, 1987, Fig. 15-4, p. 266.)

WORK OF BREATHING

The work of breathing is the amount of effort required to maintain a given level of ventilation. The respiratory pattern changes automatically to assist in the work of breathing depending on lung compliance and resistance.

Compliance. Compliance is a measure of the distensibility, or stretchability, of the lung and chest wall. It is defined as the change in volume per unit of pressure change.

$$\text{Compliance} = \frac{\text{Change in Volume}}{\text{Change in Pressure}}$$

Compliance is primarily determined by the amount of elastic recoil that must be overcome before lung inflation can occur. Elastic recoil, or elastance, refers to the ability of the lungs to return to a resting position after stretching during inspiration.

It is important to note that elastic recoil and compliance are inversely related. For example, in pulmonary fibrosis and pulmonary edema, lung tissue has greater elastic recoil that decreases distensibility. In these situations, compliance is low and the lungs are stiff and difficult to distend. High pressures are required to inflate the lungs.

In emphysema, destruction of lung tissue and enlarged air spaces cause the lungs to lose their elasticity. The decrease in elastic recoil causes compliance to be increased, or high. The lungs are more distensible in this situation, and will require lower pressures for ventilation.

Static compliance refers to compliance measured during a period of no airflow (e.g., patient holding his or her breath) and is an indicator of elastic recoil. An accurate measure of static compliance is best done in the pulmonary function laboratory. The normal static compliance value is 200 ml/cm H_2O. In the mechanically ventilated patient with normal lung function, static compliance usually ranges from 70 to 100 ml/cm H_2O (Kersten, 1989).

Dynamic compliance is measured during breathing and is an indicator of both elastic recoil and airway resistance. Static and dynamic compliance are usually equal in the normal adult. In the mechanically ventilated patient, dynamic compliance ranges from 50 to 100 ml/cm H_2O, or not more than 10 cm/H_2O greater than static compliance (Kersten, 1989). Measurement of compliance in the mechanically ventilated patient is used to identify trends in the patient's condition, not to diagnose lung disease.

Resistance. Resistance refers to the opposition to gas flow in the airways. Resistance is increased with airway spasms, mucus, and edema. Artificial airways, such as endotracheal tubes, also increase airway resistance.

LUNG VOLUMES AND CAPACITIES

The lungs have several volumes and capacities that are important in determining adequate pulmonary function. Several of these terms will be used later in the chapter when explaining methods and modes of mechanical ventilation. Volumes are measured by a device called a spirometer.

Volumes. Four different lung volumes can be measured. The total of these volumes equals the maximum volume that the lungs can expand. The values given for volumes and capacities are approximately 20 to 25% less in women (Guyton, 1986). The lung volumes and capacities are shown graphically in Figure 5-6.

Tidal Volume (V_T or TV). The V_T is the volume of a normal breath. The average V_T is 500 ml.

Inspiratory Reserve Volume (IRV). The IRV is the maximum amount of gas that can be inspired at the end of a normal breath (over and above the V_T). The average IRV is 3000 ml.

Expiratory Reserve Volume (ERV). The ERV is the maximum amount of gas that can be forcefully expired at the end of a normal breath. The average ERV is 1100 ml.

Residual Volume (RV). The RV is the amount of air remaining in the lungs after maximum expiration. The average RV is 1200 ml.

Capacities. Lung capacities consist of two or more lung volumes.

Inspiratory Capacity (IC). The IC is the maximum volume of gas that can be inspired at normal resting expiration. The IC distends the lungs to their maximum amount. The average IC is 3500 ml. IC = V_T + IRV.

Functional Residual Capacity (FRC). The FRC is the volume of gas remaining in the lungs at normal resting expiration. The average FRC is 2300 ml. FRC = ERV + RV.

Vital Capacity (VC). The VC is the maximum volume of gas that can be forcefully expired after maximum inspiration. The average VC is 4600 ml. VC = V_T + IRV + ERV.

Total Lung Capacity (TLC). The TLC is the volume of gas in the lungs at end of maximum inspiration. The average TLC is 5800 ml. TLC = V_T + IRV + ERV + RV.

Respiratory Assessment

Physical assessment of the respiratory system is an essential tool for the critical care nurse. Good assessment skills assist in identifying potential patient problems and evaluating interventions.

HEALTH HISTORY

Several questions should be asked when obtaining a patient's health history, including:

1. Tobacco use—type, amount, and number of years used
2. Occupational history, such as coal miner, asbestos worker
3. History of sputum production—type, amount, color, consistency

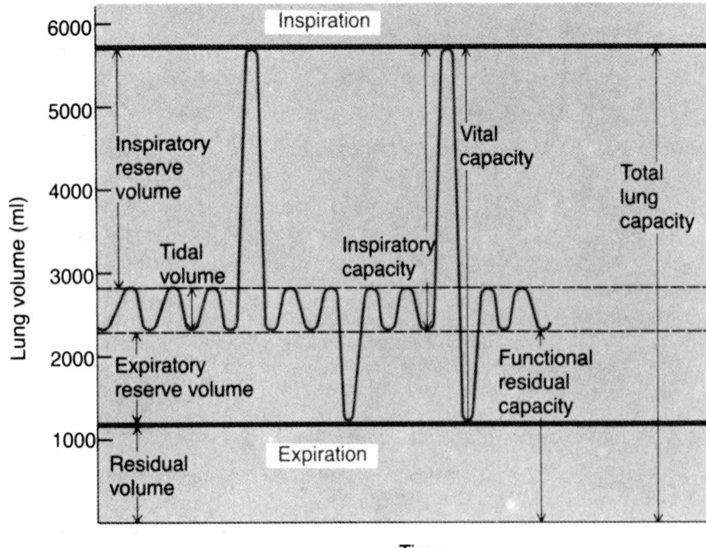

Figure 5-6. Lung volumes and capacities. (From Guyton, A.: Textbook of Human Physiology. 7th ed. Philadelphia, W. B. Saunders, 1986, Fig. 39-5, p. 470.)

4. History of shortness of breath, dyspnea, cough, or chest pain

5. Use of oral and inhalant respiratory medications, such as bronchodilators and steroids

PHYSICAL EXAMINATION

Inspection. Inspection can provide an initial clue of potential respiratory problems. The head, neck, fingers, and chest are inspected for abnormalities.

Several assessments are made when inspecting the head, neck, and fingers. Signs of respiratory distress or abnormalities include:

Pallor or cyanosis
Use of accessory muscles (e.g., shoulder or neck muscles)
Jugular venous distention
Nasal flaring
Open-mouth breathing or gasping
Pursed-lip breathing
Poor capillary refill
Clubbing of fingers

The chest is observed for abnormal breathing patterns, use of chest and abdominal accessory muscles, asymmetrical chest wall movement, and abnormal chest excursions. The respiratory rate is noted, including the ratio of inspiration to expiration (I:E ratio). The normal respiratory rate is 12 to 20 breaths per minute and expiration is usually twice as long as inspiration (I:E ratio of 1:2). Alterations from normal should be documented and reported.

Several abnormal breathing patterns are possible (Fig. 5-7). Breathing is normally regular and even with an occasional sigh. Alterations from this normal pattern should be noted. Tachypnea is defined as a respiratory rate greater than 20 breaths per minute. Tachypnea may occur with anxiety, fever, pain, anemia, and blood gas abnormalities. Bradypnea is a respiratory rate less than 10 breaths per minute. Bradypnea may occur in central nervous system disorders; it may also result from administration or ingestion of medications or alcohol, blood gas abnormalities, and fatigue. Cheyne-Stokes respirations are cyclical respiratory patterns. The patient has deep respirations that become increasingly shallow followed by a period of apnea (approximately 20 seconds). The cycle repeats after each apneic period. The apneic period may vary and progressively lengthen; therefore, the duration of the apneic period is timed for trending and reported to the physician. Cheyne-Stokes respirations may occur in central nervous system disorders and congestive heart failure. The presence of Cheyne-Stokes respirations is a finding that should be reported to the physician. Kussmaul respirations are deep, regular, and rapid (usually more than 20 breaths per minute). Kussmaul respirations commonly occur in diabetic ketoacidosis and other causes of metabolic acido-

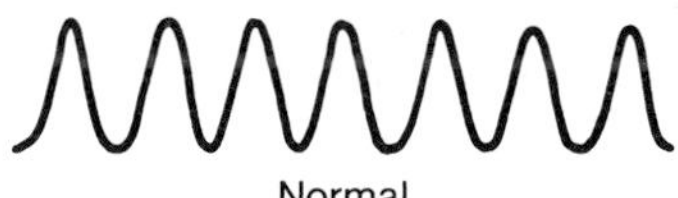

Apnea
Cheyne-Stokes respirations

Tachypnea

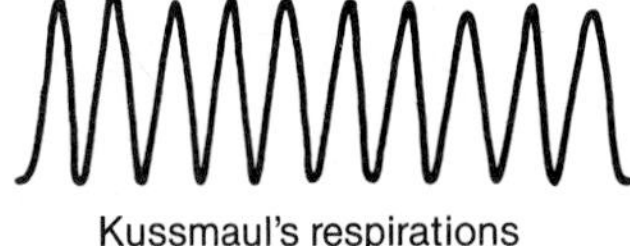

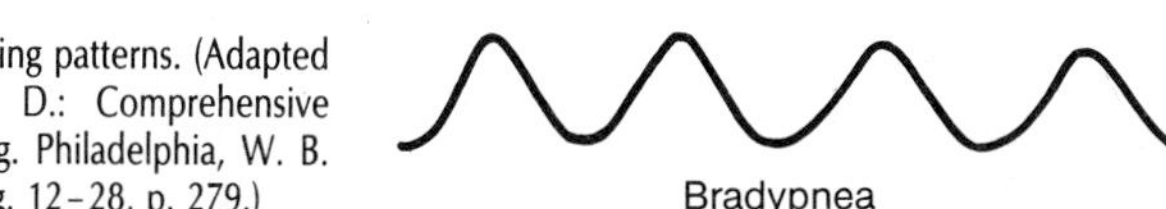

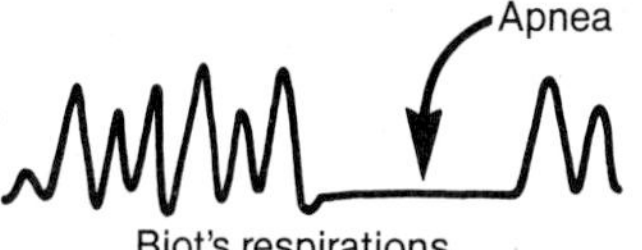

Figure 5-7. Breathing patterns. (Adapted from Kersten, L. D.: Comprehensive Respiratory Nursing. Philadelphia, W. B. Saunders, 1989, Fig. 12-28, p. 279.)

sis. Biot's respirations, or cluster breathing, are cycles of breaths varying in depth with varying periods of apnea. Biot's respirations are seen with some central nervous system disorders.

The patient should also be observed for signs of chronic obstructive pulmonary disease (COPD). Clues that might indicate COPD include wheezing, productive cough, pursed-lip breathing, barrel chest, and muscle wasting. The patient with COPD may also prefer to sit in a chair leaning forward rather than lie in bed.

Palpation. Palpation is frequently done simultaneously with inspection. Palpation is used to evaluate chest wall excursion, tracheal deviation, chest wall tenderness, subcutaneous crepitus, and tactile fremitus.

During inspiration, chest wall excursion should be symmetrical. Asymmetrical excursion is usually associated with unilateral lung problems. The trachea is normally in a midline position; a tracheal shift may occur in tension pneumothorax. The chest wall should not be tender to palpation; tenderness is usually associated with inflammation or trauma. Subcutaneous crepitus, or subcutaneous emphysema, is the presence of air beneath the skin surface. The fingertips are used to palpate for bubbles of air under the skin. Subcutaneous crepitus may occur around chest tube and tracheostomy sites. It may also result from chest trauma, such as rib fractures, and barotrauma.

Tactile fremitus is assessed by palpating the patient's chest wall with the heel of the hand while having the patient recite sounds that vibrate, such as "99." The intensity of vibrations is compared bilaterally. Tactile fremitus may be increased over consolidated areas of the lungs; vibrations may be decreased in pleural effusion and pneumothorax.

Percussion. The chest is percussed to identify respiratory disorders such as hemothorax, pneumothorax, and consolidation. In order to perform percussion, the middle finger of one hand is tapped twice by the middle finger of the opposite hand. The vibrations produced by tapping produce audible sounds depending on how the sound travels through different densities.

Five sounds may be audible upon percussion: resonance, dullness, flatness, hyperresonance, and tympany. Resonance is the sound produced by percussion of normal lung tissue. Resonance is described as sounding like a muffled drum. Dullness is heard when tissue that is denser than normal is percussed. A dull thud is the sound heard with dullness. Clinical conditions associated with dullness include pleural effusion, hemothorax, consolidation, atelectasis, tumors, and pulmonary fibrosis. Flatness is noted when air is absent in lung tissues. The sound heard with flatness is extreme dullness. Clinical conditions that may cause flatness include massive pleural effusion and lung collapse. Hyperresonance produces a slight musical sound, like a hollow drum, heard over tissue that has an increased amount of air. Clinical conditions associated with hyperresonance include emphysema, pneumothorax, and acute asthma. Tympany is a musical, drumlike sound produced by a large air-filled area. Clinical conditions that may produce tympany include tension pneumothorax or an air-filled cavity caused by an infection or abscess. Gastric distention may also produce tympany over the chest wall (Kersten, 1989).

Auscultation. Auscultation is frequently used in the critical care unit. Lung sounds are routinely assessed, often every 4 hours, in critically ill patients. Auscultation is performed to assess the character of voice sounds, quality of breath sounds, and adventitious lung sounds.

A good stethoscope is essential for proper auscultation. The stethoscope should have both a diaphragm and a bell in order to identify both high-pitched (diaphragm) and low-pitched (bell) sounds. Sounds are transmitted best through tubing that is thick and short; tubing that is too long decreases the transmission of sound. The ear pieces of the stethoscope should fit comfortably.

Several additional techniques will facilitate auscultation. A quiet environment is essential. It may be necessary to turn off television, radios, and noise-producing equipment (e.g., hypo-/hyperthermia units) during auscultation. The stethoscope should be placed directly on the chest; sounds are difficult to distinguish if auscultated through the patient's gown or clothing. If possible, auscultation over chest hair should be avoided because a crackling sound is produced by the hair. If auscultation must be done over hairy areas, wet the chest hair with water prior to auscultation. Additionally, the stethoscope tubing should be free from contact with other objects, such as sheets and bedrails, during auscultation.

Auscultation is performed systematically. The anterior, posterior, and lateral aspects of the chest are auscultated (Fig. 5–8). Auscultation is best performed with the patient sitting in an upright position. The patient is asked to breathe deeply in and out through the mouth. Compara-

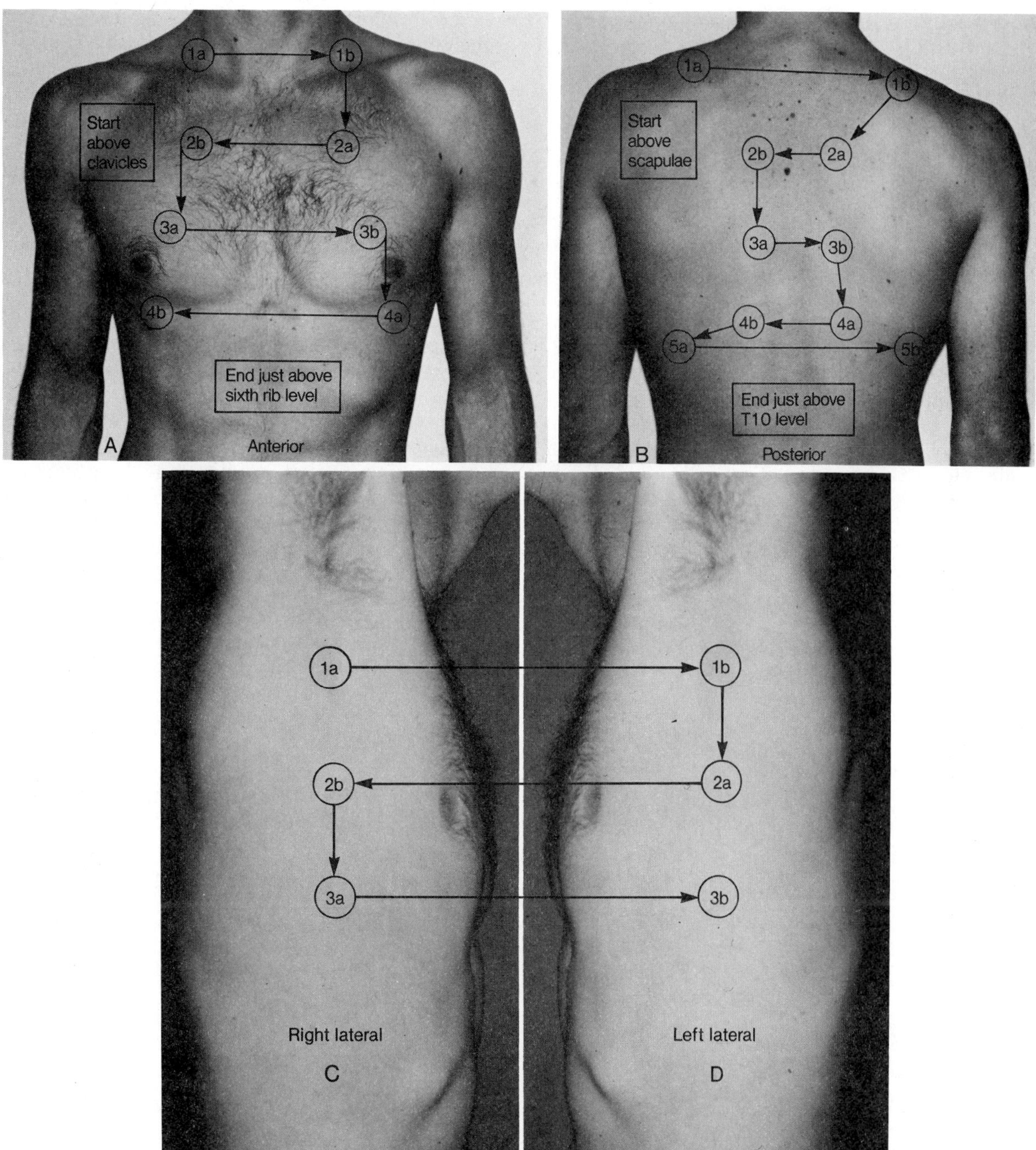

Figure 5-8. Systematic method for palpation, percussion, and auscultation of the lungs in *(A)* anterior, *(B)* posterior, and (C and *D*) lateral regions. The techniques should be performed systematically from a to b to compare right and left lung function. (From Kersten, L. D.: Comprehensive Respiratory Nursing. Philadelphia, W. B. Saunders, 1989, Fig. 12-42, p. 301.)

ble pulmonary segments are auscultated on each side of the chest; the stethoscope is moved back and forth across the chest to compare sounds.

It may not be feasible to have a critically ill patient assume a sitting position for auscultation. In this circumstance, auscultation of the posterior and lateral chest is performed when the patient is turned to the side.

Voice Sounds. In order to assess voice sounds, the chest is auscultated while the patient speaks. Voice sounds are transmitted from the larynx to the chest wall and are audible with a stethoscope. Voice sounds are normally muffled when auscultated because the vibrations are absorbed by the lung tissue.

Three abnormal voice sounds may be audible: bronchophony, egophony, and whispered pectoriloquy. Interpretation of abnormal voice sounds may be difficult and must be done in relation to the entire pulmonary assessment. Bronchophony is an increase in the intensity of sounds heard when the patient says "99." Bronchophony may be present in lung consolidation. Egophony occurs when a loud-sounding "A" is heard when the patient says "E." Egophony may be present in lung consolidation. It is also commonly heard just above the fluid level in pleural effusion. Whispered pectoriloquy is an increase in intensity of the whispered voice when the patient says "99" or "1, 2, 3." It commonly occurs in consolidation.

Breath Sounds. Types of breath sounds include vesicular, bronchial, and bronchovesicular. Vesicular sounds are the breath sounds normally heard throughout the chest with the exception of the central airways. Some texts classify vesicular sounds as "normal" breath sounds (Kersten, 1989). Vesicular breath sounds have a breezy quality, moderate intensity, and low pitch. Although the normal inspiration to expiration (I:E) ratio is 1:2, vesicular breath sounds have an audible I:E ratio of 3:1.

Bronchial sounds are normally heard over the manubrium. They have a hollow, tubular quality, loud intensity, and high pitch. The audible I:E ratio of bronchial sounds is 2:3.

Bronchovesicular sounds are normally heard over large central airways (e.g., over the sternum) and between the scapulae. They have a hollow, breezy quality, moderate to low intensity, and medium to high pitch. The audible I:E ratio of bronchovesicular sounds is 1:1.

At times, breath sounds may be decreased. The presence of fluid, air, or increased tissue can cause decreased breath sounds. Some patients normally have decreased sounds in the left upper lobe related to differences in lung anatomy (Kersten, 1989). Shallow respirations can also mimic decreased breath sounds; therefore, it is important that the patient take deep breaths during auscultation. Table 5-2 reviews types of breath sounds.

Table 5-2. TYPES OF BREATH SOUNDS

	Normal Location	Intensity	Pitch	Quality	I:E Ratio (audible)	Graphic Representation
Normal	Throughout chest except over central airways	Moderate	Low	Breezy	3:1	
Decreased	Left upper lobe posteriorly in some people	Soft	Low	Breezy	3:1	
Bronchial	Over manubrium	Loud	High	Hollow, tubular	2:3	
Bronchovesicular	Over large, central airways: sternal area, between scapulae, right upper lobe posteriorly in some people	Moderate to loud	Medium to high	Hollow, breezy	1:1	
Tracheal	Over extrathoracic trachea (not usually auscultated)	Very loud	Very high	Hollow, harsh	5:6	

From Kersten, L.D.: Comprehensive Respiratory Nursing. Philadelphia, W.B. Saunders, 1989, Table 12-5, p. 302.

Adventitious Breath Sounds. Adventitious, or abnormal, lung sounds include crackles, wheezing, and pleural friction rubs. Crackles (formerly called rales) are short, explosive, nonmusical, and discontinuous sounds. The presence of crackles usually indicates the presence of fluid in the alveoli and airways. Crackles may be audible during either inspiration or expiration. Crackles may also be audible when previously deflated airways are reinflated upon inspiration; therefore, they sometimes disappear after coughing or suctioning.

Wheezes are a continuous adventitious sound resulting from rapid passage of air through narrow airways. They are high-pitched and musical when they originate in smaller airways, and low-pitched with a snoring sound when they originate in larger airways. Wheezes are more commonly heard on expiration, but the sounds may occur during both inspiration and expiration. Airway secretions sometimes produce wheezes; in this situation, wheezes should decrease after coughing or suctioning. (The American Thoracic Society has recommended that the term *wheezes* be used to classify all continuous adventitious sounds. However, some practitioners describe the musical sounds as wheezes and the snoring sounds as rhonchi. Both of these terms are used in Table 5-3 so that the learner will better understand the associated problems and characteristics of the sounds.)

A pleural friction rub, or pleural rub, is a grating sound that occurs in the presence of inflammation of the pleura. Pleural rubs are usually heard during inspiration and expiration. If a rub is auscultated, it is important to distinguish a pleural rub from pericardial rub since both sound similar. A pleural rub is audible during respirations, whereas a pericardial rub is audible with each heartbeat. Adventitious lung sounds are reviewed in Table 5-3.

Arterial Blood Gas Interpretation

The ability to rapidly interpret arterial blood gas results (ABGs) is an essential critical care skill. The ABGs reflect oxygenation, adequacy of gas exchange in the lungs, and acid-base status. Blood for ABG analysis is obtained either from a direct arterial puncture (radial, brachial, or femoral artery) or from an arterial line. Blood gases should be interpreted in conjunction with the pa-

Table 5-3. ADVENTITIOUS BREATH SOUNDS

Type	General Location	Associated Problem(s)	Characteristics	Graphic Illustration
Crackles (rales)	Peripheral airways and alveoli	Atelectasis Inflammation Excess fluid Excess mucus	Group of discrete crackles or popping sounds Discontinuous sound Usually inspiratory, may be inspiratory and expiratory	fine coarse
Rhonchi	Large airways	Inflammation Excess fluid Excess mucus	Coarse, low-pitched sonorous sounds Continuous sound Usually expiratory, may be inspiratory and expiratory Changes in quality and timing with coughing	
Wheeze	Large and/or small airways	Bronchoconstriction (airway narrowing) from bronchospasm, fluid, mucus, inflammatory by-products, obstructive lesion Airway instability	High- (sometimes low-) pitched musical sound Continuous sound Usually expiratory, may be inspiratory and expiratory	
Pleural friction rub	Pleural surfaces	Inflamed or roughened pleural surfaces (pleuritis)	Grating sound with continuous and discontinuous qualities May appear intermittently Variable duration; usually inspiratory, may be inspiratory and expiratory Sounds the same or louder with coughing	

From Kersten, L.D.: Comprehensive Respiratory Nursing. Philadelphia, W.B. Saunders, 1989, Table 12-8, p. 310.

tient's clinical history and physical assessment findings.

OXYGENATION

The ABG values that reflect oxygenation include the partial pressure of oxygen in the arterial plasma (PaO_2) and the arterial oxygen saturation of the hemoglobin (SaO_2). Oxygen is transported from the alveoli into the plasma. Approximately 3% of the available oxygen is dissolved in plasma. The remainder of the oxygen (97%) attaches to hemoglobin in red blood cells, forming oxyhemoglobin.

***PaO_2*.** The PaO_2 is the partial pressure of oxygen dissolved in arterial blood. The normal PaO_2 (sometimes shortened to read PO_2) is 80 to 100 mm Hg at sea level. The PaO_2 decreases in the elderly; the value for individuals 60 to 80 years of age usually ranges from 60 to 80 mm Hg.

SaO_2 (O_2 Sat). The SaO_2 refers to the amount of oxygen bound to hemoglobin. The normal saturation of hemoglobin ranges from 93 to 99%. The SaO_2 is very important because the majority of oxygen supplied to the tissues is transported via hemoglobin.

Table 5-4. SIGNS AND SYMPTOMS OF HYPOXEMIA

Integumentary System
Pallor
Cool, dry
Cyanosis (LATE)
Diaphoresis (LATE)
Respiratory System
Dyspnea
Tachypnea
Use of accessory muscles
Respiratory arrest (LATE)
Cardiovascular System
Tachycardia
Dysrhythmias
Chest pain
Hypertension with increased heart rate
Hypotension with decreased heart rate
Central Nervous System
Anxiety
Restlessness
Confusion
Fatigue
Combativeness
Coma

Both the PaO_2 and SaO_2 are used to assess oxygenation. Decreased oxygenation of arterial blood (PaO_2 less than 80 mm Hg) is referred to as hypoxemia. Hypoxemia is different from hypoxia, which is a decrease in oxygen at the tissue level. Symptoms of hypoxemia are described in Table 5-4.

The relationship between the PaO_2 and SaO_2 is shown in the S-shaped oxyhemoglobin dissociation curve (Fig. 5-9). Note that the upper portion of the curve (above a PaO_2 of 60 mm Hg) is flat. In this area of the curve, large changes in the PaO_2 result in only small changes in SaO_2. For example, the normal PaO_2 is 97 mm Hg and is associated with an SaO_2 of 97%. If the PaO_2 drops to 80 mm Hg, the SaO_2 only decreases to 95%. Likewise, if the PaO_2 drops from 80 mm Hg to 60 mm Hg, the SaO_2 will decrease from 95 to 90%. Although these examples reflect a drop in PaO_2, the patient should not be immediately compromised since the hemoglobin is still well saturated with oxygen.

The critical zone of the oxyhemoglobin dissociation curve occurs when the PaO_2 falls below 60 mm Hg (see Fig. 5-9). At this point, the curve slopes sharply and small changes in PaO_2 are reflected in large changes in the oxygen saturation. These changes in SaO_2 may cause a significant decrease in oxygen delivered to the tissues.

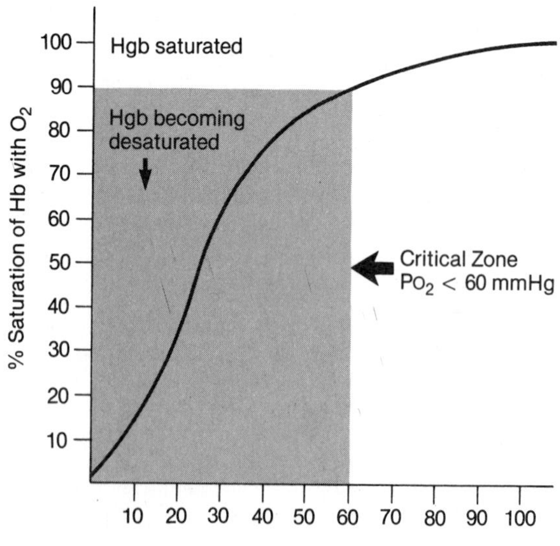

Figure 5-9. Oxyhemoglobin dissociation curve. The critical zone of the curve is noted. When the PaO_2 falls below 60 mmHg, small changes in PaO_2 are reflected in large changes in oxygen saturation. (From Kersten, L. D.: Comprehensive Respiratory Nursing. Philadelphia, W. B. Saunders, 1989, Fig. 3-6, p. 48.)

The oxyhemoglobin dissociation curve may shift in certain conditions (Fig. 5-10). When the curve shifts to the right, a decreased hemoglobin affinity for oxygen exists, resulting in more oxygen supplied to the tissues. Conditions that cause a right shift include acidemia, increased metabolism (e.g., fever), and increased levels of 2,3-DPG, which is a glucose metabolite that facilitates release of oxygen from hemoglobin. Levels are increased in anemia, chronic hypoxemia, and low cardiac output states.

When the curve shifts to the left, hemoglobin affinity for oxygen increases, and hemoglobin clings to oxygen. Conditions that cause a left shift include alkalemia, lowered metabolism, high altitudes, carbon monoxide poisoning, and decreased levels of 2,3-DPG. Common causes of decreased 2,3-DPG include administration of stored bank blood, septic shock, and hypophosphatemia.

VENTILATION/ACID-BASE STATUS

Blood gas values that reflect ventilation and acid-base include pH, $PaCO_2$, and HCO_3.

pH. The concentration of hydrogen (H^+) ions in the blood is referred to as the pH. The pH is the negative logarithm of the H^+ ion concentration. The normal pH is 7.40; the normal range for pH is 7.35 to 7.45. If the H^+ ions increase, the pH falls, resulting in acidemia. Conversely, a decrease in H^+ ions results in a high pH and alkalemia. (The suffix -emia is used to refer to the alteration in pH. The suffix -osis is used to refer to the condition or process causing the alteration in pH.)

$PaCO_2$. $PaCO_2$ (sometimes shortened to PCO_2) is the partial pressure of carbon dioxide dissolved in arterial plasma. The normal $PaCO_2$ is 35 to 45 mm Hg. The $PaCO_2$ is regulated in the lungs. A $PaCO_2 > 45$ mm Hg indicates respiratory acidosis, whereas a $PaCO_2 < 35$ mm Hg indicates respiratory alkalosis.

If a patient hypoventilates, CO_2 is retained, leading to respiratory acidosis. Conversely, if a patient hyperventilates, excess CO_2 is blown off

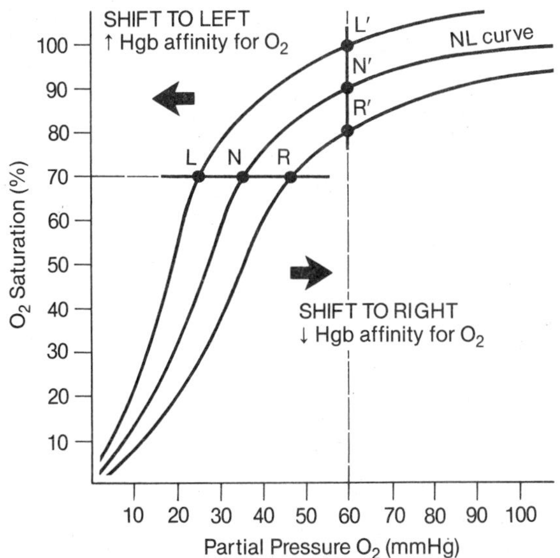

Figure 5-10. Shifts in the oxyhemoglobin curve. (From Kersten, L. D.: Comprehensive Respiratory Nursing. Philadelphia, W. B. Saunders, 1989, Fig. 3-7, p. 48.)

Table 5-5. CAUSES OF COMMON ACID-BASE ABNORMALITIES

Respiratory Acidosis: Retention of carbon dioxide
- Central nervous system disorders
- Drug overdose
- Pneumonia
- Pulmonary edema
- Pneumothorax
- Restrictive lung diseases

Respiratory Alkalosis: Hyperventilation
- Anxiety, fear
- Pain
- Fever
- Pneumonia
- Atelectasis
- Asthma
- Adult respiratory distress syndrome (ARDS)
- Congestive heart failure, pulmonary edema
- Pulmonary embolus
- Central nervous system disorders

Metabolic Acidosis: Gain of metabolic acids or loss of base
- **Increased acids**
  - Renal failure
  - Diabetic ketoacidosis
  - Anaerobic metabolism
  - Drug overdose (salicylates, methanol)
- **Loss of base**
  - Diarrhea

Metabolic Alkalosis: Gain of base or loss of metabolic acids
- **Gain of base**
  - Excess ingestion of antacids
  - Excess administration of sodium bicarbonate
- **Loss of metabolic acids**
  - Vomiting
  - Nasogastric suctioning/lavage
  - Low potassium and/or chloride
  - Increased levels of aldosterone
  - Administration of steroids and/or diuretics

Adapted from Kersten, L.D.: Comprehensive Respiratory Nursing. Philadelphia, W.B. Saunders, 1989.

by the lungs, resulting in respiratory alkalosis. In order to remember this concept, it is helpful to think of CO_2 as an "acid" regulated by the lungs. Conditions that cause respiratory acidosis and alkalosis are noted in Table 5-5.

HCO_3. The HCO_3 is the concentration of sodium bicarbonate in the blood. The normal HCO_3 is 22 to 26 mEq/L. The HCO_3 is regulated by the kidneys. An $HCO_3 > 26$ mEq/L indicates metabolic alkalosis, whereas an $HCO_3 < 22$ mEq/L indicates metabolic acidosis. It may be useful to think of HCO_3 as a substance that neutralizes acids. Therefore, a high HCO_3 would indicate metabolic alkalosis, whereas a low HCO_3 would indicate metabolic acidosis. Conditions that cause metabolic acidosis and alkalosis are noted in Table 5-5.

Buffer System. The body regulates acid-base balance through the buffer system. The buffer system can be described as a mechanism for neutralizing acids. Three buffer systems exist for maintaining acid-base status: the buffer system in the blood, the respiratory system, and the renal system (Fig. 5-11).

The blood buffer system is activated as the H^+ ion concentration changes. As H^+ ions increase, the pH falls, resulting in acidosis. Bicarbonate (HCO_3) then combines with the H^+ ions to form carbonic acid (H_2CO_3). Carbonic acid then breaks down into CO_2 (which is excreted through the lungs) and water (H_2O). The equation for this mechanism is as follows:

$$H^+ + HCO_3 \longleftrightarrow H_2CO_3 \longleftrightarrow H_2O + CO_2$$

The respiratory buffer system works by excreting excess CO_2 from the lungs. The respiratory buffer system begins to work immediately after an acid-base alteration is noted. The renal buffer system works by excreting excess H^+ ions and retaining bicarbonate. The renal buffer system activates more slowly and may take up to 2 days to regulate acid-base balance.

INTERPRETATION OF ABGS

Arterial blood gases should be interpreted systematically. Oxygenation is evaluated first. Second, the acid-base status is determined. Third, the primary imbalance is identified. Last, compensation, if any, is identified.

STEP 1. Evaluate Oxygenation

Oxygenation is analyzed by evaluating the PaO_2 and SaO_2. If the PaO_2 is below the expected normal range, hypoxemia exists. Remember that PaO_2 is normally lower in the elderly.

STEP 2. Evaluate Acid-Base Status

In order to evaluate the acid-base status, the remainder of the ABG values are evaluated individually.

1. Evaluate the pH.
   $pH < 7.35$ = acidemia
   $pH > 7.45$ = alkalemia
2. Evaluate the $PaCO_2$.
   $PaCO_2 < 35$ = respiratory alkalosis
   $PaCO_2 > 45$ = respiratory acidosis

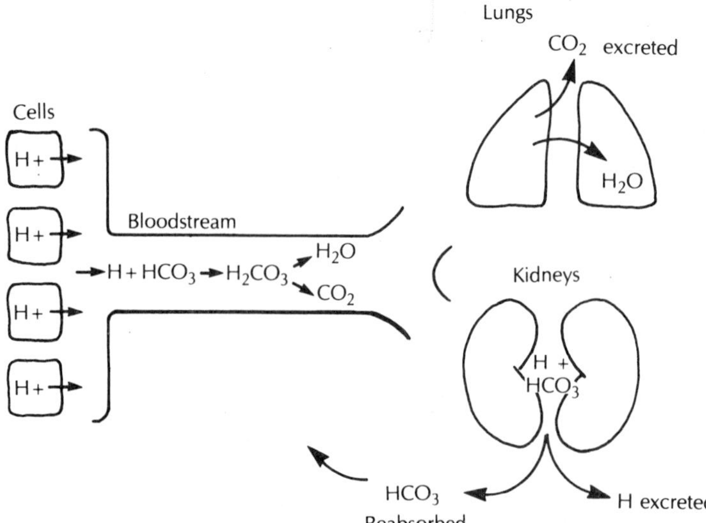

Figure 5-11. Buffer systems which regulate the body's acid-base balance. (From Harvey, M. A.: Study Guide to the Core Curriculum for Critical Care Nursing. Philadelphia, W. B. Saunders, 1986, Fig. 1-15, p. 8.)

Table 5-6. INTERPRETATION OF ARTERIAL BLOOD GASES

	$PaCO_2$ <35	$PaCO_2$ 35–45	$PaCO_2$ >45
HCO_3 <22	Respiratory alkalosis Metabolic acidosis	Metabolic acidosis	Respiratory acidosis Metabolic acidosis
HCO_3 22–26	Respiratory alkalosis	Normal	Respiratory acidosis
HCO_3 >26	Respiratory alkalosis Metabolic alkalosis	Metabolic alkalosis	Respiratory acidosis Metabolic alkalosis

3. Evaluate the HCO_3.
   $HCO_3 < 22$ = metabolic acidosis
   $HCO_3 > 26$ = metabolic alkalosis

STEP 3. Determine Primary Acid-Base Imbalance

The ABGs may reflect only one disorder. However, frequently two acid-base disorders occur simultaneously (Table 5–6). Usually one is a *primary* disorder, whereas the other is a compensatory process to restore acid-base balance. To determine the *primary* cause of the acid-base imbalance, evaluate the pH. If the pH is <7.4, the primary disorder is acidosis. Likewise, if the pH is >7.4, the primary disorder is alkalosis. Note that occasionally two primary disorders may occur simultaneously. For example, during a cardiac arrest, both respiratory and metabolic acidosis commonly occur because of hypoventilation and lactic acidosis. Figure 5–12 illustrates the concepts of acid-base imbalances.

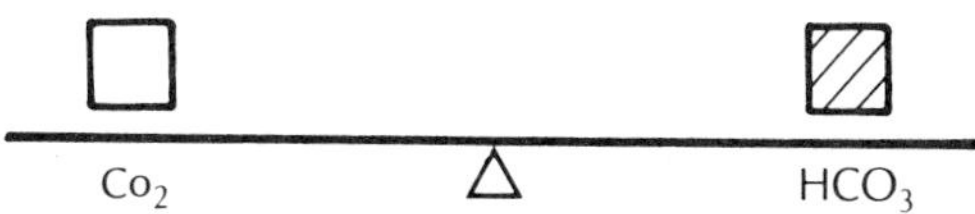

An abnormal relationship creates an imbalance.

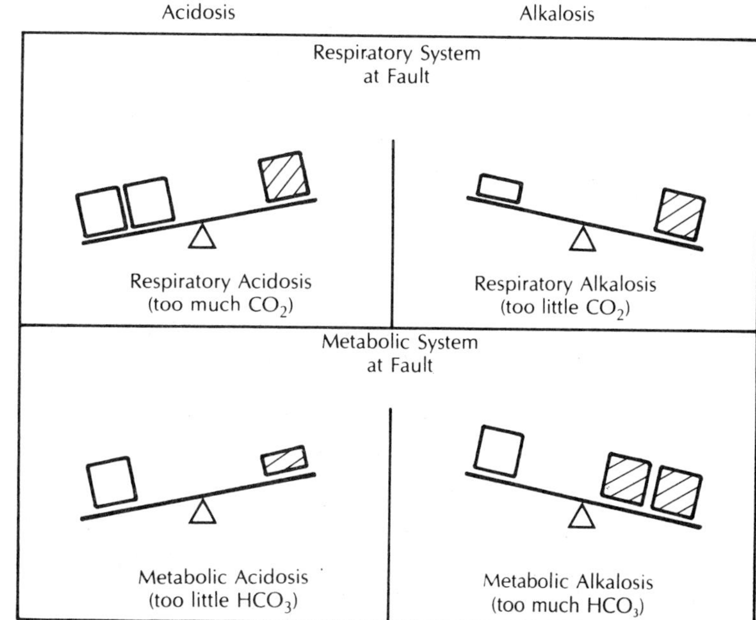

Figure 5–12. Acid-base imbalances. (From Harvey, M. A.: Study Guide to the Core Curriculum for Critical Care Nursing. Philadelphia, W. B. Saunders, 1986, Fig. 1–16, p. 9.)

Table 5-7. COMPENSATORY MECHANISMS IN ACID-BASE DISTURBANCES

Acid-Base Disturbance	Usual Compensatory Mechanism
Respiratory acidosis	Metabolic alkalosis
Respiratory alkalosis	Metabolic acidosis
Metabolic acidosis	Respiratory alkalosis
Metabolic alkalosis	Respiratory acidosis

STEP 4. Determine Compensation

As previously noted, the body has three buffer systems to maintain a constant acid-base balance. If an abnormality is present, one or more buffer systems are activated to reverse the acid-base abnormality. For example, if a patient has respiratory acidosis (low pH; high $PaCO_2$), the kidneys will respond by retaining more HCO_3 and excreting H^+ ions (metabolic alkalosis). Conversely, if a patient is in metabolic acidosis (low pH; low HCO_3), the lungs will respond by blowing off more CO_2 (respiratory alkalosis). A summary of compensatory mechanisms is shown in Table 5–7.

Compensation may be absent, partial, or complete. Compensation is absent if the usual compensatory mechanisms do not occur in response to a primary acid-base disturbance. If compensatory mechanisms are noted, but the pH is still abnormal, compensation is partial. If compensatory mechanisms are present, and the pH is within normal range, compensation is complete. Examples of ABGs and compensation are shown in Table 5–8.

Table 5–8. EXAMPLES OF ABGS AND COMPENSATION

Example 1:	
PaO_2	80 Normal
pH	7.30 Low; acidosis
$PaCO_2$	50 High; respiratory acidosis
HCO_3	22 Normal
Interpretation:	Respiratory acidosis; no compensation
Example 2:	
PaO_2	80 Normal
pH	7.32 Low; acidosis
$PaCO_2$	50 High; respiratory acidosis
HCO_3	28 High; metabolic alkalosis
Interpretation:	Partly compensated respiratory acidosis. The ABGs are only "partly compensated," since the pH is not yet within normal limits.
Example 3:	
PaO_2	80 Normal
pH	7.36 Normal
$PaCO_2$	50 High; respiratory acidosis
HCO_3	29 High; metabolic alkalosis
Interpretation:	Completely (fully) compensated respiratory acidosis. The pH is now within normal limits; therefore, complete compensation has occurred.

Noninvasive Assessment of Gas Exchange

Arterial blood gas results have been the "gold standard" for monitoring gas exchange and acid-base status. New technology now permits continuous PaO_2 monitoring through the use of an oxygen catheter and sensor inserted through an existing radial artery line. Additionally, several noninvasive techniques are available to assess gas exchange: pulse oximetry, transcutaneous monitoring of O_2 and CO_2, capnometry, and capnography.

ASSESSMENT OF OXYGENATION

Transcutaneous PO_2 ($tcPO_2$). Oxygen levels can be monitored through the use of $tcPO_2$ devices. In $tcPO_2$ monitoring, an electrode that records the oxygen level is attached to the skin. The device includes a heater that causes vasodilation under the electrode to enhance oxygen diffusion. The $tcPO_2$ reflects the PaO_2; however, the $tcPO_2$ value is usually lower than the actual PaO_2. Abnormally low values of $tcPO_2$ may be obtained if the patient has edema, subcutaneous emphysema, or decreased tissue perfusion (e.g., from hypothermia) (VonRueden, 1990).

Pulse Oximetry (SpO_2). The use of pulse oximeters has become commonplace in critical care units, the operating room, postanesthesia recovery units, and emergency departments. Pulse oximetry measures a value called SpO_2 and reflects the arterial oxygen saturation, SaO_2. Pulse oximetry uses light-emitting diodes to measure pulsatile flow and light absorption of the hemoglobin. A sensor that measures SpO_2 is placed on the finger, toe, ear, or forehead.

The oxyhemoglobin dissociation curve (see Fig. 5–9) shows the relationship between SaO_2 and PaO_2 and provides the basis for pulse oximetry. Note that an SaO_2 of 95% is equivalent to a PaO_2 of 80, whereas an SaO_2 of 90% is equivalent to a PaO_2 of 60 mm Hg, which is often considered the "critical zone." As previously discussed, when the PaO_2 falls below 60 mm Hg, small changes in PaO_2 result in large changes in SaO_2. Pulse oximetry values must be monitored with this principle in mind.

Table 5–9 assists in interpretation of SpO_2 values. Usually, parameters are specified for notifying the physician; e.g., call if SpO_2 falls below 93%. In addition to monitoring patient oxygenation, pulse oximetry may be used in weaning patients from mechanical ventilation and monitoring response to treatment (e.g., ventilator changes, pulmonary hygiene, suctioning). However, it is important to note that SpO_2 only measures oxygenation. Changes in ventilation (e.g., CO_2 retention) cannot be assessed with pulse oximetry.

ASSESSMENT OF VENTILATION

Transcutaneous Carbon Dioxide ($tcPCO_2$). Transcutaneous monitoring of CO_2 is similar to $tcPO_2$ measurement. An electrode that has the capability of measuring CO_2 is attached to the skin. Noninvasive measurement of $tcPCO_2$ may be as much as one to two times higher than $PaCO_2$; therefore, it is best used to monitor patient *trends* rather than actual values (VonRueden, 1990).

End-Tidal Carbon Dioxide ($etCO_2$). The measurement of expired CO_2 is referred to as capnometry, whereas capnography is the recording of CO_2 during the respiratory cycle. Monitoring of $etCO_2$ uses infrared light to measure CO_2 concentrations. The most common method of $etCO_2$ monitoring samples expired gas from an endotracheal tube, oral airway, or nasopharyngeal airway. The $etCO_2$ correlates well with $PaCO_2$ in patients with normal lung and cardiac functions. Uses of $etCO_2$ include monitoring the patient response to ventilator changes and respiratory treatments, determining proper position of the endotracheal tube, and weaning the patient from mechanical ventilation. It may also be useful in monitoring the effectiveness of cardiopulmonary resuscitation (VonRueden, 1990).

Table 5-9. INTERPRETATION OF PULSE OXIMETRY VALUES (SpO_2)

Value on Pulse Oximeter (%)	Probable PaO_2
97	100
95	80
94	70
90	60
85	50
75	40
57	30
32	20
10	10

Oxygen Administration

Oxygen is frequently ordered to treat or prevent hypoxemia. Oxygen may be supplied by a variety of sources: piped into wall devices in hospital rooms, oxygen tanks, and oxygen concentrators. Several devices are available to deliver oxygen to the patient. It is preferable that oxygen be humidified, since administration can dry the mucous membranes.

COMMONLY USED OXYGEN DELIVERY DEVICES

Commonly used oxygen delivery devices include the nasal cannula, face mask, face mask with reservoir, and the Venturi mask. The oxygen delivery devices are summarized in Table 5–10.

Nasal Cannula. A nasal cannula, or nasal prongs, is commonly used to deliver oxygen (Fig. 5–13). The device is relatively comfortable and provides an inexpensive method for oxygen delivery. Oxygen via a nasal cannula is usually ad-

Table 5-10. OXYGEN DELIVERY DEVICES

Device	Oxygen Flow Rate (L/min)	FIO_2
Nasal cannula	1	0.24
	2	0.28
	3	0.32
	4	0.36
	5	0.40
	6	0.44
Face mask	5–6	0.40
	6–7	0.50
	7–8	0.60
Masks with reservoirs	6	0.60
	7	0.70
	8	0.80
	9	0.80–1.00
	10	0.80–1.00
Venturi mask	4	0.24
	5	0.28
	6	0.31
	7	0.35
	8	0.40
	10	0.50

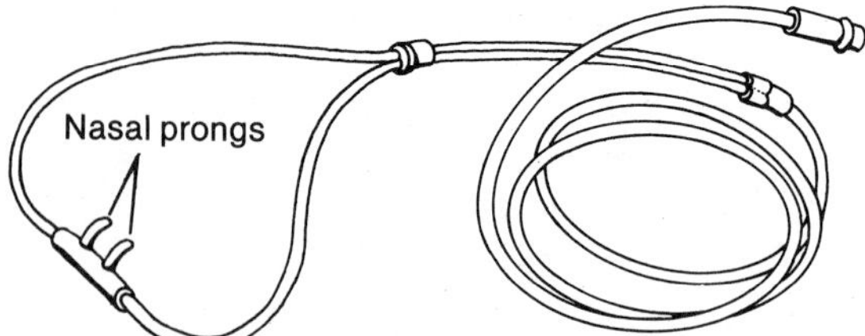

Figure 5-13. Nasal cannula. (From Kersten, L. D.: Comprehensive Respiratory Nursing. Philadelphia, W. B. Saunders, 1989, Fig. 23-10, p. 609.)

ministered at rates of 1 to 6 L/min. Oxygen administered at 1 L/min usually provides a fraction of inspired oxygen (FIO_2) of 0.24. The FIO_2 increases by 4% with each increase in liter flow. Administration at greater than 6 L/min is not effective in increasing oxygenation.

Face Mask. The face mask delivers oxygen through a simple mask device (Fig. 5-14). A mask appropriate to the size of the patient's face should be chosen in order to promote patient comfort. Oxygen is delivered at rates of 5 to 8 L/min, providing an FIO_2 of 0.40 to 0.60.

Face Masks With Reservoirs. These types of masks (Fig. 5-15) are used to provide oxygen concentrations of 60% or more and include the partial rebreathing mask and nonrebreathing mask. A reservoir is attached to the face mask. The purpose of the reservoir is to increase the amount of oxygen delivered to the patient. The partial rebreather delivers an FIO_2 of up to 0.60 at flow rates between 6 and 10 L/min. The nonrebreather delivers an FIO_2 of 0.80 to 1.00 with flow rates of 9 to 10 L/min. Either mask may be used in the critically ill patient with severe hypoxemia in an effort to prevent the need for endotracheal intubation and mechanical ventilation.

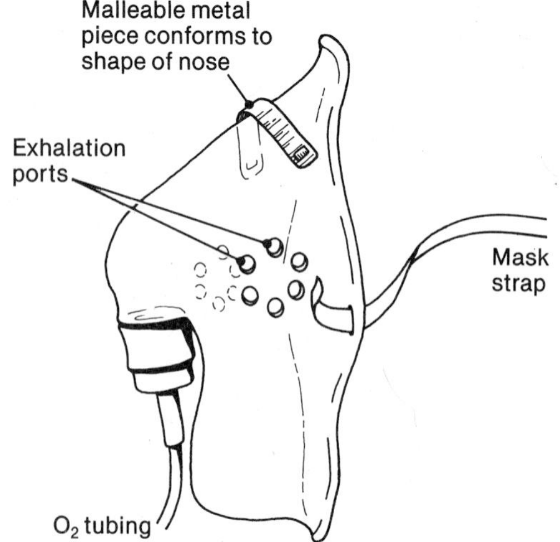

Figure 5-14. Simple face mask. (From Kersten, L. D.: Comprehensive Respiratory Nursing. Philadelphia, W. B. Saunders, 1989, Fig. 23-12, p. 609.)

Venturi Mask. The Venturi mask, or venti-mask is a device that can deliver a high flow of oxygen at a fixed concentration (Fig. 5-16). Venturi masks ensure accurate delivery of oxygen. Oxygen delivery is controlled by changing an adapter which alters the flow of oxygen. Venturi masks are commonly used in the patient with pulmonary disease so that the level of oxygen can be closely regulated to prevent complications associated with oxygen administration.

Manual Resuscitation Bag. If a patient needs assistance in breathing as well as oxygenation, a manual resuscitation bag (MRB) is used. The MRB can be used with a face mask to ventilate and oxygenate a patient who is not breathing. It can also be attached to an endotracheal tube to ventilate an intubated patient. The MRB should have a reservoir bag attached to increase the delivery of oxygen. The MRB should be connected to oxygen that is set to deliver 100% oxygen (usually 15 L/min).

■ Airway Management

POSITIONING

A patent airway is essential to survival. A primary nursing intervention with any patient is to maintain an open airway. The first method for maintaining a patent airway is proper head position. The head-tilt/chin-lift method is recommended to maintain an open airway (see Chap. 6 for greater detail).

ORAL AIRWAYS

Other methods for maintaining an open airway include oral and nasopharyngeal airways (Fig. 5-17). Oral airways are rigid tubes that prevent the tongue from falling into the pharynx (Fig. 5-18). Oral airways are used for many reasons: to facilitate secretion removal from the oropharynx; to maintain an open airway when it is necessary to ventilate a patient with an MRB and face mask; to prevent a patient from biting on an endotracheal tube; and to maintain an open airway in patients prone to seizures.

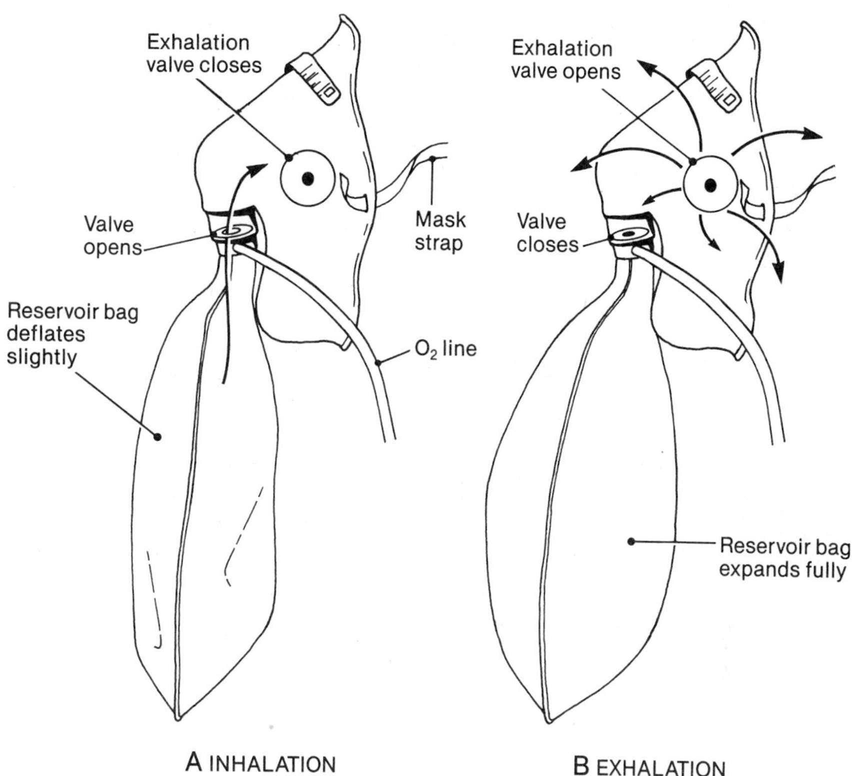

Figure 5-15. Face mask with reservoir. (From Kersten, L. D.: Comprehensive Respiratory Nursing. Philadelphia, W. B. Saunders, 1989, Fig. 23-14, p. 611.)

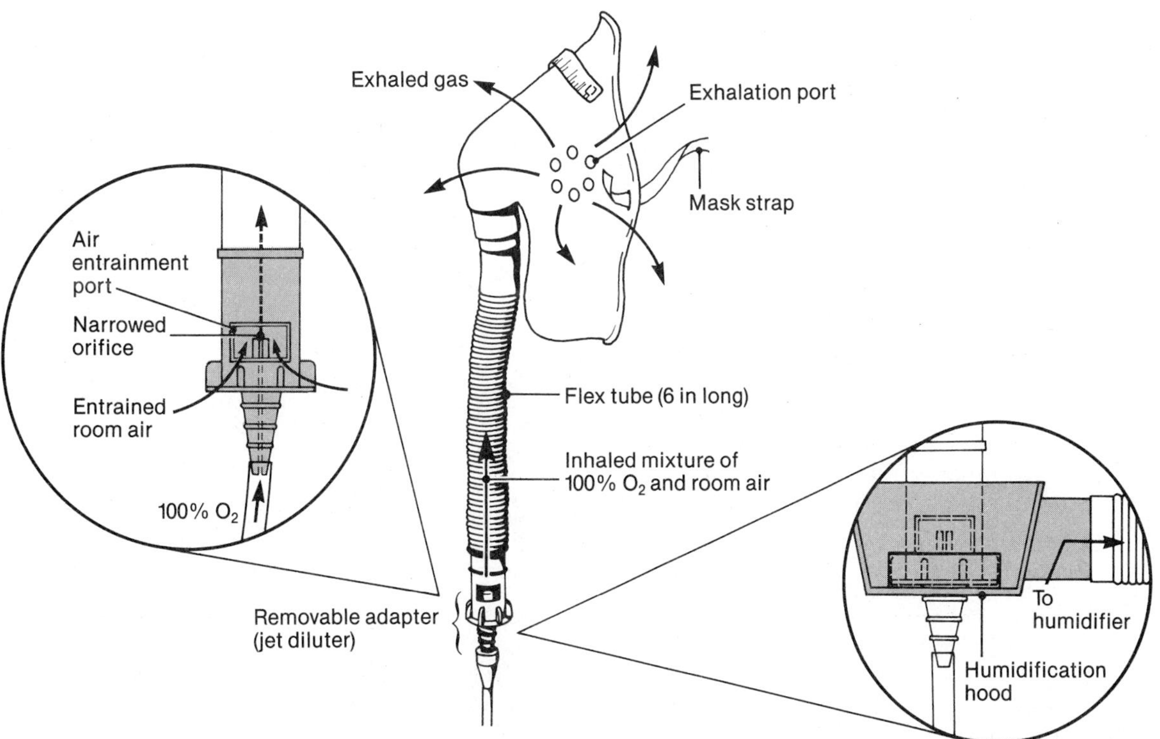

Figure 5-16. Venturi mask. (From Kersten, L. D.: Comprehensive Respiratory Nursing. Philadelphia, W. B. Saunders, 1989, Fig. 23-15, p. 611.)

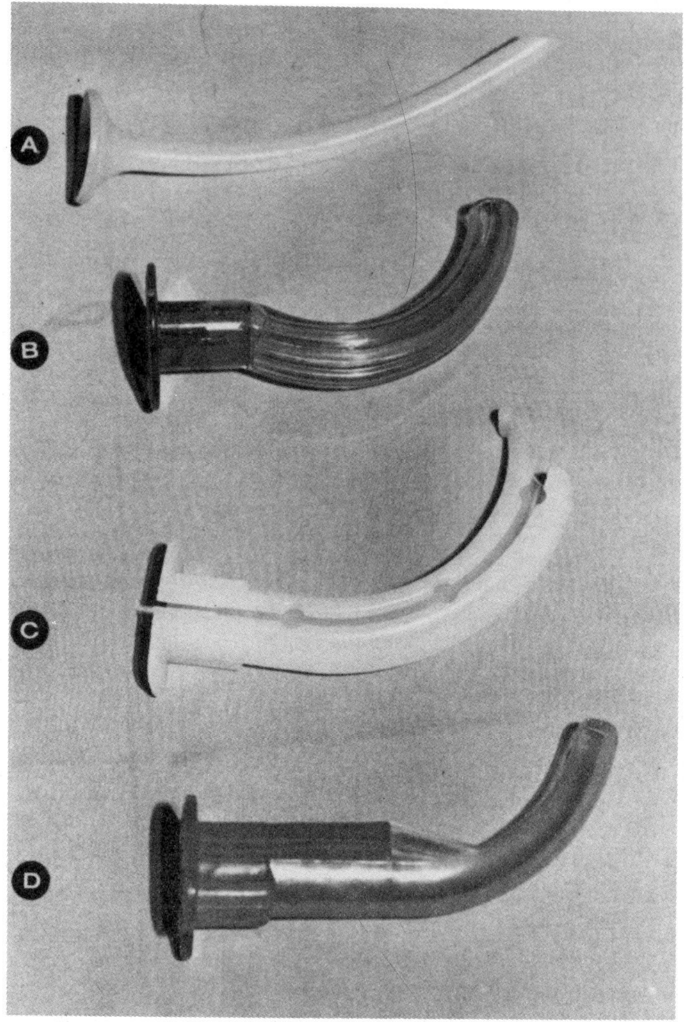

Figure 5-17. Airways: *(A)* nasopharyngeal; *(B)* oropharyngeal airway; *(C* and *D)* intubating airways. (From Chung, D. C., and Lamb, A. M.: Essentials of Anesthesiology. 2nd ed. Philadelphia, W. B. Saunders, 1990, Fig. 13-1, p. 128.)

Sizes of oral airways vary: small adult (80 mm long), medium adult (90 mm), and large adult (100 mm). Several brands are available. Some oral airways are made of a rigid plastic, whereas others are made of softer plastic materials. The configuration of the tubes also varies.

The technique for inserting an oral airway is described in Table 5-11. After insertion, the nurse looks, listens, and feels for air movement through the mouth while observing the chest rise and fall. Noises indicating upper airway obstruction should be absent. Complications of oral airways include airway obstruction if the airway is too long, accumulation of secretions, trauma to the lips and tongue, and gagging in a conscious patient.

Table 5-11. INSERTION OF ORAL AIRWAY

1. Choose the proper size. The length is determined by measuring from the corner of the mouth to the ear lobe.
2. Suction mucus from mouth using a tonsil (Yankauer) tip catheter.
3. Turn airway upside down to facilitate insertion and open the mouth. (An alternate method is to use a tongue blade to depress the tongue while the airway is inserted in the proper position.)
4. When the posterior wall of the pharynx is reached, turn (rotate) the airway into the proper position.
5. After insertion, assess patency of airway: Air movement through the airway, clear breath sounds, and chest movement.
6. Maintain proper head alignment after insertion.

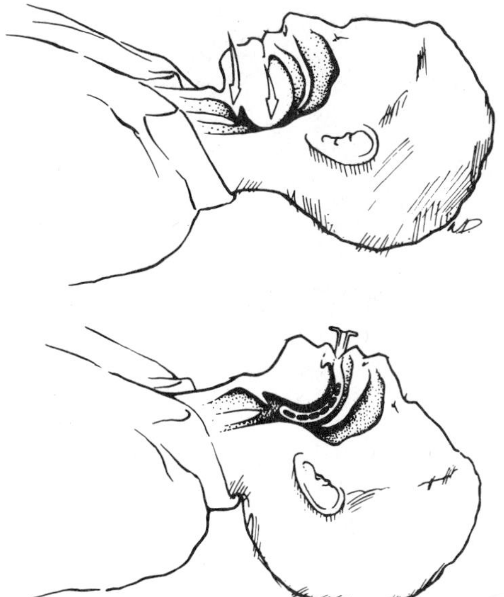

Figure 5-18. Maintaining an open airway with the use of an oral airway. (Reproduced with permission. *Textbook of Advanced Cardiac Life Support,* 2nd ed. 1990. Copyright American Heart Association, Dallas, Fig. 2, p. 28.)

NASOPHARYNGEAL AIRWAYS

Nasopharyngeal airways, also known as nasal airways or nasal trumpets, are soft rubber or latex tubes inserted into the nares and nasopharynx (Fig. 5-19). Nasopharyngeal airways are better tolerated in the conscious patient, may be left in place for longer periods of time, and facilitate nasotracheal suctioning.

The procedure for inserting a nasotracheal airway is described in Table 5-12. Complications of nasopharyngeal airways include insertion into the esophagus if the airway is too long, nosebleeds, and ulceration of the nares. Sinusitis or otitis may occur if the airway is left in place for extended periods of time.

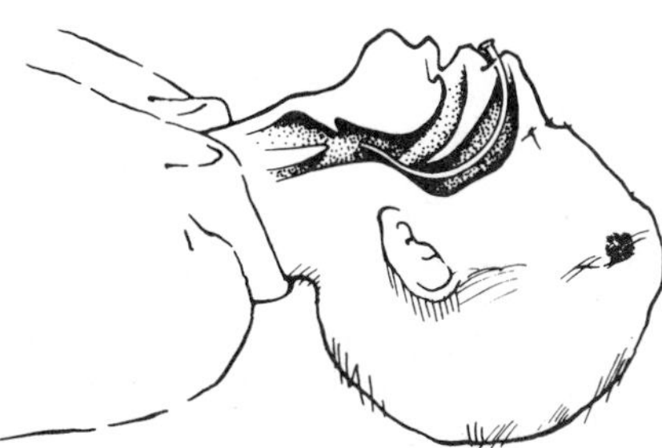

Figure 5-19. Maintaining an open airway with the use of a nasopharyngeal airway. (Reproduced with permission. *Textbook of Advanced Cardiac Life Support,* 2nd ed. 1990. Copyright American Heart Association, Dallas, Fig. 3, p. 28.)

Table 5-12. INSERTION OF NASAL AIRWAY

1. Choose the proper size. The length is determined by measuring from the nares to the ear lobe and adding 1 in.
2. Lubricate the tip and sides of the nasal airway with a water-soluble lubricant.
3. If needed, lubricate the nasal passage with a topical anesthetic.
4. Insert the airway medially and downward. It may be necessary to rotate the airway slightly.
5. After insertion, assess patency of airway: Air movement through the airway, clear breath sounds, and chest movement.

Intubation

ENDOTRACHEAL INTUBATION

Intubation refers to the insertion of an artificial airway, an endotracheal tube (ETT), into the trachea through either the mouth or nose. Advantages of oral versus nasal endotracheal intubation are listed in Table 5-13. The ETT (Fig. 5-20) is

Table 5-13. ORAL VERSUS NASOTRACHEAL INTUBATION

- Oral Intubation
  - Advantages
    - Easily and quickly performed
    - Larger tube facilitates suction and procedures such as bronchoscopy
    - Less kinking of tube
  - Disadvantages
    - Not recommended in patients with suspected cervical injury
    - Uncomfortable
    - Mouth care more difficult to perform
    - Impairs ability to gag and swallow
    - May increase salivation
    - May cause irritation and ulceration of the mouth
- Nasotracheal Intubation
  - Advantages
    - Greater patient comfort and better tolerance
    - Better mouth care possible
    - Fewer oral complications
    - Less risk of accidental extubation
    - Facilitates swallowing of secretions
    - Can administer small amounts of oral liquids if patient able to swallow
  - Disadvantages
    - More difficult to perform
    - May cause nasal hemorrhage and sinusitis
    - Secretion removal more difficult because of smaller tube diameter and longer tube length

Adapted from Kersten, L.D.: Comprehensive Respiratory Nursing. Philadelphia, W.B. Saunders, 1989.

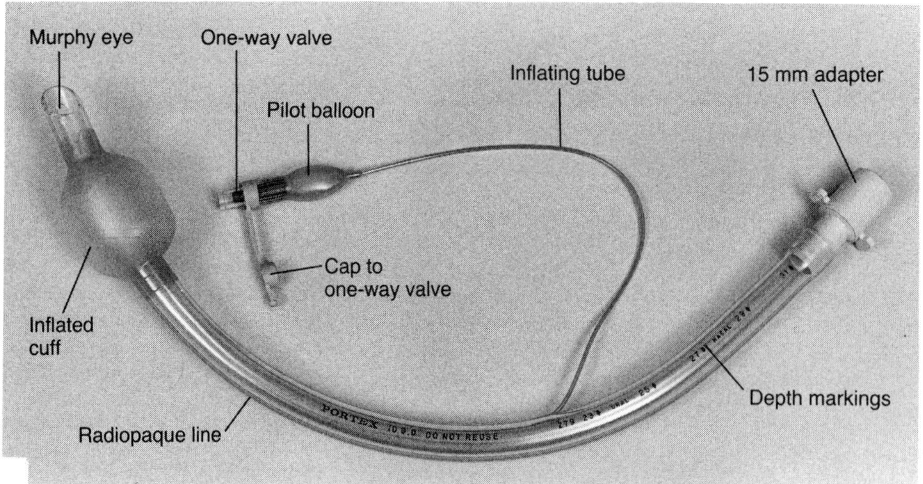

Figure 5-20. Endotracheal tube. (From Kersten, L. D.: Comprehensive Respiratory Nursing. Philadelphia, W. B. Saunders, 1989, Fig. 25-1, p. 637.)

a tube with a distal balloon, or cuff, that is inflated to facilitate ventilation of the patient. Most cuffs are high volume, low pressure. Most ETTs have cuffs that are inflated with air; however, some have foam cuffs that are passively inflated with air. (If using a foam cuff ETT, it is recommended that the manufacturer's instructions be followed for care and maintenance of the cuff.) The ETT also has a proximal adaptor that can be attached to an MRB or to a mechanical ventilator.

Intubation may be done to maintain an open airway, to assist in secretion removal, to prevent aspiration, and to provide mechanical ventilation. The procedure is done by personnel trained and skilled in the procedure, such as anesthesiologists, nurse anesthetists, emergency department physicians, and some paramedics.

Frequently, intubation is performed as an emergency procedure during a cardiopulmonary arrest. Intubation may also be performed as an "elective" procedure when a patient is having

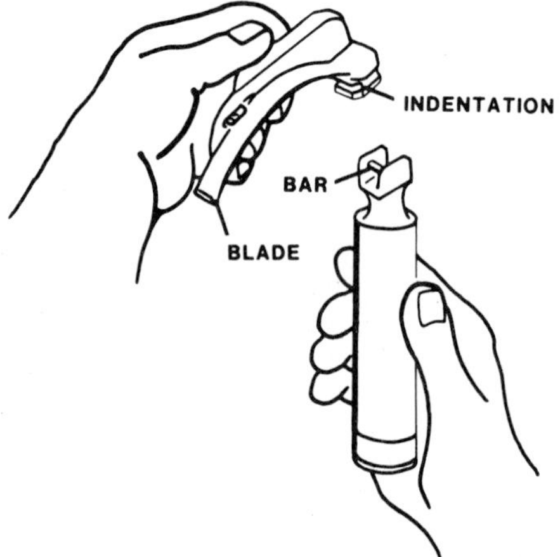

Figure 5-21. Assembly of a laryngoscope. The blade locks into place when assembled properly. (Reproduced with permission. *Textbook of Advanced Cardiac Life Support,* 2nd ed. 1990. Copyright American Heart Association, Dallas, Fig. 7, p. 31.)

Table 5-14. EQUIPMENT FOR ENDOTRACHEAL INTUBATION

- Endotracheal tube of proper size
  - Average female 7.5 to 8.0 mm
  - Average male 8.5 to 9.0 mm
- Stylet
- Laryngoscope and blade
  - Straight blade "Miller"
  - Curved blade "MacIntosh"
- Suction
  - Tonsil tip (Yankauer)
  - Suction kit
- Syringe to inflate balloon (usually 10 ml slip-tip)
- Topical anesthetic
  - Cetacaine spray, lidocaine jelly, or other agent
- Water-soluble lubricant
- Tape or device to secure tube
- Stethoscope
- Manual resuscitation bag
  - With reservoir
  - Connected to oxygen at 15 L/min
- Optional equipment
  - Magill forceps
  - Oropharyngeal airway

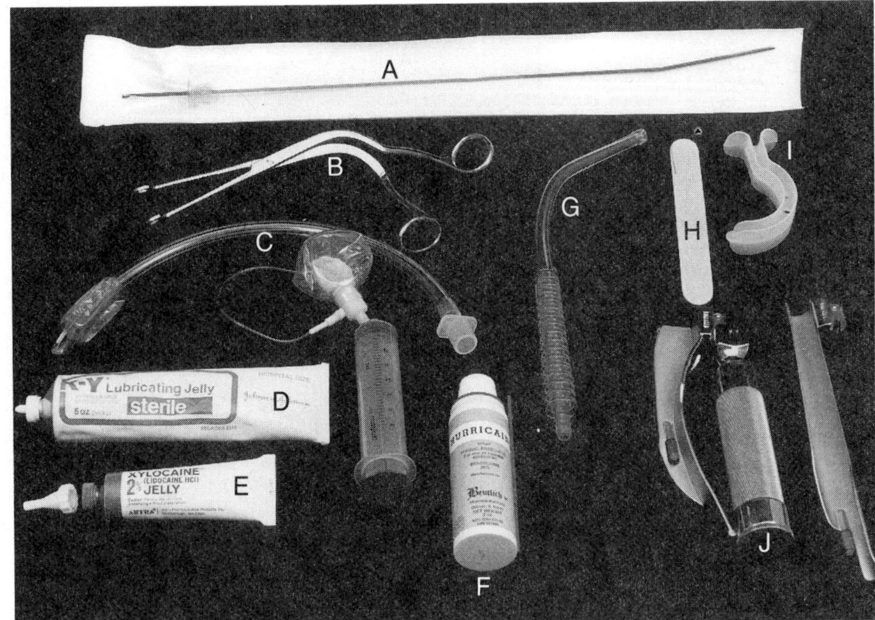

Figure 5-22. Equipment used for endotracheal intubation. *(A)* Stylet (disposable); *(B)* Magill forceps; *(C)* soft cuffed endotracheal tube with syringe for inflation; *(D)* water-soluble lubricant; *(E)* anesthetic jelly (optional); *(F)* topical anesthetic with spray stick attached to right side of cannister; *(G)* Yankauer pharyngeal suction tip (disposable); *(H)* tongue blade; *(I)* oral airway; *(J)* laryngoscope handle with a curved blade (attached) and straight blade (right). (From Kersten, L. D.: Comprehensive Respiratory Nursing. Philadelphia, W. B. Saunders, 1989, Fig. 25-3, p. 640.)

difficulty maintaining an adequate airway or oxygenation. The goal of elective intubation is to prevent cardiopulmonary arrest.

Nurses need to be familiar with equipment used for intubation and be able to gather equipment quickly prior to the procedure. Nurses also need to know how to assemble a laryngoscope (Fig. 5-21). Necessary equipment is frequently kept together on a crash cart or tray to facilitate the intubation procedure (Table 5-14; Fig. 5-22).

Procedure for Oral Endotracheal Intubation. The patient is placed in a "sniffing" position to align the airway structures (Fig. 5-23). It may be helpful to place a folded towel or bath blanket under the head to achieve this position. If the procedure is performed electively, a topical anesthetic and/or premedication with a sedative or paralytic agent may be used so that the patient better tolerates the procedure.

Prior to the procedure, the patient is hyperoxygenated and hyperventilated with 100% oxygen using an MRB with a face mask. The proper size tube is chosen. All endotracheal tubes increase the work of breathing; however, a tube that is too small substantially increases the work of breathing and may make ventilation and weaning difficult. The average size endotracheal tube for females ranges from 7.5 to 8.0 mm, whereas the average size for males ranges from 8.5 to 9.0 mm (Kersten, 1989). After the tube is selected, the cuff on the balloon is inflated to check for proper functioning and/or any leaks. The stylet is used to stiffen the ETT and facilitate insertion. The ETT is then lubricated with water-soluble lubricant. The laryngoscope is attached to the appropriate size and type of blade (straight or curved). Choice of blades varies. The straight blade elevates the epiglottis anteriorly to expose the vocal cords. The tip of the curved blade fits

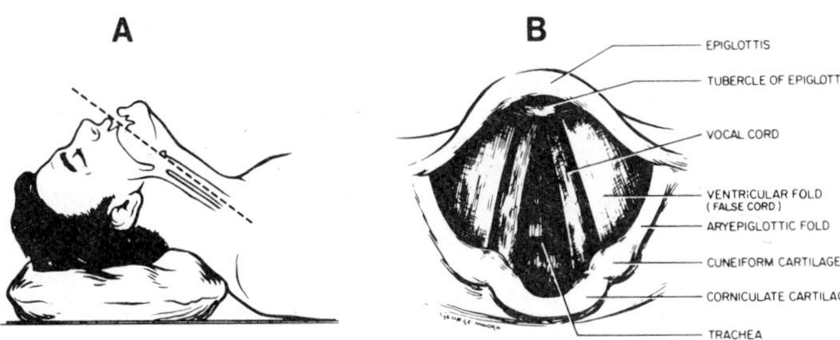

Figure 5-23. Patient positioning for endotracheal intubation. *(A)* Shows the correct position of the head and neck. *(B)* Shows the glottis as visualized through the laryngoscope. (From Chung, D. C., and Lamb, A. M.: Essentials of Anesthesiology. 2nd ed. Philadelphia, W. B. Saunders, 1990, Fig. 13-6, p. 133.)

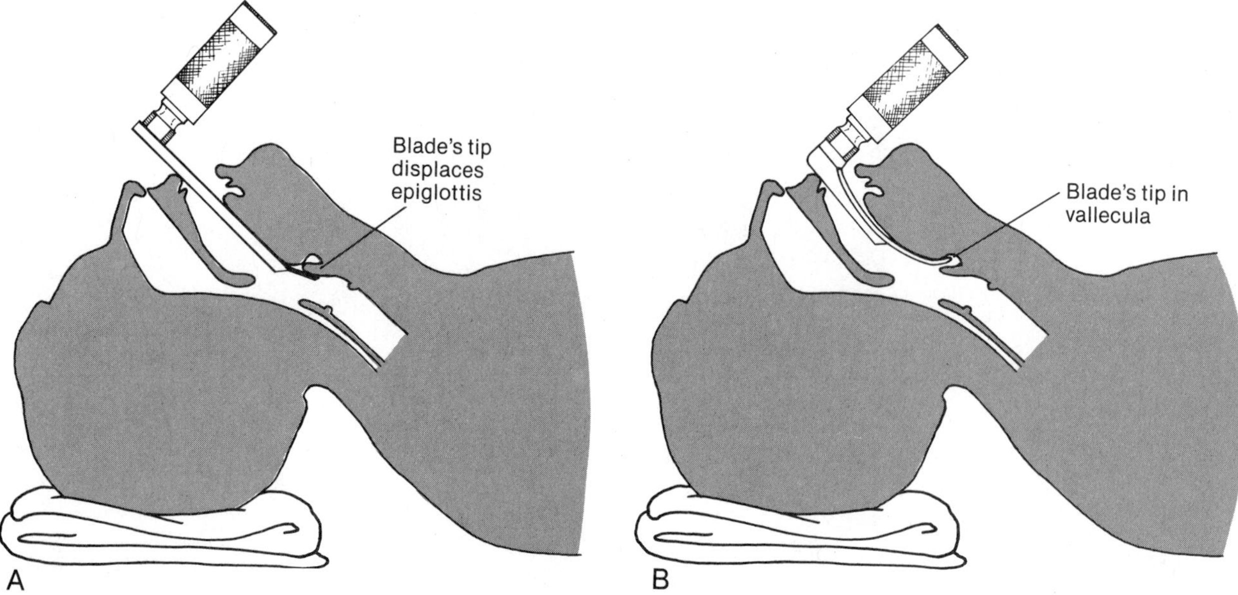

Figure 5-24. Use of a straight *(A)* versus curved *(B)* blade for endotracheal intubation. (From Kersten, L. D.: Comprehensive Respiratory Nursing. Philadelphia, W. B. Saunders, 1989, Fig. 25-6, p. 643.)

into the vallecula. When upward traction is placed on the laryngoscope, the epiglottis is displaced anteriorly. Use of the straight versus curved blade is shown in Figure 5-24.

The person doing the intubation inserts the laryngoscope into the mouth to visualize the vocal cords (see Fig. 5-22). Excess secretions and/or vomitus are suctioned to facilitate visualization of the vocal cords; the tonsil suction tip is very efficient in removing the secretions. The ETT is inserted 5 to 6 cm beyond the vocal cords and the cuff is inflated.

The procedure should be done within 30 seconds. If the intubation is difficult, the patient should be manually ventilated between intubation attempts. Frequently, the patient will require endotracheal suctioning immediately after intubation to remove excess secretions. If the patient needs assistance with breathing, ventilation is achieved with either the MRB or a ventilator. (During CPR, ventilation is provided with an MRB to facilitate an effective compression and ventilation at the recommended ratio of 5:1.) If the patient is breathing spontaneously, supplemental oxygen is delivered through the endotracheal tube via a T-piece, or Briggs device (Fig. 5-25).

Placement of the ETT is checked by feeling air moving in and out of the tube, observing bilateral chest expansion with inspiration, and auscultating bilateral breath sounds while ventilating the patient with an MRB. Another method to verify tube placement is to use $etCO_2$ monitoring. If the tube is in the trachea (versus the esophagus), CO_2 will be detected from the exhaled air. After intubation, a portable chest x-ray is always done to verify tube placement. The tip of the ETT should be approximately 2 to 5 cm above the carina.

Once proper tube placement is verified, it is secured with tape or another device to prevent dislodging. A helpful hint is to mark the endotracheal tube with an indelible marker at the lip line. The length of the tube at the lip line (e.g.,

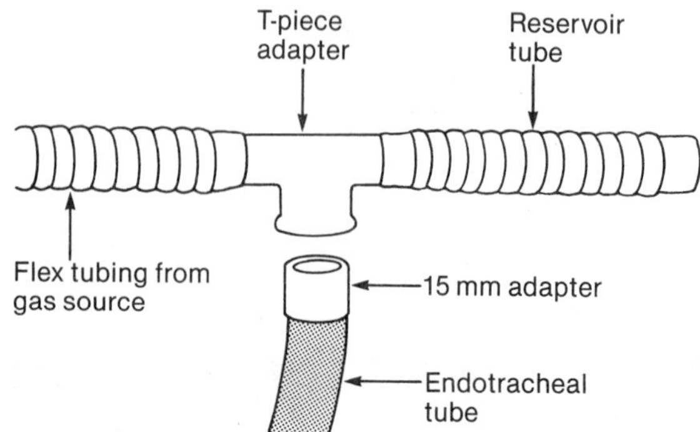

Figure 5-25. T-piece. The T-piece is used to provide supplemental oxygen through an endotracheal tube. (From Kersten, L. D.: Comprehensive Respiratory Nursing. Philadelphia, W. B. Saunders, 1989, Fig. 27-6, p. 672.)

23 cm) should also be documented in a ready reference, such as the Kardex. These nursing measures will facilitate frequent assessment of proper tube position.

Procedure for Nasotracheal Intubation. A nasotracheal ETT is usually better tolerated in an alert patient and may be easier to stabilize. Nasotracheal intubation is usually done by inserting the ETT through the nares and passing it "blindly" into the glottis during inspiration. The blind intubation method is done in the alert patient who is capable of spontaneous respirations. The nose and pharynx are anesthetized prior to the procedure.

Nasotracheal intubation can also be done by direct visualization. In this method, practitioners may use a laryngoscope and Magill forceps or fiberoptic bronchoscopy to perform the intubation.

Complications

Several complications may occur as a result of oral endotracheal or nasotracheal intubation. Complications include trauma to airway structures, hypoxia, dysrhythmias, aspiration, intubation of esophagus, laryngospasm, bronchospasm, and intubation of the right mainstem bronchus.

TRACHEOSTOMIES

A tracheostomy tube (TT) may be needed if the patient requires long-term mechanical ventilation, frequent suctioning to manage secretions, or to bypass an airway obstruction (such as a tumor). The tracheostomy procedure is usually done in the operating room; however, at times the procedure is done by the surgical team in the critical care unit. Types of TT include cuffed (low pressure or foam cuff), fenestrated, and cuffless.

Cuffed Tracheostomy Tube. A cuffed TT is inserted in the patient who requires long-term mechanical ventilation. This tube has a cuff similar to the endotracheal tube to ensure adequate ventilation and to prevent aspiration. The cuff may be a conventional low-pressure type or be constructed of foam. The foam cuff tube may prevent trauma to the airway because of the low pressure exerted. The foam cuff tube may also be used in patients who have difficulty in maintaining a good seal with conventional cuffed tracheostomy tubes. Cuffed tubes may or may not have an inner cannula. Some tubes have disposable inner cannulas that facilitate tracheostomy care and may reduce the risk of infections.

Fenestrated Tracheostomy Tube. The fenestrated TT is used to wean the patient from mechanical ventilation as well as the tracheostomy itself. This type of TT has holes that permit some air to escape from the lungs. An advantage of the fenestrated tube is that the patient is able to emit vocal sounds while the tube is in place.

Cuffless Tracheostomy Tube. A cuffless TT is used for long-term airway management in a patient who does not require mechanical ventilation and is at a low risk for aspiration. For example, some neurological patients need tracheostomies for secretion removal but do not require mechanical ventilation.

ENDOTRACHEAL SUCTIONING

Patients with either an ETT or TT frequently need to be suctioned in order to maintain a patent airway. Suctioning should be done according to a standard protocol in order to prevent complications. Complications associated with suctioning include hypoxemia, cardiac dysrhythmias, trauma to the airway, and infection. Suctioning also stimulates the cough reflex and stimulates increased mucus production.

Since suctioning is associated with complications as well as increased production of mucus, it should be performed only as indicated by the patient and *not* according to a predetermined schedule (e.g., every 2 hours). Indications for endotracheal suctioning include a change in vital signs (e.g., increased heart rate and respiratory rate), dyspnea, restlessness, visible secretions in the airway, ventilator alarms, or secretions audible on auscultation.

Several techniques have been developed to reduce complications associated with suctioning. Key points related to endotracheal suctioning are discussed in Table 5-15. Hyperinflation, hyperventilation, and hyperoxygenation are done with either the ventilator or MRB. Hyperinflation involves the delivery of breaths 1.0 to 1.5 times the tidal volume. Hyperventilation is done by giving the patient three to five quick breaths prior to and in between suctioning attempts. Hyperoxygenation is the delivery of 100% oxygen before suctioning and in between attempts. If hyperoxygenation is done via the ventilator, it is important to note that ventilators have a "washout" time that is required before 100% oxygen is delivered. The washout time varies with each ventilator; however, current research indicates that a minimum of 2 minutes is needed to achieve an oxygen concentration of 100% (Stone, 1990).

Table 5-15. KEY POINTS FOR ENDOTRACHEAL SUCTIONING

1. Suction only as indicated by patient assessment.
2. Assemble equipment. (Suction kit with 2 gloves; sterile water or saline for rinsing the catheter.)
3. Use sterile technique for the procedure.
4. Set suction vacuum at 80 to 120 mm Hg.
5. Provide three hyperoxygenation (100% oxygen) and hyperinflation (150% tidal volume) breaths to patient before, during, and after suctioning (Stone, 1990). Hyperoxygenation/hyperinflation may be accomplished via the ventilator circuit on some ventilators, or using a manual resuscitation bag.
   NOTE: If it is necessary to provide hyperoxygenation/hyperinflation with the manual resuscitation bag, two personnel should be involved in suctioning the patient: one to suction and one to manually ventilate.
6. Gently insert suction catheter until resistance is met.
7. Suction patient for no longer than 10 to 15 seconds using an intermittent suction technique.
8. Repeat endotracheal suctioning until airway is clear.
9. If secretions are thick, it may be useful to instill normal saline (without preservatives) into the trachea to loosen thick secretions. Instill 3 to 5 ml of saline and manually ventilate the patient to disperse the saline. The effectiveness of lavage is controversial (Ackerman, 1985).
10. After endotracheal suction is done, suction the mouth and oropharynx to remove excess saliva.
11. Auscultate the lungs to assess effectiveness of suctioning.
12. Document amount, color, and consistency of secretions.

Several research studies have been recently conducted to determine the most efficacious method for minimizing hypoxemia and hemodynamic consequences (e.g., increases in mean arterial pressure) associated with suctioning. Many recommendations for practice have been generated based on these studies (Stone, 1990):

1. All patients should receive hyperoxygenation prior to, during, and after suctioning.
2. All patients should be given at least three hyperoxygenation (100% oxygen) and hyperinflation (150% VT) breaths before, during, and after suctioning.
3. Hyperoxygenation/hyperinflation breaths may be given either via the ventilator or with a manual resuscitation bag.
4. Hyperoxygenation/hyperinflation breaths given via the ventilator are associated with fewer hemodynamic effects of suctioning.

Alternatives to conventional suctioning include the use of suction catheters connected to an oxygen source (oxygen insufflation catheter), adaptors, or closed tracheal suction devices. The oxygen insufflation catheter delivers oxygen to the patient via the suction catheter to prevent suction-induced hypoxemia. The use of adaptors and closed tracheal suction devices permits suctioning without disconnecting the patient from

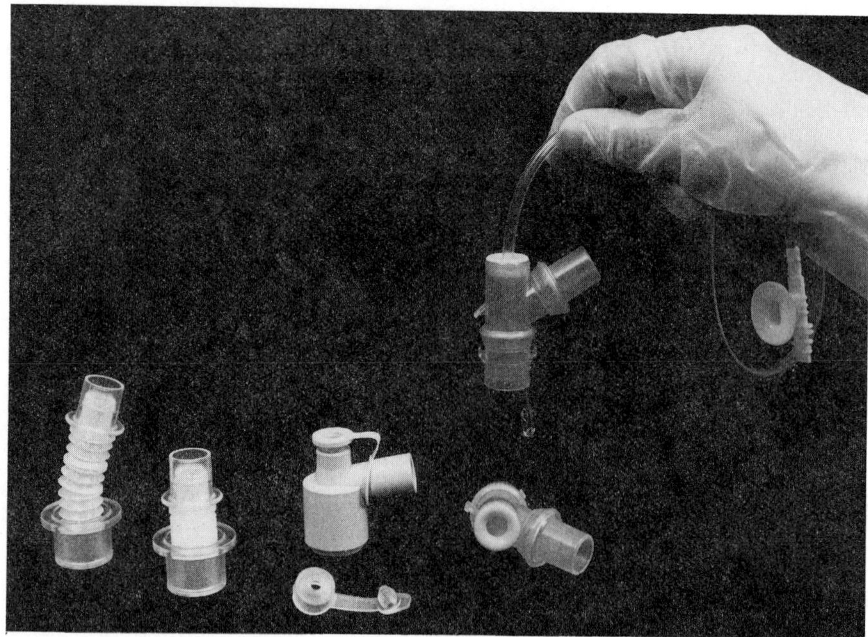

Figure 5-26. Suction adaptors. Adaptors permit suctioning of a patient without disconnecting mechanical ventilation. A suction catheter is introduced into one of the adaptors shown. (From Kersten, L. D.: Comprehensive Respiratory Nursing. Philadelphia, W. B. Saunders, 1989, Fig. 27-13, p. 690.)

the ventilator; therefore, they provide continuous oxygenation during suctioning and maintain positive end-expiratory pressure (PEEP). When an adaptor (Fig. 5–26) is employed, a conventional suction kit is used to suction the patient without removing the patient from the ventilator circuit.

The closed tracheal suction system (CTSS) consists of a suction catheter enclosed in a plastic sheath that is attached to the patient's ventilator circuit (Fig. 5–27). The closed system can also be attached to a T-piece adaptor. The CTSS maintains oxygenation during suctioning, reduces symptoms associated with hypoxemia, maintains PEEP, permits administration of respiratory medications, protects staff from patient's secretions, reduces patient anxiety, and is usually cost effective (Noll et al., 1990). Key points for using the CTSS are discussed in Table 5–16.

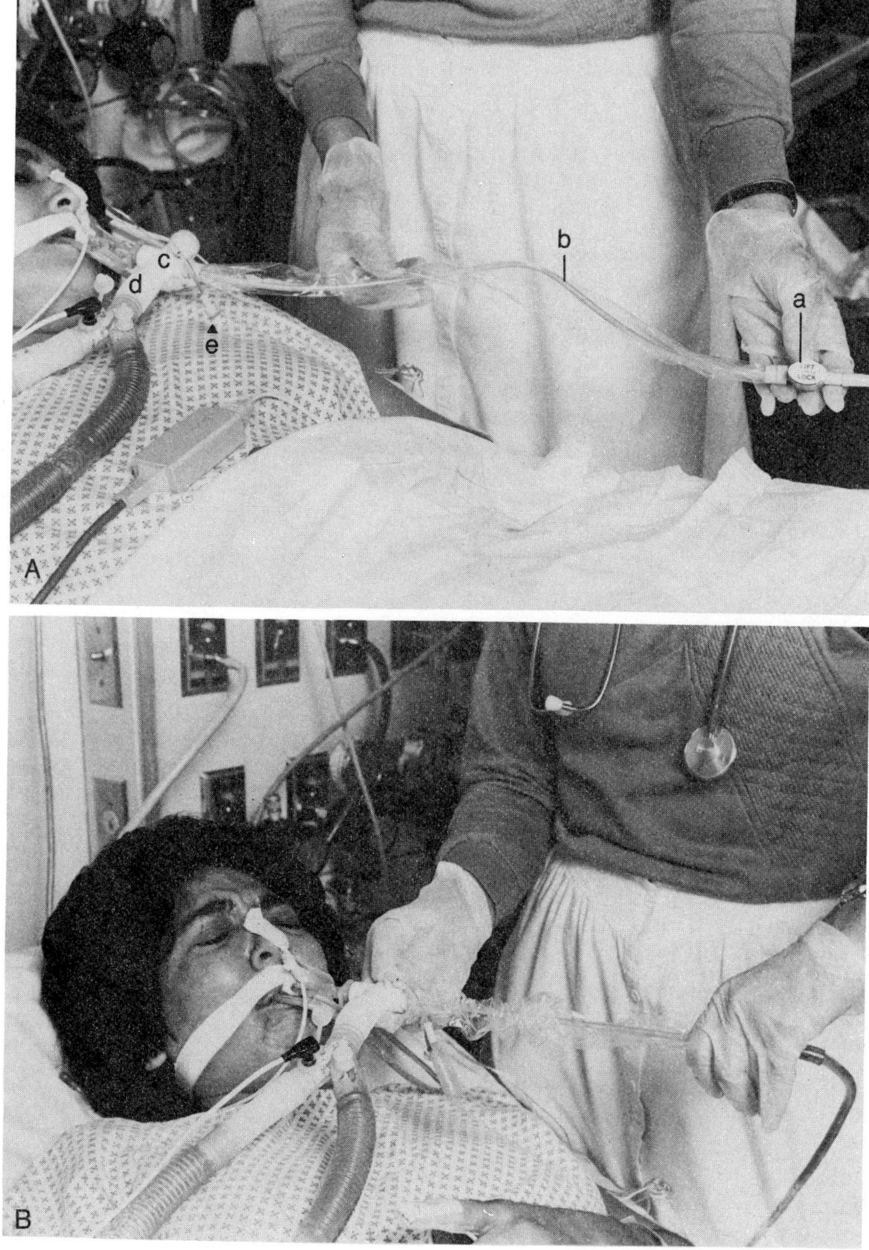

Figure 5–27. Closed-tracheal suction device. *(A)* Shows the Ballard TrachCare closed suction system: (a) suction control; (b) suction catheter enclosed in sheath; (c) sealed T-piece which connects to endotracheal tube; (d) flexible tubing which connects to ventilator, and (e) irrigation port for tracheal lavage and rinsing suction catheter. *(B)* Demonstrates use of the closed suction device. (From Kersten, L. D.: Comprehensive Respiratory Nursing. Philadelphia, W. B. Saunders, 1989, Fig. 27–11, p. 688.)

Table 5–16. KEY POINTS FOR SUCTIONING WITH A CLOSED TRACHEAL SUCTION SYSTEM (CTSS)

1. Prior to using the CTSS, review the manufacturer's instructions for use.
2. Choose the proper size CTSS. The diameter of the suction catheter should be no more than one-half the diameter of the endotracheal tube or tracheostomy tube.
3. Attach the CTSS to the ventilator circuit. (Frequently performed by the Respiratory Therapy Department.)
4. Set the suction regulator to 80 to 120 mm Hg *while depressing the suction control on the CTSS.*
5. Determine the need for hyperoxygenation prior to suction. Since the CTSS remains connected to the ventilator circuit, some institutions do not routinely hyperoxygenate the patient prior to suctioning unless the patient shows symptoms of hypoxemia, has a decrease in SaO_2 by more than 3%, or requires high PEEP (Noll et al., 1990).
   NOTE: It is recommended that the patient be hyperoxygenated via the ventilator if the *assist-control* mode is used (Craig et al., 1984).
6. Using the thumb and forefinger of the dominant hand, insert the CTSS suction catheter into the airway until resistance is met. At the same time, use the nondominant hand to stabilize the T-junction that connects the CTSS to the airway and ventilator. Withdraw the suction catheter using a steady motion while applying intermittent or constant suction for no longer than 10 to 15 seconds.
7. Ensure that the catheter has been completely withdrawn from the airway. A marking is visible on the suction catheter when it is properly withdrawn.
8. Rinse the CTSS after each use. Connect a small vial or syringe of normal saline for tracheal instillation (without preservatives) to the irrigation port of the CTSS. Simultaneously, instill the saline into the port while depressing the suction control on the CTSS.
9. If secretions are thick, saline may be instilled with the CTSS. Attach a vial of normal saline to the irrigation port of the CTSS. Insert the suction catheter 4 to 6 in into the airway. Instill 3 to 5 ml of normal saline into the CTSS. Suction the patient.
10. Change the CTSS every 24 hours, or according to manufacturer's recommendations.
11. Document effectiveness of suctioning. When the CTSS is used, some patients may require periodic conventional suctioning to remove the thick secretions.

Mechanical Ventilation

INDICATIONS FOR MECHANICAL VENTILATION

Mechanical ventilation is warranted for patients who have acute respiratory failure and are unable to maintain normal gas exchange. Respiratory failure occurs from impairment of alveolar ventilation or pulmonary vascular perfusion. The outcome of respiratory failure is life-threatening hypoxemia. Respiratory failure may result from an acute process, such as airway obstruction or pulmonary embolus, or an exacerbation of a chronic pulmonary disease. An example of the latter is a patient with chronic obstructive pulmonary disease who develops superimposed pneumonia. Respiratory failure is discussed in Chapter 10.

Assessment parameters for determining the need for intubation and mechanical ventilation include arterial blood gases, chest x-rays, and clinical signs of hypoxemia. Indications for mechanical ventilation are presented in Table 5–17.

TYPES OF MECHANICAL VENTILATORS

Mechanical ventilation is frequently used as a supportive therapy to facilitate gas exchange. Categories of mechanical ventilation include negative pressure and positive pressure types.

Negative Pressure Ventilation. Negative pressure ventilation does not require the use of an artificial airway (endotracheal tube or tracheostomy). The patient is placed in a device that applies negative pressure to the trunk or body. The negative pressure causes the chest wall to be pulled outward, causing inspiration to occur as a result of pressure changes in the pleural space. Examples of negative pressure ventilators include the iron lung, cuirass, poncho, and body wrap devices. Negative pressure devices are usually used in patients with chronic diseases who require assisted ventilation, frequently only during the night.

Table 5–17. INDICATIONS FOR MECHANICAL VENTILATION

Parameter	Normal	Ventilation
ABGs		
PaO_2 mm Hg	>80	<60
$PaCO_2$ mm Hg	35–45	>50
pH	7.35–7.45	<7.25
$PaO_2 = PaCO_2$		
Other		
Respiratory rate/minute	12–16	>35
Tidal volume ml/kg	6–8	<3.5
Vital capacity ml/kg	50–60	<10–15
NIF cm/H_2O*	>−25	<−20

* Negative inspiratory force (NIF) is the amount of negative pressure that a patient is able to generate to initiate spontaneous respirations. Normally NIF is −25 cm of H_2O or greater; i.e., −30 cm, −40 cm, etc.

Positive Pressure Ventilation. Positive pressure ventilation is more commonly used in the acute care setting. The method of mechanical ventilation "forces" air into the lung via positive pressure. Types of positive pressure ventilators include time-cycled, pressure cycled, and volume-cycled ventilators.

Time-Cycled Ventilators. These allow flow of air into the lungs until a preset amount of time has elapsed. Inspiration ends after the preset time interval. Delivered tidal volume, pressure, and flow vary according to the length of the inspiratory cycle. An example of time-cycled ventilators is the Emerson 3-PV. This type of ventilator is used more frequently with neonates and children.

Pressure-Cycled Ventilators. These ventilators allow flow of air into the lungs until a preset pressure has been reached. Once the pressure is reached, a valve closes and expiration begins. Delivered tidal volume varies widely with pressure-cycled ventilators. Examples of these ventilators are the Bird Mark series (Bird Products Corp., Palm Springs, CA) and the Bennett PR series (Puritan-Bennett Corp., Lenexa, KA). These ventilators are best for short-term use, such as in the emergency department after a patient is intubated or in the immediate postoperative patient who requires short-term ventilation. A possible disadvantage of pressure-cycled ventilators is hypoventilation.

Volume-Cycled Ventilators. These are the most commonly used type of positive pressure ventilators. They allow flow of air into the lungs until a preset volume has been reached. A major advantage of these ventilators is that they deliver the tidal volume regardless of changes in compliance or resistance. Examples of volume-cycled ventilators include the Puritan-Bennett MA-1 and MA-2 and the Bear 1 and 2. (Bear Medical Systems, Inc., Riverside, CA).

Ventilators with Flexible Capabilities. Some currently available mechanical ventilators offer flexibility in the types of ventilation they are able to provide; e.g., pressure- and volume-cycled capabilities. These include the Puritan-Bennett 7200 series and the Siemens Servo series (Siemens-Life Support Systems, Schaumburg. IL).

High-Frequency Jet Ventilation (HFJV). Initially used in children, HFJV is now used in adults who cannot be effectively ventilated with the conventional methods for mechanical ventilation. It works by using small tidal volumes at very high respiratory rates. Ventilation and oxygenation are achieved by gas diffusion and convection (Kersten, 1989). The major advantage of HFJV is a reduction in complications associated with high airway pressures in conventional mechanical ventilation; e.g., barotrauma. The major disadvantage is that the technique is still not widely used in adult patients.

MODES OF MECHANICAL VENTILATION

Various modes of mechanical ventilation may be used to ensure adequate ventilation and optimum oxygenation of the patient. These modes include controlled ventilation, assist/control (A/C) ventilation, intermittent mandatory ventilation (IMV), and synchronized IMV ventilation.

Controlled Ventilation (CMV). The control mode of mechanical ventilation delivers a preset tidal volume at a preset respiratory rate. It ventilates the patient regardless of the patient's respiratory effort. It is used in patients who have no inspiratory effort, such as patients with high cervical spine injuries, or to decrease the work of breathing in patients with chest injuries or respiratory distress. If CMV is ordered for a patient who has some spontaneous effort, it is usually necessary to medicate the patient with a neuromuscular blocking agent (e.g., pancuronium bromide or vecuronium bromide) to prevent him/her from attempting to breathe in competition with the ventilator.

Assist/Control Ventilation (A/C). The A/C mode of mechanical ventilation delivers a preset tidal volume whenever the patient exerts a negative inspiratory effort. If the patient does not spontaneously trigger the ventilator, this mode ensures that the patient receives the preset respiratory rate. For example, the A/C respiratory rate may be set at 10 breaths/minute at a tidal volume of 800 ml. If the patient initiates a negative inspiratory effort 16 times per minute, he/she will receive 800 ml of air for each of the 16 efforts. If the patient does not initiate any inspiratory effort (e.g., during sleep), he/she will still receive 800 ml tidal volume 10 times per minute. The A/C mode is useful in patients with normal respiratory drive but who are unable to sustain normal tidal volumes.

One complication of the A/C mode is respiratory alkalosis, especially if the patient hyperventilates. If respiratory alkalosis occurs, the patient may need to be sedated or changed to the IMV mode of ventilation. Another disadvantage of A/C ventilation is that the effort needed to initiate a breath may be high if associated with excessive minute ventilation (Ashworth, 1990).

Intermittent Mandatory Ventilation/Synchronized Intermittent Mandatory Ventilation (IMV/SIMV). The IMV and SIMV modes of mechanical ventilation deliver a preset tidal volume at a preset respiratory rate and permit the patient to breathe spontaneously between the ventilator breaths. The IMV mode delivers the preset breaths regardless of the patient's spontaneous effort, whereas the SIMV mode delivers preset breaths that are synchronized with the patient's spontaneous efforts. The SIMV mode prevents the patient from competing with the ventilator during spontaneous efforts. The IMV/SIMV modes are frequently used to provide ventilatory support. They may prevent the hyperventilation that may occur in the A/C mode. These modes have been used in the past to wean patients from mechanical ventilation; however, effectiveness of IMV/SIMV in weaning is controversial. The rationale for using the modes to wean patients is that they encourage spontaneous efforts from the patient. Although IMV/SIMV may be useful in weaning patients, they may increase the workload of breathing for the patient because of muscle fatigue associated with spontaneous breathing efforts and the artificial airway.

ADJUNCTS TO MECHANICAL VENTILATION

Several adjustments can be made to the modes of mechanical ventilation to enhance oxygenation and/or ventilation of the patient. Adjuncts to modes of mechanical ventilation include positive end-expiratory pressure, continuous positive airway pressure, and pressure support ventilation.

Positive End-Expiratory Pressure (PEEP). Positive airway pressure may be used in conjunction with mechanical ventilation modes. Positive end-expiratory pressure is one method for adding positive airway pressure to mechanically assisted breaths. It keeps the patient's airway open at the end of expiration and increases the functional residual capacity (FRC). It prevents the collapse of small airways at the end of expiration and increases patient oxygenation. Frequently, PEEP is used to decrease the FIO_2 needed to optimally ventilate the patient. For example, a patient may require an FIO_2 of 0.80 to maintain a PaO_2 of 85. If 10 cm PEEP is added to the ventilator settings, the FIO_2 may be able to be decreased to 0.60, while still permitting the patient to have a PaO_2 of 85. The range for PEEP is 5 to 20 cm H_2O, although higher levels have been used in patients with severe respiratory distress and hypoxemia. Complications of PEEP include a decrease in cardiac output and an increased risk for barotrauma such as a pneumothorax.

Continuous Positive Airway Pressure (CPAP). Whereas PEEP is used to increase the FRC during mechanically assisted breaths, CPAP is used to augment FRC during spontaneous breaths. Most newer mechanical ventilators can deliver CPAP (e.g., Puritan-Bennett 7200 series, Siemens Servo series [Siemens Life Support Systems, Schaumburg, IL]). For example, a patient may be on a volume ventilator in the SIMV mode at a respiratory rate of 10 breaths/minute and receive 8 cm of PEEP and 8 cm of CPAP. The PEEP is delivered with the 10 SIMV breaths. The CPAP will be applied to the patient's spontaneous breaths. The CPAP is also used as a method for weaning patients from mechanical ventilation.

Continuous positive airway pressure can also be administered via face mask. This method is sometimes used in patients to delay intubation while treatment is initiated. It is also used at night by some patients who suffer from sleep apnea.

Pressure Support Ventilation (PSV). Pressure support is a new method used in ventilatory management. In PSV, a preset level of positive pressure is used to augment or assist spontaneous breaths of the patient. The rationale for using pressure support is to facilitate spontaneous breathing by decreasing the workload of breathing. Therefore, PSV is frequently combined with IMV/SIMV. It reduces the workload associated with breathing through an endotracheal tube, may increase patient comfort, and may also provide conditioning of the diaphragm that will facilitate weaning patients from mechanical ventilation (Ashworth, 1990; Burns, 1990).

NEWER METHODS/MODES OF MECHANICAL VENTILATION

Pressure Controlled–Inverse Ratio Ventilation (PC-IRV). This is being used to ventilate patients with respiratory failure (e.g., adult respiratory distress syndrome) when conventional mechanical ventilation is not successful. The PC-IRV mode of mechanical ventilation uses prolonged inspiration to expiration (I:E) ratios ranging from 1:1 to 4:1. (Most conventional volume ventilators are set at an I:E ratio of 1:2 to mimic normal respirations.) Tidal volume is delivered via pressure rather than volume control. It is thought that PC-IRV is effective because prolonged inspiration opens and stabilizes the alveoli (St. John and LeFrak, 1990).

Mandatory Minute Ventilation (MMV). This method of mechanical ventilation ensures a constant minute ventilation regardless of the patient's respiratory rate or spontaneous tidal volume. A computer controls the ventilator and adjusts the settings on a breath-to-breath basis according to analysis of the patient's expired gases. Mandatory minute ventilation may be used as an alternative approach to mechanical ventilation or to facilitate weaning from mechanical ventilation (Toben and Lewandowski, 1988; Witta, 1990).

Differential Lung Ventilation (DLV) or Simultaneous Independent Lung Ventilation (SILV). Differential lung ventilation permits independent ventilation of each lung. The primary use of DLV is to treat unilateral lung disease such as pneumonia, atelectasis, and bronchopulmonary fistulas (Toben and Lewandowski, 1988; Traver and Flodquist-Priestly, 1986). A dual-lumen endobronchial tube (Fig. 5–28) is inserted into the patient in order to initiate DLV. A ventilator is attached to each lumen of the ETT. The ventilator settings are adjusted for each lung (e.g., different tidal volumes and oxygen concentrations can be used). The two ventilators are connected in order to synchronize inspiration and expiration.

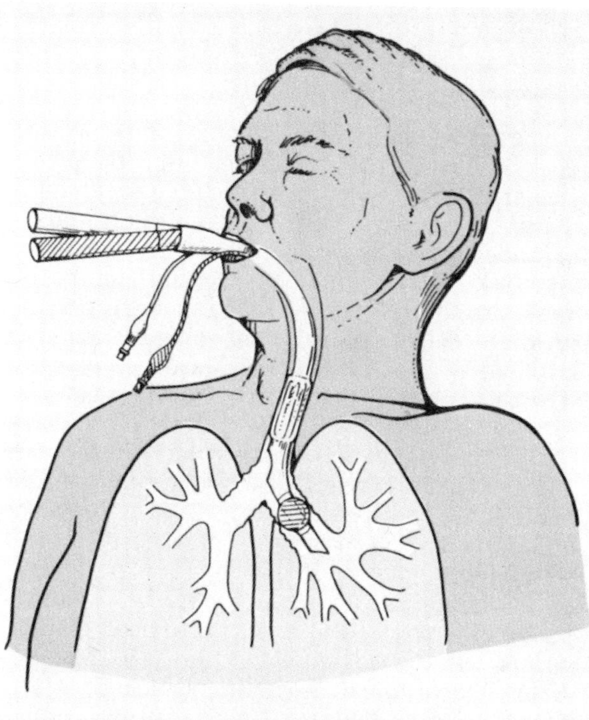

Figure 5–28. Dual lumen endobronchial tube for differential lung ventilation. (From Traver, G. A., and Flodquist-Priestly, G.: Management problems in unilateral lung disease with emphasis on differential lung ventilation. Critical Care Nurse 6(4):40–50, 1986.)

Nocturnal Nasal Positive Pressure Ventilation (NNPPV). This is a new method for providing positive pressure ventilation without an endotracheal tube or tracheostomy. In NNPPV, positive pressure ventilation is provided via a specially designed nasal mask connected to a portable ventilator. It has primarily been used in the home-care setting. It is used to treat nighttime hypoventilation in patients with pulmonary muscle weakness or chest wall deformities who have increasing symptoms of respiratory failure, increasing fatigue, or an overall decreased quality of life (Burns, 1990).

VENTILATOR SETTINGS

In most institutions, the actual ventilators are usually set up and managed by respiratory therapy personnel. However, the nurse needs to know the patient's ventilator settings and should check the ventilator for the proper settings. All ventilators have numerous buttons and dials. The nurse should be familiar with the control panel so that the ventilator mode, adjuncts to ventilation, and the settings below can be verified at least once per shift.

Tidal Volume (V_T). The amount of air delivered with each preset breath is the tidal volume. In ventilated patients, the V_T is usually set at 10 to 15 ml/kg. Therefore a patient who weighs 70 kg should have the V_T set between 750 and 1050 ml.

Respiratory Rate (RR). This is the frequency of breaths to be delivered by the ventilator.

Fraction of Inspired Oxygen (F_{IO_2}). This is the fraction of inspired oxygen delivered to the patient by the ventilator. F_{IO_2} may be set from 0.21 (21% or room air) to 1.00 (100% oxygen).

Sigh. A sigh may be included as part of the ventilator settings. A sigh is a breath that has a greater volume than the preset V_T, usually 1.5 to 2.0 times the V_T. The rationale for using the sigh mechanism is to prevent atelectasis. However, the sigh mechanism is no longer routinely used because higher than normal tidal volumes (10 to 15 ml/kg) are usually used in ventilatory management. It is also not routinely used in patients receiving PEEP because it is associated with a higher risk for complications.

Sensitivity. This is used to determine the patient's effort to initiate an assisted breath.

Inspiratory: Expiratory Ratio (I:E Ratio). In normal respiration, inspiration is shorter than expiration. When a patient is placed on mechanical ventilation, the I:E ratio is usually set at 1:2. It can be manipulated to facilitate gas exchange.

Peak Inspiratory Pressure (PIP). This is the peak pressure registered on the airway pressure gauge during normal ventilation (Fig. 5-29). The value is used to set high and low pressure alarm limits.

Pressure Limits. The high pressure limit is the maximum pressure the ventilator can generate to deliver the preset tidal volume. It is usually set 10 to 20 cm H_2O above the PIP.

RESPIRATORY MONITORING DURING MECHANICAL VENTILATION

Several respiratory parameters are routinely obtained on mechanically ventilated patients by either nurses or respiratory therapists. These parameters include spontaneous tidal volume and vital capacity, negative inspiratory force (NIF), and compliance. The tidal volume and vital capacity are measured by a spirometer. The NIF is measured with a specially designed meter.

Compliance is estimated by measuring PIP and calculating static and dynamic values. An increasing PIP may indicate increased airway resistance or decreased lung compliance.

In order to measure static compliance, a plateau pressure (PP) is measured at peak inspiration using the "inflationary hold" or "expiratory retard" dial on the ventilator. The formula for calculating static compliance is noted:

$$\text{Static compliance} = \frac{\text{Tidal volume}}{\text{Plateau pressure} - \text{PEEP}}$$

Dynamic (or effective) compliance is estimated by the following formula:

$$\text{Dynamic compliance} = \frac{\text{Tidal volume}}{\text{Peak inspiratory pressure} - \text{PEEP}}$$

As previously noted, static compliance ranges from 70 to 100 ml/cm H_2O in the mechanically ventilated patient with normal lung function. Dynamic compliance ranges from 50 to 100 ml/cm H_2O, or not more than 10 cm/H_2O greater than static compliance (Kersten, 1989).

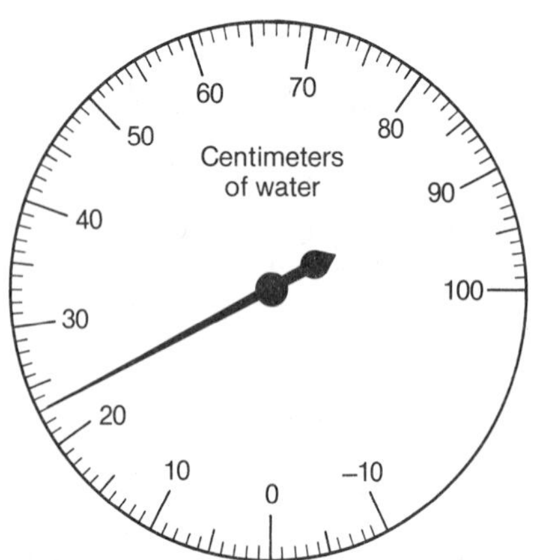

Figure 5-29. System pressure dial showing a peak inspiratory pressure of 23 cmH_2O. During expiration, the dial will return to 0 cmH_2O unless the patient is receiving positive end-expiratory pressure. (From Kersten, L. D.: Comprehensive Respiratory Nursing. Philadelphia, W. B. Saunders, 1989, Fig. 28-14, p. 717.)

COMPLICATIONS OF MECHANICAL VENTILATION

Although mechanical ventilation is a therapy used to treat respiratory failure, complications can occur.

Pulmonary System

Barotrauma. Barotrauma is the presence of extra alveolar air. This air may escape into the pleura (pneumothorax), the mediastinum (pneumomediastinum), pericardium (pneumopericardium), or under the skin (subcutaneous emphysema, or crepitus). Barotrauma may occur when the alveoli are overdistended such as with positive pressure ventilation, high tidal volumes (>15 ml/kg), and PEEP. An increased incidence of barotrauma is likely if the patient is older, has a history of chronic obstructive pulmonary disease, has an infection that destroys the alveoli, or if airway pressures are high. Signs and symptoms of barotrauma include high PIP, decreased breath sounds, high mean airway pressures, tracheal shift, and symptoms associated with hypoxemia.

A life-threatening complication is a tension pneumothorax. When a tension pneumothorax occurs, pressurized air enters the pleural space. Air is unable to exit from the pleural space and continues to accumulate. Collapse of the cardiopulmonary system occurs rapidly. Treatment is immediate insertion of a chest tube. Whenever a pneumothorax is suspected in a patient on mechanical ventilation, the patient should be removed from the ventilator and manually ventilated with an MRB until a chest tube is inserted.

Intubation of Right Mainstem Bronchus. The right mainstem bronchus is straighter than the left. If the ETT is manipulated, such as when changing the tapes or repositioning the tube in the mouth, it may move into the right mainstem bronchus. Symptoms include absent or diminished breath sounds in the left lung. Whenever the ETT is moved or manipulated, the nurse must auscultate the chest for bilateral breath sounds after completion of the procedure.

Endotracheal Tube Out of Position/Extubation. The ETT can become dislodged if not secured properly, from patient movement, or when changing tape on the ETT. The ETT may end up in the back of the throat, in the esophagus, or completely removed! Auscultation of bilateral breath sounds and/or the use of capnography can be used to verify that the ETT is in the airway.

Tracheal Damage. Damage to the trachea can occur because of pressure from the cuff. However, the risk of tracheal damage has decreased since all ETTs and TTs now have low pressure cuffs. An intervention to prevent tracheal damage is to monitor cuff pressures on a routine basis. Various commercial devices that measure cuff pressures quickly and easily are available.

Associated with Oxygen Administration. If 100% oxygen is administered, there is a lack of nitrogen in the distal air spaces. Nitrogen is needed to prevent collapse of the airway. Therefore, the patient is prone to absorption atelectasis. Other complications associated with oxygen administration include tracheobronchitis, acute lung injury (ARDS), and chronic pulmonary dysplasia.

Acid-Base Disturbances (Hypo-/Hypercapnia). If a ventilator is not set properly to maintain adequate oxygenation and gas exchange, disturbances will result. For example, if a patient is on assist/control ventilation and is breathing 30 times per minute, respiratory alkalosis will probably occur. If a patient is on IMV at a rate of six breaths per minute, and is only spontaneously breathing six breaths per minute, respiratory acidosis may occur.

Aspiration. The majority of patients who require mechanical ventilation also require tube feedings. Gastric distention, impaired gastric emptying with large amounts of gastric residue, and esophageal reflux predispose patients to aspiration.

Infection. Patients with artificial airways are at an increased risk for pulmonary infection. Normal defense mechanisms in the nose are bypassed when an artificial airway is used. Additionally, procedures such as endotracheal suction also predispose the patient to an increased risk of infection. Bacteria that frequently cause nosocomial infections include *Streptococcus, Staphylococcus, Pseudomonas, Escherichia coli,* and *Serratia.* Because of their debilitated state, patients may also acquire fungal infections, such as *Candida albicans.*

Ventilator Dependence/Inability to Wean. Patients who require long-term mechanical ventilation are usually very challenging when it is time to wean them from the ventilator. Examples of patients who fit this category include patients with underlying chronic obstructive pulmonary disease and neuromuscular disease.

Cardiovascular System

A decreased cardiac output may be associated with mechanical ventilation, especially if PEEP therapy is used. Positive pressure ventilation and PEEP increase intrathoracic pressure. This results in a decreased venous return to the heart and a decrease in cardiac output.

Gastrointestinal System

Stress ulcers and gastrointestinal bleeding may occur in patients who are mechanically ventilated. Another possible complication is a paralytic ileus. Lastly, inadequate nutrition is common in patients who are on mechanical ventilation.

Endocrine System

Fluid retention may be associated with increased humidification provided by the ventilator. Another reason for fluid retention is that increased pressure on the baroreceptors in the thoracic aorta from positive pressure ventilation stimulates the release of antidiuretic hormone, ADH. This hormone causes water retention and stimulates the renin-angiotensin-aldosterone mechanism which causes further fluid retention.

Psychosocial Complications

Several psychosocial hazards may occur as the result of being mechanically ventilated. The patient may experience stress and anxiety because of being on a machine to breathe. If the ventilator is not set properly or the patient resists breaths, "fighting" the ventilator may occur. Communication difficulties are common, since the patient cannot verbally communicate with family members and caregivers. As a result of being a patient in the intensive care unit, the patient loses autonomy and control over care. Because of the noise of the ventilator as well as the need for frequent procedures such as suctioning, alteration in sleep and wake patterns may occur. Lastly, the patient can become psychologically dependent on the ventilator even when physically able to be weaned.

NURSING CARE

Nursing care of the patient who requires mechanical ventilation is a challenge. The nurse must provide care in a holistic approach despite the use of technology. A detailed plan of care is described in the Nursing Care Plan for the Mechanically Ventilated Patient.

TROUBLESHOOTING

Individuals who care for patients receiving mechanical ventilation must be knowledgeable about the equipment and be competent at troubleshooting. In order to prevent errors, *two important rules must be followed:*

1. *Never shut alarms off.* It is acceptable to silence alarms for a preset delay while working with a patient, such as during suctioning. However, alarms should *never* be shut off.
2. *If you suspect equipment failure, or are unable to troubleshoot alarms, manually ventilate the patient with an MRB.*

Ventilator alarms vary from machine to machine. Alarms can be categorized into two common causes: volume alarms and pressure alarms. (Note: Alarm names vary from ventilator to ventilator. It is recommended that the nurse be familiar with the ventilators used in the institution.)

Volume Alarms. A volume alarm will sound if the patient is not receiving the preset tidal volume. Causes of volume alarms include disconnection of the ventilator circuit from the artificial airway, a leak in the ETT or tracheostomy cuff, displacement of the ETT or tracheostomy, and disconnection of any part of the ventilator circuit.

Pressure Alarms. Pressure alarms occur if the amount of pressure needed to ventilate a patient exceeds a preset amount. Causes of pressure alarms include excess secretions; mucus plugs; patient biting endotracheal tube; kinks in ventilator circuit; patient coughing, gagging, or attempting to talk; "fighting" the ventilator; pulmonary edema; and pressure on the chest wall.

Weaning Patients From Mechanical Ventilation

Once the decision is made to mechanically ventilate a patient, caregivers should begin to plan for weaning the patient. Generally, patients who require short-term ventilatory support (e.g., in the immediate postoperative period) can be weaned quickly. Conversely, weaning is usually a slow, tedious process for patients who require long-term ventilatory support.

CRITERIA

Criteria for patient weaning vary. Prior to weaning, the underlying disease process that necessitated mechanical ventilation should be resolved. Additionally, the patient should have a stable cardiovascular system. Table 5–18 lists criteria to be evaluated prior to weaning patients from mechanical ventilation.

Table 5–18. ASSESSMENT PARAMETERS INDICATING READINESS TO WEAN

Underlying cause for mechanical ventilation resolved
Hemodynamic stability
Adequate respiratory muscle strength
- Respiratory rate <25 breaths/minute
- Negative inspiratory force >-20 cm H_2O
- Vital capacity >15 ml/kg
- Minute ventilation <10 L/min

Adequate ABGs without a high FIO_2 and/or high PEEP
- $PaO_2 >70$ with $FIO_2 <0.5$
- $PaCO_2 <45$
- PEEP <5 cm H_2O

Adequate level of consciousness
Good nutritional status and hydration
Absence of factors which impair weaning
- Infection
- Anemia
- Fatigue
- Sleep deprivation
- Pain
- Abdominal distention

Mentally ready to wean
- Calm, relaxed
- Minimal/absent anxiety
- Motivated

NURSING CARE PLAN FOR THE MECHANICALLY VENTILATED PATIENT

Nursing Diagnosis	Expected Patient Outcome	Nursing Intervention
Ineffective breathing pattern related to disease process, artificial airway, and mechanical ventilator.	The patient will breathe effectively while mechanically ventilated, maintain normal arterial blood gas values, and have absence of symptoms of hypoxemia.	1. Maintain endotracheal tube or tracheostomy: a. Secure tubes with tape or other devices designed for ETT or tracheostomy. b. Only if necessary, restrain patient's wrists. 2. Assess respiratory status every 4 hours: a. Auscultate breath sounds. b. Assess chest excursion. c. Assess patient's ability to initiate a spontaneous breath. d. Assess for signs and symptoms of hypoxemia. 3. Monitor ventilator settings at least every 8 hours: a. Tidal volume b. FIO_2 c. Respiratory rate (machine and spontaneous) d. Mode of ventilation e. Use of PEEP, CPAP, or pressure support 4. Monitor cuff pressures of ETT or tracheostomy: a. Cuff is usually inflated with the minimum amount of air to prevent leak of air around the cuff. b. Several commercial devices are available to monitor cuff pressures. These devices attach to the pilot balloon of the ETT or TT and measure the pressure. c. Notify the physician if cuff pressures exceed 25 cm H_2O 5. Monitor oxygenation and ventilation. Notify the physician if parameters change: a. ABGs b. Continuous PaO_2 monitoring c. Pulse oximetry d. Transcutaneous oxygen and/or CO_2 monitoring e. End tidal CO_2 measurements 6. Monitor serial chest x-rays: a. Assess ETT or tracheostomy tube placement b. Assess improvement or worsening 7. Maintain PEEP: a. Avoid removing patient from the ventilator for suctioning or other procedures if PEEP is used as part of the treatment. b. Consider use of closed tracheal suction devices (Ballard Trach Care [Ballard Medical Products, Midvale, UT] or Concord/Portex Steri-Cath [Concord/Portex, Keene, NH]) or adaptors (e.g., Bodai) when suctioning patient. c. Ensure that manual ventilation bag is equipped with a PEEP valve and is set appropriately. 8. Monitor for complications associated with positive pressure ventilation: a. Barotrauma: 1. Assess for sudden increase in PIP, decreased or absent breath sounds on affected side, tracheal deviation, extreme anxiety, symptoms of shock. 2. If symptoms occur, remove patient from ventilator and manually ventilate with MRB. 3. Prepare for chest tube insertion. b. Decreased cardiac output: 1. Obtain thermodilution cardiac outputs at least every shift if pulmonary artery catheter in place.

continued

NURSING CARE PLAN FOR THE MECHANICALLY VENTILATED PATIENT *Continued*

Nursing Diagnosis	Expected Patient Outcome	Nursing Intervention
		2. Assess for hypotension, tachycardia, dysrhythmias, decreased level of consciousness. 9. Do not disconnect mechanical ventilation to perform tracheostomy care on a patient. To facilitate tracheostomy care: a. Consider use of tracheostomy *without* inner cannula. b. Consider use of tracheostomy tube with disposable inner cannula. c. Keep an extra clean inner cannula readily available for use. 10. Keep tubings free of moisture: a. Empty tubings prior to repositioning patient to avoid aspiration of moisture. b. Empty tubings as needed. Avoid draining water backwards through the ventilator circuit where the tubing connects to the patient. Do not drain water into cascade. c. Consider using devices (e.g., water traps) to facilitate drainage of moisture. 11. Medicate the patient if needed: a. Morphine—2.5 to 16 mg IV push every 1 to 2 hours. Can be reversed with naloxone hydrochloride (Narcan) if needed. b. Diazepam (Valium)—2 to 5 mg IV push every 2 to 4 hours (recommended maximum dose is 30 mg in 8 hours). c. Lorazepam (Ativan)—2 mg IV push every 6 hours (up to 4 mg can be given; however, dose should not exceed 10 mg/day) d. Pancuronium bromide (Pavulon)—0.04 to 0.1 mg/kg IV initially; then 1 to 2 mg every hour 1. Monitor patient constantly. 2. *Always* give sedatives concurrently with paralytic agents. 3. Offer reassurance to patient. 4. Protect eyes. 5. Can be reversed with neostigmine or edrophonium (Tensilon) if needed. (NOTE: Several new neuromuscular blocking agents are also being used.) 12. Monitor readiness to wean from ventilator (see Table 5-18): a. Assess spontaneous respiratory efforts. b. Assess tidal volume, vital capacity, negative inspiratory force. c. Monitor vital signs.
Ineffective airway clearance related to artificial airway, decreased ability to cough.	The patient will maintain an open airway free of secretions.	1. Assess need for suctioning (pressure alarm on ventilator, audible secretions, harsh breath sounds). 2. Suction according to hospital protocol (see Tables 5-15 and 5-16). 3. Assess breath sounds after suctioning. 4. Consider use of tracheal lavage if secretions are thick: a. Use 3 to 5 ml normal saline for tracheal instillation (do not use bacteriostatic normal saline or other preparations with preservatives). b. Instill saline into ETT or tracheostomy and manually ventilate the patient to disperse the saline.

NURSING CARE PLAN FOR THE MECHANICALLY VENTILATED PATIENT *Continued*

Nursing Diagnosis	Expected Patient Outcome	Nursing Intervention
		c. If closed tracheal suction device is used, insert suction catheter 4 to 6 in and then instill the saline. 5. If tracheal secretions are thick, assess hydration of patient. 6. Reposition the patient frequently to mobilize secretions.
Impaired verbal communication related to artificial airway and mechanical ventilation.	Patient will be able to communicate needs to caregiver.	1. Establish method for communication: a. Yes/No questions. b. Clipboard with paper and pencil. c. Magic slates. d. Picture communication boards. e. Computerized systems if available. f. Attempt lip reading if patient has nasotracheal tube or tracheostomy. 2. Speak slowly and clearly to patient. 3. Explain procedures. 4. Use significant others to assist with communication. 5. Consider use of "talking" tracheostomy tube. 6. Expect frustration from both patient and nurse.
Alteration in oral mucous membranes related to artificial airway.	Moist oral mucous membranes; absence of ulceration or other lesions.	1. Assess oral mucous membranes for ulcerations or other lesions. 2. If commercial devices are used to secure the airway, carefully inspect the mouth around and under the devices. Loosen the devices periodically as recommended by the manufacturers. 3. Provide good mouth care at least once per shift: a. Use oral swabs specifically designed for mouth care. Some institutions have kits with swabs, peroxide solution, and lip lubricant. b. Brush teeth. Use syringe to rinse mouth and tonsil suction to remove secretions. A toothbrush that attaches to suction is also commercially available c. Lubricate lips with water-soluble ointment or emollients such as Chapstick. d. *Avoid* lemon-glycerine swabs (they dry the mouth). e. Avoid mouthwashes that contain alcohol. 4. Reposition endotracheal tube according to hospital protocol (usually once per day) (may not be necessary if commercial device used.): a. Two personnel required for procedure: one to hold endotracheal tube and one for taping the tube. b. Suction endotracheal tube prior to repositioning tube. c. Move tube to opposite side of mouth and secure according to protocol. d. If an ETT is repositioned, this is an excellent time to give mouth care. e. Any time the ETT is repositioned, placement should be verified by auscultating bilateral breath sounds after completion of the procedure.
Anxiety and fear related to need for mechanical ventilation, inability to communicate needs, psychological ventilator dependence.	Relief of anxiety and fear.	1. Talk to patient frequently. 2. Explain procedures. 3. Establish communication. 4. Reassure patient that needs are being met. 5. Keep call light within reach. 6. Encourage significant others to visit with patient.

continued

NURSING CARE PLAN FOR THE MECHANICALLY VENTILATED PATIENT *Continued*

Nursing Diagnosis	Expected Patient Outcome	Nursing Intervention
Alteration in nutrition related to inability to take oral feedings, increased nutritional needs, impaired gastrointestinal function.	Adequate nutritional status.	1. Assess gastrointestinal function at least once per shift: a. Assess bowel sounds. b. Assess for gastric distention. 2. Monitor bowel habits. 3. Monitor daily weight. 4. Obtain dietary consult/nutritional evaluation. 5. Administer parenteral or enteral feedings according to hospital protocol: a. Add food color to enteral feedings to monitor for potential aspiration (controversial). b. Check gastric residual every 4 hours. 6. Observe ABGs for CO_2 retention.
Potential for pulmonary infection related to artificial airway.	Patient will remain infection free.	1. Monitor temperature every 4 hours. 2. Monitor amount, color, consistency, and odor of secretions. 3. Use good handwashing techniques. 4. Wear gloves for suctioning, oral care, and repositioning endotracheal tubes. 5. Use aseptic technique for suctioning. 6. Obtain tracheal aspirate for culture and sensitivity according to hospital protocol. 7. Administer antibiotics as ordered.
Potential for injury: gastrointestinal bleeding related to positive pressure ventilation, stress of critical illness.	Absence or prevention of bleeding.	1. Assess bowel sounds every shift. 2. Assess gastric contents for presence of occult blood. 3. Guaiac all stools. 4. Monitor bowel habits. Observe for tarry and/or bloody stools. 5. Monitor serial hemoglobin and hematocrit values. 6. Monitor gastric pH. Administer antacids as ordered to decrease acidity of gastric contents. 7. Administer histamine antagonists as ordered; e.g., cimetidine (Tagamet) and ranitidine (Zantac).
Potential for fluid volume excess related to ventilator humidification, stimulation of renin-angiotensin-aldosterone mechanism.	Absence of fluid overload.	1. Monitor intake and output every shift. 2. Monitor daily weight. 3. Assess breath sounds every 4 hours. 4. Assess vital signs every 2 to 4 hours. 5. Provide adequate nutrition.

TEAM APPROACH

A team approach is essential in the weaning of patients from long-term mechanical ventilation. Team members include nurses, physicians, respiratory therapists, dietitian, physical therapist, occupational therapist, social worker, and pastoral ministers.

METHODS FOR WEANING

Methods for weaning include the use of IMV/SIMV, T-piece (Briggs), pressure support, and CPAP. A combination of methods is frequently used.

IMV/SIMV. When IMV/SIMV is used for weaning, the respiratory rate is gradually decreased until the patient is assuming all of the work of breathing. For example, the IMV/SIMV rate is decreased by two breaths per minute at designated intervals as long as the patient tolerates the process. This method works exceptionally well in weaning postoperative patients from mechanical ventilation. The respiratory rate is frequently decreased on an hourly basis until the patient is weaned and ready for extubation. In contrast, the patient who has been on the ventilator for an extended period of time may require the IMV rate to be decreased by one breath per minute each *day*. An advantage of using the

IMV/SIMV method is that it is done on a continuous basis. It can be used during the night hours as well as during the day.

T-Piece. The T-piece, or Briggs', method requires that the patient be removed from mechanical ventilation for short periods of time, usually beginning with a 5-minute period. The ventilator is removed from the patient, and the T-piece is connected to the patient's ETT or tracheostomy tube. Supplemental oxygen is provided through the device. The patient breathes spontaneously for the predetermined amount of time. The time off the ventilator is gradually increased. For example, initially the patient may be weaned 5 minutes every 6 hours. As the patient tolerates the procedure, the weaning may occur for 15 minutes every 4 hours. If this method is used, it is important to begin the procedure in the morning after the patient is well rested. The procedure should be adequately explained to the patient. It is essential that the nurse stay with the patient during the initial weaning attempts to adequately assess tolerance to the procedure and relieve patient fear and anxiety that may be associated with the procedure. An advantage of the T-piece method is that it encourages the patient to increase the strength of the respiratory muscles.

Pressure Support. Pressure support is a newer method to assist in patient weaning. As previously noted, pressure support decreases the workload of breathing and increases the patient's ability to initiate spontaneous breathing efforts. In other words, it makes it easier for the patient to breathe. Pressure support is frequently used in conjunction with IMV/SIMV.

CPAP. CPAP is another method to facilitate weaning from mechanical ventilation. As previously noted, CPAP augments spontaneous breaths by increasing the functional residual capacity. It can be used with the newer mechanical ventilators.

WEANING PROCEDURE

During any weaning attempt, several steps should be followed. The procedure should be explained to the patient and family in a manner which reduces anxiety. The patient should be adequately rested. The patient should be positioned comfortably. Baseline parameters, including vital signs, heart rhythm, and ABGs, should be obtained prior to any weaning attempt. The patient should be observed during the weaning process for tolerance or intolerance to the procedure.

Table 5–19. CRITERIA FOR DISCONTINUING WEANING
Respiratory rate >25 breaths per minute or <8
Blood pressure increases >30 mm Hg or decreases >20 mm Hg
Heart rate increases >30 beats/minute
Dysrhythmias (e.g., premature ventricular contractions)
Use of accessory muscles
Labored respirations
Diaphoresis
Restlessness
Signs and symptoms of hypoxemia

WHEN WEANING SHOULD BE DISCONTINUED

The weaning process should be stopped if physiological changes occur (Table 5–19). If a patient exhibits signs of not tolerating the weaning process, ABGs should be drawn and the patient should be placed back on the ventilator at the previous settings.

CAUSES OF IMPAIRED WEANING

Weaning may be impaired owing to several causes: increased oxygen demand, decreased lung function, psychological causes, and because of equipment or technique. Increased oxygen demands may be caused by anemia, fever, or pain. Decreased lung function may result from malnutrition, overuse of sedatives or hypnotics, and sleep deprivation. Psychological causes include apprehension and fear, helplessness, and depression. Equipment and technique problems include the time of day, inadequate weaning periods, and inability to tolerate the technique.

Summary

Care of critically ill patients requires knowledge of normal anatomy and physiology and excellent assessment skills. Skills in establishing and maintaining an open airway and initiating mechanical ventilation are also essential. Care of the patient requiring mechanical ventilation is an everyday assignment in the critical care unit; therefore, it is essential that the nurse apply knowledge and skills to effectively care for these patients.

References

Ackerman, M. H. (1985): The use of bolus normal saline instillations in artificial airways: Is it useful or necessary? *Heart and Lung* 14:505–506.

American Heart Association (1987, 1990): *Textbook of Advanced Cardiac Life Support.* 2nd ed. Dallas.

Ashworth, L. J. (1990): Pressure support ventilation. *Critical Care Nurse* 10(7):20–25.

Burns, S. M. (1990): Advances in ventilator therapy. *Focus on Critical Care* 17:227–237.

Craig, K. C., Benson, M. S., and Peirson, D. J. (1984): Prevention of arterial oxygen desaturation during closed-airway endotracheal suction: Effect of ventilatory mode. *Respiratory Care* 29:1013–1018.

Guyton, A. C. (1986): *Textbook of Medical Physiology.* 7th ed. Philadelphia: W. B. Saunders.

Kersten, L. D. (1989): *Comprehensive Respiratory Nursing: A Decision Making Approach.* Philadelphia: W. B. Saunders.

Noll, M. L., Hix, C. D., and Scott, G. (1990): Closed-tracheal suction systems: Effectiveness and nursing implications. *AACN Clinical Issues in Critical Care Nursing* 1:318–326.

St. John, R. E., and LeFrak, S. S. (1990): Alternate modes of mechanical ventilation. *AACN Clinical Issues in Critical Care Nursing* 1:248–259.

Stone, K. S. (1990): Ventilator versus manual resuscitation bag as the method for delivering hyperoxygenation prior to endotracheal suctioning. *AACN Clinical Issues in Critical Care Nursing* 1:289–299.

Toben, B. P., and Lewandowski, V. (1988): Nontraditional and new ventilatory techniques. *Critical Care Nursing Quarterly* 11(3):12–28.

Traver, G. A., and Flodquist-Priestly, G. (1986): Management problems in unilateral lung disease with emphasis on differential lung ventilation. *Critical Care Nurse* 6(4):40–50.

VonRueden, K. T. (1990): Noninvasive assessment of gas exchange in the critically ill. *AACN Clinical Issues in Critical Care Nursing* 1:239–247.

Witta, K. (1990). New techniques for weaning difficult patients from mechanical ventilation. *AACN Clinical Issues in Critical Care Nursing* 1:260–266.

Recommended Reading

Anderson, S. (1990): Six easy steps to interpreting blood gases. *American Journal of Nursing* 90(8):42–45.

Birdsall, C. (1986): How do you use a closed suction adaptor? *American Journal of Nursing* 86:1222–1223.

Chung, D. C., and Lamb, A. M. (1990): *Essentials of Anesthesiology.* 2nd ed. Philadelphia: W. B. Saunders.

Dettenmeier, P. A. (1990): Planning for successful home mechanical ventilation. *AACN Clinical Issues in Critical Care Nursing* 1:267–279.

Geisman, L. K. (1989): Advances in weaning from mechanical ventilation. *Critical Care Nursing Clinics of North America* 1:697–705.

Grossbach, I. (1986a): Troubleshooting ventilator- and patient-related problems/Part 1. *Critical Care Nurse* 6(4):58–70.

Grossbach, I. (1986b): Troubleshooting ventilator- and patient-related problems/Part 2. *Critical Care Nurse* 6(5):64–79.

Harvey, M. A. (1986): *Study Guide to the Core Curriculum for Critical Care Nursing.* Philadelphia: W. B. Saunders.

Holloway, N. M. (1989): *Critical Care Plans.* Springhouse, PA: Springhouse.

Holtzman, G. M., Warner, S. C., Melnik, G., and Beer, W. (1990): Nutritional support of pulmonary patients: A multidisciplinary approach. *AACN Clinical Issues in Critical Care Nursing* 1:300–312.

Kersten, L. D. (1989): *Comprehensive Respiratory Nursing: A Decision Making Approach.* Philadelphia: W. B. Saunders.

Majors, M. (1988): Nutritional support of the mechanically ventilated patient. *Critical Care Nursing Quarterly* 11(3):50–61.

Mayo, J. M., and Hamner, J. B. (1987): A nurse's guide to mechanical ventilation. *RN* 50(8):18–24.

McCauley, M. D., and VonRueden, K. T. (1988): Noninvasive monitoring of the mechanically ventilated patient. *Critical Care Nursing Quarterly* 11(3):36–49.

Miracle, V. A., and Allnutt, D. R. (1990): How to perform basic airway management. *Nursing* 20(4):55–60.

Norton, L. C., and Neureuter, A. (1989): Weaning the long-term ventilator-dependent patient: Common problems and management. *Critical Care Nurse* 9(1):42–52.

Romanski, S. O. (1986): Interpreting ABG's. *Nursing* 16(9):58–63.

Rutherford, K. A. (1989): Advances in the treatment of oxygenation disturbances. *Critical Care Nursing Clinics of North America* 1:659–667.

Rutherford, K. A. (1989): Principles and applications of oximetry. *Critical Care Nursing Clinics of North America* 1:649–657.

Solomon, E. P., and Phillips, G. A. (1987): *Understanding Human Anatomy and Physiology.* Philadelphia: W. B. Saunders.

Sonesso, G. (1990): Negative pressure ventilation: New uses for an old technique. *AACN Clinical Issues in Critical Care Nursing* 1:313–317.

Vasbinder-Dillon, D. (1988): Understanding mechanical ventilation. *Critical Care Nurse* 8(7):42–56.

Weilitz, P. B. (1989): New modes of mechanical ventilation. *Critical Care Nursing Clinics of North America* 1:697–705.

Chapter

6

Anne-Marie Jones, R.N., M.S.N., CCRN
Mary Lou Noll, R.N., Ph.D., CCRN
Marilyn Lamborn, R.N., Ph.D.

Code Management

Objectives

- Compare roles of caregivers in managing cardiopulmonary arrest situations.
- Identify equipment used during a code.
- Differentiate basic and advanced life support measures employed during a code.
- Identify medications used in code management, including use, action, side effects, and nursing implications.
- Discuss treatment of special problems that can occur during a code.
- Identify information to be documented during a code.
- Describe care of patients after resuscitation.
- Identify psychosocial, legal, and ethical issues related to code management.

Code, Code Blue, Code 99, and Dr. Heart are terms frequently used in hospital settings to refer to emergency situations requiring life-saving resuscitation and interventions. Codes are called when patients suffer a cardiac and/or respiratory arrest or a life-threatening cardiac dysrhythmia that has caused loss of consciousness. (The generic term *arrest* will be used to refer to these conditions.) Whatever the cause, patient survival and a positive outcome depend on prompt recognition of the situation and immediate institution of basic and advanced life-support measures. Code management refers to the initiation of a code and the life-saving interventions performed when a patient arrests.

This chapter discusses the roles of personnel involved in a code and identifies equipment that needs to be readily available during a code. Basic and advanced life-support measures are presented, including commonly used drugs. The chapter concludes with a brief discussion of psychosocial, legal, and ethical implications of code management. For more in-depth and comprehensive information, the reader is referred to the following American Heart Association (AHA) publications:

> Standards and guidelines for cardiopulmonary resuscitation and emergency cardiac care (1986). *JAMA* 255:2843–2989. American Heart Association (1987, 1990): *Textbook of Advanced Cardiac Life Support.* Dallas: Author.

Basic Cardiac Life Support (BCLS) certification should be held by all personnel involved in hospital patient care, and is also recommended for the lay public. Advanced Cardiac Life Support (ACLS) provider certification is available through the American Heart Association (AHA) and is strongly recommended for anyone working in critical care.

Roles of Caregivers in Code Management

Prompt recognition of a patient arrest and rapid initiation of cardiopulmonary resuscitation (CPR) and advanced life-support measures are essential in order to improve patient outcomes. The first person to recognize that a patient has suffered an arrest should call for help, instruct someone to call a code, and begin CPR. One-person CPR is continued until additional help arrives.

THE CODE TEAM

Key personnel are notified to assist with code management. The overhead paging system or individual pagers may be used to contact personnel, depending on hospital policies.

Most hospitals have code teams designated to respond to codes (Table 6–1). The code team usually consists of a physician, intensive care unit (ICU) or emergency department (ED) nurse, nursing supervisor, anesthetist or anesthesiologist, respiratory therapist, pharmacist or pharmacy technician, and electrocardiogram (ECG) technician. The code team responds to the code and works in conjunction with the patient's nurse and primary physician, if present. If a code team does not exist, any available personnel usually respond.

Table 6–1. ROLES AND RESPONSIBILITIES OF CODE TEAM MEMBERS

Team Member	Primary Role
Director of the Code (usually a physician)	Make diagnoses and treatment decisions
Primary Nurse	Provide information to code director Contact attending physician Assist with medications and procedures
Nurse	"Man" the crash cart Prepare medications Assemble equipment (intubation, suction) Defibrillate
Nursing Supervisor	Control the crowd Assist with medications and procedures Ensure that a bed is available in ICU Assist with transfer of patient to ICU
Nurse or Assistant	Record events
Anesthesiologist/ Nurse Anesthetist/ Emergency Physician	Intubate patient Manage airway and oxygenation
Respiratory Therapist	Assist with ventilation Draw arterial blood gases Set up respiratory equipment
Code Management Pharmacist/ Technician	Assist with medication administration Prepare IV infusions
ECG Technician	Perform 12-lead ECG

DIRECTOR OF THE CODE

The person who directs, or "runs," the code is responsible for making diagnoses and treatment decisions. The director is usually a physician, preferably experienced in code management, such as an ED physician. However, the director may be the patient's primary physician or another physician who is available and qualified for the task. If several physicians are present, one should assume responsibility for being the code team leader, and be the only one giving orders for interventions to avoid confusion and conflict. In some small hospitals, codes may be directed by a nurse certified in ACLS. In this situation, standing physician orders are needed to guide and support the nurse's decision making.

The director of the code needs as much information about the patient as possible in order to make treatment decisions. Necessary information includes the reason for the patient's hospitalization, current treatments and medications, and events that occurred immediately prior to the code.

If possible, the code director should not be performing CPR or other tasks. Full attention should be given to assessment, diagnosis, and treatment decisions in order to direct resuscitative efforts.

CODE NURSES

Primary Nurse. The patient's primary nurse should be free to relate information to the person directing the code. The primary nurse may also start intravenous (IV) lines, give emergency drugs, or defibrillate the patient as directed by the code director. In some cases, the primary nurse may need to leave the code in order to contact the patient's attending physician or relate information to the family.

Second Nurse. An important task for the second nurse present is to "man" the crash cart. This nurse should be thoroughly familiar with the layout of the cart and location of items. This nurse locates, prepares, and labels medications and IV fluids. He/she also assembles equipment for intubation, suctioning, and other procedures such as central line insertion.

Nursing Supervisor. The nursing supervisor responds to the code to assist in whatever manner is needed. Frequently, more people respond to a code than are needed. One job of the supervisor is to limit the number of people in the code to only those necessary and those there for learning purposes. This cuts down on crowding and confusion. Maintaining communication with staff and family, and assisting with procedures such as IV insertion are other examples of how the nursing supervisor helps. If the patient needs to be transferred to the critical care unit, the supervisor can also coordinate the transfer and ensure that a critical care bed is available.

ANESTHESIOLOGIST/NURSE ANESTHETIST

The anesthesiologist or anesthetist assumes control of the patient's ventilation and oxygenation. This individual (or another trained individual) intubates the patient to ensure an adequate airway and to facilitate ventilation. The primary or secondary nurse assists with the set-up and checking of intubation equipment.

RESPIRATORY THERAPIST

The respiratory therapist usually assists with manual ventilation of the patient before and after intubation. The therapist may also draw arterial blood gases, set up oxygen and ventilation equipment, and suction the patient.

PHARMACIST/PHARMACY TECHNICIAN

In some hospitals, a pharmacist or pharmacy technician responds to codes. This individual may prepare medications and mix intravenous infusions for administration during the code. Frequently, pharmacy is also responsible for bringing additional medications. At the termination of the code, pharmacy staff may replenish the crash cart supplies and make pharmacy charges to the patient's account.

ECG TECHNICIAN

In some hospitals, an ECG technician responds to codes. This individual stands by to perform 12-lead ECGs that may be ordered.

OTHER CODE TEAM MEMBERS

Another person that may respond to a code is the hospital chaplain. The chaplain can be very helpful in comforting and waiting with the patient's family. If a chaplain is not available, the charge nurse or some other person should be available for this important task. This individual should take the family to a quiet, private area for waiting and remain with them during the code. The individual may also be able to check on the patient periodically to give the family a progress report.

Other personnel should be available to run errands, such as taking blood samples to the lab, or getting additional supplies. Meanwhile, the other patients need monitoring and care. Only staff necessary in the code should remain; otherwise, they should attend to the rest of the patients.

Equipment Used During a Code

THE CRASH CART

While the first person to recognize a code calls for help and begins life-support measures, another team member should immediately bring the crash cart to the patient's bedside (Fig. 6–1). Crash carts vary in organization and layout, but they all contain the same basic emergency equipment and medications. Many hospitals have standardized crash carts, so that anyone responding to the code is familiar with the location of items on the cart. However, the make-up and organization of the crash cart may be unique to each unit. Whether carts are standardized or unique to an individual unit, nurses responding to codes must be familiar with the cart.

Most carts have equipment stored on top as well as in several drawers. Equipment, such as back boards and portable suction machines, are frequently attached to the cart. The larger equipment is stored on the top of the cart or in a large drawer; smaller items such as medications and IV equipment are in the smaller drawers.

A back board is usually located on the back or side of the cart. It should be placed under the patient as soon as possible to provide a hard, level surface for performing chest compressions. The patient is either lifted up or log-rolled to one side in order to place the back board. Care should be taken to protect the patient's cervical spine if injury is suspected.

A monitor/defibrillator is usually located on top of the cart. The ECG leads, electrodes, and

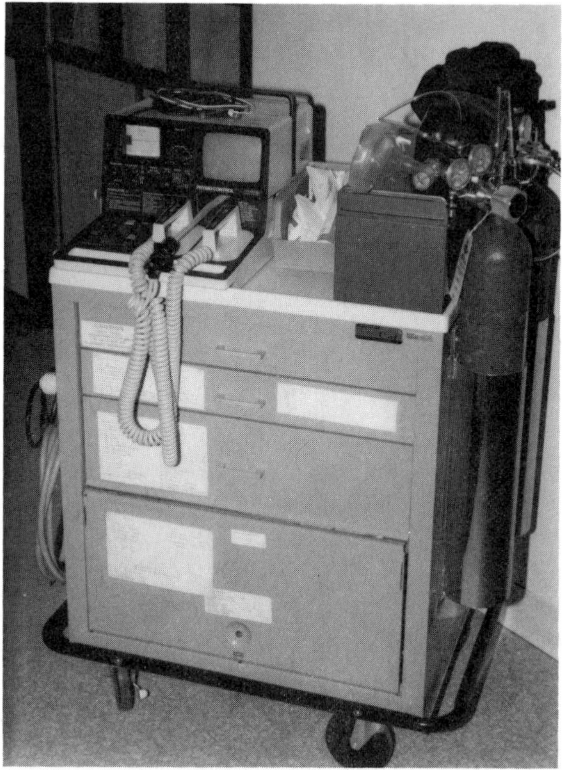

Figure 6-1. A typical crash cart.

gel or pads for defibrillation should be located with the monitor. The patient's cardiac rhythm is monitored via the leads and electrodes. Cardiac rhythm can also be noted by placing the defibrillation paddles on the chest using the "quick look" mode. In the hospital setting, continuous monitoring via the electrodes is preferable to the quick look mode. The monitor should have a recorder to document the patient's rhythm for the cardiac arrest record.

An external pacemaker may be stored on the crash cart. A combination monitor, defibrillator, and external pacemaker is also available.

A manual resuscitation bag (MRB) with a face mask and oxygen tubing attached is usually kept on top of the crash cart. The tubing should be connected either to a wall oxygen inlet or to a portable oxygen tank on the crash cart. Supplemental oxygen should always be used with the MRB.

Airway supplies are located in one of the drawers. Oral and nasal airways, endotracheal tubes, laryngoscope handles and blades, Magill forceps, lubricating jelly, 5-ml syringes, and tape are items that should be available.

Another drawer contains IV supplies, including IV needles and catheters of various sizes, IV start kits, tape, syringes, IV fluids, and IV tubing. Normal saline and 5% dextrose in 250-ml and 500-ml bags are the IV fluids most often used.

Emergency medications fill another drawer. These include IV push drugs as well as medications that must be added to IV fluids for continuous infusions. Most IV push drugs are available in prefilled syringes. Several drugs that are given via a constant infusion (e.g., lidocaine, dopamine) are also available as premixed infusions. Drugs will be discussed in more depth in the segment on pharmacological intervention.

Other important items on the cart include a suction set-up and suction catheters, nasogastric tubes, and a blood pressure cuff. Various trays are also frequently kept on the crash cart: venous cut-down, tracheotomy, and central line insertion.

The crash cart is usually checked by nursing staff every shift to ensure that all equipment and drugs are present and functional. Once the cart is fully stocked, it should be kept locked to avoid "borrowing" supplies and equipment.

The nurse can become familiar with the location of items on the cart by being responsible for checking it. Management of the code is more efficient when the nurse knows where items are located on the crash cart as well as how to use them.

■ Resuscitation Efforts

The flow of events during a code is a concentrated team effort. Basic cardiac life support is provided until the code team arrives to provide advanced life-support measures. Once help has arrived, CPR is continued using the two-person technique. Other tasks such as connecting the patient to an ECG monitor, starting IVs, and attaching an oxygen source to the manual resuscitation bag should be carried out by available personnel as soon as possible. The activities during the code are summarized in Table 6-2. It is important to note that frequently several activities are done simultaneously.

BASIC CARDIAC LIFE SUPPORT (BCLS)

The purposes of BCLS are (1) to prevent respiratory and/or cardiac arrest through prompt assessment and intervention and (2) to support respiration and circulation through CPR (AHA, 1988). Cardiopulmonary resuscitation must be initiated immediately in the event of an arrest in order to

Table 6–2. FLOW OF EVENTS DURING A CODE

Priorities	Equipment from Cart	Intervention
1. Recognition of arrest		1. Initiate CPR and call for help.
2. Arrival of resuscitation team, emergency cart, monitor-defibrillator	2a. Cardiac board b. Mouth-to-mask or bag-valve-mask unit with O_2 tubing c. Oral airway d. (oxygen and regulator if not already at bedside)	2a. Place patient on cardiac board. b. Ventilate with 100% O_2 with oral airway and mouth-to-mask or bag-valve-mask device. c. Continue chest compressions.
3. Identification of team leader		3a. Assess patient. b. Direct and supervise team members. c. Solve problems. d. Obtain patient history and information about events leading up to the code.
4. Rhythm diagnosis	4. Cardiac monitor with quick-look paddles—defibrillator (limb leads, ECG machine—12 lead)	4a. Apply quick-look paddles first. b. Limb leads, but do not interrupt CPR.
5. Prompt defibrillation if indicated		5. Use correct algorithm.
6. Venous access	6a. Peripheral or central IV materials b. IV tubing, infusion fluid	6a. Peripheral: antecubital. b. Central: internal jugular, or subclavian.
7. Drug administration	7. Drugs as ordered (and in anticipation, based on algorithms) for bolus and continuous infusion	7a. Use correct algorithm. b. Bolus or infusion.
8. Intubation	8a. Suction equipment b. Laryngoscope c. Endotracheal tube and other intubation equipment d. Stethoscope	8a. Connect suction equipment. b. Intubate patient (interrupt CPR no more than 30 seconds). c. Check tube position (listen for bilateral breath sounds). d. Hyperventilate and oxygenate.
9. Ongoing assessment of the patient's response to therapy during resuscitation		9. Assess frequently: a. pulse generated with CPR (IS THERE A PULSE?); b. adequacy of artificial ventilation; c. spontaneous pulse after any intervention/rhythm change (IS THERE A PULSE?); d. spontaneous breathing with return of pulse (IS THERE BREATHING?); e. blood pressure, if pulse is present; f. decision to stop, if no response to therapy.
10. Documentation	10. Resuscitation record	10. Accurately record events while resuscitation is in progress.
11. Drawing arterial and venous blood specimens	11. Arterial puncture and venipuncture equipment	11a. Draw specimens. b. Treat as needed, based on results.
12. Controlling or limiting crowd		12. Dismiss those not required for bedside tasks.

From American Heart Association. *Textbook of Advanced Cardiac Life Support.* Dallas: Author, 1987, 1990, 2nd ed.

prevent brain damage and improve patient outcomes. Brain damage may occur after 4 to 6 minutes without adequate oxygen.

The ABCs of cardiopulmonary resuscitation are: Airway, Breathing, and Circulation. Assessment is a part of each step, and the steps are done in order (Table 6–3). The following summary is adapted from the AHA Standards for Basic Cardiac Life Support (AHA, 1988).

Airway. An open airway is essential. The first intervention is to assess unresponsiveness by tapping or shaking a patient and shouting, "Are

Table 6–3. STEPS IN BASIC CARDIAC LIFE SUPPORT

1. Airway
   Determine unresponsiveness.
   Call for help.
   Position patient on back.
   Open airway using head-tilt/chin-lift technique.
2. Breathing
   Assess breathing.
   If breathing present, maintain airway.
   If breathing absent, give two breaths.
   Activate the cardiac arrest team, if possible.
3. Circulation
   Determine pulselessness.
   Activate cardiac arrest team, if not previously done.
   If pulse present, perform rescue breathing at 12 breaths/min.
   If pulse absent, perform chest compressions at rate of 80 to 100 beats/min.
   Alternate compressions and breaths at a rate of 15:2.

From American Heart Association. *Healthcare Provider's Manual for Basic Life Support.* Dallas, Author, 1988.

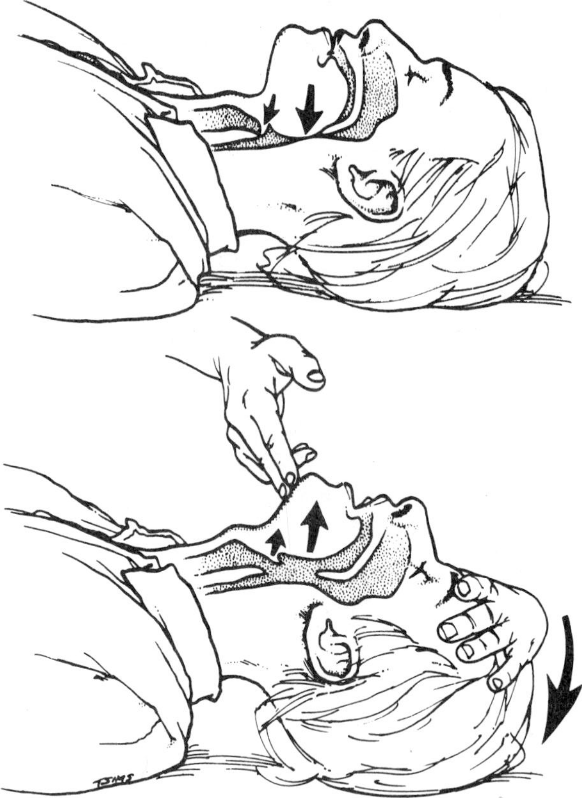

Figure 6–2. Head-tilt/chin-lift technique for opening the airway. *Top:* Airway obstruction produced by the tongue and epiglottis. *Bottom:* Relief by head-tilt/chin-lift. (Reproduced with permission. © Healthcare Provider's Manual for Basic Life Support, 1988, Fig. 22, p. 36. Copyright American Heart Association.)

you OK?" If the patient is unresponsive, the nurse calls for help by shouting to fellow caregivers or using the nurse-call system. The patient is positioned on his/her back and the airway is opened using the head-tilt, chin-lift method (Fig. 6–2). If the patient needs to be turned to the supine position, it is important to turn him/her as a unit to prevent possible injury.

Breathing. The second step of CPR is to assess breathing and initiate rescue breathing if necessary. Early initiation of rescue breathing may prevent a cardiac arrest in a patient who quits breathing but still has a pulse (e.g., patient with hypercapnia). In order to assess breathing, the nurse *looks, listens,* and *feels* for breathing while maintaining an open airway. The nurse *looks* at the chest wall to see if it is moving up and down, *listens* for air movement, and *feels* for exhaled air. Rescue breathing, ventilation, is initiated if the patient is not breathing.

If possible, the code team should be notified of the arrest at this time. The first person who arrives to help should call the code. Some critical care units and emergency departments have an emergency call system that can be activated from the patient's room by pressing a button. If this type of system is not available and the nurse is alone, he/she should press the nurse-call system and begin rescue breathing. When the call is answered, the nurse should state, "Call a code!"

In order to perform mouth-to-mouth resuscitation, the open airway is maintained, the nurse seals his/her mouth over the patient's mouth, pinches off the patient's nose, and gives two (2) breaths to the patient (Fig. 6–3). If the nurse experiences difficulty in ventilating the patient, the head should be repositioned because improper head position is the most common cause of the inability to ventilate.

If the patient has a mouth injury or the nurse has difficulty maintaining a good seal, mouth-to-nose ventilation can be done. Mouth-to-stoma ventilation is done when the patient has a tracheostomy or laryngectomy.

Alternatives to mouth-to-mouth resuscitation include mouth-to-mask techniques and ventilation with an MRB and face mask. Both of these techniques are frequently used in the hospital setting. Many hospitals have a pocket mask at every patient's bedside. Additionally, most critical care units have an MRB in every patient's room.

The mouth-to-mask technique involves placing a pocket mask over the patient's mouth and

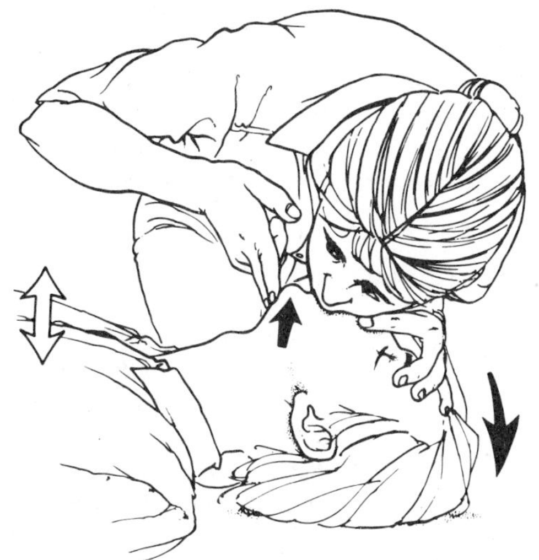

Figure 6-3. Mouth-to-mouth technique for rescue breathing (Reproduced with permission. © Healthcare Provider's Manual for Basic Life Support, 1988, Fig. 25, p. 39. Copyright American Heart Association.)

breathing through a mouthpiece connected to the mask (Fig. 6-4). Pocket masks have a one-way valve that protects the nurse from the patient's exhalation.

In order to ventilate the patient with an MRB and face mask, an open airway must be maintained. Frequently, an oral airway is used to keep the airway patent and facilitate ventilation. The MRB is connected to an oxygen source set at 15 L/min. The face mask is positioned over the patient's mouth and nose. While maintaining a good seal with the mask, the nurse manually ventilates the patient with the MRB (Fig. 6-5). Personnel should be properly trained in order to use the MRB effectively. For more information on the use of the MRB, see Chapter 5.

Circulation. The third step of CPR is to ensure adequate circulation. After the initial two breaths are given, the nurse assesses the patient to determine the presence or absence of a pulse. The pulse is assessed even if the patient is on a cardiac monitor, since artifact or a loose lead may mimic a cardiac dysrhythmia. The nurse checks the patient's carotid pulse on the side nearest him/her. The pulse is assessed for 5 to 10 seconds to detect bradycardia.

If a pulse is *present,* the nurse continues to perform rescue breathing at a rate of 12 breaths per minute, or 1 breath every 5 seconds. The pulse should be assessed periodically.

If the pulse is *absent,* the nurse begins cardiac compressions. The code team should be notified if this has not been previously done. Proper hand position is essential when performing compressions (Fig. 6-6). The location for compressions is on the lower sternum above the xiphoid process. To locate the proper area, the nurse runs his/her fingers up the rib cage to the notch where

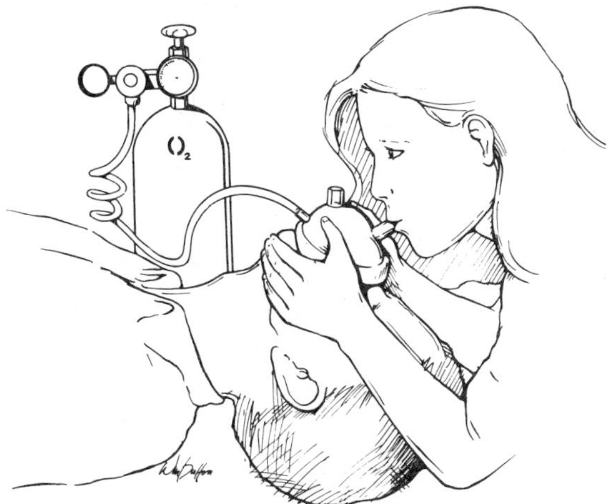

Figure 6-4. Mouth-to-mask technique for rescue breathing. (Reproduced with permission. © Textbook of Advanced Cardiac Life Support, 1987, 1990, 2nd ed. Fig. 17, p. 36. Copyright American Heart Association.)

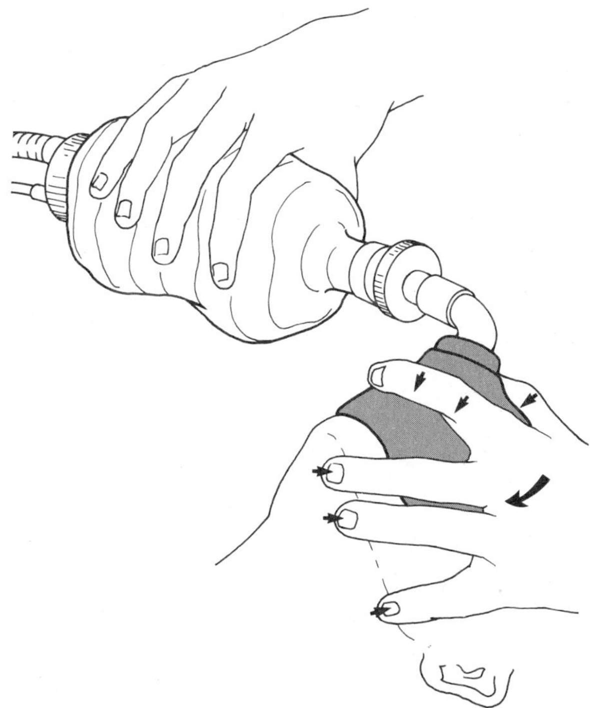

Figure 6-5. Rescue breathing with manual resuscitation bag and face mask. (From Kersten, L. D.: Comprehensive Respiratory Nursing. Philadelphia, W. B. Saunders, 1989, Fig. 24-8, p. 629.)

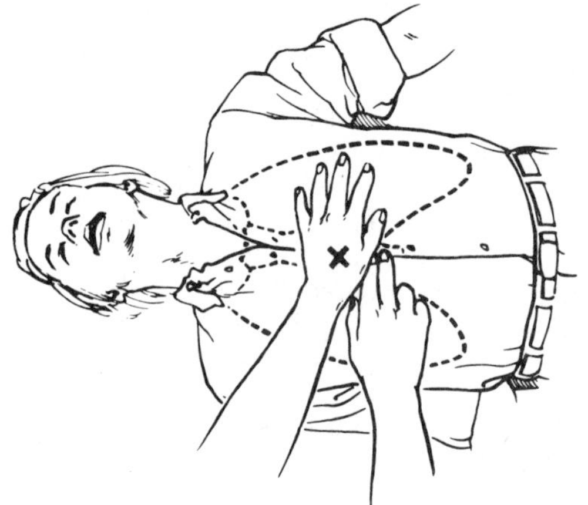

Figure 6-6. Proper hand placement for cardiac compressions during CPR. (Reproduced with permission. © Healthcare Provider's Manual for Basic Life Support, 1988, Fig. 33, p. 42. Copyright American Heart Association.)

the ribs and sternum meet. The middle finger is placed on the notch, and the index finger is aligned next to the middle finger. The heel of the opposite hand is placed next to the index finger. The first hand is then positioned on top of the hand on the sternum. Using both hands, compressions are begun by depressing the sternum 1.5 to 2.0 in for the average adult (Fig. 6-7). Compressions are performed at a rate of 80 to 100 per minute at a ratio of 15 compressions to two breaths (15:2). The carotid pulse is checked after 1 minute of CPR. If the pulse is absent, CPR is continued until additional help arrives. When there is adequate personnel to perform two-man CPR, one person maintains the airway and does rescue breathing while the other person performs compressions. During two-man CPR, the rate of compressions to breaths is 5:1.

Advanced Life Support

Basic cardiac life support is continued until the code team arrives. At that point, advanced treatment is begun to treat the cardiopulmonary arrest. Many institutions follow the AHA standards for ACLS. General principles of advanced treatment include airway management and ventilation, intravenous (IV) access and pharmacological treatment, and treatment of cardiac dysrhythmias.

AIRWAY MANAGEMENT AND VENTILATION

Rescue breathing is continued until the patient can be intubated. Endotracheal intubation is the preferred method for airway management during a code for several reasons (AHA, 1987, 1990):

1. Protects the patient from aspiration
2. Facilitates ventilation and oxygenation
3. Facilitates suctioning
4. Prevents gastric distention during ventilation

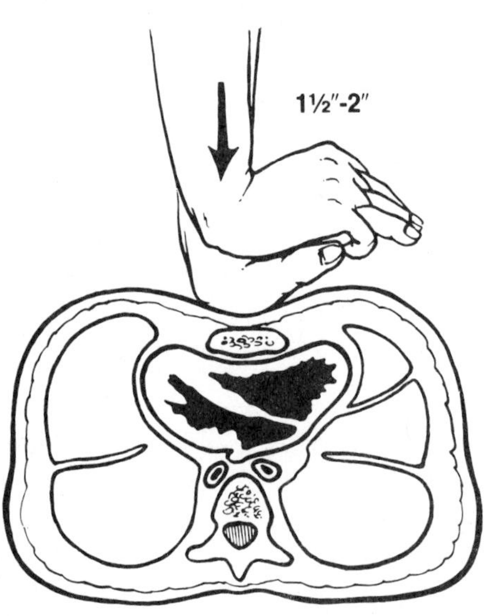

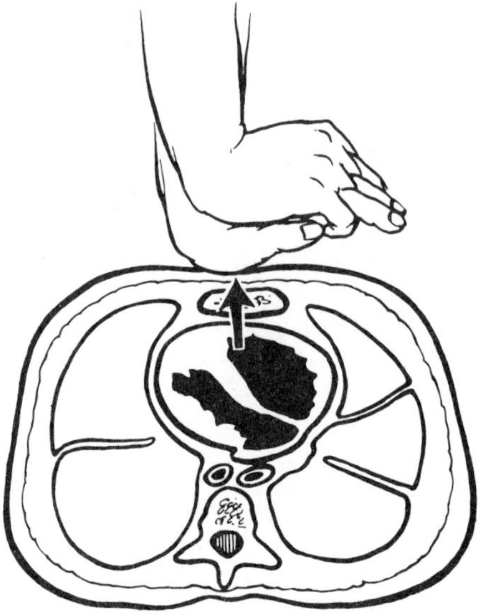

Figure 6-7. Technique for cardiac compressions. (Reproduced with permission. © Healthcare Provider's Manual for Basic Life Support, 1988, Fig. 36, p. 43. Copyright American Heart Association.)

5. Provides a route for administering some medications

Techniques of endotracheal intubation are discussed in Chapter 5. During a cardiopulmonary arrest, CPR should not be disrupted for longer than 30 seconds while intubation is attempted. Once the patient is intubated, the patient is manually ventilated with an MRB attached to the endotracheal tube (Fig. 6-8). The MRB should have a reservoir and be connected to oxygen at 15 L/min to deliver 100% oxygen to the patient. Manual ventilation is preferred over mechanical ventilation so that compressions and ventilations can be performed at a 5:1 ratio.

INTRAVENOUS ACCESS AND PHARMACOLOGICAL TREATMENT

A patent IV is necessary during an arrest in order to administer fluids and/or medications. A few drugs can be administered through the endotracheal tube until an IV access is established: epinephrine, atropine, and lidocaine (AHA, 1987, 1990).

The majority of critically ill patients have an IV infusion or heparin lock. If the patient does not have an IV, or needs an additional IV access, a large-bore IV should be inserted. Preferred areas for IV insertion include the dorsum of the hands, the wrists, and the antecubitus. During CPR, however, the only peripheral veins that should be used for drug administration are the antecubital veins (AHA, 1987, 1990). If a peripheral IV cannot be started, the physician will insert a central line for IV access.

RECOGNITION AND TREATMENT OF DYSRHYTHMIAS

Dysrhythmias are frequently the cause of an arrest; therefore, prompt recognition and treatment of dysrhythmias is essential. Most critically ill patients have continuous monitoring of cardiac rhythm. If the patient is not monitored, he/she is attached to the cardiac monitor to determine the rhythm. "Quick-look" paddles can be used to determine the rhythm or the monitor electrodes can be quickly attached. Rhythm strips should be obtained throughout the code to document the patient's rhythm and response to treatments such as medications and defibrillation.

The following dysrhythmias are often present in patients who have suffered an arrest: ventricular fibrillation, pulseless ventricular tachycardia, ventricular asystole (Fig. 6-9), and electromechanical dissociation. (See Chapter 3 to review dysrhythmias.) Other life-threatening dysrhythmias that may lead to a cardiopulmonary arrest include ventricular tachycardia with a pulse, bradycardia (including heart blocks), ventricular ectopy, and supraventricular tachycardia. Algorithms for treating these rhythm disorders have

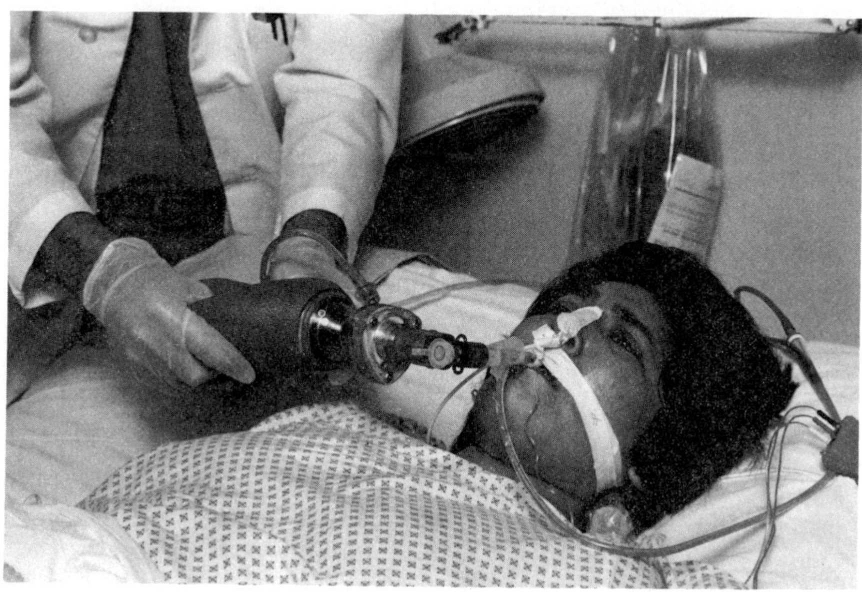

Figure 6-8. Ventilation with manual resuscitation bag connected to endotracheal tube. (From Kersten, L. D.: Comprehensive Respiratory Nursing. Philadelphia, W. B. Saunders, 1989, Fig. 24-9, p. 630.)

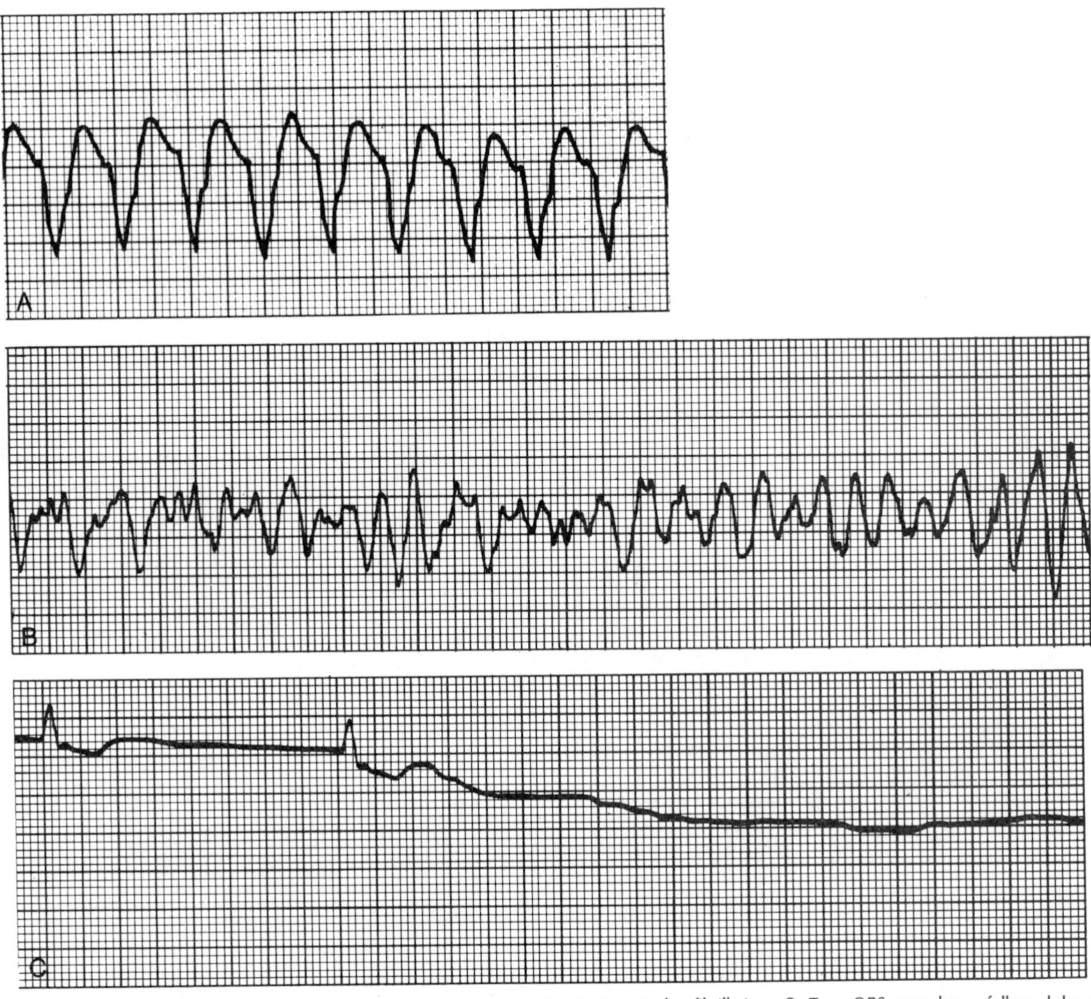

Figure 6–9. Common arrhythmias during a code. *A*, Ventricular tachycardia. *B*, Ventricular fibrillation. *C*, Two QRS complexes followed by asystole. (Reproduced with permission. © Textbook of Advanced Cardiac Life Support, 1987, 1990, 2nd ed. Figs. 51, 52, and 54, pp. 78 and 79. Copyright American Heart Association.)

been established by the AHA (1987, 1990) (Fig. 6–10 to 6–16). Key points of these algorithms are summarized.

Ventricular Fibrillation (VF) and Pulseless Ventricular Tachycardia (VT). The treatment for VF and pulseless VT is the same. If the arrest is witnessed and the patient has no pulse, a precordial thump is administered. Cardiopulmonary resuscitation is initiated until a defibrillator is available. The patient should be defibrillated as soon as possible. Up to three shocks are administered while gradually increasing the energy delivered (measured in joules, J) (e.g., 1st shock—200 J; 2nd shock—200–300 J; 3rd shock—360 J). The pulse and rhythm are assessed after *each* defibrillation attempt (AHA, 1987). If defibrillation is unsuccessful, CPR is continued and drugs and defibrillation (360 J) are alternated. Drugs include epinephrine, lidocaine, and bretylium. Arterial blood gases are frequently drawn during a code to assess the effectiveness of ventilation and determine the need for sodium bicarbonate.

Ventricular Asystole. Diagnosis of asystole should be confirmed in two different leads to rule out the possibility of VF, which is treated by defibrillation. Treatment of asystole includes CPR, epinephrine, and atropine. If these medications are unsuccessful, sodium bicarbonate and/or external pacing should be considered.

Electromechanical Dissociation (EMD). When EMD occurs, a rhythm is visible on the monitor but the patient is pulseless. In other words, electrical activity is present but mechani-

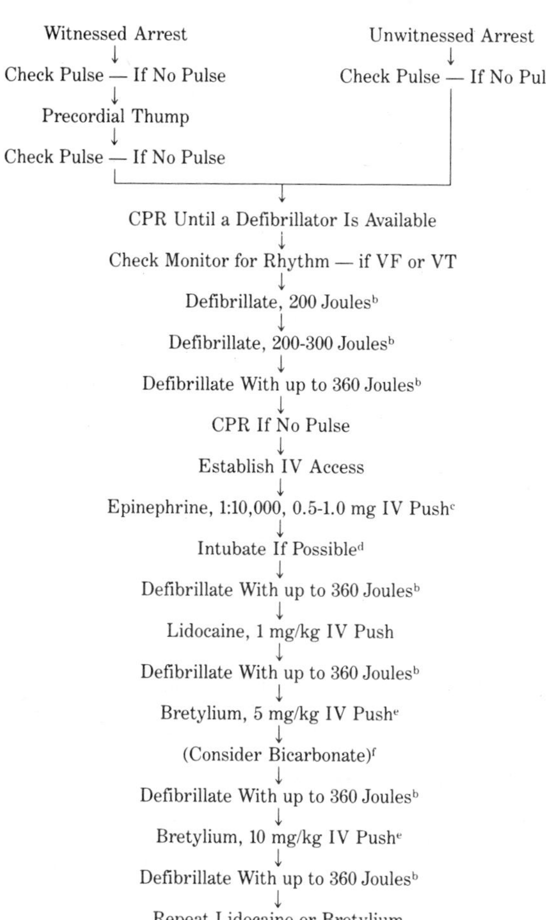

Figure 6-10. ACLS algorithm for treating ventricular fibrillation and pulseless ventricular tachycardia. This sequence was developed to assist in teaching how to treat a broad range of patients with ventricular fibrillation (VF) or pulseless ventricular tachycardia (VT). Some patients may require care not specified herein. This algorithm should not be construed as prohibiting such flexibility. Flow of algorithm presumes that VF is continuing. CPR indicates cardiopulmonary resuscitation. [a]Pulseless VT should be treated identically to VF. [b]Check pulse and rhythm after each shock. If VF recurs after transiently converting (rather than persists without ever converting), use whatever energy level has previously been successful for defibrillation. [c]Epinephrine should be repeated every 5 min. [d]Intubation is preferable. If it can be accompanied simultaneously with other techniques, then the earlier the better. However, defibrillation and epinephrine are more important initially if the patient can be ventilated without intubation. [e]Some may prefer repeated doses of lidocaine, which may be given in 0.5 mg/kg boluses every 8 minutes to a total dose of 3 mg/kg. [f]Value of sodium bicarbonate is questionable during cardiac arrest, and it is not recommended for routine cardiac arrest sequence. Consideration of its use in a dose of 1 mEq/kg is appropriate at this point. Half of original dose may be repeated every ten minutes if it is used. (Reproduced with permission. © Textbook of Advanced Cardiac Life Support, 1987, 1990, 2nd ed. Copyright American Heart Association.)

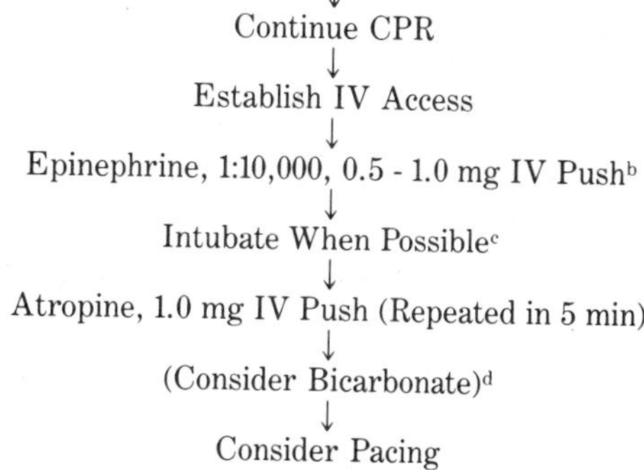

Figure 6-11. ACLS algorithm for treating asystole. This sequence was developed to assist in teaching how to treat a broad range of patients with asystole. Some patients may require care not specified herein. This algorithm should not be construed to prohibit such flexibility. Flow of algorithm presumes asystole is continuing. VF indicates ventricular fibrillation; IV, intravenous. [a]Asystole should be confirmed in two leads. [b]Epinephrine should be repeated every 5 min. [c]Intubation is preferable; if it can be accomplished simultaneously with other techniques, then the earlier the better. However, cardiopulmonary resuscitation (CPR) and use of epinephrine are more important initially if patient can be ventilated without intubation. (Endotracheal epinephrine may be used.) [d]Value of sodium bicarbonate is questionable during cardiac arrest, and it is not recommended for the routine cardiac arrest sequence. Consideration of its use in a dose of 1 mEq/kg is appropriate at this point. Half of original dose may be repeated every ten minutes if it is used. (Reproduced with permission. © Textbook of Advanced Cardiac Life Support, 1987, 1990, 2nd ed, Fig. 2, p. 239. Copyright American Heart Association.)

Continue CPR

↓

Establish IV Access

↓

Epinephrine, 1:10,000, 0.5 - 1.0 mg IV Push[a]

↓

Intubate When Possible[b]

↓

(Consider Bicarbonate)[c]

↓

Consider Hypovolemia,
Cardiac Tamponade,
Tension Pneumothorax,
Hypoxemia,
Acidosis,
Pulmonary Embolism

Figure 6-12. ACLS algorithm for treating electromechanical dissociation. This sequence was developed to assist in teaching how to treat a broad range of patients with electromechanical dissociation. Some patients may require care not specified herein. This algorithm should not be construed to prohibit such flexibility. Flow of algorithm presumes that electromechanical dissociation is continuing. CPR indicates cardiopulmonary resuscitation; IV, intravenous. [a]Epinephrine should be repeated every 5 min. [b]Intubation is preferable. If it can be accomplished simultaneously with other techniques, then the earlier the better. However, epinephrine is more important initially if the patient can be ventilated without intubation. [c]Value of sodium bicarbonate is questionable during cardiac arrest, and it is not recommended for routine cardiac arrest sequence. Consideration of its use in a dose of 1 mEq/kg is appropriate at this point. Half of original dose may be repeated every ten minutes if it is used. (Reproduced with permission. © Textbook of Advanced Cardiac Life Support, 1987, 1990, 2nd ed. Fig. 3, p. 240. Copyright American Heart Association.)

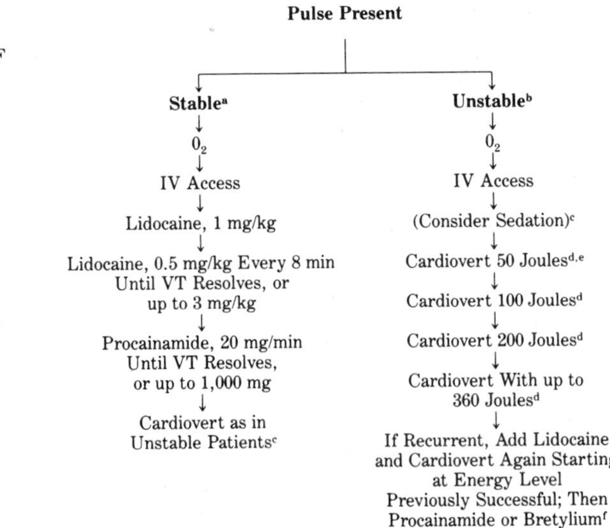

Figure 6-13. ACLS algorithm for treating sustained ventricular tachycardia (VT). This sequence was developed to assist in teaching how to treat a broad range of patients with sustained VT. Some patients may require care not specified herein. This algorithm should not be construed as prohibiting such flexibility. Flow of algorithm presumes that VT is continuing. VF indicates ventricular fibrillation. [a]If patient becomes unstable (see footnote b for definition) at any time, move to "Unstable" arm of algorithm. [b]Unstable indicates symptoms (e.g., chest pain or dyspnea), hypotension (systolic blood pressure <90 mmHg), congestive heart failure, ischemia, or infarction. [c]Sedation should be considered for all patients, including those defined in (b) as unstable, except those who are hemodynamically unstable (e.g., hypotensive, in pulmonary edema, or unconscious). [d]If hypotension, pulmonary edema, or unconsciousness is present, unsynchronized cardioversion should be done to avoid delay associated with synchronization. [e]In the presence of hypotension, pulmonary edema, or unconsciousness, a precordial thump may be employed prior to cardioversion. [f]Once VT has resolved, begin intravenous (IV) infusion of antiarrhythmic agent that has aided resolution of VT. If hypotension, pulmonary edema, or unconsciousness is present, use lidocaine if cardioversion alone is unsuccessful, followed by bretylium. In all other patients, recommended order of therapy is lidocaine, procainamide, and then bretylium. (Reproduced with permission. © Textbook of Advanced Cardiac Life Support, 1987, 1990, 2nd ed., Fig. 4, p. 241. Copyright American Heart Association.)

cal activity (i.e., pumping) is absent. Therefore, CPR must be continued until a pulse is established. The drug of choice for EMD is epinephrine. The prognosis for patients with EMD is poor unless an underlying cause can be found and treated. Causes of EMD that must be considered include the following: hypovolemia, cardiac tamponade, tension pneumothorax, hypoxemia, acidosis, and pulmonary embolism.

Ventricular Tachycardia (VT) with Pulse. Treatment for the patient who has sustained VT with a pulse is based on the stability of the patient. The patient is considered to be unstable if hypotension, pulmonary edema, and/or un-

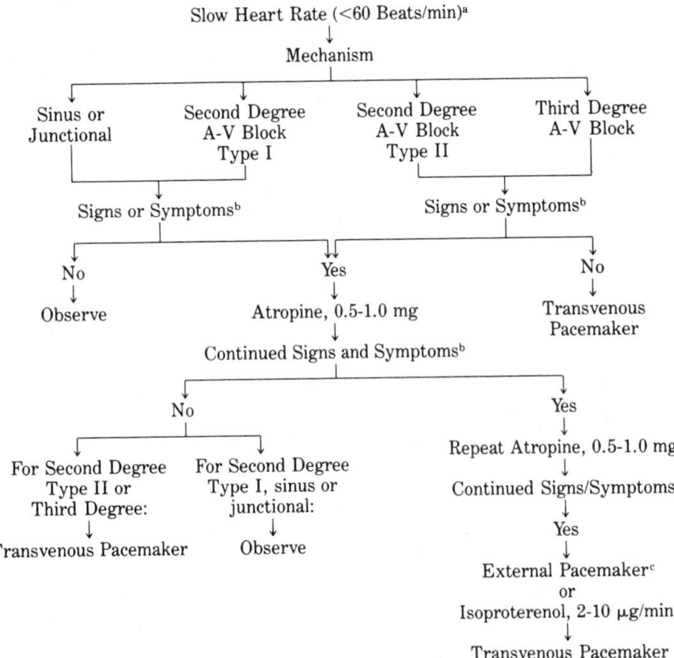

Figure 6-14. ACLS algorithm for treating bradycardia. This sequence was developed to assist in teaching how to treat a broad range of patients with bradycardia. Some patients may require care not specified herein. This algorithm should not be construed to prohibit such flexibility. AV indicates atrioventricular. [a]A solitary chest thump or cough may stimulate cardiac electrical activity and result in improved cardiac output and may be used at this point. [b]Hypotension (blood pressure <90 mmHg), premature ventricular contractions, altered mental status or symptoms (e.g., chest pain or dyspnea), ischemia, or infarction. [c]Temporizing therapy. (Reproduced with permission. © Textbook of Advanced Cardiac Life Support, 1987, 1990, 2nd ed., Fig. 5, p. 242. Copyright American Heart Association.)

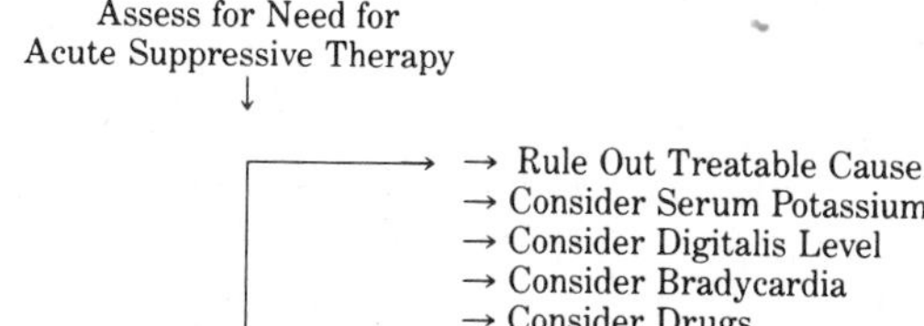

Lidocaine, 1 mg/kg
↓
If Not Suppressed,
Repeat Lidocaine, 0.5 mg/kg Every 2-5 min,
Until No Ectopy, or up to 3 mg/kg Given
↓
If Not Suppressed,
Procainamide 20 mg/min
Until No Ectopy, or up to 1,000 mg Given
↓
If Not Suppressed,
and Not Contraindicated,
Bretylium, 5-10 mg/kg Over 8-10 min
↓
If Not Suppressed,
Consider Overdrive Pacing

Once Ectopy Resolved, Maintain as Follows:
After Lidocaine, 1 mg/kg ... Lidocaine Drip, 2 mg/min
After Lidocaine, 1-2 mg/kg ... Lidocaine Drip, 3 mg/min
After Lidocaine, 2-3 mg/kg ... Lidocaine Drip, 4 mg/min
After Procainamide ... Procainamide drip, 1-4 mg/min (Check Blood Level)
After Bretylium .... Bretylium Drip, 2 mg/min

Figure 6-15. ACLS algorithm for treating ventricular ectopy. This sequence was developed to assist in teaching how to treat a broad range of patients with ventricular ectopy. Some patients may require therapy not specified herein. This algorithm should not be construed as prohibiting such flexibility. (Reproduced with permission. © Textbook of Advanced Cardiac Life Support, 1987, 1990, 2nd ed., Fig. 6, p. 243. Copyright American Heart Association.)

consciousness are present. The unstable patient is treated with oxygen and synchronized cardioversion. Cardioversion is performed up to four times while gradually increasing the energy delivered to the patient (e.g., 1st cardioversion—50 J; 2nd—100 J; 3rd—200 J; 4th—360 J). If the patient is successfully treated, an antiarrhythmic infusion (usually lidocaine) is started. If the VT is recurrent, procainamide and/or bretylium may be used.

The stable patient with VT and pulse is treated with lidocaine. If needed, procainamide can also be given and synchronized cardioversion can be performed.

Bradycardia. Bradycardia is defined as a heart rate less than 60 beats/minute. Treatment of bradycardia is based on the stability of the patient. The patient is considered to be unstable if hypotension, premature ventricular contractions (PVCs), altered mental status, chest pain, dyspnea, ischemia, and/or myocardial infarction are present. Treatment of the unstable patient with bradycardia includes atropine, external pacing, isoproterenol, and transvenous pacing. Stable

Unstable
↓
Synchronous Cardioversion 75-100 Joules
↓
Synchronous Cardioversion 200 Joules
↓
Synchronous Cardioversion 360 Joules
↓
Correct Underlying Abnormalities
↓
Pharmacological Therapy + Cardioversion

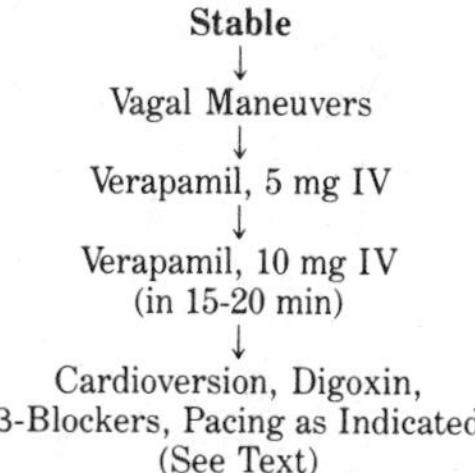

If conversion occurs but PSVT recurs, repeated electrical cardioversion is *not* indicated. Sedation should be used as time permits.

Figure 6-16. ACLS algorithm for treating supraventricular tachycardia. This sequence was developed to assist in teaching how to treat a broad range of patients with sustained PSVT. Some patients may require care not specified herein. This algorithm should not be construed as prohibiting such flexibility. Flow of algorithm presumes PSVT is continuing. (Reproduced with permission. © Textbook of Advanced Cardiac Life Support, 1987, 1990, 2nd ed., Fig. 7, p. 244. Copyright American Heart Association.)

patients with bradycardia may require transvenous pacing for type II second-degree heart block or complete heart block.

Ventricular Ectopy (PVCs). If the patient has suffered an acute myocardial infarction, PVCs should be treated with lidocaine. In other patients, lidocaine and other antiarrhythmic drugs may be given while the cause of the PVCs is assessed and treated. Causes of PVCs include hypoxemia, acid-base imbalance, electrolyte imbalance (especially hypokalemia), and digitalis toxicity.

Supraventricular Tachycardia (SVT). Emergency treatment of SVT is recommended if it causes or worsens cardiovascular problems (e.g., chest pain, dyspnea, ischemia, hypotension, or congestive heart failure) or if it occurs in patients with acute myocardial ischemia or infarction. Synchronized cardioversion is the recommended emergency treatment for SVT. In nonemergency situations, SVT may be treated with vagal maneuvers, verapamil, beta-blockers, digoxin, synchronized cardioversion, and/or overdrive pacing.

DEFIBRILLATION

The primary treatment for ventricular fibrillation and pulseless ventricular tachycardia is defibrillation. Ventricular fibrillation may occur as a result of coronary artery disease, myocardial infarction, electrical shock, drug overdose, near drowning, and acid-base imbalance.

Definition. Defibrillation is the delivery of an electrical current to the heart through use of a defibrillator (Fig. 6–17); it is sometimes referred to as countershock. The current can be delivered through the chest wall using external paddles or directly to the heart during cardiac surgery using smaller internal paddles. (External defibrillation will be emphasized in this section.) Defibrillation works by completely depolarizing the heart and disrupting the impulses causing the dysrhythmia. Since the heart is completely depolarized, the sinoatrial node or other pacemaker can resume control of the heart's rhythm.

Procedure. Two methods exist for paddle placement for external defibrillation. Transverse, or anterior, paddle placement is used most often. In the transverse method, one paddle is placed at the second intercostal space to the right of the sternum while the other paddle is placed at the fifth intercostal space, in the midclavicular line, to the left of the sternum (Fig. 6–18). The alternate method is anterior-posterior paddle placement. When this method is used, an anterior paddle is placed at the anterior precordial area

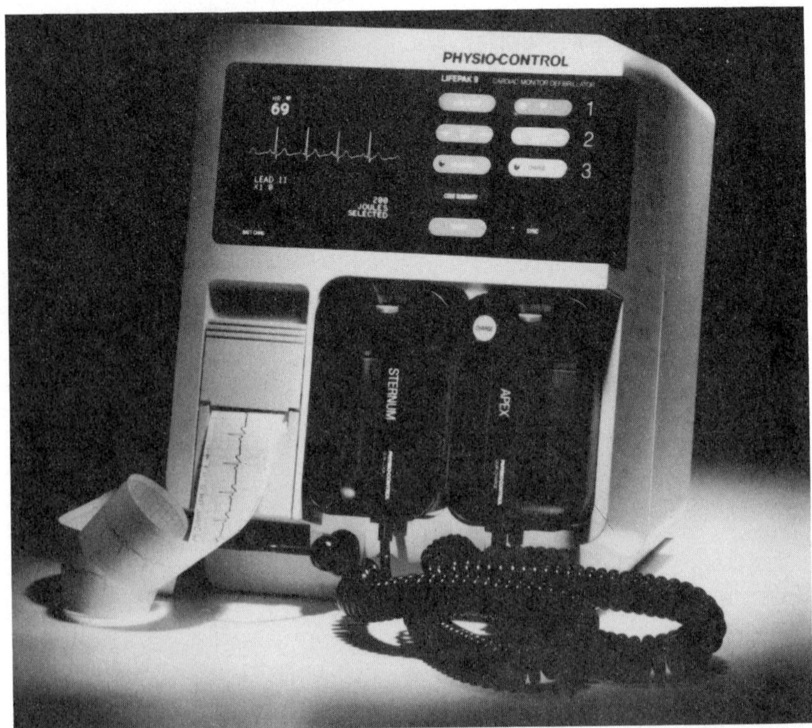

Figure 6–17. Defibrillator. (Photograph courtesy of Physio-Control, Redmond, Washington.)

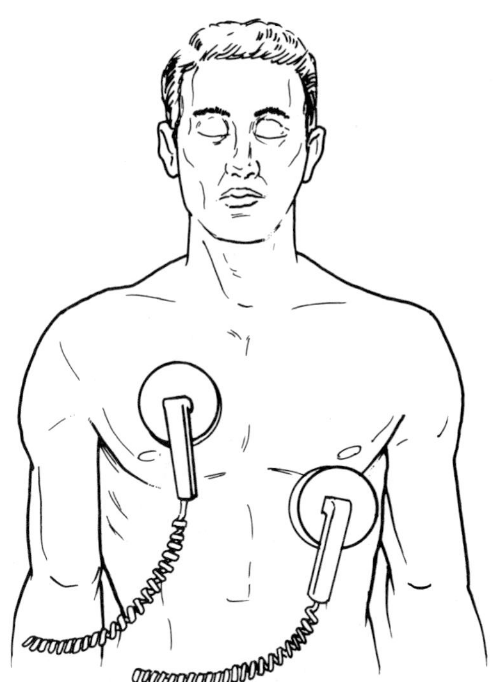

Figure 6–18. Paddle placement for defibrillation. (Redrawn from Sheehy, S. B.: Mosby's Manual of Emergency Care. St. Louis, C. V. Mosby, 1990, Fig. 3–21, p. 76.)

and the posterior paddle is placed at the posterior-infrascapular area (Fig. 6–19) (Spence, 1985a). When the anterior-posterior method is used, less energy may be needed for successful defibrillation.

Newer automatic defibrillators are undergoing trials in out of hospital settings. These defibrillators detect ventricular fibrillation and automatically deliver countershocks (AHA, 1987, 1990). Also, some newer defibrillators permit "hands-off" defibrillation. Countershocks are delivered through special electrodes attached to the patient's chest rather than to paddles.

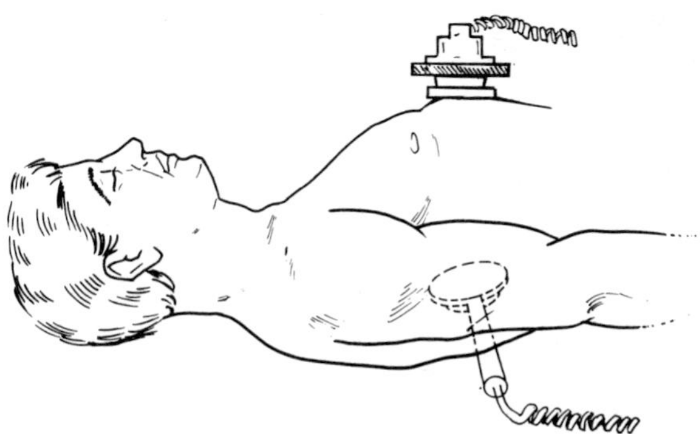

Figure 6–19. Anterior-posterior paddle placement. (Redrawn from Sheehy, S. B.: Mosby's Manual of Emergency Care. St. Louis, C. V. Mosby, 1990, Fig. 3–22, p. 77.)

Energy is delivered to the patient through the paddles. The amount of energy delivered is referred to as joules (J) or watt seconds. Most defibrillators deliver up to 360 J. The AHA (1987, 1990) recommends that three successive shocks be delivered during external defibrillation (if needed) beginning with 200 J as the initial treatment for ventricular fibrillation and pulseless ventricular tachycardia. Subsequent shocks are delivered at 200 to 300 J and 360 J. If the patient does not respond to defibrillation, CPR is continued and pharmacological management is initiated. Additional shocks at the maximum energy level (360 Js) are given if needed.

In order for the shock to be effective, some type of conductive medium is placed between the paddles and the skin. In the past, gel and saline pads have been used to conduct the electricity. If gel is used, it is important to cover the paddles completely with the gel. Commercially available defibrillator pads are now available that can be used for multiple shocks and prevent burns on the patient's skin.

The defibrillator is charged to the desired setting. The paddles are placed firmly on the patient's chest using approximately 25 lb of pressure (AHA, 1987, 1990). This amount of pressure is needed to facilitate skin contact and reduce the impedance to the flow of current.

Safety is essential during the procedure to prevent injury to the patient and the personnel assisting with the procedure. The person performing the defibrillation ensures that all personnel are standing clear of the bed by shouting, "All clear," and visually checking to see that no one is in contact with the patient or bed. The countershock is then delivered. The patient's rhythm and pulse are assessed after each defibrillation. It is helpful if one of the team members obtains rhythm strips during the procedure to document effectiveness. The procedure for defibrillation is summarized in Table 6–4.

Complications of defibrillation include burns on the skin and damage to the heart muscle. Arcing of electricity can occur if the paddles are not firmly placed on the skin and if the skin is wet. Arcing has also been noted when patients have had nitroglycerin patches on the chest; therefore, patches should be removed prior to defibrillation.

Some special situations relating to defibrillation may arise. For example, can a patient with an automatic implantable cardioverter defibrilla-

Table 6–4. PROCEDURE FOR EXTERNAL DEFIBRILLATION

1. Apply defibrillator pads to the patient's chest (*or* apply conductive gel to paddles).
2. Turn on defibrillator.
3. Charge the defibrillator to the desired setting.
4. Position paddles on chest and apply 25 lb of pressure.
5. Ensure that all personnel (including yourself) are clear of the patient, the bed, and any equipment that might be connected to the patient.
6. Shout "All clear!"
7. Deliver countershock by depressing buttons on each paddle.
8. After the defibrillation, observe patient's rhythm and feel for a pulse.

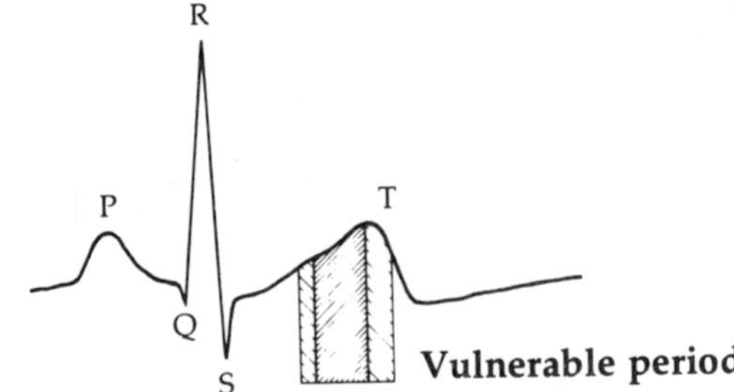

Figure 6–20. Vulnerable period during the cardiac cycle. If a countershock is delivered during this time, it may result in ventricular fibrillation. (From Higgens, S.: Defibrillation: What You Should Know. Redmond, Washington, Physio-Control, 1978, p. 12.)

tor (AICD) or permanent pacemaker be defibrillated? The answer to both questions is yes. The patient with an AICD can be defibrillated using conventional techniques, preferably with anterior/posterior paddle placement, without damaging the device. When a patient with a permanent pacemaker requires defibrillation, it is recommended that the paddles be placed at least 5 in from the pacemaker generator or battery to prevent damage to the device (AHA, 1987, 1990).

CARDIOVERSION

Definition. Cardioversion is the delivery of a countershock that is synchronized with the patient's cardiac rhythm. The purpose of cardioversion is to disrupt an ectopic pacemaker that is causing a dysrhythmia and allow the sinoatrial node to take control of the rhythm. During an emergency situation, cardioversion is used to treat patients with ventricular tachycardia or supraventricular tachycardia who have a pulse but are developing symptoms related to a low cardiac output such as hypotension, cool clammy skin, and a decreased level of consciousness. Elective cardioversion is used to treat atrial flutter and fibrillation.

Cardioversion is very similar to defibrillation with two major exceptions: (1) The countershock of cardioversion is synchronized to the patient's rhythm and (2) Less energy is used for the countershock. The countershock is synchronized with the patient's rhythm so that the shock occurs during ventricular depolarization (QRS complex). The rationale for delivering the shock during the QRS complex is to prevent the shock from being delivered during repolarization (T wave), often termed the vulnerable period. If a shock is delivered during this vulnerable period (Fig. 6–20), ventricular fibrillation may occur. Since the purpose of cardioversion is to disrupt the rhythm rather than completely depolarize the heart, less energy is required. Initially, cardioversion is done using 50 J. The amount of energy is gradually increased until the rhythm is converted.

Procedure. The procedure for cardioversion (Table 6–5) is similar to that for defibrillation. However, the defibrillator is set in the "synchronous" mode for cardioversion. The R waves are sensed by the machine and are noted by "spikes" or other markings on the monitor of the defibrillator. It is important to assess that all R waves are properly sensed. When it is time to deliver the shock, the buttons on the paddles must remain depressed until the shock is delivered, since

Table 6–5. PROCEDURE FOR SYNCHRONOUS CARDIOVERSION

1. Ensure that emergency equipment is readily available.
2. Explain the procedure to the patient.
3. Consider sedating the patient.
4. Turn on defibrillator to SYNCHRONOUS mode.
5. Observe the rhythm on the monitor to determine that the R wave is properly sensed and marked (usually with a spike).
6. Apply defibrillator pads to the patient's chest (*or* apply conductive gel to paddles).
7. Charge the defibrillator to the desired setting.
8. Position paddles on chest and apply 25 lb of pressure.
9. Ensure that all personnel (including yourself) are clear of the patient, the bed, and any equipment that might be connected to the patient.
10. Shout "All clear!"
11. Deliver synchronized countershock by depressing buttons on each paddle. Keep buttons depressed until the shock has been delivered.
12. After the cardioversion, observe patient's rhythm to determine effectiveness.

energy is discharged only during the QRS complex.

EXTERNAL NONINVASIVE CARDIAC PACING

Definition. External noninvasive cardiac pacing is used during emergency situations to treat asystole and symptomatic bradycardia. (The terms *external* and *noninvasive* will be used synonymously in the discussion.) However, it is important to note that the pacemaker may not be effective unless the underlying cause for the dysrhythmia (e.g., hypoxia, acidosis) is treated (AHA, 1987, 1990).

The noninvasive pacemaker may be a free-standing unit with a monitor and a pacemaker (Fig. 6–21). Some newer models incorporate a monitor, defibrillator, and external pacemaker into one system.

Advantages of external pacemakers include easy to perform, requires minimal training, can be initiated immediately in emergency situations, and eliminates risks associated with invasive pacemakers (Crockett and McHugh, 1988).

Procedure. The procedure (Table 6–6) for external pacing involves placing large electrodes anteriorly and posteriorly on the patient (Fig. 6–22). The electrodes are connected to the external pacemaker. The pacemaker is set in either asynchronous or demand modes. (Some devices only permit demand pacing.) In the asynchronous mode, the pacemaker generates a rhythm without regard to the patient's own rhythm. In the demand mode, the pacemaker fires only if the patient's heart rate falls below a preset limit (e.g., 50 beats/minute). The pacemaker rate is set and the output is adjusted to stimulate a paced beat.

The electrical and mechanical effectiveness of pacing is assessed. The electrical activity is noted by a pacemaker "spike" that indicates that the pacemaker is initiating electrical activity. The spike is followed by a broad QRS complex (Fig. 6–23). Mechanical activity is noted by palpating a pulse during the electrical activity. Additionally, the patient should have an increase in blood pressure, improved level of consciousness, and improved skin color and temperature (Crockett and McHugh, 1988). If the external pacemaker is effective, the patient may need to have a temporary transvenous pacemaker inserted, depending on the cause of the bradycardia.

The alert patient who requires external pacing may experience some discomfort. Because the skeletal muscles are stimulated as well as the heart muscle, the patient may experience a tin-

Table 6–6. PROCEDURE FOR EXTERNAL NONINVASIVE PACEMAKER

1. Obtain noninvasive pacemaker, pacemaker electrodes, and emergency equipment.
2. If patient is alert, explain the procedure.
3. Clip excess hair from patient's chest. *Do not* shave hair.
4. Apply anterior electrode to the chest. Electrode is centered at the 4th intercostal space to the left of the sternum.
5. Apply the posterior electrode on the patient's back in the left subscapular region.
6. Connect electrode to pacemaker generator.
7. Set pacemaker parameters for mode, heart rate, and output according to the manufacturer's instructions.
8. Turn unit on.
9. Assess adequacy of pacing:
   Heart rate and rhythm
   Blood pressure
   Level of consciousness
10. Observe for patient discomfort. May need to sedate patient.
11. Anticipate followup treatment such as insertion of a temporary transvenous pacemaker.

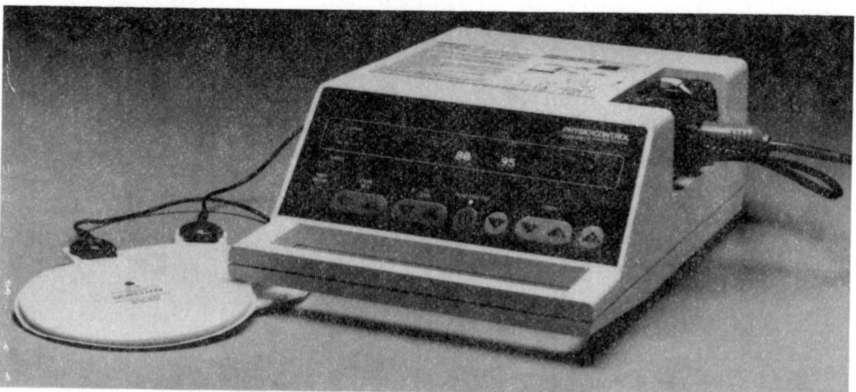

Figure 6–21. External noninvasive pacemaker. (Photograph courtesy of Physio-Control, Redmond, Washington.)

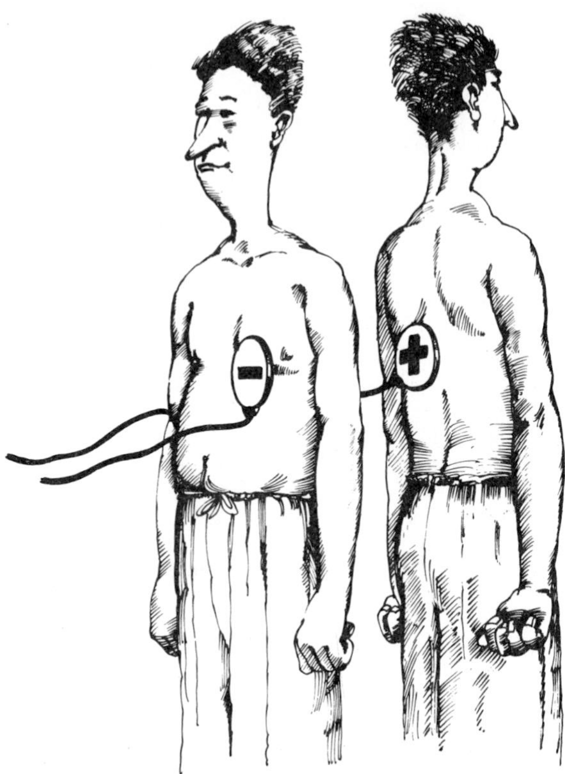

Figure 6-22. Application of pacemaker electrodes for external noninvasive pacing. Electrodes are placed anteriorly and posteriorly. (From Crockett, P., and McHugh, L. G.: Noninvasive Pacing: What You Should Know. Redmond, Washington, Physio-Control, 1988, p. 19.)

gling, twitching, or thumping feeling ranging from mildly uncomfortable to intolerable. The patient may require sedation.

Pharmacological Intervention/ Code Drugs

Medications that are administered to the patient during a code will depend on several factors: the cause of the arrest, the patient's cardiac rhythm, physician preference, and patient response. The goals of treatment with code drugs are to reestablish and maintain optimal cardiac function, correct hypoxemia and acidosis, and suppress dangerous cardiac ectopic activity. Additionally, drugs are used to achieve a balance between myocardial oxygen supply and demand, maintain adequate blood pressure, and relieve congestive heart failure. Because of the rapid and profound effects these drugs can have on cardiac activity and hemodynamic function, ECG monitoring is essential, and hemodynamic monitoring should be instituted as soon as possible after the code. Additionally, because of the precise dosages and careful administration required with these medications, volumetric infusion pumps should be used when giving continuous infusions.

The following drugs are included in ACLS guidelines (AHA, 1987, 1990) and represent those drugs most frequently used in code management. Indications, mechanisms of action, and dosages for each drug will be discussed. This information is summarized in Table 6-7.

OXYGEN

Oxygen is treated as a drug because it is essential in resuscitation and has several pharmacological considerations. Oxygen is used to treat hypoxemia, which exists in any arrest situation secondary to lack of adequate gas exchange and/or inadequate cardiac output. Artificial ventilation without supplemental oxygen will not correct hypoxemia.

Oxygen is used to improve tissue oxygenation. Additionally, the success of other medications and interventions, such as defibrillation, depend on adequate oxygenation and a normal acid-base status.

Oxygen can be delivered via mouth-to-mask, MRB with mask, MRB to endotracheal tube, or

ELECTRICAL CAPTURE

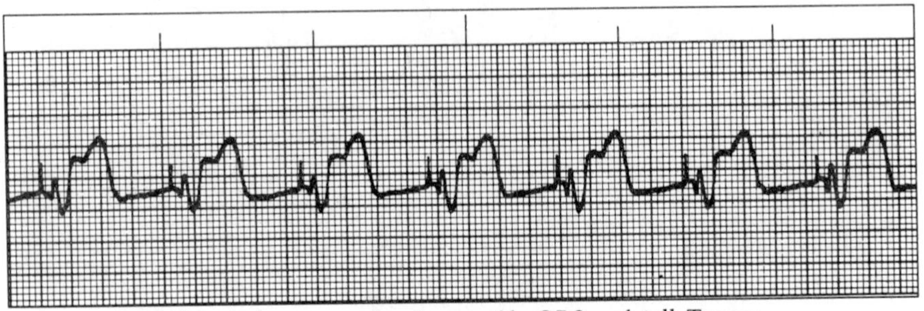

An example of electrical capture, showing a wide QRS and tall T-wave.

Figure 6-23. Electrical capture of pacemaker. Note the pacemaker spikes followed by a wide QRS complex and a tall T wave. (From Crockett, P., and McHugh, L. G.: Noninvasive Pacing: What You Should Know. Redmond, Washington, Physio-Control, 1988, p. 21.)

Table 6–7. DRUGS FREQUENTLY USED IN CODE MANAGEMENT

Drug	Indication	Mechanism of Action	Dosage/Route
Amrinone (Inocor)	Severe congestive heart failure uncorrected by other drugs	Increases contractility, decreases preload and peripheral resistance	Loading dose of 0.75 mg/kg IV push over 3 min, followed by continuous infusion of 2 to 20 μg/kg/min, titrated to effect **Dilution:** 250 mg (50 ml)/50 ml normal saline = 2500 μg/ml
Atropine	Symptomatic bradycardia, asystole, AV block	Increases SA node automaticity and AV node conduction	Bradycardia: 0.5 mg IV Asystole: 1 mg IV push or ETT May repeat every 5 min up to total of 2 mg
Beta-blockers—Propranolol, Metoprolol	Recurrent ventricular tachycardia or ventricular fibrillation; supraventricular tachycardia unresponsive to other therapy; hypertension	Reduce heart rate, blood pressure, contractility, and myocardial oxygen consumption; may control ventricular arrhythmias	Propranolol—1 to 3 mg IV push every 5 min not to exceed total of 0.1 mg/kg Metoprolol—5 mg IV push every 5 min not to exceed 15 mg
Bretylium (Bretylol)	Ventricular fibrillation or pulseless ventricular tachycardia unresponsive to lidocaine; ventricular tachycardia with a pulse uncontrolled by lidocaine and procainamide	Raises fibrillation threshold; suppresses ventricular arrhythmias	Ventricular fibrillation: initially, 5 mg/kg IV push; increase to 10 mg/kg and repeat every 15 to 30 min up to total of 30 mg/kg May follow with continuous infusion of 2 mg/min **Dilution:** 1 gm in 500 ml = 2 mg/ml
Calcium Chloride	Acute hyperkalemia, hypocalcemia, calcium channel blocker toxicity	Increases contractility	2 to 4 mg/kg of 10% solution slowly IV push; 10 ml of 10% solution = 100 mg per 1 ml; repeat in 10 min if necessary
Digitalis (Digoxin)	Atrial fibrillation or flutter with rapid ventricular response, supraventricular tachycardia	Depresses conduction through AV node	10 to 15 μg/kg IV push loading dose
Dopamine (Intropin)	Hypotension not related to hypovolemia	Low doses (1 to 2 μg/kg/min)—causes renal, mesenteric, and cerebral arteries—urine output increases Moderate doses (2 to 10 μg/kg/min)—increases contractility and cardiac output High doses (>10 μg/kg/min)—causes vasoconstriction and increased systemic vascular resistance	Continuous IV infusion, initially 2 to 5 μg/kg/min and titrated as needed **Dilution:** 400 mg in 250 ml 5% DW = 1600 μg/ml Extravasation may cause necrosis and sloughing
Dobutamine (Dobutrex)	Low cardiac output, pulmonary congestion	Increases contractility and cardiac output without increasing myocardial oxygen consumption	Continuous IV infusion at 2.5 to 20.0 μg/kg/min, and titrated as needed **Dilution:** 250 mg in 250 ml 5% DW = 1000 μg/ml
Epinephrine (Adrenalin)	Ventricular fibrillation, pulseless ventricular tachycardia, electrical mechanical dissociation, asystole	Increases contractility, automaticity, systemic vascular resistance and arterial BP; vasoconstriction improves coronary and cerebral perfusion	0.5 to 1.0 mg IV push or 1.0 mg ETT q 5 min. Follow ETT administration with 10 ml NS and several forceful ventilations Occasionally used as continuous infusion to treat hypotension **Dilution:** 1 mg/250 ml 5% DW; start infusion at 1 μg/min and titrate as needed
Furosemide (Lasix)	Pulmonary congestion from left ventricular dysfunction	Inhibits sodium and chloride reabsorption in nephron, causing diuresis; decreases venous return and central venous pressure	20 to 40 mg IV push over 1 to 2 min

continued

Table 6–7. DRUGS FREQUENTLY USED IN CODE MANAGEMENT *Continued*

Drug	Indication	Mechanism of Action	Dosage/Route
Isoproterenol (Isuprel)	Symptomatic bradycardia when atropine has failed and external pacing is not available	Increases contractility and heart rate; also greatly increases myocardial oxygen demand	Continuous IV infusion at initial dose of 2 μg/min, titrated to maintain heart rate of 60 **Dilution:** 1 mg in 500 ml 5% DW = 2 μg/ml
Lidocaine (Xylocaine)	Ventricular fibrillation, ventricular tachycardia, PVCs	Suppresses ventricular arrhythmias; raises fibrillation threshold	Ventricular fibrillation: 1 mg/kg IV push followed by 0.5 mg/kg IV push q 8 to 10 minutes (to a total of 3 mg/kg or approximately 225 mg). Bolus doses may be given ETT May be followed with continuous IV infusion of 2 to 4 mg/min **Dilution:** 1 g lidocaine in 250 ml 5% DW = 4 mg/ml
Morphine	Myocardial infarction, pulmonary edema	Analgesic effects; vasodilates and decreases systemic vascular resistance, which relieves pulmonary congestion and decreased myocardial oxygen consumption	2 to 5 mg IV push every 5 to 30 min as needed
Nitroglycerin (Nitrol, Tridil)	Unstable angina, congestive heart failure	Relaxes vascular smooth muscle; decreases preload; coronary vasodilator so increases myocardial oxygen supply	50 μg bolus IV followed by continuous infusion started at 10 to 20 μg/min; titrated up by 5 to 10 μg/min every 5 to 10 min to desired effect; dose range of 50 to 500 μg/min. **Dilution:** 50 mg/250 ml = 200 μg/ml Use IV tubing especially made for nitroglycerin drips
Norepinephrine (Levophed)	Hypotension uncorrected by other drugs	Arterial and venous vasoconstriction	Continuous IV infusion at 2 μg/min, titrated upward as necessary. **Dilution:** 4 mg in 500 ml = 8 μg/ml Administer through central line if possible; extravasation may cause necrosis and sloughing
Oxygen	Cardiopulmonary arrest, chest pain, hypoxemia	Increases arterial oxygen content and tissue oxygenation	100% in a code Mask, manual resuscitation bag
Procainamide (Pronestyl)	PVCs, ventricular tachycardia uncontrolled with lidocaine	Reduces automaticity of ectopic pacemakers; slows intraventricular conduction	100 mg IV push every 5 min (at 20 mg/min) until arrhythmia controlled, hypotension occurs, QRS widens by 50% of original width, or total of 1 g has been given May be followed by infusion at 1 to 4 mg/min **Dilution:** 1 g/250 ml 5% DW = 4 mg/ml
Sodium Bicarbonate ($NaHCO_3$)	Metabolic acidosis in cardiopulmonary arrest uncorrected by defibrillation, effective CPR, oxygenation, and other drugs	Counteracts metabolic acidosis by binding with hydrogen ions to produce water and carbon dioxide	Initial dose 1 mEq/kg IV push; if necessary, can be repeated every 10 min in doses of 0.5 mg/kg—Administration should be dictated by ABG results
Sodium Nitroprusside (Nipride)	Hypertensive crisis, severe heart failure	Peripheral vasodilator; decreases preload and peripheral arterial resistance	Begin with 0.5 μg/kg/min continuous IV infusion; titrate upward to effect **Dilution:** 50 mg/250 ml 5% DW = 200 μg/ml Protect solution from light
Verapamil (Calan, Isoptin)	Supraventricular tachycardia not requiring cardioversion	Calcium channel blocker—negative inotrope, slows AV nodal conduction, vasodilates vascular smooth muscle	Initially, 0.075 to 0.15 mg/kg (or 5 mg-10 mg) IV push over 2 min; repeat dose 0.15 mg/kg (or 10 mg) after 30 min if needed

other airway adjuncts. During an arrest, 100% oxygen is administered.

EPINEPHRINE (Adrenalin)

Epinephrine is a potent vasoconstrictor. Because of its alpha- and beta-adrenergic effects (Table 6–8), epinephrine increases systemic vascular resistance and arterial blood pressure as well as heart rate, contractility, and the automaticity of cardiac pacemaker cells. Because of peripheral vasoconstriction, blood is shunted to the heart and brain. Epinephrine also increases myocardial oxygen requirements.

Epinephrine is indicated in an arrest to restore cardiac electrical activity. In addition, epinephrine increases automaticity and force of contraction, which makes the heart more susceptible to successful defibrillation. Epinephrine is used to treat ventricular fibrillation, pulseless ventricular tachycardia, asystole, and electromechanical dissociation.

During a code, epinephrine may be given IV or through an endotracheal tube (ETT). The IV dosage is 0.5 to 1.0 mg (5 to 10 ml of a 1:10,000 solution), and is repeated every 5 minutes as needed. When given through the ETT, epinephrine should be diluted in 10 ml of normal saline or sterile water. (Either diluent should be preservative free to prevent injury to the lungs.)

Occasionally, epinephrine is administered by continuous infusion. Dilution is 1 mg in 250 ml 5% dextrose/water (5% DW). The infusion is started at 1 μg/min and is titrated according to the patient's response.

ATROPINE

Atropine is used to increase the heart rate by decreasing vagal tone. It is indicated for patients with symptomatic bradycardia. In an arrest, atropine may be used for asystole as it may initiate electrical activity or restore conduction through the AV node.

For symptomatic bradycardia, atropine is given in 0.5-mg doses IV and repeated every 5 minutes as needed (until a total of 2 mg has been given) to maintain the heart rate greater than 60, or until adequate tissue perfusion is achieved (as indicated by blood pressure, level of consciousness, and so forth.) In asystole, a 1-mg dose is given and repeated once if necessary. Doses lower than 0.5 mg can cause a paradoxical bradycardia and may precipitate ventricular fibrillation. If necessary, atropine may be given via the ETT. The dose for ETT administration is 1 to 2 mg diluted in 10 ml of normal saline or sterile water (without preservatives).

Table 6–8. EFFECTS OF ADRENERGIC RECEPTOR STIMULATION

Alpha
- Vasoconstriction
- Increased contractility

$Beta_1$
- Increased heart rate
- Increased contractility

$Beta_2$
- Vasodilation
- Relaxation of bronchial, uterine, and GI smooth muscle

Dopaminergic
- Vasodilation of renal, mesenteric, and cerebral vessels

LIDOCAINE (Xylocaine)

Lidocaine is an antiarrhythmic drug that suppresses ventricular ectopic activity. It depresses the ventricular conduction system and reduces automaticity.

Lidocaine is the drug of choice for ventricular ectopy (PVCs), ventricular tachycardia, and ventricular fibrillation. It is also recommended for prevention of ventricular ectopy in patients with acute myocardial infarctions.

During a code, 1 mg/kg of lidocaine is administered IV push (also known as a bolus). Additional boluses of 0.5 mg/kg are administered every 8 to 10 minutes, as needed, until a total dose of 3 mg/kg has been given. If IV access is not available, lidocaine may be given through the ETT using the same dose schedule.

If lidocaine is successful in treating the cardiac dysrhythmia, a continuous infusion should be started at 30 to 50 μg/kg/min (2 to 4 mg/min). One gram of lidocaine is mixed in 250 ml 5% DW or 2 g can be mixed in 500 ml. Both solutions deliver 4 mg/ml, the standard dilution.

In a nonarrest situation, an initial bolus of 1.0 mg/kg of lidocaine is administered. It is followed by a continuous lidocaine infusion at 2 to 4 mg/min, with a second bolus of 0.5 mg/kg given after 10 minutes.

Dosages of lidocaine should be decreased in patients with impaired hepatic blood flow (congestive heart failure, acute myocardial infarction, shock) and in elderly patients. Blood levels should be monitored, and the patient assessed for central nervous system disturbances that may indicate lidocaine toxicity. Common side effects of lidocaine include lethargy, confusion, tinnitus, and paresthesias.

BRETYLIUM TOSYLATE (Bretylol)

Bretylium is a second-line antiarrhythmic drug that is used to treat ventricular dysrhythmias unresponsive to other treatments (such as lidocaine and procainamide). In a code, it is used after lidocaine and repeated shocks fail to convert ventricular fibrillation, or if the fibrillation is recurrent.

With initial administration, bretylium causes a transient hypertension and tachycardia. Following this initial sympathetic-like response, adrenergic (sympathetic) blockade occurs resulting in significant hypotension.

In ventricular fibrillation, a dose of 5 mg/kg of undiluted bretylium is given rapidly IV. After administration, defibrillation is again attempted. The dose may be increased to 10 mg/kg and repeated every 15 to 30 minutes if ventricular fibrillation persists.

In ventricular tachycardia unresponsive to other treatment, 500 mg of bretylium is diluted in 50 ml, and 5 to 10 mg/kg is injected over 8 to 10 minutes. This dose may be repeated in 1 to 2 hours if necessary. A continuous infusion of 2 mg/min may also be administered. One gram of bretylium is mixed in a 500 ml of solution when a continuous drip is needed; this solution will deliver 2 mg/ml.

Postural hypotension is very common with the administration of bretylium. Nausea and vomiting may occur in the awake patient.

PROCAINAMIDE (Pronestyl)

Procainamide is an antiarrhythmic drug that reduces the automaticity of ectopic pacemakers and slows intraventricular conduction. It is used to treat ventricular ectopy and ventricular tachycardia uncontrolled by lidocaine. It may also be used to treat supraventricular dysrhythmias. Procainamide is ineffective in ventricular fibrillation because of the length of time needed to achieve adequate blood levels.

Procainamide is given IV in 100-mg doses (diluted in 10 ml of sterile water for injection) every 5 minutes at a rate of 20 mg/min until the dysrhythmia is controlled, the patient becomes hypotensive, the QRS widens by 50% of its original width, or a total of 1 g has been given. If procainamide successfully controls the dysrhythmia, a continuous infusion is given at a rate of 1 to 4 mg/min for maintenance. In order to prepare the infusion, 1 g of procainamide is mixed in 250 ml of fluid, yielding 4 mg/ml. As with lidocaine, the drug's level should be monitored. It should be administered in reduced dosages to patients with left ventricular dysfunction or renal failure.

Hypotension may occur after rapid injection of procainamide. Procainamide may also cause widening of the QRS interval and prolongation of PR or QT intervals, resulting in atrioventricular conduction disturbances and/or cardiac arrest.

VERAPAMIL (Calan, Isoptin)

Verapamil is a calcium channel blocker that has vasodilating and negative chronotropic effects (i.e., causes the heart rate to slow). Verapamil slows conduction through the AV node, making it useful in the treatment of supraventricular dysrhythmias. In addition, verapamil slows ventricular conduction in atrial fibrillation and atrial flutter with fast heart rates. Verapamil is indicated in stable supraventricular tachycardia (which does not require cardioversion). Verapamil is contraindicated in the Wolff-Parkinson-White (WPW) syndrome, which is a tachycardia with a wide QRS. Verapamil may actually increase the ventricular rate in WPW (AHA, 1987, 1990). Verapamil is not effective and should not be used in the treatment of ventricular tachycardia. Severe hypotension and/or ventricular fibrillation may result.

The initial dose of verapamil is 0.075 to 0.15 mg/kg (or 5 to 10 mg) given over 1 minute. A repeat dose of 0.15 mg/kg (or 10 mg) may be repeated in 30 minutes if needed. In older patients, verapamil should be given more slowly. Since verapamil is also a vasodilator, arterial blood pressure should be monitored closely during and after administration. Verapamil is contraindicated in patients with preexisting severe heart failure as hemodynamic compromise may result.

SODIUM BICARBONATE

A patient who has suffered an arrest quickly becomes acidotic. The acidosis results from two sources: (1) retention of carbon dioxide from inadequate ventilation and (2) the build-up of lactic acid from anaerobic metabolism induced by hypoxia. Effective ventilation with supplemental oxygen may correct these causes of acidosis.

Sodium bicarbonate is indicated in the treatment of metabolic acidosis *only* after interventions such as defibrillation, intubation and hyperventilation with 100% oxygen, and pharmacological agents have been instituted. Administration of sodium bicarbonate should be based on arterial blood gas results.

If indicated, the initial dosage of sodium bicarbonate is 1 mEq/kg IV push. Subsequent doses of half this amount may be repeated every 10 minutes, as determined by arterial blood gas results. Sodium bicarbonate should not be mixed or infused with any other drug because it may precipitate or cause deactivation of other drugs.

DOPAMINE (Intropin)

The primary use of dopamine during a code is vasoconstriction; however, the drug's effects are dose related. For instance, at low doses of 1 to 2 μg/kg/min, vasodilation of renal, mesenteric, and cerebral arteries occurs through stimulation of dopaminergic receptors (see Table 6–7). This will increase urine output without affecting the blood pressure or heart rate. At rates of 2 to 10 μg/kg/min, myocardial contractility increases from beta-adrenergic stimulation, and cardiac output increases (Chernow, 1989). At rates above 10 μg/kg/min, systemic vascular resistance markedly increases owing to generalized vasoconstriction produced from alpha-adrenergic stimulation, which predominates in this dosage range. Above 20 μg/kg/min, marked vasoconstriction and increases in myocardial contractility occur. Myocardial workload is increased without an increase in coronary blood supply, which may cause myocardial ischemia.

Dopamine is indicated for hypotension that is symptomatic (e.g., changes in mental status or oliguria) and not caused by hypovolemia. Dopamine is administered by continuous IV infusion starting at 2 to 5 μg/kg/min, and is titrated upward. A dilution of 400 mg dopamine in 250 ml of fluid will deliver 1600 μg/ml. The lowest dose necessary for blood pressure control should be used to minimize side effects and ensure adequate perfusion of vital organs. Vasodilators (e.g., nitroprusside) may be used in conjunction with dopamine to lower vascular resistance while improving cardiac output.

In addition to causing myocardial ischemia, dopamine may also cause cardiac dysrhythmias such as tachycardia and PVCs. Necrosis and sloughing of tissue may occur if the drug infiltrates; therefore, it should be infused into a central line if possible. Phentolamine, 5 to 10 mg in 10 to 15 ml of normal saline, can be injected into the infiltrated area to prevent necrosis.

DOBUTAMINE (Dobutrex)

Dobutamine increases cardiac output by increasing myocardial contractility and causing mild vasodilation. $Beta_1$- and alpha-adrenergic receptors are stimulated in the heart, which increase contractility; $beta_2$ stimulation causes the mild vasodilation (see Table 6–8). Coronary blood flow is actually increased with dobutamine. This drug is indicated in the treatment of patients with low cardiac output, pulmonary congestion, or hypotension when vasodilators cannot be used. Adverse effects include tachycardia, dysrhythmias, and myocardial ischemia, especially when administered in high doses.

Dobutamine is given as a continuous infusion of 2.5 to 20 μg/kg/min, although lower doses may be effective. After reconstituting the 250-mg vial of dobutamine with 10 to 20 ml diluent, it is mixed in 250 ml of fluid to deliver 1000 μg/ml. The lowest dose necessary to maintain desired hemodynamic parameters should be used.

AMRINONE (Inocor)

Amrinone is another inotropic agent that increases contractility and decreases systemic vascular resistance and preload. Amrinone is used to treat severe congestive heart failure when conventional drugs (e.g., dopamine, dobutamine) have failed.

A loading dose of 0.75 mg/kg IV push is given over 3 minutes, followed by a continuous infusion at 2 to 20 μg/kg/min. The infusion is titrated to the desired hemodynamic response. By mixing 250 mg (50 ml) in 50 ml of fluid, a concentration of 2500 μg/ml is achieved. Normal saline should be used for dilution rather than dextrose. The lowest possible dose should be used, since tachycardia and myocardial ischemia may occur with higher doses. A precipitate will form if furosemide is injected into the same IV line as amrinone.

NOREPINEPHRINE (Levophed)

Norepinephrine is a potent vasoconstrictor that also increases myocardial contractility. Norepinephrine's $beta_1$-adrenergic effects increase myocardial contractility; vasoconstriction results from its potent alpha-adrenergic effects (see Table 6–8). Despite the increase in contractility, cardiac output rarely improves because of the marked increase in systemic vascular resistance. Myocardial oxygen requirements are increased, and ischemia can result. Norepinephrine is indicated in hemodynamically significant hypotension when other vasopressors have failed.

Doses start at 2 μg/min IV and are increased to achieve adequate blood pressure. Though higher doses may be required, the average dose is 2 to 12 μg/min. The standard dilution of 4 mg in 500 ml delivers 8 μg/ml. Fluid used for dilution should contain dextrose.

As with dopamine, extravasation of this drug can cause necrosis and sloughing of tissue. Phentolamine is used as a local antidote.

ISOPROTERENOL (Isuprel)

Isoproterenol increases the heart rate and contractility through stimulation of beta-adrenergic receptors. Cardiac output may increase because peripheral vasodilation occurs (decreased afterload). However, myocardial oxygen demand is markedly increased with the use of isoproterenol, and ischemia and cardiac dysrhythmias may result.

Isoproterenol is indicated in symptomatic bradycardia that is unresponsive to atropine. If possible, external cardiac pacing should be used to treat bradycardia rather than using isoproterenol because of the drug's side effects. Isoproterenol is contraindicated in cardiac arrest because it lowers coronary artery perfusion pressure and could cause additional myocardial ischemia.

The initial dose of isoproterenol is 2 μg/min via continuous IV infusion. The dose is titrated upward to achieve a heart rate of 60. The standard solution is 1 mg of isoproterenol in 500 ml solution, yielding 2 μg/ml.

CALCIUM CHLORIDE

Calcium increases the force of myocardial contraction. The only use of calcium chloride in a code is to treat underlying hypocalcemia, hyperkalemia, or calcium channel blocker toxicity that may be a cause of the arrest. Unless these conditions are present, calcium chloride should not be used in resuscitation efforts.

When indicated during a code, 2–4 mg/kg of a 10% solution is administered via IV push. (A 10-ml prefilled syringe of 10% calcium chloride yields 100 mg/ml.) This dose may be repeated at 10-minute intervals. Calcium must be administered slowly to prevent a decrease in the heart rate (when the heart is beating). Ventricular irritability and coronary or cerebral vasospasm may also occur after administration.

Calcium gluceptate and calcium gluconate may also be used in doses of 5 to 7 ml and 5 to 8 ml, respectively.

BETA-BLOCKERS

Propranolol (Inderal) and metoprolol (Lopressor) are beta-blocking agents that decrease the heart rate, blood pressure, myocardial contractility, and myocardial oxygen consumption. In addition, these drugs are used to treat a variety of dysrhythmias: recurrent episodes of ventricular tachycardia and ventricular fibrillation when other antiarrhythmics fail, atrial fibrillation, atrial flutter, and some supraventricular tachycardias. Beta-blockers that are cardioselective, such as metoprolol, have predominant effects on the heart. Noncardioselective beta-blockers, such as propranolol, must be avoided in patients with COPD; their use may cause bronchospasm in these patients.

In an emergency situation, low doses of beta-blockers are administered slow IV push. Propranolol is given in doses of 1.0 to 3.0 mg every 5 minutes, not to exceed a total dose of 0.1 mg/kg. The dose for metoprolol is 5 mg every 5 minutes until 15 mg has been given.

DIGOXIN (Lanoxin)

Digoxin is used to increase myocardial contractility and decrease the heart rate. It is especially useful in controlling rapid heart rates that may occur in atrial fibrillation and atrial flutter. It may also be used to convert supraventricular tachycardia to sinus rhythm in the hemodynamically stable patient who does not require immediate cardioversion.

Digoxin may be given IV push or by mouth. The IV route has a more rapid onset. A loading dose of 10 to 15 μg/kg is given, followed by a maintenance dose based on the patient's response.

Digoxin toxicity is common and can cause dysrhythmias as well as other systemic effects. Cardioversion should be avoided in the presence of digitalis toxicity as fatal ventricular dysrhythmias may result.

NITROGLYCERIN (Nitrol, Tridil)

Nitroglycerin relaxes smooth muscle, causing coronary arterial and systemic venous dilatation. These effects improve the myocardial oxygen supply and reduce myocardial oxygen demand. It is the drug of choice for emergent congestive heart failure and unstable angina.

In these situations, nitroglycerin is administered by a continuous IV infusion. Nitroglycerin can be diluted by adding 50 mg to 250 ml of fluid, which delivers 200 μg/ml. Another standard dilution is 8 mg in 250 ml, delivering 32 μg/ml.

The nitroglycerin infusion is started at 5 μg/min. This infusion can be increased 5 to 10 μg/min every 3 to 5 minutes as needed for the relief of pain or desired hemodynamic effects. Normal dosages range from 50 to 200 μg/min, but may be as high as 500 μg/min.

Nitroglycerin must be used cautiously in patients with acute myocardial infarction. Hypotension may occur, resulting in reduced coronary blood flow to the ischemic myocardium.

SODIUM NITROPRUSSIDE (Nipride)

Sodium nitroprusside is a potent arterial and venous smooth muscle vasodilator. It is used to treat hypertensive crisis and congestive heart failure. Immediate reduction of peripheral resistance occurs with its administration, which makes it the drug of choice for hypertensive emergencies. In congestive heart failure, it decreases preload and afterload, thereby improving stroke volume and cardiac output. Nitroprusside is often used in combination with dopamine for the treatment of heart failure.

Sodium nitroprusside is given by a continuous IV infusion at an initial rate of 0.5 μg/kg/min. It is titrated until the desired clinical response is achieved. The average dose is 0.5 to 8.0 μg/kg/min. The infusion is mixed by adding 50 mg of sodium nitroprusside to 250 ml of fluid, which delivers 200 μg/ml. The solution should be protected from light.

Hypotension may occur with the use of this drug. It may also cause myocardial ischemia.

FUROSEMIDE (Lasix)

Furosemide is a potent diuretic that acts by inhibiting sodium and chloride reabsorption in the nephron. It is used in emergency situations to relieve pulmonary congestion.

Furosemide is given initially in bolus doses of 20 to 40 mg IV over 1 to 2 minutes. Adverse effects of furosemide include hypotension from dehydration and electrolyte disturbances. A precipitate will form if furosemide is injected into the same IV line as amrinone.

MORPHINE

Morphine is an analgesic used to treat ischemic chest pain. It is also used in pulmonary edema because it increases venous capacitance and decreases systemic vascular resistance. These effects reduce pulmonary congestion and myocardial oxygen demand.

Morphine is given IV push in small increments of 2 to 5 mg every 5 to 30 minutes, as necessary. Respiratory depression and/or hypotension may result from the use of morphine.

Special Problems During a Code

In addition to electrical and pharmacological interventions carried out in a code, it may be necessary to immediately treat the underlying cause of the arrest. Tension pneumothorax and cardiac tamponade are two such problems that require rapid invasive therapeutic techniques.

TENSION PNEUMOTHORAX

A tension pneumothorax occurs when air enters the pleural space but cannot escape. Pressure increases in the pleural space, causing the lung to collapse. Tension pneumothorax is a life-threatening emergency. It may be caused by barotrauma from mechanical ventilation, blunt or penetrating trauma, or invasive procedures that inadvertently cause air to enter the pleural space. Symptoms of a tension pneumothorax include dyspnea, chest pain, tachypnea, tachycardia, and jugular venous distension. On assessment, breath sounds on the affected side will be diminished, and the trachea may be shifted to the opposite side. If left untreated, the tension pneumothorax may progress and cause cardiovascular collapse and cardiac arrest. Because little time exists for x-ray confirmation, a needle may be inserted into the second or third anterior intercostal space on the affected side to relieve a tension pneumothorax. If air is under pressure in the pleural space, it will escape through the needle, making a hissing noise.

PERICARDIAL TAMPONADE

Pericardial tamponade is the accumulation of fluid in the pericardial sac. The fluid causes a decrease in cardiac output and may cause electromechanical dissociation or cardiac arrest. Tamponade can be caused by such things as trauma, pericarditis, CPR, or invasive procedures.

The patient with cardiac tamponade will have an increased central venous pressure, hypotension with narrowing of the arterial pulse pressure, and paradoxical pulse. Paradoxical pulse is the exaggerated fluctuation of arterial pressure during the respiratory cycle. It is defined as a peak systolic blood pressure drop of greater than 10 mm Hg during normal inspiration (Sulzbach, 1989). Further assessment may reveal distant or muffled heart tones. Pericardiocentesis, or needle aspiration of pericardial fluid, is done to alleviate the pressure around the heart. Additionally, rapid administration of IV fluids (to increase preload and stroke volume) and drugs such as epinephrine or isoproterenol may be used.

Documentation of Code Events

A detailed chronological record of all interventions must be maintained during the code. This task is sometimes forgotten; therefore, the nurse team leader or nursing supervisor should ensure that someone is assigned to record information throughout the code. Recording may be done by anyone, even nursing students or nonlicensed personnel.

Documentation should include the time the code is called, time CPR is started, any actions taken, and patient response (e.g., pulse, blood pressure, cardiac rhythm). Intubation and defibrillation (with energy used) must be documented with patient response. Time and sites of IV starts, types and amounts of fluids administered, and medications given to the patient should all be accurately recorded. Many hospitals have standardized Code Records (Fig. 6–24) that list actions and medications and include spaces to enter the time of interventions and any comments. It is best if information can be recorded directly on the Code Record during the code to ensure that all information is obtained. However, simply writing down information on any available piece of paper will suffice as the information can be transcribed to the Code Record after the code. Code Records become part of the patient's permanent record.

Care of the Patient After Resuscitation

The survivor of a cardiac or respiratory arrest requires intensive monitoring and care. If not already in a critical care unit, the patient is transferred to one as soon as possible. Postresuscitation care includes airway and blood pressure maintenance, oxygenation, and control of dysrhythmias. Underlying abnormalities that may have caused the arrest, such as hypokalemia or myocardial ischemia, are corrected.

Oxygen is given at a concentration of 100%. It is adjusted according to blood gas and pulse oximeter values. Dopamine or other pharmacological intervention may be needed to maintain systolic blood pressure at or above 90 mm Hg. Blood pressure and heart rate should be recorded every 15 minutes during continuous infusion of vasoactive medications. If antiarrhythmic drugs were used successfully in the code, boluses may be repeated to achieve adequate blood levels, or continuous infusions may be administered for 24 hours. Other drugs may be given to improve cardiac output and myocardial oxygen supply. Arterial lines and pulmonary artery catheters are frequently inserted after a code to facilitate patient treatment.

Cardiopulmonary cerebral resuscitation (CPCR) is a term used for the interventions that are carried out to optimize cerebral recovery following an arrest. When a patient suffers a cardiac arrest, blood flow to the brain is interrupted, causing a lack of oxygen and glucose. Even with correct CPR, blood flow may not be sufficient. Hypoxemia and a lack of an energy source result, leading to ischemia, lactic acid accumulation, and leaky cell membranes. Cerebral edema may occur, causing further damage and impedance to cerebral blood flow (CBF). Much research is being done in this area to determine which interventions and pharmacological agents improve cerebral recovery, since brain injury results frequently from cardiac/respiratory arrest (Rolfsen and Davis, 1989).

The goal of CPCR is promotion of cerebral perfusion. This is accomplished through maintenance of blood pressure and prevention or reduction of increased intracranial pressure (ICP). Mean arterial pressure should be maintained between 60 and 150 mm Hg through the use of plasma volume expanders and/or vasopressors. Hemodilution, an experimental technique, may be used to decrease blood viscosity and improve flow. The goal is a hematocrit of 30 to 35% (Hunter, 1987).

Increased intracranial pressure should be prevented or decreased because it can impede cerebral perfusion. Hyperventilation is one measure used to prevent an increase in ICP. The patient is frequently hyperventilated to maintain a $Paco_2$ of

SANTA ROSA MEDICAL CENTER
CARDIOPULMONARY RESUSCITATION RECORD

DATE:	TEAM RESPONSE	TIME
TIME ARREST NOTED:	ER PHYSICIAN:	
TIME CPR STARTED:	RESPIRATORY CARE:	
TIME "DR. HEART" CALLED:	SUPERVISOR:	
TIME MONITOR ON:	EKG TECH:	
INITIAL RHYTHM:	PASTORAL MINISTRY:	

(Addressograph)

IV THERAPY			
TIME	SITE/NEEDLE	AMOUNT/SOLUTION	RATE

RESPIRATORY MANAGEMENT			
METHOD	TIME	BY	INTUBATION
ORAL AIRWAY			TIME:
MOUTH/MOUTH			SIZE:
AMBU/MASK			BY:
AMBU/ET			PLACEMENT CK:

IV PUSH MEDICATIONS					
DRUG	DOSE	TIME			
ATROPINE					
BICARBONATE					
BRETYLIUM					
CALCIUM CHLORIDE					
DEXTROSE 50%					
EPINEPHRINE		IV IC ET	IV IC ET	IV IC ET	IV IC ET
LIDOCAINE					

NOTIFICATION OF:	TIME(S) CALLED	TIME OF ARRIVAL
FAMILY		
DR.		
DR.		

DEFIBRILLATION/CARDIOVERSION			
TIME	ARRHYTHMIA	JOULES	RESPONSE

IV INFUSIONS	
DRUG	TIME/RATE
BRETYLIUM Gm in ml D5/W	
DOPAMINE Mg in ml D5/W	
ISUPREL Mg in ml D5/W	
LIDOCAINE Gm in ml D5/W	

VITAL SIGNS				
TIME				
BP				
PULSE				
RESP.				
PUPILS				
RHYTHM				

PROCEDURES/TIME(S)	PROCEDURES/TIME(S)
ABG's:	CENTRAL LINE:
LAB:	FOLEY:
CXR:	NG:
EKG:	PACER:

Resuscitation stopped at ____________ am/pm by order of

Dr.____________________ Survived: ________ Expired: ______

Transferred to ____________ at ______ am/pm with

______ % O_2, IV, cardiac monitor & accompanied by:

____

OBSERVATIONS ON REVERSE SIDE

SIGNATURES: ____________________ ____________________ ____________________

RECORDER NURSE TEAM LEADER PHYSICIAN IN CHARGE

34008-P 1/87 Rev.

Figure 6–24. Sample of a flowsheet used to document activities during a cardiac arrest. (Flowsheet reproduced with permission of Santa Rosa Hospital, San Antonio, Texas.)

25 to 30 mm Hg (Sullivan, 1989). Decreased carbon dioxide levels cause vasoconstriction, which decreases cerebral blood volume and ICP. High concentrations of oxygen are used to assure adequate oxygenation and prevent increases in ICP (Rolfsen and Davis, 1989).

Straining, restlessness, and seizures as well as nursing measures such as turning and suctioning the patient can increase ICP. Events that increase ICP should be minimized; medication to control or prevent restlessness and/or seizures, such as phenytoin, may be used (Hunter, 1987). Mannitol, an osmotic agent, and furosemide, a loop diuretic, may be used to decrease ICP by eliminating excess fluid.

Other drugs may be used in CPCR, including steroids, barbiturates, and calcium channel blockers. The use of steroids and barbiturates is controversial and needs research (Rolfsen and Davis, 1989; Sullivan, 1989). Calcium channel blockers such as nimodipine appear to improve cerebral perfusion, though more research is needed (Rolfsen and Davis, 1989).

Other nursing measures in CPCR include maintaining normal body temperature, monitoring for glucose and electrolyte abnormalities, and thorough neurological assessments. Cooling blankets and/or antipyretic drugs should be used to maintain normothermia. Glucose and electrolyte monitoring is essential, since disturbances can alter cerebral functioning (Rolfsen and Davis, 1989). Neurological assessment should include the patient's level of consciousness, orientation, motor function, pupillary response, and respiratory patterns.

Emotional support is an important aspect of care following an arrest. Fear of death or a recurrence of the arrest is common. Some patients have out-of-body experiences during the code. Although this phenomenon is poorly understood, it may have a significant impact on the patient. Survivors often feel the need to discuss their experience in depth, and they should be listened to objectively.

Psychosocial/Legal/Ethical Implications

PSYCHOSOCIAL CONCERNS

Besides the patient, many other people are affected when a code occurs. Family members, roommates and other patients, and staff members are all impacted by the emergency.

If the family is with the patient when the arrest occurs, they should be tactfully removed from the scene as quickly as possible. A staff member, chaplain, volunteer, or friend should try to remain with the family during this time and keep them informed of the patient's progress. Honesty is crucial, and it is important that they know that their family member is receiving the best possible care. If the family is not present, the next of kin should be called as soon as possible and informed of the patient's critical status.

If the patient is successfully resuscitated, the family should be allowed to see the patient as soon as is feasible. If the patient does not survive, the family should be encouraged to see the patient; this may facilitate the grief process.

All efforts should be made to remove a roommate or alert patients from the scene. If this is not feasible, the curtains should be drawn. These patients may experience fear and will probably want to talk about the experience. As with the survivor and family members, they will require emotional support. Patient privacy must also be protected; it will suffice to tell curious patients that an emergency is in progress. Also, it is easy to overlook other patients and their needs during a code. If staff members are not performing a specific role in the code, they should clear the area and tend to other patients.

Staff members are also affected by a code. Besides the grief that may be felt over the loss of a patient, guilt, anger, and anxiety may be felt. It is helpful for the staff involved in a code to be "debriefed," not only to evaluate how well the code went, but to discuss feelings about the events. Here, too, emotional support is needed.

LEGAL AND ETHICAL CONCERNS

In the critical care setting and in the absence of a written order from a physician to withhold resuscitative measures, CPR must be initiated when a patient arrests. The physician generally makes the decision as to whether or not a patient will be resuscitated. Likewise, it is the physician who makes the decision to terminate CPR in progress. At times, this can present quite an ethical dilemma for the nurse, patient, and family. In situations of terminal or prolonged catastrophic illness, it may be the wish of the patient not to be resuscitated. When the patient is comatose or otherwise unable to make that decision (such as from irreversible brain damage), the family may express wishes as to what they do or do not want done for their loved one. The patient and/or family members need to express their wishes to the physician and discuss these issues. Often it is the nurse who must approach a physician regarding a "do not resuscitate" order, and encourage open communication with the patient and family. The patient and the patient's family should understand and agree with the decision whether it be to withhold CPR or do everything possible to sustain life. Orders related to treatment in the event of an arrest should be clearly documented in the medical record. Federal law, the Patient Self-Determination Act, now mandates that patients make informed decisions about medical care in advance of terminal medical illness.

Summary

Positive patient outcomes depend on the health care team members' ability to recognize problems and intervene effectively. When a patient suffers a cardiac or respiratory arrest or both in the hospital, basic and advanced life support measures must be initiated immediately. How the code team functions and how interventions are carried out will affect the patient's potential for recovery. Thus, code management is an important topic for anyone involved in caring for patients, especially those in critical care areas.

References

American Heart Association (1987, 1990). *Textbook of Advanced Cardiac Life Support.* 2nd ed. Dallas: American Heart Association.

American Heart Association (1988): *Healthcare Provider's Manual for Basic Life Support.* Dallas: American Heart Association.

Chernow, B. (1989): *Essentials of Critical Care Pharmacology.* Baltimore: Williams & Wilkins.

Crockett, P., and McHugh, L. G. (1988): *Noninvasive Pacing: What You Should Know.* Redmond, WA: Physio-Control.

Higgens, S. (1978): *Defibrillation: What You Should Know.* Redmond, WA: Physio-Control.

Hunter, C. (1987): Cardiopulmonary cerebral resuscitation: Nursing interventions. *Critical Care Nurse* 7(3):46–54.

Kersten, L. D. (1989): *Comprehensive Respiratory Nursing.* Philadelphia: W. B. Saunders.

Rolfsen, M., and Davis, W. R. (1989): Cerebral function and preservation during cardiac arrest. *Critical Care Medicine* 17(3):283–292.

Spence, M. I. (1985a): Cardioversion. In: S. Millar, L. K. Sampson, and S. M. Soukup (eds.). *AACN Procedure Manual for Critical Care.* 2nd ed. Philadelphia: W. B. Saunders, pp. 29–35.

Spence, M. I. (1985b). Defibrillation. In: S. Millar, L. K. Sampson, and S. M. Soukup (eds.). *AACN Procedure Manual for Critical Care.* 2nd ed. Philadelphia: W. B. Saunders, pp. 36–40.

Sullivan, J. (1989): Nursing interventions. *Critical Care Nursing Clinics of North America* 1(1):155–164.

Sulzbach, L. M. (1989): Measurement of pulsus paradoxis. *Focus on Critical Care* 16(2):142–145.

Recommended Reading

American Heart Association (1988): *Healthcare Provider's Manual for Basic Life Support.* Dallas: American Heart Association.

American Heart Association (1987, 1990): *Textbook of Advanced Cardiac Life Support.* 2nd ed. Dallas: American Heart Association.

Britt, J. (1990): What to do when your patient codes. *Nursing '90* 20(1):42–43.

Budney, J., and Anderson-Drevs, K. (1990): IV inotropic agents: Dopamine, dobutamine, and amrinone. *Critical Care Nurse* 10(2):54–62.

Campbell, C. D., and Newsome, J. A. (1990): Detecting life-threatening arrhythmias. *Nursing* 20(12):34–39.

Ellstrom, K., and Bella, L. D. (1990): Understanding your role during a code. *Nursing* 20(5):37–43.

Feeney-Stewart, F. (1990): The sodium bicarbonate controversy. *Dimensions of Critical Care Nursing* 9(1):22–28.

Jones, S., and Bagg, A. M. (1988): LEAD drugs for cardiac arrest. *Nursing '88* 18(1):34–41.

Padilla, M. C. O., and Purcell, J. A. (1990): Using a structured cardiopulmonary resuscitation flow sheet. *Focus on Critical Care* 17:490–494.

Willens, J. S., and Copel, L. C. (1989): Performing CPR on adults. *Nursing* 19(1):34–43.

PART

III

Nursing Care During Critical Illness

Chapter 7

Mary G. McKinley, M.S.N., R.N., CCRN
Catherine F. Robinson, M.S., R.N., CEN, CCRN

Shock

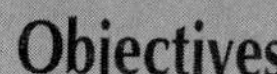

Objectives

- Understand the basic pathophysiological principles of shock.
- Compare and contrast the various classifications of shock.
- Identify the stages and symptoms of shock based on characteristics of the various clinical manifestations that may be seen in shock patients.
- Discuss nursing assessment activities and criteria for determining cause, classification, stage, and treatment of shock.
- Discuss nursing diagnosis, varied treatment, and potential outcome for patients experiencing shock.
- Develop a patient-centered care plan for the patient in shock.

Overview

There are common denominators in all cases of illness that must be dealt with at some point in time. Because of its potential occurrence in any patient, one such common denominator is the syndrome of shock (Rice, 1991a). The effects of shock are not isolated in any one organ system; it affects all systems of the body (Emmanuelson and Rosenlicht, 1986). The syndrome is a complication of a myriad of disease states. So what exactly is shock?

Shock has been defined as a decrease in the blood pressure, a drop in the urinary output, or a loss of cardiac output. Shock is best described by symptoms because of the complex nature of the process. Shock is a clinical syndrome characterized by inadequate tissue perfusion that results in impaired cellular metabolism. There may be differences in how the syndrome occurs, but the endpoint of poor nutritional blood flow and impaired cellular metabolism is the same. The process of patient responses to the syndrome and its treatment can vary. Nursing care of patients with shock requires skill, knowledge, and judgment based on research.

Shock can be an insurmountable challenge for the patient and the nurse. This challenge can be met only if one considers the source of the problem and is aware of the needs of the patient.

The purpose of this chapter is to introduce the nurse to the complex syndrome of shock and its management. The syndrome of shock is explored and examined, and the etiological factors and pathophysiology of shock are reviewed. Nursing assessment and diagnosis that may be appropriate for the patient are reviewed to provide a guide for nursing care. The complex management of the patient in shock is also discussed, including fluids, pharmacological and mechanical modalities, and supportive nursing care. An overview of complications and a comprehensive nursing care plan complete the chapter on shock.

Definition

Shock is a clinical syndrome characterized by inadequate tissue perfusion that results in impaired cellular metabolism.

Etiological Factors

BASIC MECHANISMS

The cardiovascular system continually provides cells with the oxygen and nutrients necessary for survival, and rids the body of the waste products of metabolism. It is a closed, interdependent system composed of the heart, blood, and vascular bed. Arteries, veins, and the capillary network or microcirculation (i.e., arterioles, venules, and capillaries) make up the vascular bed. The microcirculation is the most significant portion of the circulatory system for cell survival (Fig. 7-1). It includes over 90% of the blood vessels and consists of that portion of the vascular bed between the arterioles and venules (Potter, 1983). Its functions are to deliver nutrients to, and remove wastes from, cells, regulate blood volume, and adjust blood flow to tissues in relation to their metabolic needs. Whereas the heart, arteries, and veins increase cardiac output in response to sympathetic nervous system stimulation, the microcirculation responds to local tissue needs. The vessels of the microcirculation constrict or dilate in order to selectively regulate blood flow to cells in need of oxygen and nutrients while bypassing those not in demand.

The microcirculation differs according to the function of the tissues and organs it supplies; however, all of these vascular beds have common structural characteristics (Potter, 1983). This arrangement allows for changes in the amount and course of blood flow.

As blood leaves the aorta it flows through progressively smaller arteries until it flows into an arteriole (see Fig. 7-1). Arterioles are lined with smooth muscle that allows these small vessels to change diameter, and as a result direct and adjust blood flow to the capillaries. From the arteriole blood then enters a metarteriole, a smaller vessel that branches from the arteriole at right angles. Metarterioles are partially lined with smooth muscle, allowing them to also adjust diameter size and regulate blood flow into capillaries.

Blood next enters the capillary network by passing through a muscular precapillary sphincter. Capillaries are narrow, thin-walled vascular networks that branch off the metarterioles. This network configuration increases the surface area to allow for greater fluid and nutrient exchange, and decreases the velocity of the blood flow to prolong transport time through the capillaries.

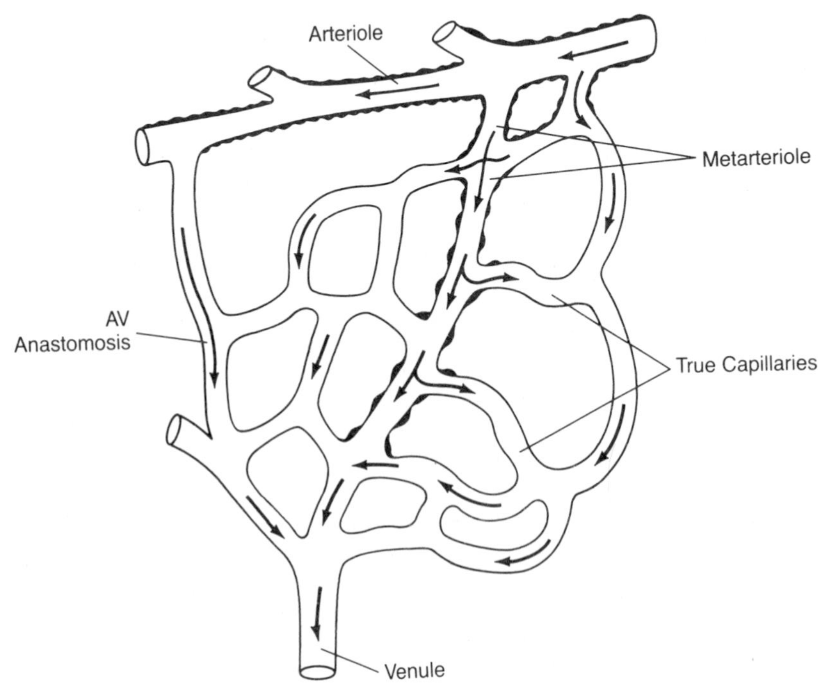

Figure 7-1. Microcirculation. Redrawn from Perry AG, Potter PA (1983): *Shock: Comprehensive Nursing Management.* St. Louis: C.V. Mosby, p. 43.

Capillaries have no contractile ability, and are not responsive to vasoactive chemicals, electrical or mechanical stimulation, or to pressure across their walls. The precapillary sphincter is the only means of regulating blood flow into a capillary. When the precapillary sphincter constricts, blood flow is diverted away from a capillary bed and directed to one that supplies tissues in need of oxygen and nutrients.

Once nutrients are exchanged for cellular waste products in the capillaries, blood then enters a venule. These small muscular vessels are able to dilate and constrict, offering postcapillary resistance to regulate blood flow through capillaries. Blood then flows from the venule and enters the larger veins of the venous system.

Another component of the microcirculation is the arteriovenous anastomoses that connect arterioles directly to venules (see Fig. 7–1). These muscular vessels are able to shunt blood away from the capillary circulation, sending it directly to tissues in need of oxygen and nutrients.

Shock begins when the cardiovascular system fails to function properly owing to an alteration in at least one of the three essential circulatory components: blood volume, myocardial contractility, and/or vascular resistance. Under healthy circumstances these three function together to maintain circulatory homeostasis. When one of these components fails, the remaining parts will compensate. However, as compensatory mechanisms fail, or more than one of the circulatory components are affected, a state of shock will ensue. Shock is not a single clinical entity but a life-threatening response to alterations in circulation, and consequently tissue oxygenation and cellular metabolism.

CLASSIFICATIONS OF SHOCK

A variety of diverse events may initiate the shock syndrome. These events may be classified according to the altered or affected circulatory component (Table 7–1) (Niedringhaus, 1983a; Rice, 1991a).

Regardless of the causative etiology, the deadly common denominator in any shock state is that of inadequate tissue perfusion occurring as a result of the marked reduction in nutritional blood flow through the microcirculation.

Pathophysiology

HYPOVOLEMIC SHOCK

Causes

Hypovolemic shock occurs when there is inadequate circulating blood volume to fill the vascular network. Intravascular blood volume deficits may be due to either external or internal losses (Table 7–2) (Rice, 1991a). In either case, the blood volume is depleted and, therefore, unable to transport oxygen and nutrients to tissues.

External volume deficits of blood, plasma, and/or body fluids can result in hypovolemic shock. The most common cause of hypovolemic shock is hemorrhage with the loss of whole blood (Niedringhaus, 1983b; Rice, 1991a). Hypovolemia due to hemorrhage is classified according to the volume of blood lost and the resultant effects on the level of consciousness, vital signs, capillary refill, and urine output (Table 7–3) (*Advanced Trauma Life Support,* 1989; Siskind, 1984; *Trauma Nurse Core Course,* 1987). External hemorrhage may be seen after traumatic injury, surgery, delivery of a baby, or with coagulation alterations (i.e., hemophilia, thrombocytopenia, disseminated intravascular coagulation, anticoagulant medications). External plasma losses may be seen with exudative lesions or burn injuries. Burn shock occurs as plasma rapidly shifts from the intravascular compartment through heat-damaged capillaries into the interstitial space or burned surface area. The loss of proteins with the plasma causes colloidal osmotic pressure to decrease, causing a further reduction of intravascular volume. Excessive external loss of fluid may result in dehydration shock if not corrected. This may be seen with losses via the gastrointestinal

Table 7–1. CLASSIFICATION OF SHOCK

Altered Circulatory Component		Classification of Shock
Blood volume	=	Hypovolemic shock
Myocardial contractility	=	Cardiogenic shock
Vascular resistance	=	Distributive shock

Table 7–2. CAUSES OF HYPOVOLEMIC SHOCK

External Losses	Internal Losses
Blood	Third-space sequestration
Plasma	Fluid loss into intestinal lumen
Body fluid	Internal hemorrhage

Table 7-3. CLASSIFICATION OF HYPOVOLEMIC SHOCK AND ESTIMATED FLUID AND BLOOD REQUIREMENTS*

	Class I	Class II	Class III	Class IV
Blood Loss (ml)	up to 750	750–1500	1500–2000	2000 or more
Blood Loss (%BV)	up to 15%	15–30%	30–40%	40% or more
Pulse Rate	<100	>100	>120	140 or higher
Blood Pressure	Normal	Normal	Decreased	Decreased
Pulse Pressure (mmHG)	Normal or increased	Decreased	Decreased	Decreased
Capillary Refill Test	Normal	Delayed	Delayed	Delayed
Respiratory Rate	14–20	24–30	30–40	>35
Urine Output (ml/hr)	30 or more	24–30	5–15	Negligible
CNS–Mental Status	Slightly anxious	Mildly anxious	Anxious and confused	Confused-lethargic
Fluid Replacement (3:1 Rule)	Crystalloid	Crystalloid	Crystalloid + blood	Crystalloid + blood

* For a 70-kg male.

From Advanced Trauma Life Support, 1989. Adapted with permission from the American College of Surgeons Committee on Trauma ATLS® Student Manual, 1988 Edition.

tract (i.e., wound drainage, suctioning, vomiting, diarrhea, reduction in oral fluid intake, fistulas), the genitourinary tract (i.e., diuresis, diabetes mellitus with polyuria, diabetes insipidus, diabetic ketoacidosis, hyperglycemic hyperosmolar nonketotic coma, diuretic therapy, Addison's disease), and/or through the skin (diaphoresis without fluid and electrolyte replacements).

Internal volume deficits due to third-space sequestration, fluid leakage into the intestinal lumen, and/or internal hemorrhage may also result in hypovolemic shock. Third-space sequestration, or the pooling of fluid in interstitial spaces, is seen with ascites, cirrhosis, peritonitis, and edema. Intestinal obstruction causes fluid to leak from the intestinal capillaries into the lumen of the intestine. This results in a decreased venous return. Internal hemorrhage may be seen with a ruptured spleen or liver, hemothorax, hemorrhagic pancreatitis, fractures of the femur or pelvis, and lacerations of the great vessels.

Consequences

Hypovolemic shock results in a reduction of intravascular volume and decreased venous return to the right side of the heart. Ventricular filling pressures are reduced and consequently there is a decrease in stroke volume and cardiac output. As the cardiac output falls, the blood pressure decreases and there is a reduction in tissue perfusion. The end result is impaired cellular metabolism as a result of the decrease in nutritional blood flow through capillaries that supply the cells with oxygen and nutrients.

CARDIOGENIC SHOCK

Causes

Cardiogenic shock is the failure of the heart to act as an effective pump. A decrease in myocardial contractility results in decreased cardiac output and impaired tissue perfusion. This type of shock occurs with any condition that interferes with the pumping action of the heart. Rice (1991a) concludes that there are coronary and noncoronary causes of cardiogenic shock. The majority of cases of cardiogenic shock are those that are coronary in nature. This is seen in the patient with an acute myocardial infarction (AMI). It can occur when there are diseased coronary arteries that are no longer capable of meeting the oxygen demand of the working myocardial cells. There is a correlation between the amount of myocardial damage and the likelihood of the individual developing cardiogenic shock. If 40% or more of the myocardium is damaged there is a good chance that the patient may develop cardiogenic shock (Huang et al., 1983).

The noncoronary causes of cardiogenic shock include those conditions that result in ineffective myocardial cell function that is not related to diseased coronary arteries. These include cardiac tamponade, cardiomyopathy, myocarditis, metabolic derangements, valvular disease, structural disorders, and vitamin deficiencies (Emmanuelson and Rosenlicht, 1986; Whitman, 1988). Cardiogenic shock is one of the most difficult types of shock to treat and carries a mortality of 80 to 85% (Emmanuelson and Rosenlicht, 1986).

Consequences

The specific pathophysiology of cardiogenic shock can be understood by reviewing cardiac dynamics. Contractile force is responsible for the amount of blood ejected from the heart. The amount of blood ejected is called the stroke volume. The ventricular filling pressure is the pressure in the ventricles as they fill. Therefore, when the contractile force is reduced by some damage to the myocardium, as in myocardial infarction, the two basic factors of stroke volume and ventricular filling pressure are upset. The stroke volume is decreased as the heart is unable to pump effectively and eject adequate amounts of blood. The ventricular filling pressures begin to rise as the stroke volume declines. This occurs because blood that is not being pumped into the periphery remains in the cardiac chambers and increases the pressure in the ventricles. As these two things occur, the cardiac output decreases and causes hypotension. This hypotension brings about a reflex compensatory peripheral vasoconstriction, resulting in an increase in the afterload or the workload the heart must pump against. At the same time, the backup of blood into the pulmonary circulation causes a decrease in the perfusion of oxygen across the alveolar membranes, reducing the oxygen tension in the blood.

The already failing heart is now in a real crisis situation (Fig. 7–2). There is an increased demand placed on the myocardium owing to the increased blood that the cells require. The heart may increase its rate to compensate, which only increases the oxygen demand on an overworked myocardium. Coronary circulation is reduced, adding to myocardial ischemia and injury. This compounds the problem. In those patients whose cardiogenic shock is coronary in nature, this may cause an increase in infarction size.

Thus, cardiogenic shock becomes a vicious circle. There is reduced myocardial contractility, a decreased coronary artery blood flow, increased myocardial ischemia, and reduced cardiac output. This cycle leads to the common thread of decreased cellular perfusion to the myocardium.

The nurse must understand the consequences of cardiogenic shock in order to implement appropriate management of the syndrome. Management for cardiogenic shock will focus on the manipulation of afterload, preload, and contractility of the heart.

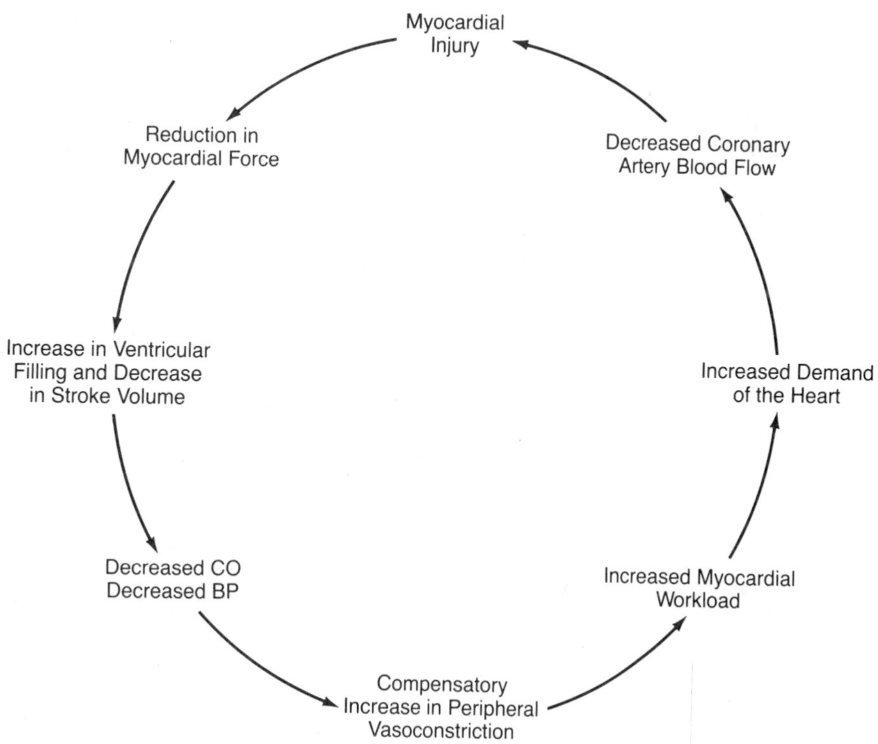

Figure 7–2. Cycle of cardiogenic shock.

DISTRIBUTIVE SHOCK

Causes

Distributive shock is a term used to describe several different types of shock that have in common widespread vasodilation with a decrease in peripheral vascular resistance. Vasodilation increases the vascular capacity; however, the blood volume that remains normal is abnormally distributed in the circulatory system. Neurogenic, anaphylactic, and septic shock are forms of distributive shock.

Neurogenic Shock

Neurogenic shock occurs when a disturbance in the nervous system affects the vasomotor center. In healthy individuals, the vasomotor center in the medulla initiates sympathetic stimulation of nerve fibers that travel down the spinal cord and out to the periphery. There they innervate the smooth muscles of the blood vessels to cause vasoconstriction. In neurogenic shock, specific disturbances interrupt sympathetic nerve impulses from the vasomotor center and consequently vasodilation and decreased peripheral vascular resistance result. Causes of neurogenic shock include injury or disease of the upper spinal cord, spinal anesthesia, and vasomotor depression (Rice, 1991a). Patients who suffer from cervical spinal cord injury or disease may experience a permanent or temporary interruption in sympathetic nerve stimulation. Spinal anesthesia may extend up the spinal cord and block sympathetic nerve impulses from the vasomotor center. Vasomotor depression may be seen with deep general anesthesia, injury to the medulla, drugs, severe pain, and hypoglycemia.

Anaphylactic Shock

A severe allergic reaction may precipitate a second form of distributive shock known as anaphylactic shock. Antigens, or foreign substances to which the individual is sensitive, initiate an antigen-antibody response. Antigens are classified by the route by which they enter the body (Table 7–4) (Myers, 1983).

Once an antigen enters the body, antibodies are produced and attach to mast cells and basophils. The greatest concentrations of mast cells are found in the lungs, around blood vessels, in connective tissue, and in the uterus. To a lesser extent, they are also found in the kidney, heart, skin, liver, spleen, and the omentum of the gastrointestinal tract. Basophils circulate in the blood. Both mast cells and basophils contain histamine and histamine-like substances.

Table 7–4. CLASSIFICATIONS OF ANTIGENS

Route	Substance
Injection	
Drugs	Antibiotics, Analgesics, Anesthetics, Vaccines, Hormones
Contrast Media	Iodine based radiologic dye
Blood Transfusions	Sensitivity to antigens in donor blood
Ingestion	Antibiotics, Milk, Egg, Egg whites, Oranges, Mangos, Bananas, Beans, Soybeans, Sesame and Sunflower Seeds, Seafood, Shellfish
Bites/Stings	Venomous snakes, Wasps, Bees, Hornets, Yellow jackets

The initial exposure to the antigen may not cause any harmful effects. However, subsequent exposures to the antigen cause the anaphylactic reaction. From this point on, when there is contact with the antigen, the antigen attaches to the antibodies on the mast cells and basophils. The antigen-antibody reaction causes cellular breakdown with the release of vasoactive substances from the cells (i.e., histamine, bradykinin, serotonin, prostaglandins, leukotrienes, heparin, and eosinophil chemotactic factor of anaphylaxis) (Dickerson, 1988). These substances cause vasodilation, increased capillary permeability, and contraction of smooth muscles. The combined effects are a decrease in blood pressure and a relative hypovolemia due to the vasodilation and fluid shifts as well as symptoms of anaphylaxis that primarily affect the skin, respiratory, and gastrointestinal systems. (See Assessment section below.)

Septic Shock

A third type of distributive shock, septic shock, is caused by an overwhelming systemic infection known as sepsis. Septicemia, an infection in which bacteria rapidly multiply in the blood stream, often precludes the development of sepsis and septic shock. In healthy individuals, the body is protected from bacterial invasion by the reticuloendothelial system, which ingests bacteria, and by the inflammatory response, which delivers defense components to the injured site. Predisposing factors, however, increase the risk for developing septic shock. It is commonly seen in individuals who have compromised immunity and/or have undergone invasive medical or surgical procedures that interrupt their defense system and create portals of entry for invading microorganisms (Table 7–5) (Littleton, 1988; Rice, 1991a and b; Smith-Collins, 1983).

Many illnesses, therefore, can be complicated by localized or systemic infections. Those that develop into septicemia and may progress to septic shock often begin at a primary site in the blood or urinary, respiratory, or gastrointestinal tract (Smith-Collins, 1983). Each of these systems has unique properties that bacteria require in order to survive and reproduce. The blood can be a primary site of infection, particularly in debilitated patients who require multiple invasive intravenous lines and catheters. The highly vascular renal tissue and the culture medium provided by the urinary tract make it a common portal for bacterial growth. The respiratory system is directly exposed to air and has the warm, dark, moist environment that bacteria need to proliferate. Surgery, abscesses, or perforations of the gastrointestinal tract can provide a route for the many microorganisms found in this system to enter the blood stream.

Gram-negative bacteria are the most common cause of septic shock, and infection with these microorganisms results in high mortality rates (Rice, 1991a, 1984a; Smith-Collins, 1983). The cell wall of gram-negative bacteria contains endotoxins that when released at the death of the cell cause deleterious effects. Gram-negative bacteria include *Escherichia coli, Klebsiella pneumoniae, Enterobacter, Proteus, Pseudomonas, Serratia marcescens,* and *Bacteriodes* (Rice, 1984a; Smith-Collins, 1983). These bacteria are normally found in the gastrointestinal and genitourinary tracts, the nose, throat, and skin, and in wounds and abscesses. They are also prevalent in hospital environments and are resistant to disinfectants.

Table 7–5. PREDISPOSING RISK FACTORS FOR SEPTIC SHOCK

Compromised Immunity	Invasive Procedures
Chronic Debilitating Diseases	Surgical Procedures
Neoplastic Disease, Leukemia, Cirrhosis, Diabetes Mellitus, Cardiovascular Disease, Pulmonary Disease, Renal Failure, Lupus, Alcoholism, AIDS	Invasive Diagnostics
Anemia, Malnutrition	Urologic Procedures
Skin Alterations	Bronchoscopies
Burns, Ulcerations	OB/GYN Procedures
Drug Therapy	Septic Abortions, Cesarean Sections
Antibiotics, Immunosuppressives	Hysterectomy for Pelvic Inflammatory Disease
Cytotoxics, Corticosteroids	Invasive Lines/Tubes
Extremes of Age	Indwelling Catheters
Less than 1 year	Pulmonary Artery Catheters
More than 65	Central Venous Lines
	ET Tube/Tracheostomy

Gram-positive bacteria may also cause septic shock, but the clinical presentation is less severe and the incidence and mortality rates are lower in comparison (Rice, 1991a, 1984a; Smith-Collins, 1983). Gram-positive bacteria include *Staphylococcus, Streptococcus, Pneumococcus, Clostridium,* and *Meningococcus* (Rice, 1991a, 1984a).

Septic shock may also be caused by viral, yeast, rickettsial, and fungal infections (Rice, 1984a; Smith-Collins, 1983).

Septic shock caused by gram-negative bacteria progresses through two distinct clinical patterns due to the effects of endotoxins (Holt et al., 1985; Rice, 1991a, 1984a). The first stage is a hyperdynamic cardiovascular and metabolic state known as warm, high-output, or hyperdynamic shock. The invading bacteria multiply faster than the body can kill them. As the bacteria are destroyed, endotoxins are released into the blood stream, damaging tissues and altering cellular metabolism. The cells are unable to use the oxygen and other nutrients, and consequently cellular hypoxia and a reduction in energy production results. In addition, endotoxins cause the release of histamine, a vasoactive substance that causes vasodilation. As a result, there is a decrease in peripheral vascular resistance, a fall in blood pressure, and venous pooling, all of which reduce the amount of blood returned to the heart (i.e., preload). The cardiac output may be normal to high because of a compensatory tachycardic response and the heart does not have to pump as hard against the low peripheral vascular resistance and blood pressure (i.e., afterload); however, the blood is shunted away from the hypoxic cells. This early stage of shock may go undetected as this hyperdynamic state presents a clinical picture of high urinary output, hyperventilation with respiratory alkalosis, vasodilation with warm, dry, flushed skin, hyperthermia, and a cardiac output that exceeds 7 L/min. Patients usually remain in this hyperdynamic phase for 30 min to 16 hours.

As septic shock progresses, the patient presents with hypodynamic, low-output, or cold shock, which is also due to the effects of endotoxins. Histamine now causes increased capillary permeability. Third spacing occurs as fluid leaks from the intravascular space, causing a relative hypovolemia and stagnation of blood in the vasculature. Systemic vascular resistance increases in an attempt to compensate for the reduction in blood pressure, but this intense vasoconstriction aggravates tissue ischemia and organ failure. Venous return to the heart is diminished and the patient presents with a clinical picture of poor tissue perfusion, decreased cardiac and urinary output, hypotension, pulmonary congestion, depressed level of consciousness, and vasoconstriction with cold, clammy skin.

Septic shock caused by gram-positive bacteria also results in vasodilation and increased vascular permeability; however, the clinical picture is less severe. The decreased peripheral vascular resistance and fluid shifts cause a decrease in the venous return to the right side of the heart. Stroke volume and cardiac output fall, and decreased tissue perfusion and cellular hypoxia are the end results. Toxic shock syndrome is one form of septic shock caused by a gram-positive bacteria, *Staphylococcus aureus.* The bacteria release a potent toxin that exerts its effects within hours. It is commonly associated with the use of tampons in menstruating women; however, toxic shock syndrome is also seen in patients with surgical wounds, deep and superficial abscesses, infected burns, abrasions, insect bites, herpes zoster, cellulitis, septic abortion, osteomyelitis, after vaginal and cesarean delivery, and in some newborns in whom the bacteria were transmitted from the mother.

Consequences

Distributive shock results in a relative hypovolemia. Blood volume remains normal but the blood is abnormally distributed in this "increased" vascular space because of massive vasodilation and decreased peripheral vascular resistance. The result is a decreased venous return to the right side of the heart and a reduction in ventricular filling pressures. Anaphylactic shock and the hypodynamic, or cold stage, of septic shock are also complicated by an increase in capillary permeability that decreases intravascular volume, contributing further to the decrease in venous return. Eventually in all forms of distributive shock, there is a decrease in stroke volume and cardiac output. The blood pressure decreases and with that there is a reduction in tissue perfusion. The end result is impaired cellular metabolism due to a decrease in nutritional blood flow through capillaries that supply the cells with oxygen and nutrients.

Clinical Manifestations

OVERVIEW OF THE STAGES OF SHOCK

The diminished supply of oxygen and nutrients that occurs in shock eventually disrupts cellular metabolism and the production of energy. The cells then convert to anaerobic metabolism, producing lactic acidosis. As acids accumulate, they cause the cell to release powerful enzymes that destroy the cell membrane. Once this occurs, the cellular changes are irreversible and the state of shock ensues. While the response to shock is highly individualized according to the patient's circumstances, the clinical picture presents in stages that progress at unpredictable rates (Bullock and Rosendahl, 1988; Luckmann and Sorenson, 1987; Niedringhaus, 1983a; Rice, 1991b). These stages of shock result regardless of whether the clinical syndrome is due to alterations in blood volume, cardiac contractility, or vascular resistance.

Stage I: The Initial Stage

During the initial stage, observable clinical symptoms are absent, but cellular metabolism may be altered in response to the reduction in cardiac output and the subsequent decrease in tissue perfusion (Rice, 1991b). At this stage, shock may be reversed by infusion of blood, fluids, and/or pharmacological therapy (Niedringhaus, 1983a).

Stage II: Early, or Compensatory, Stage

As shock progresses, the sustained reduction in cardiac output initiates a set of neural, endocrine, and chemical compensatory mechanisms in an attempt to restore homeostasis (Rice, 1991b).

Neural Compensation. Baroreceptors (sensitive to pressure changes) and chemoreceptors (sensitive to chemical changes) located in the carotid sinus and aortic arch detect the reduction in arterial blood pressure. Impulses are relayed to the vasomotor center in the medulla oblongata that stimulate the sympathetic branch of the autonomic nervous system to release epinephrine and norepinephrine from the adrenal medulla. In response to these catecholamines, the heart increases the rate and force of contractions in order to supply the heart muscle with more oxygen.

Vasoconstriction occurs with arterial vasoconstriction, improving blood pressure, whereas venous vasoconstriction augments return to the heart, increasing cardiac output. Additionally, vasoconstriction of blood vessels that supply the kidneys, gastrointestinal tract, and skin shunts blood flow to vital organs such as the heart and brain. Bronchial smooth muscles are relaxed and respiratory rate and depth are increased, thus improving oxygen and carbon dioxide gas exchange in the lungs. Additional catecholamine effects are an increase in blood sugar (as the liver is stimulated to convert glycogen to glucose), dilation of pupils, cool, moist skin (due to increased sweat gland activity), and vasodilation of blood vessels to skeletal muscle. The overall effects of sympathetic nervous system stimulation attempt to combat shock by vasoconstriction, increased cardiac output, improved blood pressure, and increased perfusion to the heart and brain.

Endocrine Compensation. In response to the reduction in blood pressure (detected by the baro- and chemoreceptors), messages are also relayed to the hypothalamus that stimulate the anterior pituitary gland to release adrenocorticotropic hormone (ACTH) and the posterior pituitary gland to release antidiuretic hormone (ADH). The ACTH acts on the adrenal cortex to release gluco- and mineralocorticoids. Glucocorticoids increase the blood sugar by increasing the conversion of glycogen to glucose (glycogenolysis). Mineralcorticoids act on renal tubules to reabsorb sodium and chloride, which causes water to be reabsorbed, thus conserving intravascular volume. Aldosterone is also released in response to a reduction of pressure in the renal arterioles that supply the glomeruli of the kidneys, and/or by the increase in sodium levels as sensed by the kidneys' juxtaglomerular apparatus. This reduction in renal perfusion is a consequence of decreased cardiac output and vasoconstriction that shunts the blood away from the kidneys. In response, the juxtaglomerular apparatus releases renin. Renin circulates in the blood and reacts with angiotensinogen to produce angiotensin I. Angiotensin I circulates through the lungs, where it forms angiotensin II, a potent arterial and venous vasoconstrictor, which increases blood pressure and improves venous return to the heart. Angiotensin II also activates the adrenal cortex to release the mineralcorticoid aldosterone, which exerts the effects on renal tubular reabsorption described above. Antidiuretic hormone (ADH) is secreted by the posterior pituitary in response to the increased osmolality of the blood (which occurs with an increase in sodium reabsorption due to the aldosterone effects just described) and to the dehydration state seen in shock (due to the loss of intravascular volume as a consequence of increased capillary permeability and fluid shifting). The overall effects of endocrine compensation attempt to combat shock by providing the body with glucose for energy and increasing the intravascular blood volume.

Chemical Compensation. As cardiac output decreases, pulmonary blood flow is reduced. This results in ventilation perfusion imbalances. The alveoli may be adequately ventilated with oxygen, but the perfusion of blood through the alveolar capillary bed is decreased. Chemoreceptors, located in the aorta and carotid arteries, are stimulated in response to this low oxygen tension in the blood. Consequently, the rate and depth of respirations increases, but as the patient hyperventilates respiratory alkalosis occurs and carbon dioxide is blown off during expirations. A reduction in carbon dioxide levels and the alkalotic state cause vasoconstriction of cerebral blood vessels. This vasoconstriction, coupled with the reduced oxygen tension, leads to cerebral hypoxia and ischemia. The overall effects of chemical compensation attempt to combat shock by increasing oxygen supply; however, in doing so, they cause negative effects on cerebral perfusion.

During the early or compensatory stage of shock the patient begins to present with clinical signs and symptoms (see Assessment section below). At this stage, shock may still be reversed if appropriate interventions are initiated (see Management section below) (Niedringhaus, 1983a).

Stage III: Intermediate, or Progressive, Shock

If the cause of shock is not corrected and/or compensatory mechanisms continue without reversing the shock, they now begin to contribute to the deteriorating condition of the patient. Whereas during the compensatory stage the systemic circulation and microcirculation worked together with vasoconstriction to increase venous return, they now begin to function independently and in opposition (Luckmann and Sorensen, 1987; Rice, 1991b).

The systemic circulation continues to vasoconstrict. While this shunts blood to priority organs, the decrease in cutaneous blood flow may lead to ischemia in peripheral extremities, weak or absent pulses, and altered body defenses. Prolonged vasoconstriction results in decreased capillary blood flow and eventually results in cellular hypoxia. The cells convert to anaerobic metabolism, which leads to a local metabolic acidosis. At this point, the microcirculation exerts the opposite effect and dilates in order to obtain the limited blood supply for local tissue needs. While the arterioles remain constricted in an attempt to keep vital organs perfused, the precapillary sphincters relax, allowing blood to flow into the capillary bed. Meanwhile, postcapillary sphincters remain constricted. As a result, blood flows freely into the capillary bed but becomes bottled up in the capillaries as blood flow from the capillary bed is impeded. Capillary hydrostatic pressure increases and fluid is pushed from the capillaries into the interstitial space, causing edema. Additionally, fluid shifting from the intravascular space is further aggravated as histamine increases capillary permeability and the loss of proteins through enlarged capillary pores lowers colloidal osmotic pressure. As intravascular blood volume decreases, the blood becomes more viscous and blood flow is slowed. This causes capillary sludging, and red blood cells, platelets, and proteins clump together. This further impairs blood flow, and later contributes to coagulation alterations. The loss of intravascular volume along with capillary pooling further reduces the venous return to the heart and cardiac output. At this point, the patient presents with classic shock signs and symptoms affecting all body systems (See Assessment section below).

This phase of shock responds poorly to fluid replacement alone, and requires aggressive medical and nursing management if it is to be reversed (Niedringhaus, 1983a).

Stage IV: Refractory, or Irreversible, Shock

Prolonged inadequate tissue perfusion that is unresponsive to therapy ultimately contributes to multiple organ failure and the inevitable death of the patient. A large volume of the blood remains pooled in the capillary bed, and the arterial blood pressure is too low to support perfusion of the vital organs with oxygen and nutrients. Poor renal function, respiratory failure, and impaired cellular function aggravate the existing state of acidosis, which in turn contributes to further fluid shifts, loss of vasomotor tone, and relative hypovolemia. Coronary artery perfusion and oxygen delivery to the heart muscle are reduced, causing myocardial ischemia and dysrhythmias. This reduction, coupled with the dysrhythmias, continued acidosis, and the accumulation of myocardial depressant factor, reduces the heart rate and impairs cardiac contractility and cardiac output. Acidosis, decreased intravascular fluid volume, and sluggish blood flow through the capillaries leads to clumping of platelets and red blood cells. These aggregates form fibrin clots that occlude small vessels and further impede blood flow. This cycle depletes clotting factors and may result in disseminated intravascular coagulation (DIC) (see Complications section below). Cerebral ischemia occurs because of the reduction in cerebral blood flow. Consequently, the sympathetic nervous system is stimulated, which aggravates the existing vasoconstriction, increasing afterload and decreasing cardiac output. Prolonged cerebral ischemia eventually causes the loss of sympathetic nervous system response and vasodilation and bradycardia result. The patient's decreasing blood pressure and heart rate cause a lethal decrease in tissue perfusion, and ultimately brain death and cardiopulmonary arrest result.

Clinical Manifestations

ASSESSMENT

The most important step of the nursing process is assessment. This is particularly true in the patient in shock. It is from this information that the nurse identifies goals that provide the direction for the definitive care of the patient (Rice, 1991c). If the nurse is unclear as to the type of shock or the mechanisms that are occurring in the patient, then care may be misdirected or perhaps inappropriate. Assessment is also important in considering the prodromal aspects of the syndrome. It would be much better to prevent shock from occurring rather than focus on how to treat it. Therefore, continuous assessment of the patient at risk can mean the difference between life and death. If problems are not treated as they arise, the patient may suffer because of this deficit.

As was noted earlier, shock is a common threat to the cells of all organ systems. If there is a decrease in tissue perfusion occurring in the shock syndrome, then all tissues suffer—shock is not selective in its effects. So in considering the assessment of the individual in shock, the nurse must look at how the cells and the organ systems in which they exist are affected by the decrease in tissue perfusion. Assessment should focus on three areas: history, clinical picture, and laboratory diagnosis. The logical framework for assessment to follow is to first examine the history of the patient and then look at the systems most sensitive to a lack of needed nutrients.

History

As previously discussed, history is vital to identifying the appropriate nursing approaches to patients in shock. The nurse must look at such patients with a high index of suspicion and obtain specific data regarding the causative incident. A clearly documented history may be the key to successful treatment of the patient.

Clinical Picture

Central Nervous System

The central nervous system (CNS) is the most sensitive to changes in the supply of oxygen and nutrients. Thus, it is the system first affected by changes in cellular perfusion. The initial response of the CNS to shock includes agitation, anxiety, nervousness, and restlessness. This symptomology can be related to the sympathetic nervous stimulation that is occurring. As the shock state progresses, the patient becomes drowsy, confused, and lethargic because of the decreased blood flow to the brain. This can continue to progress with increased lethargy, drowsiness, and stupor until in the late phase the patient becomes unresponsive.

Cardiovascular System

Blood Pressure. A major concern and focus of assessment for years has been the blood pressure in shock states. Today, this remains a cardinal symptom of shock but with some cautions. In general, initial blood pressures are normal to hypertensive. This occurs as a result of the effects of the sympathetic nervous system. As the shock state progresses, however, the patient's blood pressure will drop. It is important for the nurse to know a baseline blood pressure. Texts will vary in listing blood pressure parameters, but a drop in systolic blood pressure below 80 mm Hg can be used as a guide. People who have hypertension may differ in these values. For a hypertensive patient, a drop of 100 mm Hg from his/her average pressure may be considered severe hypotension.

A key point to consider in assessing the blood pressure is that cuff pressures may be very inaccurate. Remember that one of the chief compensatory mechanisms that occurs early in the shock state is vasoconstriction initiated by the sympathetic nervous system, which generally assists in maintaining perfusion to the vital organs. This vasoconstriction can also lead to inaccuracies in peripheral blood pressure readings. For this reason, it is often recommended that if the pressure is not heard via auscultation, a blood pressure reading should be attempted by palpation or ultrasound (Doppler) devices.

Intra-arterial lines may also be considered an accurate method to assess the blood pressure changes that the patient in shock may exhibit. Arterial lines provide a direct source for obtaining blood samples when frequent laboratory determinations are needed.

The location of palpable pulses can give an approximation of the blood pressure if instrumentation is not available. If the brachial pulse is readily palpable, the approximate systolic pressure is 80 mm Hg. Corresponding blood pressures for the femoral and carotid pulses are 70 and 60 mm Hg respectively (McQuillan and Wiles, 1988).

One other assessment of the blood pressure to consider is the tilt test. With this technique, the patient is taken from a lying to a sitting position very quickly and blood pressures pre- and postpositioning are compared. If the pressure drops 10 mm Hg, it is correlated with a mild degree of shock. Decreases of 25 to 50 mm Hg approximate a moderate degree of shock, and a loss of 50 mm Hg or greater indicates a marked or severe state of shock.

Pulse. The rate, quality, and character of the pulse should be evaluated. The nurse should include major pulses in the assessment. These are carotid, radial, femoral, dorsalis pedis, and posterior tibial. In shock states, the heart rate is tachycardic, generally over 100 beats per minute, weak, thready, and of short duration (Emmanuelson and Rosenlicht, 1986; Rice, 1991c). The rhythm of the pulse is dependent upon the presence of dysrhythmias. The pulse is elevated in a compensatory response to the decreased cardiac output and the demand of the cells for increased oxygen. In the later stages of shock, the pulse will slow and the patient will be further compromised as far as the cardiovascular status is concerned (Emmanuelson and Rosenlicht, 1986). This slowing of the pulse may be related to the myocardial depressant factor that is released in severe cases of metabolic acidosis (Alspach, 1991).

Capillary Refill. An indicator that can reveal the ability of the cardiovascular system to maintain perfusion to the periphery is capillary refill.

The normal response to pressure on the nail bed is blanching. The color of the nail bed returns to a normal pink hue 1 to 2 seconds following release of pressure. A longer delay in the return of color indicates peripheral vasoconstriction. Capillary refill is a quick reference assessment of the patient's overall cardiovascular status.

Central Venous Pressure (CVP). Central venous lines may be put in place to aid in the differential diagnosis of shock, monitor therapies, and provide an evaluation of the preload of the heart. Normally, the CVP is 4 to 12 cm H_2O or 0 to 4 mm Hg (Dailey and Schroeder, 1989). In the presence of a decreased blood volume (i.e., hypovolemic shock), the CVP will fall. With cardiogenic shock, however, the CVP may be high owing to the poor myocardial contractility and high filling pressure in the ventricles.

Pulmonary Artery Pressure. A pulmonary artery line (PA line) is one of the most useful tools available for helping with the diagnosis and the treatment of the patient in shock. The flow-directed, balloon-tipped catheter can give information regarding fluid balance, the pumping ability of the heart, and the effects of vasoactive agents. In general, a quadruple-lumen catheter is used to get the most information. Specifically, this catheter aids in measuring the hemodynamic parameters (Table 7–6).

The primary indicators of cardiovascular functioning are examined with use of the pulmonary artery catheter. Preload, measured by the mean right atrial pressure for the right ventricle and by the pulmonary capillary wedge pressure for the left ventricle, is the value that can be examined in looking for problems in the fluid balance of an individual. The systemic vascular resistance (SVR) is a primary numerical value that offers specific information on the afterload or the workload of the left ventricle, and the pulmonary vascular resistance (PVR) measures right ventricular workload or afterload. The cardiac output (CO) and the cardiac index (CI) are the values that give information regarding the contractility of the heart and how it is handling the cell's demands for nutrients.

Using a pulmonary artery line can facilitate the care of the patient in shock. It aids in both the diagnosis (Table 7–7) and treatment because the nurse can readily see the effects of fluids, vasoactive drugs, and any agents used to improve contractility.

Table 7–6. HEMODYNAMIC PARAMETERS WITH NORMAL VALUES

Parameter	Normal
Right Atrial Pressure (RAP)	0–7 mm Hg
Pulmonary Artery Systolic (PASP)	0–7 mm Hg
Pulmonary Artery Diastolic (PADP)	15–25 mm Hg
Pulmonary Capillary Wedge (PCWP)	6–12 mm Hg
Cardiac Output (CO)	4–6 L/min
Cardiac Index (CI)	2.5–4 L/min
Systemic Vascular Resistance (SVR)	800–1200 dyne/sec
Pulmonary Vascular Resistance (PVR)	250 dyne/sec/cm

Respiratory System

Respirations in the early stage of shock are rapid and deep. The respiratory center responds to the shock state and the metabolic acidosis that occurs with an increase in rate to eliminate the built up CO_2. It is a direct stimulation of the medulla by the chemoreceptors that is responsible for the alteration of the respiratory pattern. The chemoreceptors are sensitive to the increased acid level in the blood. In an effort to maintain acid-base balance, the response is to blow off CO_2. Two things occur that may cause a change in this pattern. As the shock state progresses, metabolic wastes build up and cause generalized muscle weakness and the respiratory muscles are affected. This leads to shallow breathing that does not exchange air. These two mechanisms account for the changes in respirations that occur and result in hypoventilation; respiratory failure will follow.

Pulse oximetry is frequently used to measure the saturation of arterial blood with oxygen. A probe is placed on a digit and a fiberoptic sensor evaluates the saturation of the red blood cell with oxygen. This tool can be useful to evaluate the patient's overall oxygenation, but it must be used with caution in the patient in shock. Pulse oximeters require peripheral pulsations to calculate the oxygen levels. In shock, the peripheral circulation is the first to suffer a decrease, and therefore pulse oximetry may not provide the best information on the patient's oxygen status.

Renal System

At one time, the urinary output was considered a prime indicator for the patient in shock. It remains a valued indicator but it is not the early sign used to identify the patient in shock. The urinary output drops in shock because of the re-

Table 7-7. HEMODYNAMIC ALTERATIONS IN SHOCK STATES

Parameter	Shock Type	Early or Compensated	Late or Decompensated
Right Atrial Pressure	Cardiogenic	↑	↑
	Hypovolemic	↓	↓
	Distributive	↓	↑
Pulmonary Artery Systolic	Cardiogenic	↑	↑
	Hypovolemic	↓	↓
	Distributive	↓	↑
Pulmonary Artery Diastolic	Cardiogenic	↑	↑
	Hypovolemic	↓	↓
	Distributive	↑	↑
Pulmonary Capillary Wedge	Cardiogenic	↑	↑
	Hypovolemic	↓	↑
	Distributive	↓	↑
Cardiac Output	Cardiogenic	↓	↑
	Hypovolemic	↓	↑
	Distributive	↑	↓
Cardiac Index	Cardiogenic	↓	↑
	Hypovolemic	↓	↑
	Distributive	↑	↓
Systemic Vascular Resistance	Cardiogenic	↑	↑
	Hypovolemic	—	↑
	Distributive	↓	↑

duction in renal perfusion. The kidneys try to compensate by reducing excreted fluids and concentrating urine. There is also a response from hormones released to aid the body in the shock state. Aldosterone promotes the retention of sodium and, therefore, the reabsorption of water. It is considered a definite sign of shock when the urinary output falls below 30 ml/hr. If not treated, and the output continues to fall, renal shutdown will occur and the patient will be in renal failure.

Skin, Mucous Membranes, and Musculature

Skin and Mucous Membranes. Skin color, temperature, texture, turgor, and moisture level should be evaluated when assessing the patient in shock or at risk for the development of shock. There can be characteristic changes in the skin depending upon the type of shock involved. In septic shock, the skin will often be moist, flushed, and hot to touch. In hypovolemic or cardiogenic shock, the skin will likely be pale, cool, and moist. The mucous membranes will be dry and pale in shock owing to the decreased perfusion. In toxic shock, the patient will display a red macular rash and desquamation of the skin and the mucous membranes may be bright red in color (i.e., strawberry tongue, pharyngitis, or conjunctivitis) (Broscious, 1991). In general, the patient in shock will suffer from neuromuscular fatigue occurring in all muscle systems. In the gastrointestinal system, this will result in a slowing of intestinal activity with problems such as a paralytic ileus. Patients with toxic shock will also exhibit neuromuscular symptoms such as arthralgia, general aching, malaise, abdominal discomfort, and neck stiffness (Broscious, 1991).

Skin assessment also includes observing for cyanosis. It must be noted that this is a late and unreliable sign. It is not a primary indicator of tissue perfusion and is subject to misinterpretation. Cyanosis is present when there is deoxygenated hemoglobin circulating in the blood stream. Deoxygenated hemoglobin has a bluish tint. Hypoxia is one reason why one might see cyanosis. There can be other conditions that result in deoxygenated hemoglobin being circulated. In the patient with polycythemia, for example, there are abnormally high levels of hemoglobin present, and since not all of the hemoglobin is saturated with oxygen, it is therefore characteristically blue in color. This patient will look cyanotic but has no deficit of oxygen. There are cases in which the

Table 7–8. LABORATORY VALUES COMMON IN SHOCK

Test	Normal Value	In Shock
Blood Glucose	70–100 mg/100 ml	Early: Increased Late: Decreased
Blood Urea Nitrogen	5–20 mg/100 ml	Increased
Creatinine	0.6–1.2 mg/100 ml	Increased
Sodium	136–142 mEq/L	Increased
Chloride	95–103 mEq/L	Decreased
CO_2	21–28 mEq/L	Early: Increased Late: Decreased
Arterial Blood Gases		
pH	7.35–7.45	Early: Increased Late: Decreased
Pco_2	35–45 mm Hg	Early: Decreased Late: Increased
Po_2	80–100 mm Hg	Decreased
HCO_3	22–28 mEq/L	Late: Decreased

patient has thick skin and this may alter the perception of the color of the skin. If the patient does exhibit cyanosis, it can be one of two types. The patient may exhibit central cyanosis seen in the mucous membranes of the mouth and nose or peripheral cyanosis evident in the nails and ear lobes.

Musculature. In assessing the musculature of the patient in shock, generalized weakness and fatigue are the major complaints. Alterations in perfusion to the gastrointestinal musculature causes symptoms of decreased bowel sounds, distention, nausea, and constipation. Prolonged decrease in perfusion can lead to ulceration.

Laboratory Diagnosis

Included in the diagnosis of shock are many laboratory tests that can aid in assessing the patient. As can be seen in Table 7–8, the laboratory testing done can be focused on those tests that have a general impact on the whole body. Tests that can give more of an idea of the differential diagnosis of shock are included in Table 7–9. It must be remembered that by the time many of the laboratory test results are altered, it is late in the staging of shock. The clinical picture is more heavily relied upon for rapid diagnosis and immediate treatment.

Other Diagnostics and Assessments

There are additional diagnostic tests and assessment parameters that may be used to assist in the care of the patient in shock or with the differential diagnosis of shock. These tests include urine studies, chest x-rays, heart sounds, peritoneal lavage, and computed tomography (CT).

Urine studies may be ordered to follow through on the renal status of the patient. One study that may be considered would be the specific gravity. This will be elevated in the patient suffering from shock owing to the decreased perfusion and increased retention of water that occurs as a defense mechanism secondary to the release of antidiuretic hormone. The urine osmolarity would also be increased because of the ADH release.

Chest x-rays are helpful for establishing the respiratory status of the patient in shock. They can be used to identify pulmonary edema in the

Table 7–9. LABORATORY TESTS FOR DIFFERENTIAL DIAGNOSIS OF SHOCK

Test	Normal Value	In Shock
Blood Culture	No Growth	Positive in Septic Shock
Hemoglobin	14.5–16.5 g/100 ml men 12.6–14.2 g/100 ml women	Decreased in Hypovolemic Shock Due to Hemorrhage
Hematocrit	42–52% men 37–47% women	Decreased in Hypovolemic Shock Due to Hemorrhage
Red Blood Cells	4.6–6.2 mil/ml men 4.5–5.4 mil/ml women	Decreased in Hypovolemic Shock Due to Hemorrhage
Cardiac Enzymes		
CPK	18–22 μ/L men 14–78 μ/L women	All Enzymes May Be Increased in Cardiogenic Shock Due to Coronary
CPK MB	0–1.4 μ/L <3% of Total	
LDH 1	25–33%	
LDH 2	35–41%	

patient in cardiogenic shock. Pulmonary edema can further compromise the patient's cellular oxygenation. Chest x-rays are also helpful in the early recognition of adult respiratory distress syndrome (ARDS), which is a common complication of the shock syndrome. In the patient admitted with chest injuries, the pleural space is often a source of bleeding. This may lead to shock, since a large volume of blood can be held in this cavity.

Cardiac auscultation will reveal abnormal heart sounds if the patient is in cardiogenic shock. A third heart sound (S_3) indicates filling of a flabby ventricle which occurs with myocardial muscle damage. A fourth heart sound (S_4) reflects a noncompliant ventricle (Rice, 1991c). Murmurs may be present in the patient with valvular diseases.

For the identification and confirmation of abdominal bleeding, a peritoneal lavage may be done. This is indicated in cases of severe trauma and is generally completed in the emergency department. Another assessment parameter that may be done is to measure the abdominal girth of the individual. An increase in the girth may also be an indicator of abdominal bleeding or fluid loss into the abdomen.

Computed tomography can be very helpful in assisting with the differential diagnosis of shock. It can pinpoint sources of bleeding in the abdomen. Computed tomography may reveal an area where abscess formation may be the cause of sepsis. It can also show spinal injuries that can precipitate spinal shock.

It cannot be reinforced enough that nursing assessment is key to treating the patient in shock. Assessment can help to identify the underlying causes and assure the appropriate treatment of the patient.

■ Nursing Diagnosis

Alteration in tissue perfusion (cellular) related to either decreased blood volume, myocardial contractility, or vascular resistance; or a combination of these.

■ Management Care Plan

The risk for shock is a common threat for many patients. Therefore, the primary goal is to identify those at risk and initiate early preventive interventions. Accurate assessments and early recognition of the signs and symptoms of impending shock are critical in order to prevent shock's progression or to reverse this life-threatening condition. See the Nursing Care Plan for the Patient with Hypovolemic Shock.

INDEX OF SUSPICION

One of the first things to take into consideration is the type of patients who might be more prone to developing the syndrome. If the nurse is alert for the patient who has the potential to develop shock, there is a greater likelihood that preventive steps can be taken (Bordick, 1980; Emmanuelson and Rosenlicht, 1986; Rice, 1991a). Once symptoms develop, the shock response has already begun to produce cellular alterations—alterations that may be fatal.

Generally speaking, those patients who are at high risk to develop shock are those who require frequent assessment. Any patient with traumatic injury, those with burns, or those who have required major surgery may be prone to develop hypovolemic shock. Patients with acute myocardial infarctions (AMIs), especially large infarcts involving the left ventricular wall, are susceptible to developing cardiogenic shock (Rice, 1991c). Anaphylactic shock must be considered for those patients with documented allergies. Septic shock may be averted by giving consideration to the use of invasive lines, Foley catheters, or endotracheal tubes. These patients can be susceptible to infections, and therefore sepsis can ensue. Patients with spinal injuries or those who have received spinal anesthesia must be monitored for the development of neurogenic shock. In summary, awareness of the potentiality of shock is the first step. It is here that shock may be prevented from occurring. The role of nursing is key in monitoring the patient to allay the occurrence and progression of shock. Nursing can be the first line of defense against death.

PREVENTION

As noted, awareness of the potential for shock is the first step in assessing the patient at risk. Following is a discussion of the types of shock and methods that may be taken by the nurse that may assist in reducing the patient's risk to develop shock.

Hypovolemic Shock

In preventing hypovolemic shock, the key is to monitor the fluid balance of the patient (Rice, 1991d). Fluid losses can occur in very frank or

NURSING CARE PLAN FOR THE PATIENT WITH HYPOVOLEMIC SHOCK		
Nursing Diagnosis	**Outcome**	**Intervention**
Alteration in tissue perfusion (cellular) related to decreased blood volume, myocardial contractility or vascular resistance, or a combination of these	Optimize tissue perfusion Fluid intake and output levels will balance Frank bleeding or fluid loss will be controlled Serum lab values and arterial blood gases will approximate patient normal Vital signs, cardiac and respiratory status will be normal for patient status Fluid and nutrition will be obtained orally rather than through infusion lines Mentation and cognition levels will be consistent with patient status Urinary and bowel elimination will be normal for patient Ambulation and mobility will begin to approximate normal for patient status Verbalizes comfort and cognition of events and surrounding environment	Monitor fluid balance (intake and output) every hour. Include chest drainage, N/G tube, dressings, etc. Daily weights Measure abdominal girth daily Apply pressure to control bleeding as needed Use of military anti-shock trousers (MAST) as needed Control frank fluid or blood loss Administer fluids as ordered; e.g., crystalloids, colloids, plasma expanders, blood and/or blood products Establish peripheral and central line access to vascular system Assess respiratory status, including airway status, breath sounds every 2 hr Administer oxygen as prescribed Monitor serum lab values and arterial blood gases every 4 hr or as needed Monitor chest x-ray for correct intubation and chest tube placement daily Assess cardiovascular status Monitor vital signs, capillary refill time, skin color, and temperature every hour Monitor ECG rhythm continuously Type and cross match for potential blood replacement Prepare patient for autotransfusion Assess neurological status every 4 hr Monitor level of consciousness constantly Insert Foley cathether and monitor urinary output every hour Test urine for hematuria and specific gravity every 4 hr Prepare patient for insertion of invasive monitoring lines and pulmonary artery catheters Administer medications as prescribed, particularly inotropic agents Monitor CVP, PCWP to determine volume and need for fluid replacement every 2 hr or as needed Frequent assessment of patient receiving blood transfusion Prepare patient for potential insertion of intra-aortic balloon pump (IABP) Constant monitoring and assessing of patient status while on IABP Cautious use of the Trendelenburg position Cautious use of warming blankets and heavy blankets for patients in shock Assess skin color, turgor, texture, temperature, and intactness every hour Provide psychological and physiological support for patient, family, and others
Potential for continued fluid volume deficit related to hemorrhage secondary to coagulopathy	Prevent, minimize, or correct clotting disorders Lab values will return to normal Verbalizes comfort and cognition of events and environment surrounding patient Respiratory, cardiac, neurological, and renal assessments are normal for patient status	Monitor pulmonary, cardiovascular, neurological, and renal status every hour Assess cognition and mentation every 2 hr Monitor serum lab values frequently; e.g., prothrombin time, partial thromboplastin time, platelets, and fibrinogen Administer blood or blood products as prescribed; e.g., RBCs, platelets, fresh frozen plasma, and cryoprecipitate Warm all blood before transfusing Administer calcium as needed and prescribed Monitor arterial blood gases and prepare for administration of sodium bicarbonate when blood pH level indicates

NURSING CARE PLAN FOR THE PATIENT WITH HYPOVOLEMIC SHOCK *Continued*

Nursing Diagnosis	Outcome	Intervention
		Prepare patient for use of autotransfusion Provide psychological and physiological support for patient, family, and others
Potential for hypothermia related to decreased tissue perfusion and rapid infusion of IV fluids	Maintain a normothermic state Body temperature approximates normal Respiratory, cardiac, neurological, and renal assessments are normal for patient status Skin is clear, cool without abnormal discoloration and abrasions Verbalizes comfort and cognition of events and surrounding environment	Monitor core body temperature continuously Provide warming devices as needed but cautiously; e.g., warming blankets, heavy blankets, warming lights, blood warmer Cautious use of the Trendelenburg position Monitor respiratory, cardiovascular, neurological, and renal status hourly Assess skin for color, turgor, temperature, discolorations, and intactness

Data from Doenges, M., et al.: Nursing Care Plans: Guidance for Planning Patient Care. 2nd ed. Philadelphia, F.A. Davis, 1989; Strange, J.M.: Shock Trauma Care Plans. Springhouse, PA, Springhouse Corp., 1987; and Swearingen, P., and Keen, J.H.: Manual of Critical Care: Applying Nursing Diagnosis to Adult Critical Illness. St. Louis, C.V. Mosby, 1991.

very subtle ways. Monitoring must include the measurement of any drainage such as a chest tube or nasogastric tube, dressings being weighed, and consideration of insensible losses such as perspiration. Abdominal girth may be taken periodically in patients in whom a hidden bleed may be suspected or in whom ascites may account for fluid losses.

Daily weights must be obtained using the same scale with the same clothing at approximately the same time each day in order to give the most accurate weight of the patient. The more accurate the weight, the more likely preventive measures can be instituted.

Bleeding from trauma may be controlled with pressure applied on or above the site to decrease the blood loss. Use of military anti-shock trousers (MAST) may also be indicated as a preventive step in decreasing blood loss (see Mechanical Management section below). Surgical intervention may be required to ligate or cauterize vessels that may be causing the blood loss.

Cardiogenic Shock

Prevention of cardiogenic shock is aimed at those measures that can decrease the myocardial oxygen demand and those that can increase oxygen supply to the damaged tissue (Rice, 1981c). By using aggressive therapy, the size of the infarction may be minimized. Thrombolytic agents, beta-blockers, and percutaneous transluminal angioplasty (PCTA) may help to reduce the size of the infarction. The nurse must be cautious in the use of positive inotropic agents such as digoxin that will increase the force of contraction of the heart, and thereby increase the myocardial oxygen requirement. The nurse can be key in assuring rest for the patient both physically and emotionally. Rest can be significant in reducing the workload of the heart, and therefore reduce infarct size. Another helpful treatment may be to reduce the amount of sodium in the diet of the patient, which will decrease the workload on the myocardium. Oxygen administration will increase the supply of oxygen to ischemic muscle and may help to save myocardial tissue from death.

Distributive Shock

Shock involving alterations in the vascular tree may also be prevented (Rice, 1991d). Prevention of septic shock can be accomplished through the maintenance of proper handwashing and the use of strict aseptic technique. The critical care patient is often one who is debilitated by an overwhelming disease process. This disease process may also require the insertion of multiple IV lines and catheters to adequately care for the patient. The combination of a weakened patient with many potential portals of entry for pathogens can often result in serious infectious processes and sepsis. Frequent monitoring of temperature as well as laboratory findings of white cell and differential counts are important to identify general responses to infection. Judicious use of appropriate antibiotics must be considered for the patient at risk.

Emphasis on a complete nursing history is essential in preventing anaphylactic shock. This part of a nursing database must be as detailed as possible with regard to drug reactions and possible allergies that the patient might have. Assessment for allergic responses must include questions about drugs with similar chemical structure or make-up. For example, drugs in the penicillin or lidocaine family may cause problems for the patient. Intravenous administration of drugs must be cautiously monitored. Injecting small amounts of the drug before the entire dosage is given is recommended. This may assist in detecting a possible reaction before an overwhelming dose is administered. Care must be taken in the administration of blood or blood products that can result in allergic reactions. The patient receiving any of these products should be observed closely for any signs of an allergic reaction such as flushing, rashes, pruritus, redness, swelling, or an increased temperature.

By constant immobilization of spinal injuries, the nurse may assist in preventing severe neurogenic shock. This may include traction devices such as skull tongs or halo brace (to maintain alignment), or surgical intervention to stabilize the injury. Administration of spinal anesthesia may also result in neurogenic shock, so the nurse must be aware that it can occur. The patient who has received a spinal anesthetic agent may be kept with the head of the bed at a 20-degree elevation to prevent the spread of the agent up the cord.

It is a conscious awareness that can aid in the prevention of shock. Consideration of the history and clinical presentation of the patient will give clues as to the potential to develop shock. Once the nurse has identified this potential, then actions can be taken to forestall the process.

DEFINITIVE CARE RELATED TO ETIOLOGICAL FACTORS

Management of the patient in shock requires definitive care specific for the causative etiology and directed toward correcting and/or reversing the altered circulatory component (i.e., blood volume, cardiac contractility, or vascular resistance). This care will include a combination of fluid, pharmacological, and mechanical therapies implemented to maintain tissue perfusion.

Hypovolemic Shock

Definitive care priorities for patients in hypovolemic shock include locating and controlling the source of fluid loss while restoring circulatory blood volume. A combination of crystalloids, colloids, plasma expanders, and blood and/or blood products may be used depending on whether the hypovolemic state is due to hemorrhage, plasma losses, or dehydration.

Cardiogenic Shock

Definitive care priorities for patients in cardiogenic shock are interventions to protect the ischemic myocardium. A combination of pharmacological agents, mechanical assist devices, and surgery may be used to reestablish circulation to the myocardium, increase cardiac output, decrease workload of the left ventricle (afterload), and increase oxygenation to the myocardium.

Distributive Shock

Definitive care priorities for patients in distributive shock are interventions to restore vascular tone. Vasopressor therapy and/or measures to correct the specific cause of the vascular alteration are directed to reverse the relative hypovolemia caused by massive vasodilation. The etiology of shock in patients with spinal cord injury must be determined in order to intervene appropriately. Vasopressor therapy and/or eliminating a physiological irritant such as a full bladder or gastric distention is indicated for neurogenic shock due to spinal cord injury. However, these patients frequently have multiple system injuries, both obvious and occult, and altered host defenses with portals of entry for microorganisms either because of injuries or therapeutic measures (e.g., central lines, endotracheal tubes, indwelling catheters). Therefore, shock due to hypovolemia or sepsis must be ruled out. The definitive treatment for each of these differs and necessitates accurate assessment as to the cause in order to intervene appropriately. Interventions to treat distributive shock caused by anaphylaxis are to prevent further introduction of the antigen and to reverse the allergic reaction with medications to restore vascular tone, neutralize the effects of histamine, promote bronchial dilation, and stabilize capillary walls. In septic shock, the infection is located by obtaining cultures from potential sites (i.e., urine, blood, sputum, and/or wounds), and sensitivity studies are done to guide administration of appropriate antibiotic therapy to eradicate the causative organism.

COLLABORATIVE CARE

Fluid Therapy

Shock, regardless of the etiology, produces profound extremes in fluid derangements that ultimately affect tissue perfusion. Therefore, patients experiencing an absolute (i.e., hypovolemic) or relative (i.e., distributive) hypovolemia require the administration of intravenous fluids to correct the volume deficit, restore intravascular volume, maintain oxygen-carrying capacity, and establish the hemodynamic stability necessary for optimum tissue perfusion (Rice, 1984b). The choice of fluid as well as the volume and rate of infusion will depend upon the individual patient circumstances. According to Rice (1984b), the benefits of parenteral fluid administration are (1) an increase in intravascular volume that increases venous return to the right side of the heart (i.e., preload), (2) optimal stretching of the ventricle that results in improved myocardial contractility and increased cardiac output, and (3) the end result of enhanced tissue perfusion.

These "benefits," however, are dangerous in the patient experiencing cardiogenic shock as large volumes of fluid will overwork an already failing heart. Cardiogenic shock is instead managed primarily through pharmacological therapy that aims to reduce both preload and afterload. Intravenous access is, therefore, established in these patients to provide a route for the administration of medications.

Establishing IV routes in a patient in shock presents a particular challenge as peripheral vasoconstriction and venous collapse make accessibility difficult. Yet, the patient in shock requires a minimum of two intravenous lines, one in a peripheral vein and one in a central vein. A peripheral line started with a large-gauge catheter (i.e., no. 14 or 16) provides a route for immediate, rapid fluid and/or medication administration. Initially, until fluid volume is replaced and the veins become more prominent, it may be necessary to use the large veins in the antecubital fossa (i.e., the basilic, cephalic, or accessory cephalic vein), the internal jugular vein, or in extreme emergencies the physician may perform a venous cutdown. A central line is established for large volume replacement and can be used to monitor central venous pressure or to place a pulmonary artery catheter. These central lines provide significant information to guide further fluid replacement (see Assessment section above). The veins commonly used as insertion sites for a central line are the subclavian or internal jugular vein, and to a lesser extent the femoral vein. A central line can be inserted in the external jugular, basilic, cephalic, or saphenous veins; however, the disadvantages of these routes include difficulties with catheter placement, spasms, interference with blood flow, and greater risk for thrombophlebitis and infection. Multilumen catheters, which provide multiple access ports via one insertion site, are often used for fluid, medication, and blood administration via a central line.

Once the intravenous access is established, an initial fluid challenge may be prescribed to assess the patient's hemodynamic response to the rapid administration of a specific amount of fluid. There are various methods for administering a fluid challenge, but typically the physician orders a volume of intravenous fluid, 10 to 20 ml/min, to be given via an infusion pump over a prescribed period of time, e.g., 10 minutes. The nursing responsibilities include obtaining baseline hemodynamic measurements (i.e., central venous pressure, pulmonary wedge pressure, cardiac output) and vital signs, giving the fluid challenge, and assessing the patient's response by monitoring changes in hemodynamic measurements, vital signs, breath sounds, urinary output, and level of consciousness. According to Rice (1984b), the following responses should guide the administration of the fluid challenge:

1. The fluid challenge should be discontinued if at any time during the infusion the PWP (pulmonary wedge pressure) increases by more than 7 mm Hg or the CVP (central venous pressure) has increased by more than 5 cm H_2O.
2. Repeat the fluid challenge if the PWP has increased by less than 3 mm Hg or the CVP has increased by less than 2 cm H_2O.
3. Observe the patient if at the end of the challenge the PWP has increased by more than 3 but less than 7 mm Hg or the CVP has increased by more than 2 but less than 5 cm H_2O. During this observation, if the PWP falls to within 3 mm Hg or the CVP falls to within 2 cm H_2O of the baseline measurements, the fluid challenge should be repeated. On the other hand, discontinue the fluid challenge if the PWP does not fall to within 3 mm Hg or the CVP does not fall to within 2 cm H_2O of the baseline measurements.

An increase in PWP or CVP without an improvement in blood pressure indicates ineffective myocardial contractility. In such a case, the patient's heart cannot tolerate additional fluid administration, and the patient may need interventions to decrease cardiac workload. Additional fluid is administered if the PWP or CVP increases only slightly, or increases and then rapidly decreases, as this indicates hypovolemia.

Parenteral fluid therapy is essential in the treatment of shock in order for other therapeutic modalities to be effective in supporting vital functions and restoring tissue perfusion. While the nurse is not responsible for selecting the infusion or transfusion, it is imperative that the nurse understands the rationale for the prescribed fluid therapy as well as the expected and unexpected effects in order to assess patient outcomes. A return to normal of the laboratory and hemodynamic values as found in Tables 7–6 and 7–8 as well as the desirable patient outcomes found in Table 7–10 are the goals of fluid therapy (Meyers and Hickey, 1988; Niedringhaus, 1983b, Rice, 1991c). Blood, blood products, plasma expanders, and crystalloids may be used alone or in combination to restore intravascular volume. Initially, crystalloids and/or colloids are infused until diagnostics, typing, and cross matching are completed to guide further treatment. The choice of fluid(s) depends upon the cause of the volume deficit, the patient's clinical status, and the physician preference. Patients in severe shock may require rapid volume replacement. The flow rate can be increased by infusing the parenteral fluid under pressure using a blood pump, and/or large-bore trauma infusion tubing, or using a rapid infusion device. The use of infusion pumps to accurately administer the volume and rate of crystalloid solutions (i.e., Ringer's lactate, normal saline) is also indicated for the patient in shock. Consideration should be given to running fluids through a warmer when administering rapid, massive parenteral infusions or transfusions in order to prevent complications associated with hypothermia.

Table 7–10. DESIRABLE OUTCOMES AS A RESULT OF FLUID THERAPY

1. Alert and responsive (in the absence of head injury)
2. Warm, dry, normal-colored skin with good turgor
3. Pink, moist mucous membranes
4. Capillary refill less than 2 sec
5. Nondistended, not collapsed jugular veins
6. BP ± 20 mm Hg as compared to preshock
7. Mean arterial pressure 80 mm Hg
8. Heart rate 60–100, strong and regular
9. Respirations 10–20, regular and unlabored
10. Balanced intake and output
11. Stable weight
12. Urinary output 30–60 ml/hr, specific gravity = 1.010–1.025

Crystalloids. Ringer's lactate and 0.9% normal saline are electrolyte solutions used initially to expand intravascular volume. They are inexpensive and readily available. Crystalloid solutions move freely from the intravascular space into the tissues; therefore, a ratio of 3 ml of crystalloid solution is used to replace each 1 ml of blood loss (Meyers and Hickey, 1988). Ringer's lactate, generally the fluid of choice for shock, closely resembles plasma, rarely causes side effects, and may be the only fluid replacement required if the blood loss is less than 1500 ml (Niedringhaus, 1983b). Normal saline is an isotonic solution; however, its side effects include hypernatremia, hypokalemia, and metabolic acidosis. D5W and 1/2 normal saline (0.45% normal saline) are hypotonic solutions that should only be used temporarily to establish an IV line because these fluids rapidly leave the intravascular space, causing interstitial and intracellular edema. D5W may be used as the fluid of choice to treat shock caused entirely by water deprivation. If large volumes of crystalloids are the only parenteral fluids infused, the patient is at risk for the development of edema and hemodilution of red blood cells and plasma proteins. Hemodilution of red blood cells may impair delivery of oxygen to the cells if the hematocrit is decreased to such an extent that the cardiac output cannot increase enough to compensate. Hemodilution of plasma proteins decreases the colloidal osmotic pressure, which places the patient at risk to develop pulmonary edema.

Blood and Blood Products. Whole blood, packed red blood cells, washed red blood cells, fresh frozen plasma, platelets, albumin, and plasmanate are given to treat major blood or plasma loss. Typing and cross matching are done for some of these products to identify the patient's blood type (A, B, AB, O), determine the presence of the Rh factor, and to assure compatibility with the donor blood in order to prevent transfusion reactions. In extreme emergencies, the patient may be transfused with O negative blood, considered to be the universal donor.

Transfusions require an IV access with at least a 20-gauge and preferably an 18-gauge or larger catheter (a 22- or 23-gauge needle or catheter may be used in neonates, children, or adults with small veins). The use of a multiple lead tubing (i.e., Y-set) allows you to piggyback the blood with an IV solution to run concurrently, or allows you to stop the transfusion and still keep the vein open. Blood transfusions may be piggybacked into an IV infusion of 0.9% normal saline, or 50 to 100 ml of this solution may be injected directly into the unit of blood. This decreases the viscosity of the blood and allows for a more rapid infusion rate. (A pressure device such as a blood pump may also be used to increase the flow rate of transfusions.) D5W solution should never be used as it causes red blood cells to clump, swell, and burst. Ringer's lactate should also not be used as it can cause clots. Intravenous medications are never infused in the same line in which blood is infusing. Blood transfusions place the patient at risk for the development of allergic reactions and adult respiratory distress syndrome. Using a micropore blood filter that traps the debris and tiny clots found in blood may prevent some of these complications. Hospital protocols should be followed in regards to obtaining baseline vital signs prior to the transfusion and repeat vital signs and assessments during the transfusion. Before starting any transfusion, hospital policy should be followed for crosschecking the patient and transfusion information. Usually, the blood product must be double checked (generally by two nurses) for the following:

1. Verify that the blood product matches the order on the patient's chart.
2. Match the name and donor unit ID number on the transfusion form to that on the patient's wristband/blood bracelet (if the patient can respond, ask his/her name).
3. Verify that the ABO group, Rh type, and the donor unit ID number on the transfusion form matches those on the donor unit with its compatibility tag and blood bag label.
4. Check the expiration date on the blood bag.
5. Inspect the blood product for clots, bubbling, or purplish tinge, which indicates bacterial contamination.

Frequent assessment of the patient receiving a blood transfusion is necessary to identify the onset of an adverse reaction. Baseline vital signs are obtained as changes in the pulse, blood pressure, temperature, and respirations are early indications of a reaction. Assess the patient frequently during the transfusion for any unusual sensations or signs and symptoms. Table 7–11 lists the types of reactions, the causes, signs and symptoms, prevention measures, and the collaborative interventions to take in the event of a reaction (Querin and Stahl, 1983). In general, the nurse should discontinue the transfusion and disconnect the transfusion tubing from the IV access site, keep the vein open with an IV of normal saline solution, assess and stay with the patient, notify the physician and the lab, send to the lab all transfusion equipment (bag, tubing, solutions) and any blood or urine specimens obtained, and document the events of the reaction and the patient's response to interventions.

Table 7–11. COMMON ADVERSE REACTIONS TO BLOOD TRANSFUSIONS

Type of Reaction	Symptoms
Hemolytic transfusion reaction	Fever Chills Chest pain Burning sensation along vein Headache
Allergic reaction	Anaphylaxis Urticaria Pruritus Rare: Facial or glottal edema, asthma, pulmonary edema
Febrile reaction	Chills and fever Headache Flushing Tachycardia
Circulatory overload	Tightness in chest Dry cough Labored breathing Pulmonary edema
Bacterial reactions	Fever Hypotension Dry, flushed skin Pain

Data from Dolan, J. T.: Critical Care Nursing: Clinical Management Through the Nursing Process. Philadelphia: F. A. Davis, 1991, (p. 1050); and Jennings, B. M.: Nursing role in management of hematologic problems. In: S. M. Lewis and I. C. Collier (eds.) Medical-Surgical Nursing: Assessment and Management of Clinical Problems. New York: McGraw-Hill (pp. 699–700).

Blood and blood products are given until the hematocrit returns to 30% or higher (Niedringhaus, 1983b; Rice, 1984b). The transfusion administration time varies with the particular blood product and the individual patient circumstances. Documentation of the transfusion includes the blood product administered, baseline vital signs, time the transfusion was started and completed, volume of blood and fluid administered, assessment of the patient during the transfusion, and any nursing actions taken.

Whole blood is indicated for the treatment of both rapid and slow bleeding conditions. It restores blood volume and oxygen-carrying capacity; however, side effects include volume overload. Additionally, acidosis, hyperkalemia, and coagulation problems are associated with transfusions of banked blood over 24 hours old. Typing and cross matching of whole blood are required.

Packed red blood cells (PRBCs) have increased red blood cell concentrations so they are able to increase the blood volume and oxygen-carrying capacity without the problems of volume overload frequently seen with the administration of whole blood. One unit of PRBCs should increase the hematocrit by 3% and the hemoglobin by 1 gm in a 70-kg patient (Rice, 1984b). Typing and cross matching of packed red blood cells are required. (Red blood cells tend to aggregate because of the fibrinogen coating; therefore, washed red blood cells may be given to decrease capillary sludging.)

Fresh frozen plasma (FFP) acts as a plasma expander that contains all clotting factors except platelets. Repeated blood transfusions wash out coagulation factors; therefore, when massive transfusions are being infused, FFP (1 U of FFP for every 4 to 5 U of blood transfused) should be given rapidly to restore coagulation factors. Typing and cross matching of fresh frozen plasma are required.

Platelets are given rapidly to help control bleeding when it is due to low platelet counts (less than 50,000). Typing of platelets, but not cross matching, is required.

Albumin and plasmanate are naturally occurring colloid solutions given to increase the colloidal osmotic pressure in the intravascular space. Plasmanate is given when the volume loss is due to plasma rather than blood loss (i.e, burns, peritonitis, bowel obstruction). Colloidal osmotic pressure holds and attracts fluid into blood vessels, expanding plasma volume. Colloids are given rapidly and remain in the intravascular space longer as compared to crystalloids, so smaller volumes of this more expensive therapy are required. Typing and cross matching of albumin and plasmanate are not required. Pulmonary edema may be seen as a complication of colloid administration because of increased pulmonary capillary permeability (seen in some stages of shock), or due to increased capillary hydrostatic pressure in the pulmonary vasculature created by rapid plasma expansion.

Pharmaceutical Plasma Expanders. Dextran is a hypertonic synthetic colloid used as a plasma expander. Low molecular weight dextran (dextran 40, Rheomacrodex) has a duration of effectiveness for 12 hours. Its use is contraindicated in shock due to hemorrhage because it causes a decrease in platelet adhesiveness and consequently may increase bleeding from wounds. Low molecular weight dextran has a lower incidence of allergic reactions as compared to high molecular weight dextran. High molecular weight dextran (dextran 70, Macrodex) is effective for 24 hours, but it increases platelet aggregation and blood viscosity and interferes with blood typing and cross matching (therefore, this should be done prior to infusing dextran 70). No more than 1 L of dextran should be given in a 24-hour period. Additional complications associated with this plasma expander include allergic reactions and renal damage. Hespan (Hetastarch) is a synthetic colloid that acts as a plasma expander but with less risk for the development of pulmonary edema as compared to albumin. As compared to dextran, hespan has no apparent effect on renal function and is less likely to cause allergic reactions. Its side effects include prolonged PT and PTT times, decreased colloidal osmotic pressure, and the potential for circulatory overload. For this reason, it is recommended that no more than 1 L be given in a 24-hour period.

New Therapies for Shock Management. Stroma-free hemoglobin, fluorocarbons, and hypertonic saline are among the newest therapies introduced to manage shock (Feola and Canizaro, 1988). Stroma-free hemoglobin is a solution with oxygen-carrying capacity indicated for use in the treatment of massive hemorrhage. It does not require typing and cross matching, is compatible with IV solutions and blood, is easily administered, and does not cause antigen reactions. Additionally, it exerts an osmotic effect to hold fluid in blood vessels, increasing intravascular volume. However, the stroma-free hemoglobin resists releasing oxygen to tissues, especially when arterial oxygen levels are already low (as in hypovolemic shock).

Fluorocarbons are oxygen-carrying solutions that remain in the circulation for 12 to 24 hours. This product is acceptable to persons whose religious beliefs prohibit the transfusion of blood products. Disadvantages of flurocarbons include limited availability and the accumulation of chemicals in the body.

Hypertonic saline increases cardiac output by increasing extracellular volume. Less fluid is required initially, thereby decreasing the incidence of interstitial and pulmonary edema. However, with increased volumes of hypertonic saline, hypernatremia and cellular dehydration occur.

Pharmacological Management of Shock

The pharmacological management of the shock syndrome is based upon the manipulation of four variables: contractility, preload, afterload, and heart rate (Rice, 1985). It is important when considering the pharmacological treatment of shock that the pathophysiological basis of a decreased cardiac output with a concurrent impairment in cellular nutrition be considered. There are no drugs that can magically restore cellular nutrition, but there are agents available that can assist in the manipulation of the four circulatory variables that make nutrients available to the cells. Pharmacological management, therefore, is aimed at the alteration of the heart and the blood vessels, whereas the administration of fluids is aimed at increasing the volume. Drugs that are used in treating shock are those that can influence the variables identified above. Each variable will be discussed and specific drugs in each category included.

Drugs That Affect Contractility

Inotropic agents are used frequently in the treatment of shock. These are drugs that affect the contractility of the heart. Positive inotropic agents are those that increase the contractile force of the heart (Table 7–12). These drugs make the heart pump more effectively. As the contractility increases, two things occur. First, ventricular emptying increases and the filling pressure of the heart decreases. Second, the stroke volume improves, increasing cardiac output, which in turn increases the blood pressure. The increase in blood pressure improves perfusion to the tissues and provides much-needed nutrition to the cells. Thus, positive inotropic agents can be very useful in the treatment of shock. They do have a negative effect, which is to increase the myocardial oxygen demand (Rice, 1985). They do this by increasing the workload of the heart and by increasing the vascular resistance. In patients with an ischemic heart or in cases of cardiogenic shock, this can be a serious detriment. Therefore, these drugs have a limit to their usefulness, which must be taken into consideration when administering inotropic agents. It does not mean that they will not be used, but caution in administration and close monitoring of the effects of inotropic agents is required.

Table 7–12. PHARMACOLOGICAL MANAGEMENT OF SHOCK

- Commonly Used Positive Inotropic Agents
  - Dopamine (in mid range doses—5–10μg/kg/min)
  - Dobutamine
  - Amrinone
  - Norepinephrine
  - Epinephrine
  - Isoproterenol
  - Digoxin
- Commonly Used Drugs to Reduce Preload
  - Diuretics—Furosemide
  - Nitroprusside
  - Nitrates
  - Morphine Sulfate
- Commonly Used Agents to Increase Afterload
  - Dopamine (in high doses—10–20 μg/kg/min)
  - Norepinephrine
  - Phenylephrine
  - Metaraminol
- Commonly Used Agents to Decrease Afterload
  - Amrinone
  - Nitroprusside
  - Hydralazine
  - Captopril
  - Nifedipine
- Commonly Used Positive Chronotropic Agents
  - Atropine
  - Isoproterenol
- Commonly Used Negative Chronotropic Agents
  - Verapamil
  - Propranolol
  - Adenosine
  - Digitalis
- Commonly Used Antiarrhythmic Agents
  - Lidocaine
  - Procainamide
  - Bretylium

Inotropic agents are more frequently used in cases of distributive and cardiogenic shock. The problem in these types of shock is either decreased vascular resistance or decreased pumping ability of the heart. These agents can influence both of these problems. In cardiogenic shock, the heart has lost its contractile force and cardiac output declines. In distributive shock, the problem is a loss of vascular resistance, which leads to a subsequent decrease in the cardiac output. Positive inotropic agents increase the contractility of the heart and are useful drugs in treating distributive and cardiogenic shock.

There are negative inotropic agents that are not used in the treatment of shock, but need to be addressed because of the widespread use of these agents in the treatment of angina, hypertension, and dysrhythmias (Rice, 1985). These agents work primarily by blocking the effects of the beta branch of the sympathetic nervous system, causing a decrease in the cardiac output. Obviously this is undesirable in shock where the problem is already a decrease in the output. These drugs decrease the contractile force of the heart with their negative inotropic effect. They also exert a negative chronotropic effect that decreases the rate of the heart. It is important that the nurse know the effects of these medications because the patient who is taking them will have an altered ability to respond to the stress of shock and may not exhibit typical signs and symptoms.

Drugs That Reduce Preload

The primary treatment to increase preload is to administer fluids. This was addressed earlier. There are some drugs that can be used, however, to manipulate this variable. This may be a factor in the treatment of the patient in cardiogenic shock. Such a patient does not need volume. In these patients, the fluid volume is adequate but the problem is that the heart cannot pump that volume. In fact, in cardiogenic shock, if more volume is given, the patient will get worse. In these cases, drugs are administered that can reduce preload. Drugs given are those that reduce the venous return to the heart. Table 7–12 lists drugs used to reduce preload.

It must be noted that the administration of agents that reduce the preload on the myocardium must be closely evaluated with regard to the effects. It is generally considered good practice to evaluate the patient's response with hemodynamic monitoring tools such as a pulmonary artery line. The measure of right ventricular preload—the right atrial pressure—can be obtained and identification of the effect of agents can be accomplished. A serious side effect of these drugs is that they may reduce the preload to such an extent that the patient will suffer from an extreme loss of volume, increasing hypoperfusion to the cells, and the results may be seriously detrimental to the patient.

Drugs That Increase Afterload

This variable is the force that the heart must overcome in order to pump nutrient-rich blood to the periphery. This parameter is directly affected in distributive shock states. When the peripheral vascular resistance has been altered, blood is trapped in the periphery as a result of the poor vascular resistance. Cardiac output is reduced because of the pseudoreduction in volume or decreased venous return. What is needed is an increase in the vascular tone to improve venous return and consequently increase cardiac output (see Table 7–12).

As with other agents, there is a negative side. Although the individual needs an increase in vascular resistance, such an increase can put too much of a workload on the heart, causing an increase in the myocardial oxygen demand. Accurate measurement of afterload is essential and the pulmonary artery line provides the tool for precise measures. The primary numbers used to evaluate vascular resistance are the SVR (systemic vascular resistance) and the PVR (pulmonary vascular resistance).

There are cases in which consideration may be given to reduce the afterload. Cardiogenic shock is a prime example. In these patients, increased afterload is a real danger and can cause an already ischemic heart to suffer more insults. In patients with cardiogenic shock, a reduction in afterload is appropriate. Monitoring is essential to the care of these patients. (See Table 7–12 for agents that reduce afterload.)

Drugs That Alter Heart Rate

Heart rate (chronotropism) is the fourth variable that can be altered in the treatment of shock. (See Table 7–12 for drugs that alter the heart rate.) Extremes in heart rate and dysrhythmias can have deleterious effects on the patient in shock. A very slow heart rate can reduce cardiac output by decreasing the number of times per minute that the heart produces a pulse. Fast rates do not allow the heart to fill properly, which reduces the stroke volume; and diastole is decreased, which impairs coronary artery perfusion, and increases the myocardial oxygen demand. Dysrhythmias can cause problems with perfusion to the tissues.

Bradydysrhythmias are treated with atropine as the first-line agent. This is a vagolytic drug that increases the heart rate (Jeffries and Whelan, 1989). The other pharmacological agent used to increase the heart rate is isoproteranol. The increased heart rate may be desired, but it can also cause more problems in the patient in shock. Therefore, these drugs must be used with caution.

Rapid rates and dysrhythmias can be treated using various drugs. For the suppression of tachydysrhythmias that are ventricular in nature, drugs such as lidocaine, procainamide, or bretylium may be considered. Atrial tachydysrhythmias, including atrial flutter, fibrillation, and tachycardia, may be treated by verapamil, propranolol, adenosine, or digitalis. In using these drugs the nurse must monitor the patient carefully. The agent that is most appropriate but has the least side effects should be used. Lidocaine, for example, can cause alterations in the CNS and impair the neurological function of the patient. Such alterations may make neurological assessment difficult. Procainamide and bretylium can cause hypotension. This is not a desirable effect in the patient who already has problems maintaining an adequate blood pressure. Verapamil and propranolol can overdepress the myocardium and reduce contractility, which is not always a positive effect. Digitalis can increase the oxygen demands of the myocardium. Therefore, the use of these agents must be very cautiously calculated and very carefully monitored. In some cases, electrical management may be chosen to correct the dysrhythmias.

In summary, four variables can be altered through the use of pharmacological agents. In treating the patient with shock, the balance of myocardial oxygen supply and demand must be maintained while trying to reach the ultimate goal of increased tissue perfusion. This balance can be difficult to achieve but is the goal of pharmacological treatment.

Other Pharmacological Therapy

There are additional agents that may be useful in the management of the patient in shock. Each of these will be reviewed below.

Steroids. These have a controversial place in the treatment of shock because their exact effect is not fully understood (Shatney, 1986). Some of the effects under consideration include increases in visceral organ blood flow, increased cardiac index, and increased glucose and lactic acid metabolism. Steroids also cause a decrease in platelet aggregability and arteriolar and venous resistance (Shatney, 1986). The increase in membrane stabilization assists in the reduction of complications in shock. Steroids are used primarily in septic shock. However, there are indications for their use in the cardiogenic and hypovolemic types of shock.

Sodium Bicarbonate. Acid-base balance is of major concern in caring for the patient in shock. Sodium bicarbonate reacts with hydrogen ions to form water and carbon dioxide to buffer metabolic acidosis. Metabolic acidosis can reduce the effectiveness of the cell's ability to function. Care must be taken with cautious administration of sodium bicarbonate, since the carbon dioxide produced crosses rapidly into the cells and may cause a paradoxical worsening of intracellular hypercardia and acidosis (*Textbook of Advanced Cardiac Life Support,* 1987, 1990). Other methods of reducing the hydrogen ion concentration may be considered before the use of sodium bicarbonate. This includes maximizing the ventilatory function of the patient. Measurements of the patient's acid-base status can be obtained to guide the administration of sodium bicarbonate.

Oxygen. One agent that is of primary importance in the treatment of the patient in shock is oxygen. Oxygen administration elevates the arterial oxygen tension and increases the arterial oxygen content of the blood, thereby improving tissue oxygenation (*Textbook of Advanced Cardiac Life Support,* 1987, 1990). Oxygen may be administered via any of the full range of respiratory therapy devices from simple nasal cannula to mechanical ventilation. Oxygen toxicity is of concern in patients who require long-term high-dose therapy. In general, acute episodes of shock can be short term in management and toxicity will not be a problem.

Antibiotics. Antibiotic therapy may be used in patients who have septic shock. The antibiotic to be used is determined by the results of a blood culture and sensitivity tests that pinpoint the drug that will be most successful in treating the infective organism. Patients who experience the shock syndrome are susceptible to infections and may be on prophylactic antibiotic therapy.

Naloxone, a narcotic antagonist, has also been used in patients with septic shock (Schumann and Remington, 1989). It has been experimentally used to reverse the hypotension that occurs in this type of shock. It is thought that naloxone may block the effects of endogenous opiates that contribute to the cardiovascular collapse associated with septic shock. This is an experimental use of naloxone and is recommended for early in septic shock and in conjunction with the traditional therapy of antibiotics and vasoactive drugs.

In summary, there is no single agent that has all the effects needed in all cases of shock. Pharmacological therapy utilizes a wide range of agents which may be useful but may also have deleterious effects. It is astute nursing observation and evaluation that contribute to the survival of the patient when faced with the complex syndrome of shock and its equally complex pharmacological management.

Mechanical Management of Shock

The management of shock can include the use of mechanical devices that can aid the patient in restoring perfusion to the cells. These devices focus on specific etiological factors and may assist in various ways. The mechanical devices are the intra-aortic balloon pump (IABP), external ventricular assist devices (EVAD or LVAD), and the military anti-shock trouser (MAST). Each of these tools will be discussed.

Intra-Aortic Balloon Pump

One method of mechanically assisting the heart and its pumping is through the use of counterpulsation via the IABP (Whitman, 1988). This device is most often used in the patient with cardiogenic shock, but it may be useful in other types of shock as well. It is a dual-chambered balloon that is inserted into the aorta via the femoral artery (Rice, 1981d). The tip of the balloon is positioned just distal to the left subclavian artery (Fig. 7–3). The IABP may be inserted using fluoroscopy to visualize placement or may be inserted and placement verified via chest film after insertion.

The balloon pump can assist the patient in shock in several ways. It can directly improve the coronary artery perfusion, reduce afterload, which can serve to reduce myocardial oxygen demand, and can assist in improving tissue perfusion to other vital organs.

IABP works by inflating during diastole and deflating prior to systole. Inflation during diastole aids the heart by increasing coronary artery perfusion and the perfusion to the periphery. This increase in perfusion is based on the increase in intravascular pressure. The inflation cycle displaces a like amount of blood and forces it forward and backward simultaneously (Rice,

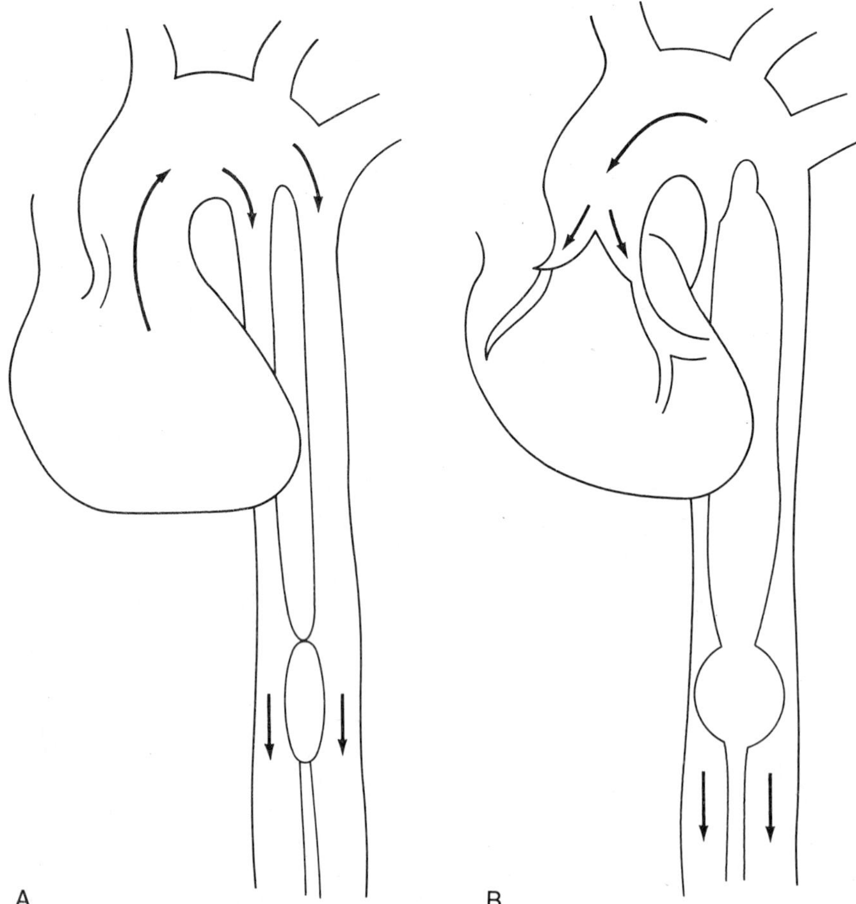

Figure 7–3. *A*, Diastole. *B*, Systole.

1981d). The forward flow increases the perfusion to vital organs and the backward flow forces an increased amount of blood into the coronary arteries.

The balloon pump also assists the heart in the systolic phase. In systole, the balloon deflates just prior to contraction. This sudden deflation reduces the pressure in the aorta. The reduction in aortic pressure decreases afterload and makes the work of the heart less (Rice, 1991d). This decrease in afterload subsequently reduces myocardial oxygen demand.

The IABP is not without its problems. Because it is a highly technical piece of equipment, it requires a high degree of nursing skill. It is often instituted late rather than early in the course of circulatory collapse and, therefore, is not effective.

There is the likelihood of limb ischemia related to placement of the catheter and embolic phenomena. Other complications include dissection of the aorta, infection, inappropriate timing, leakage of gas, and technical problems. The use of the balloon pump is contraindicated in patients with aortic insufficiency and thoracic aneurysms.

The use of the IABP is concurrent with a definitive measure such as pharmacological therapy. There can be problems with its long-term use and patients can become pump dependent. Weaning is required by gradually decreasing the pump to patient ratio from 1:1 to 1:4, and so forth.

External Ventricular (Circulatory) Assist Devices (EVADs)

These devices are used in cases of refractory ventricular response to other methods of treatment. The devices vary tremendously in design and technology. In general, they consist of an external pump that pulls blood from the heart and then reinfuses it to the major vessels.

External ventricular assist devices may be used for either the left or the right ventricle depending upon the need of the patient. If the left side requires support, the pump removes blood from the left atrium or ventricle and reinfuses it into the aortic root. If the right side of the heart is failing, then the device will remove blood from the right atrium or ventricle and infuse it into the pulmonary artery (Rutan, et al., 1989). This will bypass the ventricle and consequently requires no ventricular activity. The EVAD will aid the patient in shock by providing the needed pumping action while allowing the ventricles to recover.

Research is being done on the use of EVADs in the treatment of shock. They are not typically available in community hospitals. Extensive training and advanced nursing care are required to use EVADs.

Military Anti-Shock Trousers

Military anti-shock trousers (MAST) are another mechanical device that may be used in the care of the patient in shock (Fig. 7–4). These may also be called pneumatic anti-shock garments (PASG), anti-shock garments, external counterpressure devices, or G suits. These raise the mean arterial pressure by increasing the peripheral vascular resistance in the lower portion of the body. They consist of a one-piece inflatable bladder that when inflated can maintain a high internal pressure. Most models have three separate compartments that can be inflated individually to compress the lower extremities and the abdomen. The suits usually are inflated with a foot pump and have pop-off valves that assist in regulating the internal pressure.

The trousers work primarily by increasing peripheral vascular resistance. Secondary considerations in the use of the trousers are that the pressure improves hemostasis and provides a splinting action and decreased blood flow to torn vessels under the garment (*Textbook of Advanced Cardiac Life Support,* 1987, 1990). Thus, in examining the primary and secondary effects, it can be seen that this garment is most useful in the case of those suffering from the hypovolemic types of shock. It may be useful particularly in patients with traumatic injury to the lower half of the body.

A major disadvantage is that MAST can cause a compromise of blood flow and tissue perfusion to the lower half of the body. The garment is a stop-gap measure that is only temporary and definitive measures must be instituted as soon as possible (*Textbook of Advanced Cardiac Life Support,* 1987, 1990). These measures may include, e.g., fluid, blood administration, and surgery.

In most instances, MAST will be instituted in emergency situations in the field or emergency department and may be removed prior to admission to the critical care unit. Therefore, the nurse may not be involved in the care of the patient. It is an important part of the history, however, to be aware that the garment was used. The nurse should closely monitor the vascular status of the lower extremities and watch for the reappearance

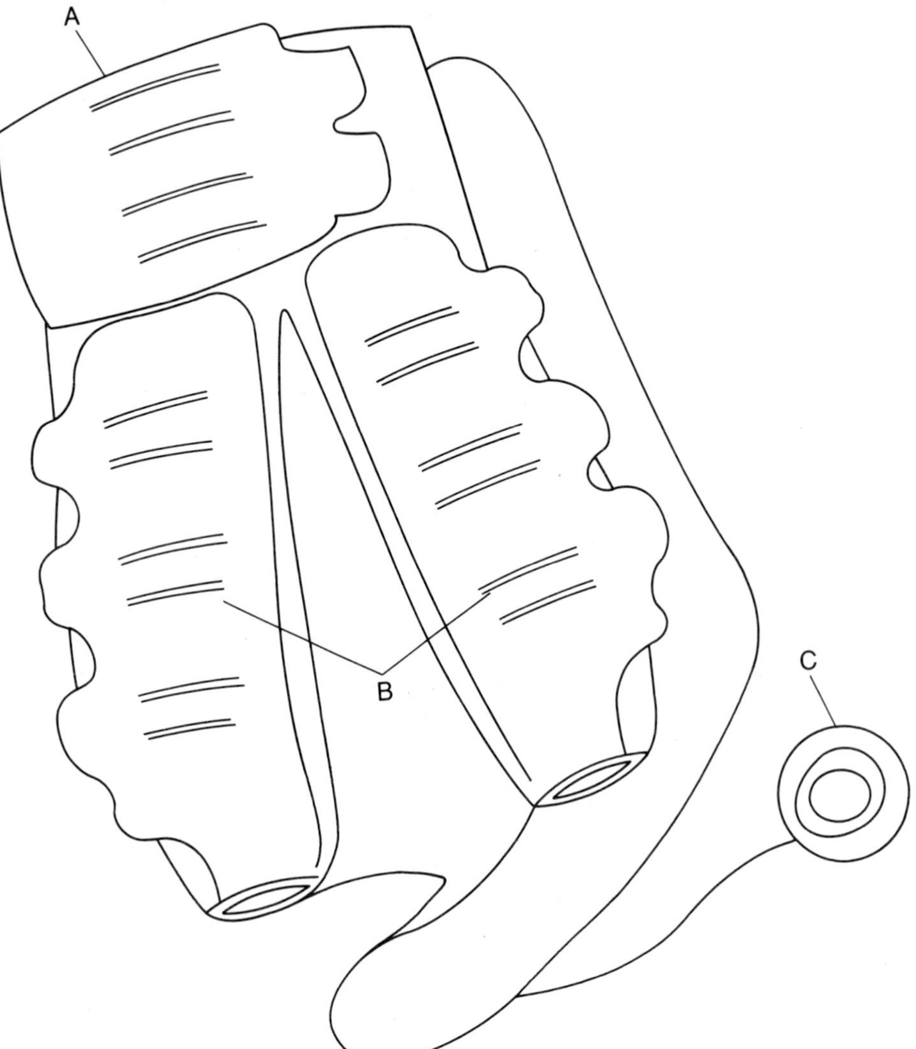

Figure 7-4. Military anti-shock trousers—MAST.

of the signs and symptoms of shock. If the patient is admitted to the unit with MAST in place, the nurse should monitor the circulatory status of the patient closely. Assistance with removal of the device is required as the patient stabilizes. Removal requires gradual reduction of the pressure in the compartments. The abdominal section is deflated first to allow gradual redistribution of blood volume and to avoid trapping of large volumes of blood in the lower extremities. The vital signs of the patient must be closely monitored. Removal of MAST in a patient who is not fully stabilized may cause sudden relapse into the shock syndrome.

These are the current mechanical adjuncts used in the treatment of the patient in shock. Technology is constantly increasing and more and more advances in mechanical devices may be made to treat this most complex syndrome.

SUPPORTIVE CARE

The nurse must also consider the aspects of care that will support the tissue perfusion of the patient in shock until efforts of definitive care are effective. Supportive care is aimed at maintenance of organ function and the interventions that are included are primarily nursing directed.

Maintenance of a Patent Airway

The priority action in shock is maintenance of a patent airway. This can be achieved by proper positioning of the head and neck so that the airway will be open. The best position for this is to tilt the head backward and to lift the chin upward. This simple maneuver serves to lift the soft tissues from the upper airway and allow for clear air passage. If this is not adequate, adjunctive airways may be required such as oropharyngeal, nasopharyngeal, endotracheal, or tracheostomy to provide for an open airway. These adjuncts provide control of the airway and allow for the easy removal of secretions. Removing secretions to keep the air passage open is an essential part of airway maintenance. Chest physical therapy may also be indicated to facilitate removal of secretions and maintain pulmonary function. Once an airway is established, the next step is to provide oxygen therapy via the best route for the patient. This may range from a simple nasal cannula to mechanical ventilation in order to provide for oxygen administration.

Position of the Patient

In supportive care, the nurse must also consider the overall position of the patient. Traditionally, the Trendelenberg position (Fig. 7-5) has been used for the patient in shock. This position was thought to increase venous return to the heart and thereby increase cardiac output. The Trendelenberg's position has some detrimental effects, however, that can actually worsen the shock state. By raising the legs, diaphragmatic movement is restricted and this may cause a decrease in the tidal volume and ventilation. This is most certainly not wanted in a patient in shock. There also can be a reflex inhibition of the baroreceptors by the dramatic increase in venous return caused by the elevation of the legs. The increased venous return is interpreted by the baroreceptors that there is adequate blood volume and this, in turn, can cause the blood pressure to fall even more. The position that is best for the patient in shock is one that does not cause a large increase in venous return and yet does not compromise ventilation. The position recommended is to elevate the lower extremities slightly. This elevation can increase venous return without compromising the ventilatory status of the patient.

Maintenance of Body Temperature

Another area of concern in the care of the patient is to maintain the body temperature. Patients need to be kept warm and comfortable and yet not be overly warmed. Excessive warmth can serve to the detriment of the patient by increasing the metabolic needs of the patient and placing a larger demand on an already stressed cardiovascular system. Light blankets and frequent checks of the patient's temperature should be done.

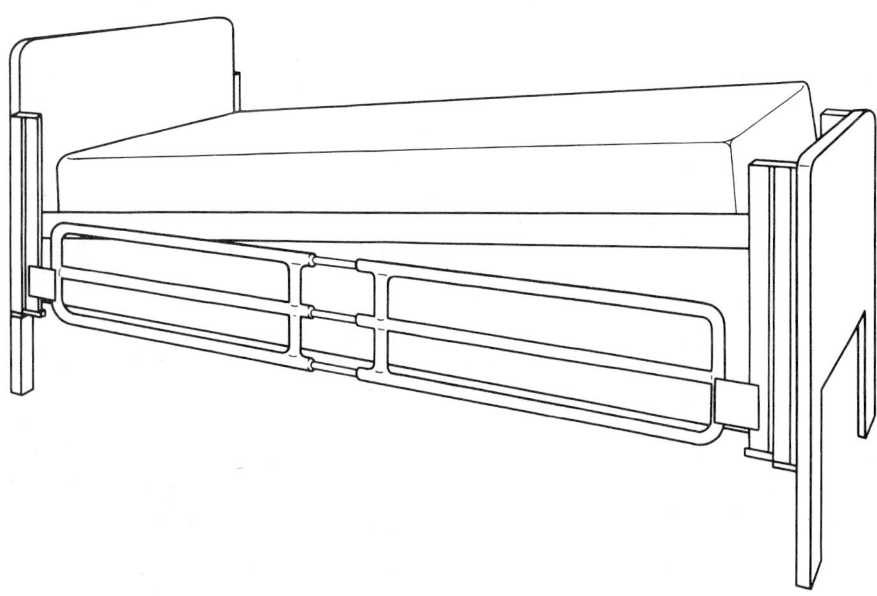

Figure 7-5. Trendelenberg's position—bed with head down.

Maintenance of Skin Integrity

Another concern of the patient in shock is maintenance of the first line of defense—the skin. As noted previously, the skin will suffer from a decreased perfusion early in the shock syndrome. This decreased perfusion can precipitate injury to this all-important defense mechanism. Meticulous skin care is required to assure that no breaks occur in the patient's skin. This will include the nursing measure of turning and applying lotion to the patient at frequent intervals. Devices such as egg crate or air pressure mattresses may be indicated to reduce the risk of injury to the skin. Newer devices have been developed that may assist in the maintenance of the skin in very difficult cases. These include airflow mechanical beds that automatically regulate pressure so that the circulation to the skin is not compromised.

Psychological Support

A section on supportive care would be remiss if it did not address the area of psychological support. The patient and family must receive direct, active support from the nurse. Nursing interventions for the patient and family who are experiencing a life-threatening situation such as shock must identify the impact of the illness on the patient and the family. Nursing interventions at this point in the process can include the provision of information; information about the patient's status, the necessity for procedures, explanations of tests and test results, and an understanding of routines within the unit. All of this information is essential for the psychological equilibrium of the patient and the family. These items of information may help to give the patient and family a sense of understanding and control of the situation. It may also be important to include information about the hospital and the community to help the family in the development of coping mechanisms.

Psychological support may include nursing actions such as providing time, space, and privacy for family discussion, allowing ventilation, encouragement, and acceptance. This intervention may also include assurance of social support structures. This may be through the social service department or by simply providing contact of significant others for the individual or family. There are countless examples of cases in which the nurses themselves become the social support for patients or families who need them.

Psychosocial aspects are essential to both the patient and the family. Working in critical care, the nurse is continuously faced with the difficult task of meeting the overwhelming physiological and psychosocial needs of the patient and family undergoing a life-threatening illness. Nursing must demonstrate the commitment to providing holistic, individualized care. It is through the provision of psychosocial support that the nurse can maintain that which is the heart of nursing—caring.

Complications of Shock

INDIVIDUAL SYSTEMS AFFECTED

The complications of shock can be related to the metabolic and tissue changes that result from the syndrome. If the normal compensatory mechanisms are not assisted with effective therapeutic interventions, the pathological consequences will perpetuate a vicious circle that will end with the death of the patient. The ischemia to the cells initiates this cycle. Ischemia enhances incomplete oxidation and the anaerobic metabolism of glucose that leads to an accumulation of lactic acid and an ensuing metabolic acidosis. This acidosis leads to irreversible changes in the cells (Emmanuelson and Rosenlicht, 1986). It is best to address complications as they occur in the organ systems that are affected first.

Central Nervous System

Once the brain has become ischemic and hypoxic secondary to the shock syndrome, it turns to anaerobic metabolism like all the other tissues. Lactate levels begin to rise and as glucose consumption falls the availability of energy for the cells in the CNS declines. As the energy levels decrease and cellular function falters, the cells begin to retain sodium and water and cerebral edema ensues. This initiates a vicious cycle in the cerebral cells and further compromise of the tissue will occur. Neurological deficits can be the end result of severe and prolonged episodes of shock.

Cardiovascular System

The major mechanisms for failure of the heart in shock are thought to be (1) a fall in cardiac output, (2) a decrease in coronary blood flow, and (3) a marked decrease in myocardial contractility (Shatney, 1986). The factors that contribute to these processes in shock are the decreased oxygen availability and the production of myocardial depressant factor (MDF). Studies have shown that the MDF does not seem to have the major impact on the myocardium that it was once thought to have, though it seems to play a role in decreasing the efforts of the myocardium (Shatney, 1986). Whatever the factors, the continued decreased perfusion to the myocardial working cells causes frank heart failure and the organism will die.

A part of the cardiovascular system is the blood itself. There are alterations in the clotting process that are common complications of the shock syndrome. The most frequent occurrence is disseminated intravascular coagulation (DIC). This results in coagulation in the microcirculation and a paradoxical hemorrhage. The patient develops multiple clots, whereas being unable to form a clot where it is needed. In general, DIC is a late occurrence in the shock syndrome.

Also in dealing with alterations that occur in the blood stream, the white blood cells are affected by the shock syndrome. Leukopenia is a common occurrence, with shock leaving the host susceptible to lethal infections (Huang et al., 1983).

Respiratory System

The major complication that involves the respiratory system is adult respiratory distress syndrome (ARDS) (Emmanuelson and Rosenlicht, 1986; Huang et al., 1983; Whitman, 1988). This occurs secondary to the reduced pulmonary blood flow and the increased pulmonary vascular resistance. The exact mechanisms by which this occurs are not yet identified. There is some consideration given to the role that the complement system may have to play in the syndrome (Whitman, 1988). Whatever the pathology, the result is respiratory failure that is refractory to oxygen therapy. There is an increase in the pulmonary capillary permeability and a decrease in surfactant. These two processes interfere with the absorption of oxygen and the elasticity of the tissue, decreasing pulmonary compliance. Respiratory failure ensues.

Renal System

The kidneys play a major role in the shock syndrome and are susceptible to major complications. Decreased renal perfusion leads to acute tubular necrosis (ATN). Ischemic injury extends to the basement membrane of the nephron. Once this injury occurs, the tissue sloughs off and tissue collects in the tubular space (Alspach, 1991). This tissue collection leads to necrosis and renal failure.

Liver

Impairment of the hepatic cells results in a decreased ability to produce energy and detoxify circulating toxins (Shatney, 1986). Ischemic hepatic cells release lysosomes into the circulation and damage the capillary walls in the liver. This results in multiple problems for the patient in shock. Hormones and circulating toxins cannot be detoxified and continue to cause problems for the individual. Energy reduction is already a problem and increases in this lead to further cellular damage.

Gastrointestinal System

The ischemia of the intestines causes two distinct problems. The first is a reduction in blood supply affecting the protective mechanism of the GI tract. This leads to mucosal damage and ulceration of the intestines. Second, ischemia increases the likelihood of bacteria and toxins crossing the intestinal barrier and entering the circulation, leading to sepsis and more problems (Huang et al., 1983).

MULTIPLE ORGAN FAILURE

The syndrome of multiple organ failure (MOF) is the latest in the series of complications of the shock syndrome that is currently undergoing intensive research (Rutan et al., 1989). Multiple organ failure has been identified as a complication of shock and/or severe injury. The syndrome of MOF is one that will require continued research into the mechanics of why it occurs. It occurs whenever more than one organ is unable to maintain its own function. Sepsis is generally considered a contributing factor to this syndrome. The process of MOF is initiated by generalized tissue injury. This is followed by an activation of available defenses that attempt to contain the injury. If the defenses fail or suffer dysfunction, invasive infection occurs and MOF follows.

Summary

The risk for shock is a common threat for all patients. Its causes are many, and the treatment varied and complex. Prevention is the primary goal, accomplished through identification of high-risk patient conditions and early interventions to avert this complication. The patient in shock is critically ill. Successful management relies heavily on accurate nursing assessments, data analysis, implementation of definitive interventions, evaluation of patient response to treatment, and attainment of expected outcomes. Shock is a crisis for the patient, family, nurse, and the health care team. A collaborative approach of clinical expertise while never sacrificing the caring element, will do much to assist the patient to reach a positive outcome from shock, the common threat.

References

Advanced Trauma Life Support for Physicians (1989): Chicago: American College of Surgeons.

Alspach, J. (1991): *AACN Core Curriculum for Critical-Care Nursing.* 4th ed. Philadelphia: W. B. Saunders.

Bordick, K. (1980): *Patterns of Shock.* 2nd ed. New York: Macmillan.

Broscious, S. (1991): Toxic shock syndrome and its potential complications. *Critical Care Nurse* 11(4):28–35.

Bullock, B., and Rosendahl, P. (1988): *Pathophysiology Adaptations and Alterations in Function.* Glenview, Illinois: Scott, Foresman. Little, Brown.

Dailey, E., and Schroeder, J. (1989): *Bedside Techniques in Hemodynamic Monitoring.* 4th ed. St. Louis: C. V. Mosby.

Dickerson, J. (1988): Anaphylaxis and anaphylactic shock. *Critical Care Nursing Quarterly* 11(1):68–74.

Doenges, M., Moorhouse, M., and Geissler, A. (1989): *Nursing Care Plans: Guidelines for Planning Patient Care.* 2nd ed. Philadelphia: F. A. Davis.

Emmanuelson, K., and Rosenlicht, J. (1986): *Handbook of Critical Care Nursing.* New York: John Wiley & Sons.

Feola, M., and Canizaro, P. C. (1988): Stroma-free hemoglobin solution: The potentially ideal blood substitute. In: R. M. Haldaway (ed.). *Shock: The Reversible Stage of Dying.* Littleton, MA: PSG Publications, p. 467–470.

Huang, S., Dasher, L., Larson, C., and McCulloch, C. (1983): *Coronary Care Nursing.* Philadelphia: W. B. Saunders.

Jeffries, P., and Whelan, S. (1989): Cardiogenic shock: current management. *Critical Care Nursing Quarterly* 11(1):48–56.

Littleton, M. (1988): Pathophysiology and assessment of septic shock. *Critical Care Nursing Quarterly* 11(1):30–47.

Luckmann, J., and Sorensen, K. C. (1987): *Medical-Surgical Nursing: A Psychophysiologic Approach.* 3rd ed. Philadelphia: W. B. Saunders.

McQuillan, K., and Wiles, C. (1988): Initial management of traumatic shock. In: V. Cardona, P. Hurn, P. Mason, A. Scanlon-Schlipp, and S. Veise-Berry (eds.). *Trauma Nursing from Resuscitation Through Rehabilitation.* Philadelphia: W. B. Saunders, pp. 160–183.

Meyers, I., and Hickey, M. (1988): Nursing management of hypovolemic shock. *Critical Care Nursing Quarterly* 11(1):57–67.

Myers, J. (1983): Anaphylactic shock. In: A. Perry and P. Potter (eds.). *Shock Comprehensive Nursing Management.* St. Louis: C. V. Mosby, pp. 194–212.

Niedringhaus, L. (1983a): Classifications of shock. In: A. Perry and P. Potter (eds.). *Shock Comprehensive Nursing Management.* St. Louis: C. V. Mosby, pp. 91–100.

Niedringhaus, L. (1983b): Hypovolemic shock. In: A. Perry and P. Potter (eds.). *Shock Comprehensive Nursing Management.* St. Louis: C. V. Mosby, pp. 126–151.

Potter, P. (1983): Microcirculation. In: A. Perry and P. Potter (eds.). *Shock Comprehensive Nursing Management.* St. Louis: C. V. Mosby, pp. 42–63.

Querin, J., and Stahl, L. (1983): 12 Simple, sensible steps for successful blood transfusions. *Nursing, 83* 13(11):34–44.

Rice, V. (1991a): Shock; A clinical syndrome: An update. part 1. An Overview of Shock. *Critical Care Nurse* 11(4):26–7.

Rice, V. (1991b): Shock; A clinical syndrome: An update. part 2. The Stages of Shock. *Critical Care Nurse* 11(5):74, 76, 78–9.

Rice, V. (1991c): Shock; A clinical syndrome: An update. part 3. Therapeutic Management. *Critical Care Nurse* 11(6):34–9

Rice, V. (1991d): Shock; A clinical syndrome: An update. part 4. Nursing Care of the Shock Patient. *Critical Care Nurse* 11(7):28–32, 35–40.

Rice, V. (1984a): The clinical continuum of septic shock. *Critical Care Nurse* 4(5):86–109.

Rice, V. (1984b): Shock management part I. *Critical Care Nurse* 4(6):69–82.

Rice, V. (1985): Shock management part II. *Critical Care Nurse* 5(1):42–58.

Rutan, P., Roundtree, W., Myers, K., and Barker, L. (1989): Initial experience with the hemopump. *Critical Care Nursing Clinics* 1(3):527–534.

Siskind, J. (1984): Handling hemorrhage wisely. *Nursing '84* 14(1):34–41.

Smith-Collins, A. (1983): Septic shock. In: A. Perry and P. Potter (eds.). *Shock Comprehensive Nursing Management.* St. Louis: C. V. Mosby, pp. 172–193.

Strange, J. M. (1987): *Shock Trauma Care Plans.* Springhouse, PA: Springhouse Corp.

Swearingen, P., and Keen, J. H. (1991): *Manual of Critical Care: Applying Nursing Diagnosis to Adult Critical Illness.* St. Louis; C. V. Mosby.

Textbook of Advanced Cardiac Life Support. Dallas: American Heart Association, 1987, 1990 (2nd ed.).

Trauma Nursing Core Course (1987): Chicago: Award Printing Corp.

Whitman, G. (1988). Tissue perfusion. In: M. Kinney, D. Packa, and S. Dunbar (eds.). *AACN Reference for Critical-Care Nursing.* 2nd ed. New York: McGraw-Hill, pp. 115–159.

Recommended Readings

Borzott, A., and Polk, H. (1983): Multiple system organ failure. *Surgical Clinics of North America* 63(2):315–336.

Holt, J., McKenny, S., and Pribyl, C. (1985): Shock. *Nursing Life* 5(1):33–40.

Jillings, C. (1990): Shock psychosocial needs of families and patients. *Critical Care Nursing Clinics of North America* 2(2):325–330.

Kuhn, M. M. (1991): Colloids vs. crystalloids. *Critical Care Nurse* 11(5):37–44, 46–51.

Lancaster, L. (1990): Renal response to shock. *Critical Care Nursing Quarterly* 2(2):221–234.

McCormac, M. (1990): Managing hemorrhagic shock. *American Journal of Nursing* 90(8):22–27.

McMenemin, I. M. (1987): Acute circulatory failure in intensive care—basic physiology, monitoring and therapeutic techniques. *Intensive Care Nursing* 3(1):34–40.

Peter, N. K. (1988): Care of patients with traumatic pelvic fractures. *Critical Care Nurse* 8(3):62–66, 68, 70.

Physiologic shock (1987): In: J. Luckmann and K. Sorenson (eds.). *Medical-Surgical Nursing: A Psychophysiologic Approach.* 2nd ed. Philadelphia: W. B. Saunders, pp. 214–257.

Rice, V. (1987): Acid-base derangements in the patient with cardiac arrest. *Focus on Critical Care* 14(6):53–61.

Rice, V. (1987): Septic shock: Nursing implications of current medical research. *NITA* 10(5):326–333.

Schumann, L., and Remington, M. (1989): The use of naloxone in treating endotoxic shock. *Critical Care Nurse* 10(2):63–71.

Shatney, C. (1986): Pathophysiology and treatment of circulatory shock. In: D. Zschoche (ed.). *Mosby's Comprehensive Review of Critical Care.* 3rd ed. St. Louis: C. V. Mosby, pp. 177–217.

Sommers, M. S. (1990): Fluid resuscitation following multiple trauma. *Critical Care Nurse* 10(10):74–81.

Textbook of Advanced Cardiac Life Support (1987): Dallas: American Heart Association, pp. 41–44, 97–109.

Urban, N. (1986): Integrating hemodynamic parameters with clinical decision making. *Critical Care Nurse* 6(2):48–61.

Chapter

8

Marilyn L. Lamborn, Ph.D., R.N.
Marsha E. Fonteyn, Ph.D., R.N., CCRN

Cardiac Alterations

Objectives

- Contrast various pathological cause/effect mechanisms producing acute cardiac disturbances.
- Discuss the nursing care responsibilities related to selected laboratory, electrocardiographic, radiological, and nuclear studies used in the diagnosis of cardiac disease.
- Compare and contrast pharmacological, operative, and electrical treatment modalities used in the management of cardiac disease addressing:
  a. Rationale and therapeutic effect of treatment
  b. Complications of treatment
  c. Nursing responsibilities related to treatment
- Identify specific nursing interventions designed to prevent or minimize physiological or psychological disturbances or complications of patients with critical cardiac disease.
- Develop and use fact-related and patient-centered nursing care plan for the acutely ill cardiac patient involving: assessment, inferential nursing diagnosis, measurable patient goals, nursing priorities and actions, and evaluations of patient outcomes and nursing actions.

The care of the patient with alterations in cardiac status encompasses care for the seriously ill cardiac patient who is at risk and whose outcome is uncertain. The critical care nurse must have both a theoretical knowledge and practice-related understanding of the common cardiac diseases and must possess the clinical judgment skills necessary to make rapid and accurate decisions in a variety of life or death situations. The purpose of this chapter is to identify and explore some of the more common serious cardiac alterations likely to be encountered by critical care nurses when caring for patients with compromised cardiac status, and to describe the type of nursing care that is most likely to bring about a positive outcome.

Normal Structure and Function of the Heart

An essential component of effective nursing care is a comprehensive knowledge of the normal structure and function of the heart. The heart muscle is composed of cells that are connected to each other end-to-end as well as side-to-side, giving the shape and appearance of a lattice fence (Fig. 8–1). The myocardial fibers or myofibril can contract and expand lengthwise as well as widen and narrow in an accordion-type movement. The heart muscle itself is approximately the size of a person's closed fist and lies within the mediastinal space of the thoracic cavity between the lungs, directly under the lower half of

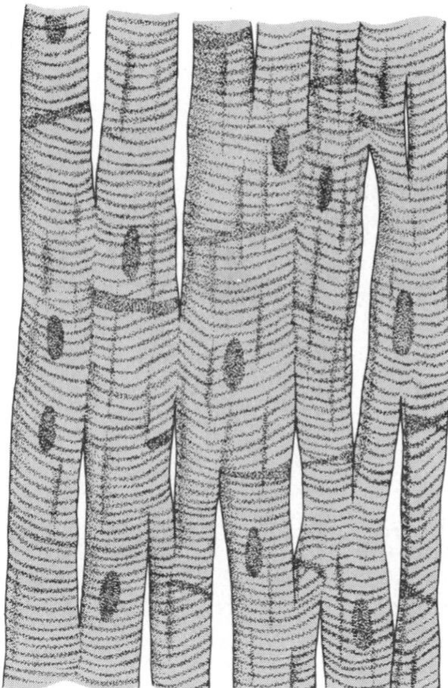

Figure 8-1. The "syncytial," interconnecting nature of cardiac muscle. (From Guyton, A. C.: *Textbook of Medical Physiology*. 7th ed. Philadelphia, W. B. Saunders, 1986.)

the sternum, and above the diaphragm (Fig. 8-2) (Thibodeau, 1990). It is covered by the pericardium, which has an inner visceral layer and an outer parietal layer. Certain diseases can cause this covering to become inflamed and subsequently diminish the effectiveness of the heart as a pump. There is a small amount of lubricating fluid between these layers. There are pathological conditions that can increase the amount and consistency of this fluid and this can also effect the pumping ability of the heart (Canobbio, 1990). The heart muscle itself is composed of three layers: the outer layer, or epicardium; the middle, muscular layer, or myocardium; and the inner endothelial layer, or endocardium (Fig. 8-3) (Thibodeau, 1990). It is these layers that are damaged or destroyed when a patient has a heart attack.

Functionally, the heart is divided into right- and left-sided pumps separated by a septum. The right side is generally considered to be low pressure, whereas the left side is high pressure. Each side has an atrium that receives blood and a ventricle that pumps it out. The right atrium (RA) receives deoxygenated blood from the body through the superior and inferior venae cavae (SVC and IVC). Blood travels by gravity from the atrium to the ventricles when the valves separating these chambers open. The right ventricle (RV) pumps the deoxygenated blood to the lungs through the pulmonary artery for oxygen and carbon dioxide exchange. The left atrium (LA) receives the newly oxygenated blood by way of the pulmonary veins from the lungs, and the left ventricle (LV) pumps the oxygenated blood through the aorta to the systemic circulation (Fig. 8-4) (Vander et al., 1985; West, 1991).

The four cardiac valves maintain the unidirectional blood flow through the chambers of the heart. There are two types of valves: the atrioventricular (AV) valves, which separate the atria from the ventricles, and the semilunar valves, which separate the pulmonary artery from the RV and the aorta from the LV (Fig. 8-5). The atrioventricular valves include the tricuspid valve, which lies between the right atrium and right ventricle, and the mitral valve, which is located between the left atrium and left ventricle. Each AV valve is anchored by chordae tendineae to the papillary muscles on its ventricular floor. The semilunar valves are the pulmonic valve, which lies between the right ventricle and the pulmonary artery, and the aortic valve, which is between the left ventricle and the aorta. These semilunar valves are not anchored by the chordae tendineae. Instead, their closing is caused by the blood pressing against their cusp-like valve flaps (Thibodeau, 1990; West, 1991).

HEART SOUNDS

The vibrations produced by vascular walls, flowing blood, heart muscle, and heart valves create sound waves known as heart sounds. Auscultating these sounds with a stethoscope over the heart provides valuable information about valve and cardiac functions (Fig. 8-6). Systole occurs when the pulmonic and aortic valves open to allow blood to be pumped to the lungs (right ventricle-pulmonic valve) and systemic circulation (left ventricle-aortic valve). This sound has been described as "lubb." Diastole produces the second heart sound (sounds like "dup") when the tricuspid and mitral valves open to allow the ventricles to fill with blood (Braunwald et al., 1988; Dossey et al., 1990; Underhill, 1989).

The first heart sound is known as S_1. It is caused by closure of the mitral and tricuspid valves. It is best heard at the apex (lower point of the heart muscle) of the heart and represents the beginning of ventricular systole.

The second heart sound is known as S_2 and is caused by the closure of the aortic and pulmonic valves. It is best heard at the second intercostal space and represents the beginning of ven-

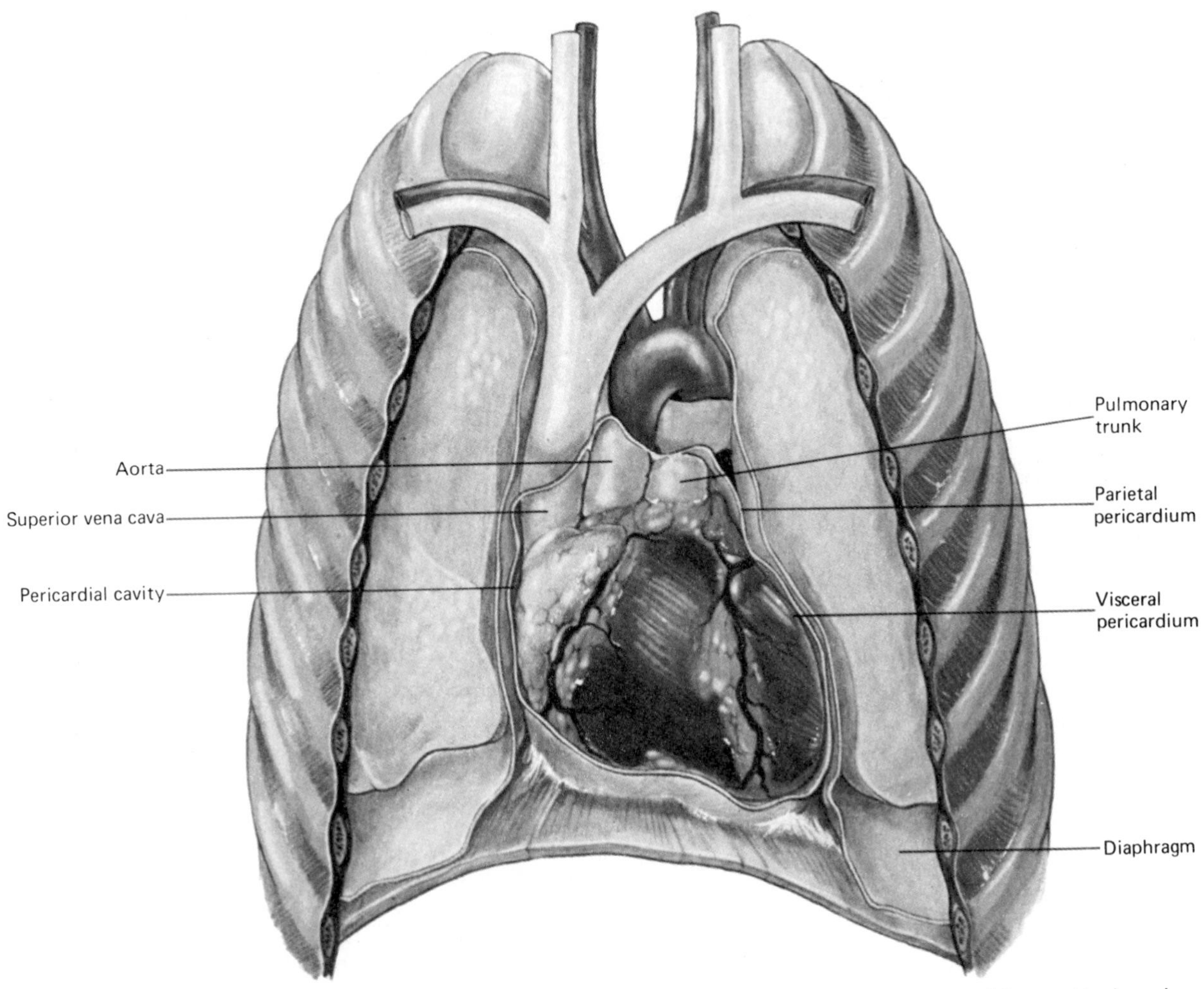

Figure 8–2. The heart lies in the mediastinum between the lungs. Its apex rests on the diaphragm. The heart and the roots of the great blood vessels are loosely enclosed by the pericardium. (From Solomon, E. P., and Phillips, G. A.: *Understanding Human Anatomy and Physiology*. Philadelphia, W. B. Saunders, 1987.)

tricular diastole. The first and second heart sounds are best heard with the diaphragm of the stethoscope.

A third heart sound, S_3, can be normal in a child, but it usually represents pathology in the adult. It is caused by a rapid flow of blood into a nonpliable ventricle. The S_3 sound can best be heard with the bell of the stethoscope at the apex of the heart. It occurs immediately after the second heart sound (S_2). Together with S_1 and S_2, S_3 produces a sound like "lubb-dup-a" or "ken-tuk'e." A fourth heart sound, S_4, is produced from atrial contraction that is more forceful than normal. Together with S_1 and S_2, S_4 produces a sound like "te-lubb-dup" or "ten-ne'se." S_4 can be normal in the elderly, but is often a sign of early failure, when the atria contract more forcefully against ventricles distended with blood. In the severely failing heart, all four sounds (S_1, S_2, S_3, and S_4) may be heard, producing a "gallop" rhythm, so named because it sounds like the hoof beats of a galloping horse (Braunwald et al., 1988; Underhill, 1989). It can best be heard with the bell of the stethoscope at the lower end of the sternum or the apex.

HEART MURMUR

A heart murmur is a sound caused by a turbulence of blood flow through the valves of the

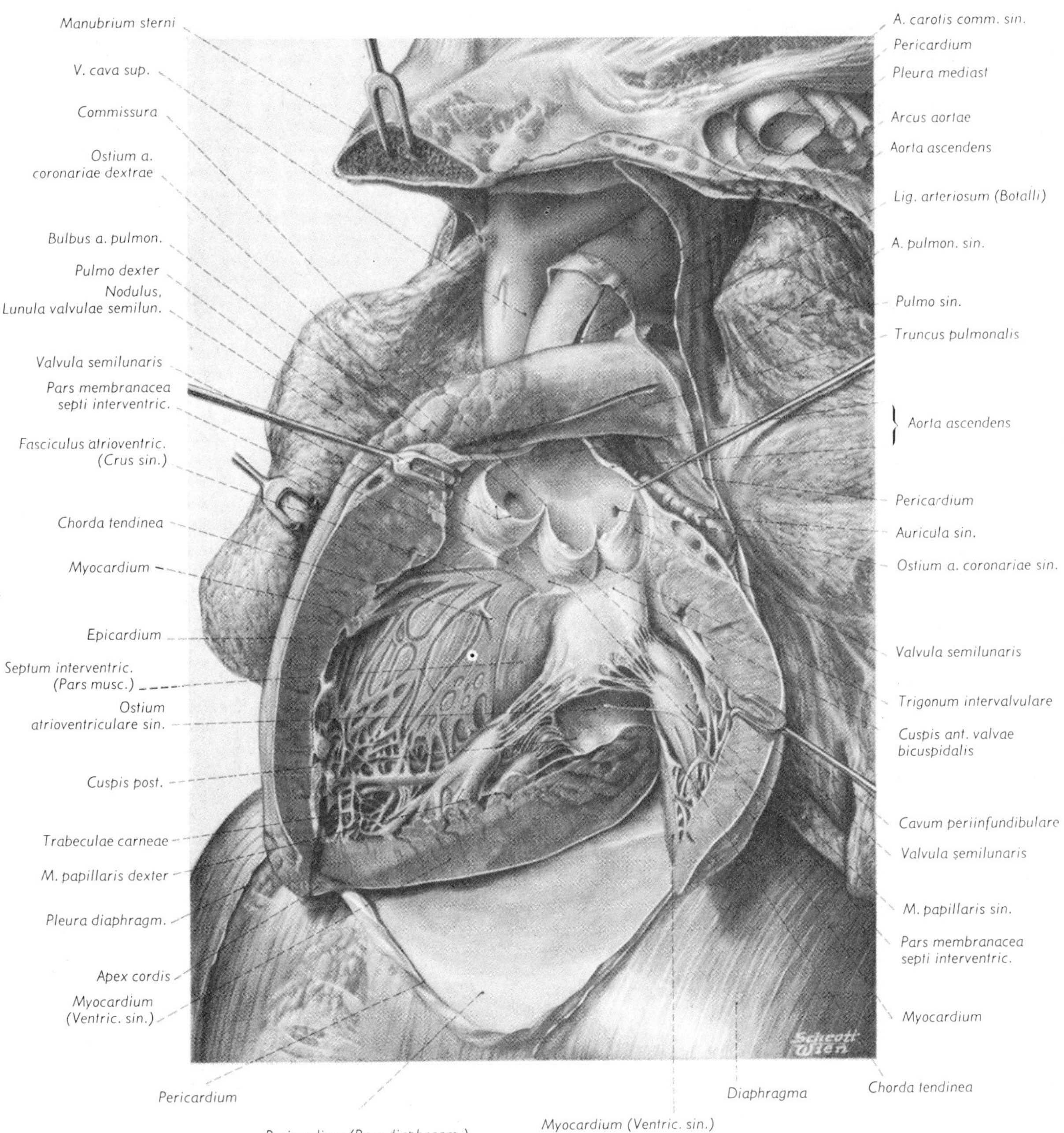

Figure 8-3. View into left ventricle showing layers of heart muscle and other anatomical landmarks. (From Pernkopf, E.: *Atlas of Topographical and Applied Human Anatomy*. Vol. 2. Philadelphia, W. B. Saunders, 1964.)

heart. In children and adults, murmurs can also be heard when there is a septal defect. In adults, murmurs can be heard when a valve, usually aortic or mitral, is either narrow, inflamed, stenosed, or incompetent, or there is failure of the valve leaflets to approximate (insufficiency). The presence of a new murmur warrants special attention, particularly in a patient with an acute myocardial infarction (MI). A papillary muscle may have ruptured, causing the valve to not approximate correctly and can be indicative of severe damage and impending complications (such

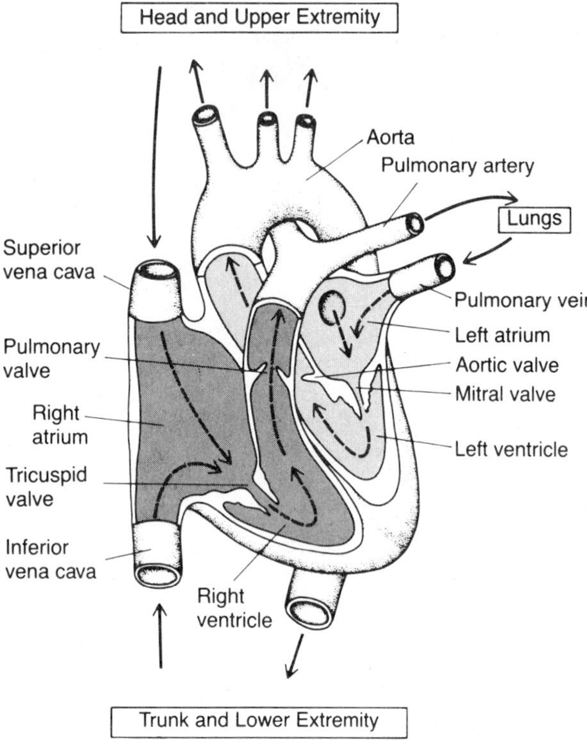

Figure 8–4. Structure of the heart, and course of blood flow through the heart chambers. (From Guyton, A. C.: *Textbook of Medical Physiology.* 7th ed. Philadelphia, W. B. Saunders, 1986.)

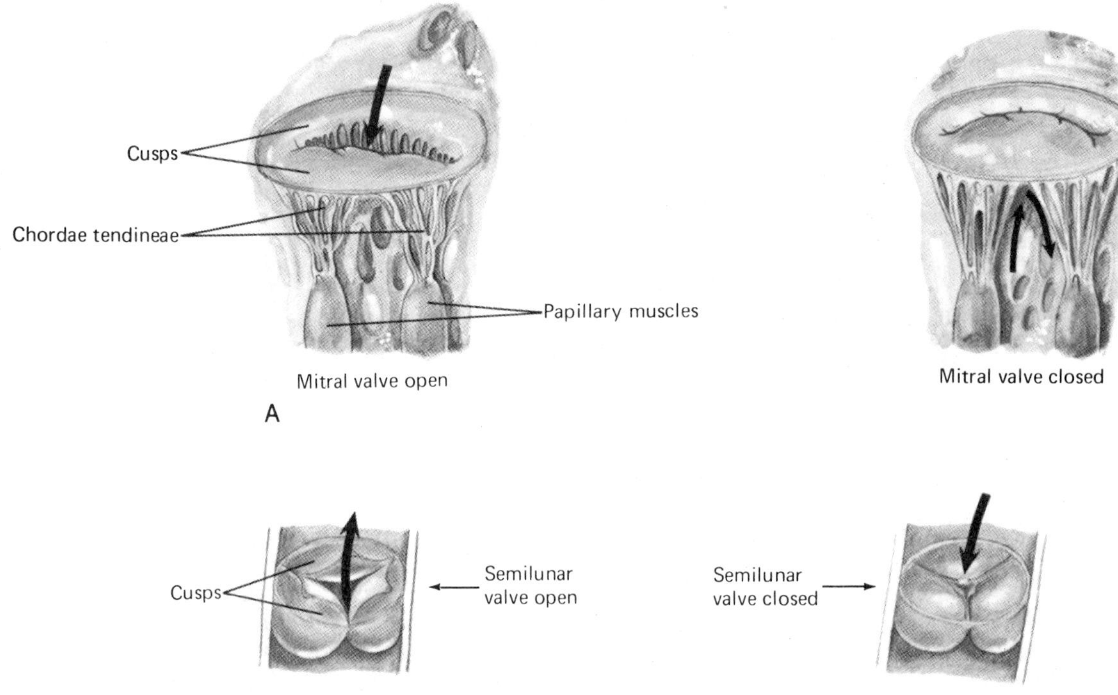

Figure 8–5. How the valves of the heart work. (*A*), The mitral valve in the open and closed position. (*B*), A semilunar valve in the open & closed positions. (From Solomon, E. P., and Phillips, G. A.: *Understanding Human Anatomy and Physiology.* Philadelphia, W. B. Saunders, 1987.)

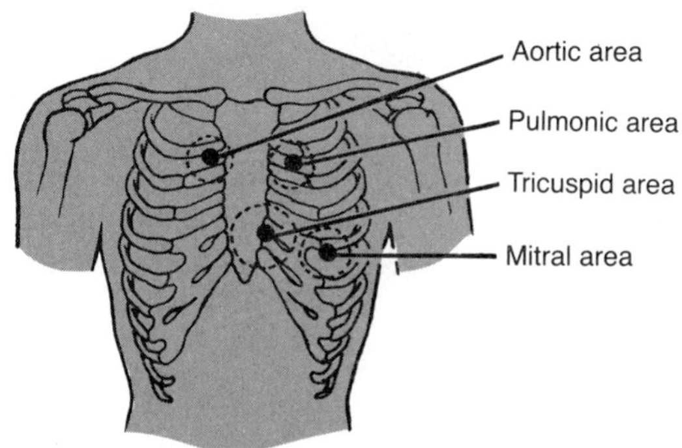

Figure 8-6. Chest areas from which each valve sound is best heard. (From Guyton, A. C.: *Textbook of Medical Physiology*. 7th ed. Philadelphia, W. B. Saunders, 1986.)

as congestive heart failure and pulmonary edema). A murmur is usually a rumbling, blowing, or harsh sound. It is important to distinguish the sound, location, loudness, and intensity of a murmur and the extra heart sounds (Dossey et al., 1990). This skill is developed from practice listening to many different patients' hearts and correlating the sounds heard with the patients' pathological conditions.

The autonomic nervous system exerts control over the cardiovascular system. The sympathetic nervous system releases norepinephrine, which has two effects: alpha-adrenergic, which causes arterial vasoconstriction; and beta-adrenergic, which increases sinus node discharge (positive chronotrope), increases the force of contraction (positive inotrope), and accelerates the arterioventricular (AV) conduction time (dromotrope).

The parasympathetic nervous system releases acetylcholine and occurs through stimulation of the vagus nerve. It causes a decrease in the sinus node discharge and slows AV conduction (Braunwald et al., 1988; Thibodeau, 1990; Vander et al., 1985; West, 1991).

In addition to this innervation, there are receptors that help to control cardiovascular function. These are chemoreceptors that are sensitive to changes in PO_2, PCO_2, and pH blood levels. These stimulate the vasomotor center in the medulla that controls vasoconstriction and vasodilation. The baroceptors are those that are sensitive to stretch and pressure. If blood pressure increases, these cause the heart rate to decrease. If the blood pressure decreases, these stimulate an increase in the heart rate (Vander et al., 1985; West, 1991).

CORONARY CIRCULATION

Since many cardiac problems arise because of an occlusion or partial occlusion of a coronary artery, an understanding of the coronary blood supply is necessary. The blood supply to the myocardium is derived from the coronary arteries that branch off the aorta immediately above the aortic valve (Fig. 8-7). There are two major branches: the right coronary artery (RCA) and the left coronary artery (LCA), which splits into two branches: the left anterior descending (LAD) branch and the left circumflex (LCX) branch. Knowledge of what portion of the heart receives its blood supply from a particular coronary artery allows the nurse to anticipate problems related to occlusion of that vessel. The right coronary artery generally supplies the major portion of the right atrium and right ventricle, the SA and AV nodes, and the inferior portion of the LV. The left anterior descending artery passes behind the pulmonary artery and provides the blood supply to the septum, and the anterior and apical sections of the left ventricle. The left circumflex artery provides blood supply to the left atrium and lateral and posterior left ventricle. Please note that variations in the branching and exact placing of the coronary arteries are common (Thibodeau, 1990; Vander et al., 1985; West, 1991).

Blood flow to the coronary arteries occurs during diastole when the aortic valve is closed and the sinuses of Valsalva are filled with blood. Myocardial fibers are relaxed at this time, promoting blood flow through the coronary vessels. The coronary veins return blood from the coronary arteries back to the heart through the coronary sinuses to the right and left atria (Bates and Hockelman, 1983; Hurst and Logue, 1990).

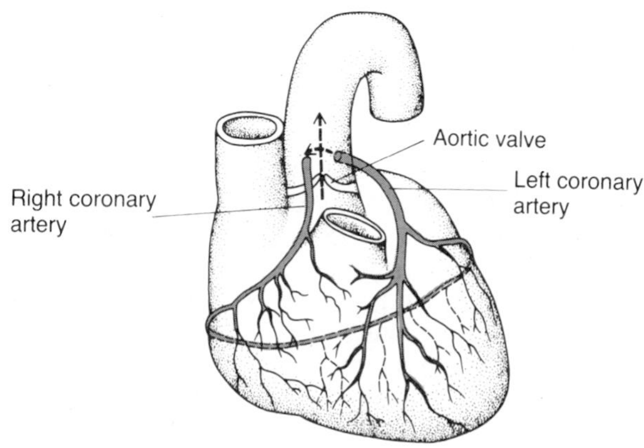

Figure 8-7. The coronary vessels. (From Guyton, A. C.: *Textbook of Medical Physiology*. 7th ed. Philadelphia, W. B. Saunders, 1986.)

PROPERTIES OF THE CARDIAC MUSCLE

Contractility is the ability of muscle fibers to shorten when stimulated, providing the pumping mechanism of the heart. This results in a consistent amount of blood volume (known as stroke volume, SV) being delivered to the pulmonic and systemic circulation with each heart beat.

Rhythmicity is the ability of the heart muscles to depolarize rhythmically.

Conductivity is the heart cell's ability to transmit electrical impulses rapidly and efficiently to all areas of the heart.

Automaticity is the ability of the heart cell to beat spontaneously and to generate an impulse without external stimulation.

Excitability is the cell's ability to respond to electrochemical stimulation (Marriott and Conover, 1989).

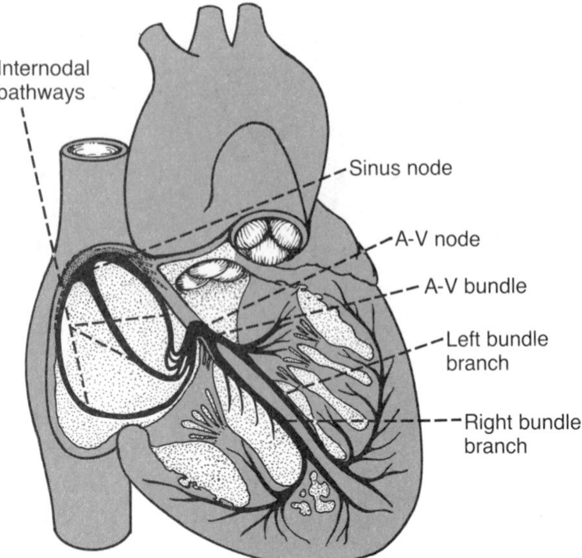

Figure 8–8. The SA node and the Purkinje system of the heart, showing also the AV node, the atrial internodal pathways, and the ventricular bundle branches. (From Guyton, A. C.: *Textbook of Medical Physiology*. 7th ed. Philadelphia, W. B. Saunders, 1986.)

CONDUCTION SYSTEM

As a consequence of the aforementioned properties of the cardiac muscle, the heart spontaneously and rhythmically initiates impulses. The cardiac impulse normally originates in the SA node, which is referred to as the natural pacemaker of the heart. These impulses travel through internodal tracts to the AV node, which is the normal route for transmission of impulses from the atria to the ventricles.

From the AV node, the impulse spreads to the bundle of His, which divides into right and left branches. These branches terminate in a band of fibers, Purkinje fibers, which spreads impulses through the ventricles (Fig. 8–8) (Marriott and Conover, 1989).

FACTORS OF CIRCULATION

The primary function of the heart is to pump blood through the pulmonary and systemic circulations. Circulation must be adequate to meet the fluctuating demands of the body. If the heart fails to perform, there is a compromise in cardiac output. Cardiac output is the traditional measure of cardiac function and is equal to heart rate (HR) times stroke volume (SV). The average heart rate = 70 beats per minute and the average stroke volume = 70 milliliters (ml) per beat. Thus, the average cardiac output = 70 × 70 = 4900 ml, or about 5 liters (L) per minute. Since adequate cardiac output is dependent on body size, a more specific measure of cardiac function is the cardiac index, which is calculated by dividing the cardiac output by the body surface area (BSA) obtained from a table taking into account height and weight (Gardner, 1989). The normal cardiac index is 2.8 to 4.2 L/min/m^2. A value of less than 2 is considered incompatible with life (Dossey et al., 1990).

Stroke volume is the amount of blood ejected with each ventricular contraction; normally 60 to 100 ml. Stroke volume is determined by three variants: preload, afterload, and contractility. Preload is the amount of blood remaining in the LV at the end of diastole (left ventricular end-diastolic pressure, LVEDP). It is measured by the pulmonary capillary wedge pressure (PCWP) or the left atrial pressure. The normal PCWP is approximately 8 to 12 mm Hg, but it rises considerably in heart failure. If the failing heart is moderately distended with blood at the end of diastole (due to less efficient pumping by the heart), then the subsequent contraction will be more forceful. This phenomena is known as Starling's law of the heart, which states that, within limits, the greater the stretch or length of the myocardial fiber (and the stretch will be greater if the heart is distended with blood), the greater the force of contraction, thereby increasing cardiac output (Patterson et al., 1914). Optimal contractility occurs at a PCWP of 12 to 18 mm Hg. Further stretch in cardiac muscle fibers beyond this PCWP will ultimately result in poor contractile function analogous to the effect of overstretching a rubber band.

Afterload refers to the resistance to blood flow during ventricular ejection (Dossey et al., 1990). Afterload affects the rate of contraction by affecting the force-velocity relationship; i.e., the less force or resistance the fiber must overcome, the more rapidly and efficiently it can contract. Therefore, a decrease in afterload (vasodilation) will cause an increase in the CO, and an increase in the afterload (hypertension, vasoconstriction, aortic stenosis) will decrease the CO. Systemic vascular resistance (SVR) is the force opposing blood flow within the vessels, and is the measurement of afterload. It is the product of three factors: vessel radius, vessel length, and blood viscosity. The third factor in determining stroke volume is contractility, which has been discussed earlier in this chapter (Thibodeau, 1990; Underhill, 1989; West, 1991).

Cardiac reserve is the capacity of the heart to adjust to increased demands of the body, such as an elevated temperature or stress, by increasing the cardiac output and raising the blood pressure to meet these demands.

Blood pressure is the pressure exerted by the blood on the arterial wall, and is a reflection of the function of the ventricles as pumps. Blood pressure is represented by systolic pressure (which is the peak pressure and occurs during contraction of the ventricles) and diastolic pressure (which is the residual pressure or point of least pressure in the arterial system). It is at this point (diastole) in the cardiac cycle that the myocardial muscle fibers lengthen, the heart dilates, and the ventricles fill with blood.

The mean arterial pressure (MAP) is the average pressure of blood flow to the tissues during a given cardiac cycle. To calculate the MAP:

$$\frac{\text{systolic} + 2\ (\text{diastolic})}{3}.$$

For instance, a pressure of 120/80, the MAP is 93 mm Hg (systolic + 2 diastolic/3 = 120 + 160/3 = 93). Please note that this is a value and not an arithmetic mean, which would be calculated by adding the systolic and diastolic and dividing by 2. Because diastole is longer than systole, the MAP is closer to the diastolic reading (Hurst and Logue, 1990; Price and Wilson, 1986).

Coronary Artery Disease

The heart muscle requires a substantial flow of blood that can increase when physical or emotional demands on the heart increase activity. When coronary artery disease compromises the supply of coronary blood flow, the efficiency and function of the heart muscle is jeopardized. Coronary artery disease (CAD) is a partial or total occlusion of the coronary arteries by atherosclerosis. The terms *coronary artery disease* and *arteriosclerotic heart disease* (ASHD) are used synonymously.

PATHOPHYSIOLOGY

Arteriosclerosis produces degeneration, hardening, or thickening of the arterial walls. Atherosclerosis is the most common form of arteriosclerosis, and is characterized by lipid deposits on the intimal layer of the artery, which can progress to partially or totally occlude the lumen. Atherosclerosis is a disease that involves the aorta, its branches, and medium-sized arteries such as those supplying blood to the brain, heart, and major internal organs (Price and Wilson, 1986). Atherosclerosis does not seem to involve the arterioles or the venous circulation.

The atherosclerotic lesion, atheroma, or atherosclerotic plaque, consists of an elevated mass of fatty streaks that are lipid-filled smooth muscle cells, and may have secondary deposits of calcium salts and blood products. These raised fibrous plaques create changes in the arterial wall caused from chronic endothelial injury. They generally form at points where the arterial tree branches. This is especially true of the carotid and iliac arteries (Kinney et al., 1991). Coronary arteries are particularly susceptible to atherosclerosis, which is most commonly seen in individuals who also have coronary artery disease with a history of a high-fat diet, smoking, and sedentary life style.

The atheromas are derived from the lipids, cholesterol, triglycerides, and free fatty acids. An elevated level of cholesterol (above 200 mg) is associated with an increased risk of coronary artery disease (NIH, 1989). Cholesterol and triglycerides are insoluble in plasma and must be transported by lipoproteins, which are soluble. These lipoproteins can be separated and measured. Lipoproteins are composed of lipids and proteins. High-density lipoproteins (HDLs) are composed mostly of protein and carry 10 to 50% of total plasma cholesterol. The lipids are removed during circulation through the liver. Because an increase in HDLs means a decrease in the incidence of coronary artery disease, a higher level of HDLs is desired in proportion to low-density lipoproteins (LDLs), which carry most of the cholesterol in the plasma and deposit lipids and cholesterol in the vessels, particularly the coronary arteries. Thus, an increase in LDL levels can indicate an increased risk of coronary artery disease. Very low-density lipoproteins (VLDLs) carry mostly triglycerides and lesser amounts of cholesterol and deposit them in the coronary arteries. Increased triglyceride levels also contribute to the process of atherosclerosis, particularly in the coronary arteries (Kinney et al., 1991; LaRosa, 1991: NIH, 1989).

During the atherosclerotic process, a thickening occurs of the intima of the coronary artery vessel wall. This thickening along with the adherence of lipids, collagens, and elastic fibers to the wall of the damaged vessel produces the atherosclerotic lesion. Lipids, calcium, and thrombi can be found obstructing the affected vessel, decreasing blood flow and oxygen delivery to the heart muscle and causing coronary insufficiency and ischemia that results in coronary artery disease (Guzzetta and Dossey, 1984).

ASSESSMENT

Patient Assessment

A thorough, basic cardiovascular assessment is imperative in the understanding of the individual cardiac patient and inherent to planning nursing care for that patient.

An adequate and pertinent history, including subjective data, should reveal previous medical history regarding both pediatric and adult illnesses. Of particular interest would be a positive history for rheumatic fever, diabetes mellitus, hypertension, asthma, renal diseases, or cerebrovascular accident (CVA). Knowledge of prior hospitalizations is also important so records can be obtained for review. Information regarding the patient's current medications, both prescription and over-the-counter (OTC) drugs, should include an identification of the patient's understanding and use of these medications. It is also important to determine any drug or food allergies of the patient. A medical history of the patient's family can provide insight into real or potential risk factors.

A psychosocial or personal history is also important to plan the patient's care. This would include possible stress events or everyday stressors. What, if any, is the individual's exercise routine? What type, how much, what regularity? What is the patient's daily food pattern and intake? What is his/her sleep pattern? What are the patient's habitual patterns in using tobacco, alcohol, drugs, coffee, tea, and caffeinated sodas?

Before beginning the physical examination, the nurse should try to determine recent and recurrent symptoms that may be related to the patient's current problems. Such information gathering should include the presence or absence of fatigue, fluid retention, dyspnea, irregular heart beat (palpitations), chest pain (including location, intensity, provocation, alleviating factors). The physical examination itself should encompass all the body systems and not be limited to only the cardiovascular system because all of the body systems are interrelated and interdependent on one another. Although, it is imperative that a total picture is completed regarding the physical status of the patient, a patient whose primary problems are cardiovascular will most commonly exhibit alterations in circulation and oxygenation. Thus, all systems should be examined from this perspective.

The examination should be done in an orderly, organized manner and should involve the techniques of inspection, auscultation, percussion, and palpation. A baseline assessment is provided in Table 8–1.

Medical Assessment

Risk Factors

Until the late 1960s, the incidence for the occurrence of CAD and its complication increased at a steady and alarming rate. During the late 1960s research evidence began being published that linked certain risk factors to the increased likelihood of the development of CAD. Much of the early research comes from a study begun in the 1940s and 1950s when the population of Framingham, Massachusetts, was studied for the determination of risk factors for CAD. The study has spanned over many years, and involves a wide variety of families and life styles. With the advent of the Framingham study and other similar research, the public has become progressively more aware and knowledgeable of the recognized risk factors and what measures can be taken hopefully to edify the occurrence of CAD and its complications (Kannel and Gordon, 1978; National Research Council, 1989).

Table 8–1. BASELINE ASSESSMENT OF THE CARDIOVASCULAR PATIENT

Neurology	Level of consciousness, orientation to time, place events; hallucinations, depression, withdrawal, trembling; pupils (size, equality, response); paresthesias; eye movements (nystagmus, focus, directional movement); restlessness, apprehensiveness, irritability, cooperative; hand grips; leg movement; response to tactile stimuli; location of pain, type; relieved by; patient's complaints
Skin	Color, temperature, dryness, turgor, rashes, broken areas, pressure areas, urticaria, incision site, wounds
Cardiology	BP; apical and radial pulses; pulse deficit; lead patient on; rhythm, frequency of ectopics; PR and QRS intervals; heart sounds—presence of abnormalities (e.g., rubs, gallops); neck vein distention with head of bed at what angle; edema (sacral and dependent; calf pain; varicosities; presence of pulses—bilateral carotid, radial, femoral, posterior tibial, dorsalis pedis; capillary refill in extremities; presence of invasive pressure monitoring devices; CVP; temporary pacemaker settings; specifics as to medication drips to maintain BP or rhythm.
Respiratory	Rate and quality of respirations; O_2; accessory muscles used; cough, sputum—type, color, suctioning frequency; symmetry of chest expansion and breath sounds; describe breath sounds; note current ABGs; chest tube with description of drainage, fluctuation in water seal, bubbling, suction applied; tracheostomy or endotracheal tube; ventilator used; ventilator settings; ventilator rate vs patient's own breaths; patient's own TV if possible
GI	Abdominal size and softness, bowel sounds, nausea and vomiting, bowel movement, dressing and/or drainage, NG tube with description of drainage, feeding tube—type and frequency of feedings, drains, T-tube.
GU	Foley or voiding, urine color, quantity; C&A, specific gravity, vaginal or urethral drainage.
IV	Size of bottle or bag, solution, rate; IV site condition.
Wounds	Dry or drainage, type, color, amount, odor; hematoma, inflamed, drains, hemovac, dressing changes, cultures.

Risk factors are divided into two areas: unmodifiable and modifiable. The unmodifiable risk factors are those over which we have no control. They include age over 55, gender (males show greater incidence than females until menopause), race (blacks have higher incidence), and a family history of CAD, hyperlipidemia, or diabetes mellitus. The modifiable, or those we can control or modify, are increased LDL levels, hypertension, (BP $>$140/90), smoking, obesity, sedentary life style, and stress/behavior. The first three of the "modifiable" risk factors are considered to be the most important and most easily modified risk factors. The latter three are also important, but the impetus of research and impact of the first three risk factors are of primary importance for the control of CAD (Castelli et al., 1986; Wenger, 1985).

Diagnostic Studies. In determining the management of the patient with CAD, certain diagnostic studies are fundamental for patient care and treatment. Below is a listing and brief description of some of the more common diagnostic studies the cardiac patient may encounter.

12-Lead Electrocardiogram (ECG/EKG). This is a noninvasive test and is usually preliminary to most any other testing done. It is used as a baseline for many other tests and for comparison pre- and posttest or procedures. This test is useful in identifying rhythm disturbances, ischemia, myocardial injury, and detection and confirmation of infarct.

Holter Monitor. This is a noninvasive test that is used to detect suspected dysrhythmia. The patient is connected to a small portable recorder (about the size of a pocket radio) by three to five electrodes that is worn for 12 to 24 hours. The patient goes about the normal daily activities, keeps an activities log, returns to the laboratory after the designated period of time, and the recording is analyzed.

Exercise Tolerance Test (ETT) or Stress Test. This is a noninvasive test that involves the patient being connected to an ongoing ECG machine while the patient is exercising (putting stress on the heart and vascular system). Physical stress causes an increase in myocardial oxygen consumption exceeding the supply, thereby inducing ischemia. The stress test is used to document exercise-induced ischemia under a closely monitored and controlled situation (Kinney et al., 1991). The exercising usually involves walking on a treadmill that progresses in speed and incline, and/or walking up and down steps or stairs. The patient is constantly monitored, the pulse and blood pressure checked at intervals, and the ECG readout analyzed at the end of the testing period. The patient usually rests in the lab to ensure a return to the normal state before returning to his/her room or going home.

Chest X-Ray. This is a noninvasive procedure and is usually taken in the anterior-posterior view. The chest x-ray is used to detect cardiomegaly, cardiac positioning, degree of fluid infiltrating the pulmonary space, and other structural and positional situations that may affect the physical ability of the heart to function in a normal manner.

Phonocardiogram. This is a noninvasive test involving the use of a microphone recording of the heart sounds that are converted to electrical activity. This procedure is used to time events of the cardiac cycle, to measure systolic time intervals, and in determining the timing and characteristics of murmurs and abnormal heart sounds. The patient may be asked to perform certain activities or may be exposed to certain medications during the recording time. The procedure usually lasts 1 to 2 hours.

Echocardiogram. This is a noninvasive procedure and involves the use of ultrasound to visualize cardiac structures and the motion and function of cardiac valves and chambers. A transducer is placed on the chest wall and sends ultrasound waves at short intervals. The reflected sound waves are termed "echoes" and are displayed on a graph for interpretation. Echocardiography is used to assess valvular function, evaluate congenital defects, measure size of cardiac chambers, evaluate cardiac disease progression, evaluate ventricular function, diagnose myocardial tumors and effusions, and, to a lesser degree, measure cardiac output.

Radioisotope Studies. These are noninvasive studies involving the use of two radioactive isotopes, thallium 201 (^{201}Tl) and technetium pyrophosphate (^{99m}Tc) along with a scintillation gamma camera that follows the progression of the radioisotopes. An increase or decrease in the uptake of a radioisotope will occur in abnormal myocardial cells. An area of increased uptake is known as a "hot spot." Technetium is used to detect hot spots that may indicate a suspected myocardial infarction (MI). An area of decreased uptake is known as a "cold spot." Thallium is used to detect cold spots that assess decreased myocardial perfusion secondary to coronary stenosis or previous MI.

Cardiac Catheterization/Arteriography. This is an invasive procedure and can be divided into two stages. Cardiac catheterization is used to confirm and evaluate the severity of lesions of the heart muscle, assess left ventricular (LV) function, measure pressures within the chambers of the heart, measure cardiac output, and measure blood gas content. The procedure is done by placement of a catheter in the femoral or brachial vein and carefully advanced into the RA and progressed to the RV and pulmonary artery. A second catheter is placed in a femoral or brachial artery and is advanced through the aorta into the LV. Blood samples drawn from these two lines can be analyzed to determine oxygen saturation levels. Cardiac output can also be measured.

Coronary Arteriography. This is done to visualize coronary arteries, note the area and extent of lesions within the vessels' walls, evaluate CAD and anginal-related spasms, locate areas of infarct along with the radioisotopes, and perform a percutaneous coronary angioplasty (PTCA) or intracoronary thrombolysis. The procedure entails repositioning of the left ventricular catheter through the aorta into the proximal end of the coronary arteries. Dye is then injected into the arteries and an x-ray picture is recorded as the dye progresses or fails to progress through the coronary circulation. Finally, dye is injected into the heart chamber and the amount of dye ejected with the next systole is measured to determine the ejection fraction; i.e., the fraction of the total end-diastolic volume that is ejected during systole.

Nursing care for a patient having a cardiac catheterization for a coronary arteriogram procedure involves: the preprocedure instruction—the procedure will be done under local anesthesia, and that the patient may feel a warm or hot "flush" sensation or flutter of the catheter as it moves about; and instruction for the postprocedure routine. The postprocedure routine encompasses: bedrest for 8 hours, the extremity used for catheter insertion is kept immobile, observe for bleeding or hematoma at the catheter insertion site, the head of the bed must not be raised above 30 degrees, check peripheral pulses, check color and sensation of extremities, encourage fluids, and if an arteriogram is done, observe for an adverse reaction to dye (Dossey et al., 1990).

Magnetic Resonance Imaging (MRI). This is a noninvasive test that is relatively new when used in the area of cardiac diagnostic studies. The MRI is a technique using radio frequencies to produce a variation in the normal magnetic field of the body. As these radio frequencies are emitted, they are picked up and fed into a computer that reconstructs the image and can differentiate between healthy and ischemic tissue (Braunwald et al., 1988; Epstein et al., 1982; Kinney et al., 1991; Swan, 1975).

Diagnostic Measures. This term encompasses serum electrolyte studies and cardiac enzymes. As there are a number of competent manuals available on reading and interpretation of laboratory values, this section will present a brief overview of the more important blood studies.

SERUM ELECTROLYTES (TABLE 8–2)
Potassium: Normal levels 3.5 to 5.0 mEq/L

- Hypokalemia (low potassium) is probably the most common electrolyte abnormality and can be associated with vomiting, diarrhea, prolonged digitalis and diuretic therapy, prolonged nasogastric suctioning, alkalosis, and excessive steroid administration. This may be detected by the presence of a U wave on the ECG. A U wave follows the T wave, which may be flattened, and precedes the P wave. Untreated hypokalemia can result in PVCs, ventricular tachycardia, ventricular fibrillation, and death.
- Hyperkalemia (high potassium) is often caused by overtreating hypokalemia. Other causes can include Addison's disease, acute renal failure, acidosis, and traumatic injuries, and can be detected by tall, peaked T waves. Untreated hyperkalemia can result in a widening of the QRS until ventricular fibrillation or sudden death occurs.

Calcium: Normal levels 9 to 11 mg/dl

- Hypocalcemia can occur in patients with renal failure, hypoparathyroidism, and malabsorption syndromes. Hypocalcemia can be detected by the occurrence of tetany, which begins with tingling and numbness of the mouth and extremities and progresses to muscle spasms and seizures. Two measures to identify a decreased serum calcium level are: Chvostek's sign—tapping the facial nerve below the temple anterior to the ear produces facial spasm; and Trousseau's sign—inflating the BP cuff approximately 20 mm Hg > systole causes flexion and inward rotation of the hand and wrist (McCance and Huether, 1990). The QT interval can become lengthened and the T wave may become inverted.
- Hypercalcemia can be seen in patients with hyperparathyroidism, neoplastic processes, and osteoporosis. Hypercalcemia may be detected by the presence of muscle weakness, irritability, and generalized peripheral neuropathy. The QT interval will become shortened and U waves may be present or accentuated.

Sodium: Normal levels 135 to 145 mEq/L

- Sodium concentration depends on the body's state of fluid balance as governed by release of ADH (antidiuretic hormone) and water intake. Sodium has implications for the sodium-potassium exchange in the polarization of the heart muscle (see Chap. 3) and the peripheral edema found in congestive heart failure. Generally, for sodium changes to be visualized on an ECG, the serum levels are incompatible with life, and therefore are rarely seen (Thibodeau, 1990; West, 1991).

Table 8–2. RELATION OF ELECTROLYTE ABNORMALITIES TO ECG CHANGES

Electrolyte Abnormality	Results
Hypokalemia	Increased ectopic activity Prominent U wave with prolonged T wave, ventricular tachycardia
Hyperkalemia	Increased block in the conduction system
Hypocalcemia	Prolonged QT interval, ventricular tachycardia
Hypercalcemia	Shortened QT interval

From Shoemaker, W. C.: *Textbook of Critical Care*. 2nd ed. Philadelphia, W. B. Saunders, 1989.

SERUM ENZYMES. Enzymes are proteins that are produced by all living cells and released into the blood stream. Injured or diseased cells increase the release of the particular enzyme into the serum. Because each cell in an organ produces a different enzyme, the identification of the particular enzyme and its elevation can suggest where in the body the damage has occurred and how extensive that damage may be. The three major cardiac enzymes are creatine phosphokinase (CPK, also known as creatine kinase, CK), lactic dehydrogenase (LDH), and serum glutamic oxaloacetic transaminase (SGOT).

1. CPK (or CK) is the fastest rising and fastest falling of the cardiac enzymes. Onset is 4 to 6 hours after infarction with a peak of 5 to 12 times normal values within 12 to 20 hours. Serum levels will usually return to normal within 2 to 3 days. The CPK enzyme is second only to the LDH isoenzyme for being specific for cardiac damage. The isoenzyme of CPK-MB is reported to be 100% specific (6 to 10% of the total CPK value) for myocardial infarction (MI) or other heart muscle damage, and peaks in 12 to 24 hours.

2. LDH is another enzyme released after a MI. Abnormally high levels are seen in the serum 12 to 24 hours after the MI. A peak is reached in 48 to 72 hours and returns to normal in 7 to 10 days. Since LDH is present throughout the body in the heart, kidney, skeletal muscles, lung, liver, and red blood cells, five LDH isoenzymes have been identified. LDH_1 is the isoenzyme present in the cardiac muscle and is the isoenzyme of consequence when determining cardiac damage.

3. SGOT is the third cardiac enzyme that becomes elevated with myocardial damage. Its levels begin to rise in 6 to 8 hours, peaks in 18 to 36 hours, and returns to normal within 4 to 6 days. SGOT is present in many tissues of the body such as the liver, skeletal muscles, renal tissue, red blood cells, the brain, pancreas, and lung tissue. Because it is fairly prevalent throughout the body and there is no identifiable isoenzyme specific to cardiac damage, this test tends to be not as specific and not as highly significant as the other two serum enzyme studies (Braunwald et al., 1988; Guzzetta and Dossey, 1984; Hudak et al., 1986; Price and Wilson, 1986).

NURSING DIAGNOSIS

Since coronary artery disease (CAD) is a very broad diagnostic area, several nursing diagnostic categories may apply. It is with the complications of CAD, e.g., angina, myocardial infarction, and congestive heart failure, that the diagnostic categories will be more specific. Nursing diagnosis of patients with coronary artery disease include:

1. Pain related to decreased coronary artery tissue perfusion
2. Fear related to treatments and invasive procedures used for diagnostic testing
3. Knowledge deficit related to understanding of anatomy and pathophysiology of the heart and its functions
4. Health-seeking behaviors related to desire for information to decrease or alter ongoing disease process
5. Role performance, altered, potential, related to possible change in physical activity secondary to illness (McFarland and McFarland, 1989; Thelan et al., 1990).

INTERVENTIONS

Nursing Interventions

Nursing interventions are client centered and developed around three areas: health assessment, patient education, and the nursing process. The format and necessity of a complete health assessment have been covered in detail earlier in this chapter. It is important to emphasize the utilization of the psychosocial and family support assessment as well as the patient's history and physical examination findings. Education of and information sharing with the patient, the family, and/or support group must begin upon entry into the health care system. If a patient enters the health care system through admission to a critical care unit, there may be a sense of fear, frustration, anger, and loss of control for the patient and members of the family or support system. Informing the patient and family of what is happening physiologically to the patient, the need and method of procedures and tests and equipment used, medication and dietary orders, and modification of risk factors will help alleviate some of the tension and fear that is normal for this situation. Again, communication and uncomplicated explanations are the key elements to patient and family education.

To tie the two elements of health assessment and education together, the astute nurse may use the nursing process as a means of organizing and facilitating patient care. Assessment must be ongoing and ever observant to changes; the plan of care must be organized but flexible to change as the status of the patient changes; implementation of care must be accurate and yet encompass change according to the evolving assessment; and evaluation of care and interventions should lend to constant updating and mobilizing care to facilitate the patient's recovery and rehabilitation.

Medical Interventions

Medical interventions or management for the patient with CAD should also encompass risk factor modification through patient education, related dietary management, assistance with cessation of smoking, and interpretation of diagnostic studies. Pharmacological agents such as antilipid agents may also be ordered:

1. To restrict lipoprotein production; e.g., nicotinic acid (niacin) or clofibrate (Atromid-S)
2. To increase lipoprotein removal; e.g., cholestyramine, colestipol
3. To control cholesterol production; e.g., lovastatin (Mevacor).

Antiplatelet agents are used to inhibit platelet adhesion, to prevent problems with CAD, and for long-term therapy for angina, transient ischemic attacks (TIAs), and valve replacement. Examples of these are dipyridamole (Persantine) and aspirin. If more than one antilipid agent is ordered, they should never be given together, but separately and the patient monitored for adverse reactions (Underhill et al., 1990).

OUTCOMES

Expected outcomes are that the patient will

1. Verbalize the absence or relief of pain
2. Actively participate in health behaviors prescribed or desired (such as those behaviors required in preparation for diagnostic tests, surgery, or physical examination, or those behaviors related to recovery from illness and prevention of recurrence or complications)
3. Experience less anxiety, related to fear of the unknown, fear of loss of control, role performance, misconceptions, or previously given misinformation
4. Describe disease process, causes, and factors contributing to symptoms and the procedures for disease or symptom control (Carpenito, 1989; Holloway, 1989; Moorhouse et al., 1987).

■ Angina

Angina is chest pain or discomfort due to myocardial ischemia that results from an imbalance between myocardial oxygen supply and demand.

PATHOPHYSIOLOGY

Angina (from Latin meaning "squeezing") is the chest pain associated with myocardial ischemia, is transient in nature, and does not cause cell death, but it may be a precursor to cell death from myocardial infarction. The neural pain receptors are stimulated by accelerated metabolism, chemical changes and imbalances, and/or local mechanical stress resulting from abnormal myocardial contractions. There is a decrease of oxygen circulating to the myocardial cells, causing ischemia to the tissue, and resulting in pain.

Myocardial oxygen requirements are dictated by myocardial contraction. The factors that influence myocardial oxygen demand include heart rate, the force of cardiac contraction, and myocardial wall tension (determined by afterload, preload, and wall thickness). An increase in any of these factors will increase myocardial oxygen demand. A heart at rest will use only a fraction of the oxygen that an active or stressed heart will demand. Thus, an essential intervention to teach patients with anginal pain is to stop their activity and rest at the onset of pain (Enger and Schwertz, 1989; Greenspon and Goldberg, 1983).

ASSESSMENT

Patient Assessment

Assessment of the patient with actual or suspected angina involves continual observation of the patient, with monitoring of signs, symptoms, and diagnostic findings. The patient must be monitored for the type and degree of pain: chest pain or pressure; mild to severe aching of the chest, left arm, or left shoulder; a sharp tingling, burning sensation in the jaw or epigastric and substernal regions; a squeezing feeling in the chest; and "heartburn" lasting from 1 to 5 minutes.

The precipitating factors that can be identified as bringing on an episode of anginal pain include physical or emotional stress (including exercise), exposure to temperature extremes (particularly cold, or going suddenly from hot to cold), and ingestion of a heavy meal, particularly one rich in LDL and cholesterol. It is important to know what factors alleviate the anginal pain, including cessation of activity or exercise, and taking nitroglycerine (NTG) sublingual tablets (Enger and Schwertz, 1989).

Patient assessment also involves an ongoing observation and evaluation of the patient as he/she progresses through the diagnostic process as well as a complete history and physical and psychosocial examinations. Some specific consideration are as follows.

Etiology and precipitating factors

1. CAD
2. Coronary artery spasm
3. Activity or stress
4. Hypertension
5. Anemia
6. Dysrhythmia
7. Congestive heart failure (CHF)

Signs and Symptoms

1. Pain is usually substernal, lower sternal or retrosternal. It may radiate to the jaw, left shoulder, or left arm.
2. Pain can be described as burning, squeezing, heaviness, or smothering.
3. Usually last 1 to 4 minutes.

4. Classic placing of clenched fist against chest (sternum) may be seen or may be absent if confused with indigestion.

5. Pain usually begins with exertion and subsides with rest.

Types of Angina. There are three types of angina: stable, unstable, and Prinzmetal's. Stable angina occurs over several months with no changes in symptoms, severity, or frequency, and is controlled each time by NTG or rest. Unstable, or "crescendo," angina shows a definite change in quality, severity, frequency, and duration, usually occurring over a 3-month period. The pain may precipitate at rest and can last as long as 20 minutes. Two NTG tablets will not be sufficient to relieve the pain. During an unstable attack the ECG may show ST segment depression. The patient has an increased risk for MI within 18 months. Prinzmetal's (variant) angina usually occurs at rest and without other precipitating factors because it is a coronary artery spasm. The ECG will show a marked ST segment elevation (usually seen only in an MI) during the episode. Myocardial infarction can occur as a result of prolonged coronary artery spasm even when the arteries are normal (Enger and Schwertz, 1989; Guzzetta and Dossey, 1984).

Diagnostic studies for angina will include history and physical, looking specifically for patterns of pain and precipitating risk factors; laboratory data, including blood studies for anemia (H&H), cardiac enzymes (CPK-MB, SGOT), and cholesterol and triglyceride levels; ECG studies during resting periods, precipitating events (exercise), and anginal pain episodes; exercise tolerance test (ETT) or stress testing; thallium 201 scan; and coronary angiography.

Complications from untreated or unstable angina may include MI, CHF, dysrhythmia, and psychological depression (Bates and Hockelman, 1983; Holloway, 1989; Hudak et al., 1986).

NURSING DIAGNOSIS

Nursing diagnosis and intervention for patients with angina include the following.

Alteration in Comfort: Pain Related to Myocardial Ischemia

1. Maintain rest during episodes of pain.
2. Record description of pain and activity prior to onset of pain.
3. Administer nitroglycerin (NTG); up to three NTG sublingually, one every 5 minutes.
4. Administer O_2 as ordered.
5. Maintain diet (soft, low-sodium, low-fat and, cholesterol); if chest pain occurs while eating, encourage several small meals a day rather than three larger ones.

Anxiety: Related to Knowledge Deficit Regarding Disease Process. Provide patient and family education through

1. Discussion of nature of angina, etiology, risk factors, and importance of modifying those risk factors.
2. Discussion of possible denial of critical episode by patient or family, and assist in support and counseling.
3. Discussion of nature and characteristics of chest pain, and assist in identifying precipitating factors.
4. Discussion of activity level: Avoid isometric-type exercise; avoid heavy lifting and pushing; exercise regularly; encourage regular home exercise program.
5. Remind patients to avoid sexual activity when fatigued. If chest pain does occur during sex, stop and take nitrates (NTG) as ordered, usually up to three NTG tablets, one every 5 minutes. If chest pain is unrelieved, call emergency medical service (EMS), and do not attempt to drive oneself to the emergency room (ER).
6. Self-management during episodes of pain: Stop the activity and rest, take nitrates as ordered, 3 NTG tablets, one every 5 minutes; if pain persists, call EMS.
7. Diet as ordered; avoid caffeine.
8. Explain importance of controlling any related diseases or problems that may aggravate atherosclerosis; i.e., hypertension, diabetes, and hyperlipidemia.
9. Explain importance of controlling weight and avoiding obesity.
10. Explain role of stress in aggravating heart disease and identify individual stress-producing factors and methods of stress management, including relaxation techniques.
11. Discuss medications; name, dosage (amount and times), purpose, and side effects.

Other related nursing diagnoses

1. Sleep pattern disturbances related to present status and unknown future
2. Potential constipation related to bed rest, change in lifestyle, and medications
3. Activity intolerance related to fear of recurrent angina

4. Potential self-concept disturbance related to perceived or actual role changes

5. Possible impaired home maintenance management related to angina or fear of angina

6. Potential altered family processes related to impaired ability of person to assume role responsibilities

7. Potential sexual dysfunction related to fear of angina and altered self-concept

Nursing interventions may include:

1. Oxygen; 2–10 l/min on a Venturi mask depending on the patient's history for COPD

2. Rest; the patient is instructed to cease all activity until pain subsides

3. Vital signs monitored (including apical pulse) every 4 to 6 hours; more frequently during pain and SOB episodes

4. A diet low in saturated fat, low in cholesterol, and low in sodium content will be ordered (Carpenito, 1989; Govoni and Hayes, 1985; Holloway, 1989).

MEDICAL INTERVENTIONS

Medical interventions and management of the patient experiencing angina should also include:

Vasodilators are used to relax smooth muscles in arteries, arterioles, and/or veins because this causes relief of pain and lowering of blood pressure. Examples are nitroglycerine (NTG; sublingual, intravenous, transdermal, spray, or ointment), isorbide (Isordil), pentaerythritol (Peritrate), and erythrityl (Cardilate). Side effects of these vasodilators include headaches, flushing, dizziness, and orthostatic hypotension. The patient should be instructed to take NTG prior to activity; replace the NTG every 3 months; be cautious of NTG patches near microwave ovens (leaking waves may cause an explosion of the patch!). If an acute attack of angina occurs, tell the patient to take up to three tablets NTG sublingual, one every 5 minutes—if there is no relief, seek medical attention immediately (EMS or ER).

Beta-adrenergic blocking agents may also be used to treat angina. They block catecholamine–induced sympathetic effects, and reduce BP by decreasing CO, and decreasing renin secretion. Examples include propranolol (Inderal); nadolol (Corgard); timolol (Blocadren); atenol (Tenormin). The side effects of these agents include bradycardia, AV blocks, asthma attacks, depression, hypotension, memory loss, and they may mask hypoglycemia attacks. Teach the patient to take these agents as prescribed, not to abruptly stop taking them, and to monitor heart rate and BP at regular intervals while on them.

Calcium channel blockers alter the electrochemical properties of myocardial cells, block the movement of calcium, resulting in decreased myocardial oxygen demand and decreased afterload. They are used in tachyarrhythmias, vasospasms, CHF, and hypertension as well as to treat angina. Examples include verapamil (Calan, Isoptin); nifedipine (Procardia); diltiazem (Cardizem). The side effects of calcium channel blockers include dizziness, flushing, headaches, decreased heart rate, hypotension. Teach the patient to monitor BP for hypotension, especially if taken in combination with nitrates and beta-blockers (Hurst and Logue, 1990; Kinney et al., 1991; Underhill et al., 1990).

OUTCOMES

The outcomes for the patient with angina are:

1. The patient will verbalize the absence of chest discomfort.

2. The patient will actively participate in health behaviors prescribed.

3. The patient will experience less anxiety related to fear of the unknown, fear of loss of control, misconceptions, or previously given misinformation.

4. The patient will describe the disease process, causes, and factors contributing to symptoms, and the procedure for symptom control through rest, medication, progressive activity, diet, stress control, and controlling related physiological problems (Carpenito, 1989; Johanson et al., 1988).

■ Myocardial Infarction

A myocardial infarction (MI) is ischemia and death of the myocardium due to lack of blood supply from the occlusion of a coronary artery and its branches. Twenty-five percent of all deaths in the United States are due to MIs (approximately 1.5 million). Despite emergency services and the use of advanced technology to treat these patients, there is still a 30 to 40% mortality rate, with over half dying before reaching an acute care facility. Most deaths related to MIs occur during the first hour (American Heart Association, 1989); therefore, it is imperative that the person having a MI be accurately and quickly diagnosed and transported to a hospital for immediate treatment and care.

PATHOPHYSIOLOGY

An acute MI is caused by an imbalance between myocardial oxygen supply and demand. This imbalance is the result of decreased coronary artery perfusion, which is usually due to artherosclerosis, coronary artery vasospasm, coronary artery thrombus, dysrhythmias, or a combination of any of these factors. Atherosclerotic coronary artery disease is the most common cause of the acute myocardial infarction (AMI). Reduced blood flow to an area of the myocardium causes significant and sustained oxygen deprivation to myocardial cells. Normal functioning is disrupted as ischemia and injury lead to eventual cellular death. Myocardial dysfunction occurs as more cells are involved.

Prolonged ischemia lasting 30 to 45 minutes causes irreversible cellular damage and muscle death (necrosis) (Fig. 8–9). Permanent cessation of contractile function occurs in the necrotic or infarcted area of the myocardium. The infarct is surrounded by a zone of ischemic, potentially viable tissue. The ultimate size of the infarct depends upon the fate of this ischemic zone. If unsuccessfully treated, this margin will increase as tissue death occurs. If successfully treated, the residual necrosis can be minimized (see Fig. 8–9). There are two types of MIs: transmural, which involves the entire thickness of the heart muscle; and subendocardial, which involves a partial thickness of inner half of the myocardial muscle thickness. The severity of the MI will be determined by the success or lack of success of the treatment, as stated above, and the degree of collateral circulation that is present at that particular part of the heart muscle. Collateral circulation is the alternative routes or channels that can develop in the myocardium in response to chronic ischemia or regional hypoperfusion. Through this small, tiny network of "extra" vessels, blood flow can be improved to the threatened myocardium (Braunwald et al., 1988; Hurst and Logue, 1990; Price and Wilson, 1986).

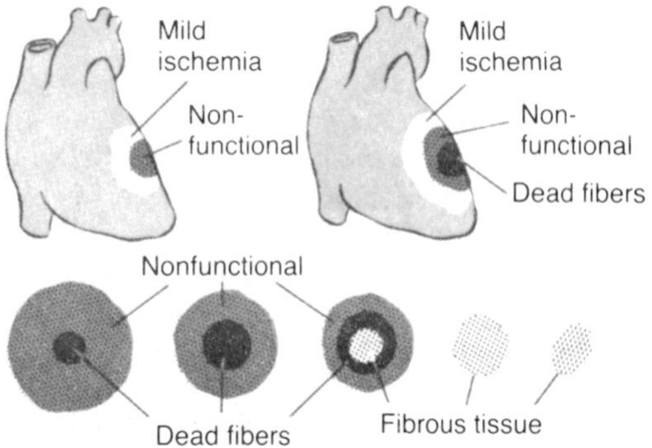

Figure 8–9. *Top*: Small and large areas of coronary ischemia. *Bottom*: Stages of recovery from myocardial infarction. (From Guyton, A. C.: *Textbook of Medical Physiology*. 7th ed. Philadelphia, W. B. Saunders, 1986.)

ASSESSMENT

Patient Assessment

Patient assessment includes close observation to identify classic signs and symptoms of an AMI. Chest pain is the paramount sign and symptom. It may be severe, crushing, tightness, squeezing, or simply a feeling of pressure. It can be precordial, substernal, or in the back; radiating to arms, neck or jaw; and/or unrelated to exertion and respirations. It will not cease with rest or nitrates, and thus can be distinguished from the pain of an angina attack. Chest pain does not always occur, but when it does, it is usually associated with the lumen of the involved coronary artery being 75% or more occluded (Von Rueden, 1989). The longer the duration and the more severe the pain, the greater the likelihood that an MI is occurring.

The skin may be cool, clammy, pale, and diaphoretic; color may be dusky or ashen; there may also be slight hyperthermia. The patient may be short of breath, dyspenic, and tachypenic (hyperventilating), may feel faint, or have intermittent loss of sensorium. There may be hypotension, often accompanied by dysrhythmias, particularly ventricular ectopy, bradycardia, or tachycardia, and heart blocks of varying degrees. The type of dysrhythmia will depend on the area of the MI. The patient may be anxious, restless, or exhibit certain behavior responses, including denial, depression, sense of "impending doom." Nausea and vomiting are other common features.

Note: Silent MIs can occur with no presenting signs or symptoms (Bates and Hockelman, 1983; Guzzetta and Dossey, 1984).

The types of MIs can be determined by the particular coronary artery involved and the blood supply to that area (Table 8–3).

Assessment of a MI patient takes all of the above signs and symptoms into account when doing a history and physical. Risk factors for a MI (CAD, coronary spasm, and embolism) are also considered when determining a diagnosis. Other areas of assessment imperative for accurate diagnosis include:

Table 8–3. MYOCARDIAL INFARCTION BY SITE, ECG CHANGES, AND COMPLICATIONS

Location of MI	Primary Site of Occlusion	Primary ECG Changes	Complications
Inferior MI Note: accounts for 40 to 50% of AMI; may also have RV infarct; AV block—Wenckebach or complete	RCA (80–90%) L Circumflex (10–20%)	Leads: II, III, aVF	First- and second- degree heart block
Inferolateral MI	L Circumflex	II, III, aVF, V_5, V_6	Third-degree heart block, left CHF, cardiomyopathy, left ventricular rupture
Posterior MI	RCA or L Circumflex	No lead truly looks at posterior surface; therefore, look at referred changes in anterior leads of V_1 and V_2; note tall, broad R waves, ST depression, and tall T waves.	First, second- and third-degree heart blocks, CHF, bradyarrhythmias
Right Ventricular Infarct	RCA	$V_4 - V_6$	Increased CVP, decreased cardiac output, bradyarrhythmia, heart blocks, hypertension, cardiogenic shock
Anterior MI	LAD	$V_2 - V_4$	Third-degree heart block, left CHF, left bundle branch block
Anterior-Septal MI	LAD	$V_1 - V_3$	Second- and third-degree heart block
Anterior-Lateral and Lateral	LAD or L Circumflex	V_5, V_6, aVL, I	CHF, cardiomyopathy

Medical Assessment

ECG Changes

- Ischemia—T wave inversion
- Injury—ST segment elevation
- Infarct—pathological or well-defined and deep Q wave

Cardiac Enzymes

	Onset	*Peak*	*Return to Normal*
CPK	4–6 hr	12–20 hr	2–3 days
SGOT	6–8 hr	18–36 hr	4–6 days
LDH	12–24 hr	48–72 hr	7–10 days

Isoenzymes specific for cardiac damage: CPK-MB and LDH_1 (see CAD section of this chapter).

Diagnostic Studies

1. Almost all MI patients eventually undergo coronary angiography to visualize the coronary anatomy to determine if other areas of myocardium are in jeopardy, and ventriculography to determine the function of the myocardium (Ochsner, 1989). Indications for coronary angiography and its timing after an AMI change as experience evolves and have set different criteria for three separate phases: evolving MI, completed MI, and convalescent MI (Subcommittee on Coronary Angiography, 1987).

2. Multiple-gated acquisition (MUGA) scan. The procedure utilizes radioisotope tagging of RBCs with technetium (^{99m}Tc) and images of cardiac volumes are collected during the cardiac cycle. The purpose of a MUGA scan is to collect information about the ejection fraction (EF) and left ventricular (LV) wall motion. Ejection fraction is a measurement of left ventricular systolic pump performance. The normal EF is $>65\%$; EF $<50\%$ indicates ventricular dysfunction.

3. Myocardial infarct scan also uses technetium to detect the infarcted area by showing increased radioactivity as a "hot spot" on a scan. The purpose is to detect areas of infarct when no ECG or cardiac enzyme changes have occurred.

4. Myocardial perfusion imaging is a radioisotope study using thallium 201. Ischemic areas will show decreased radioactivity or "cold spot." This is sometimes used in conjunction with exercise tolerance testing (ETT) to initiate the ischemic process. It is used to detect areas of infarct when there are no ECG changes or normal enzymes.

5. Other diagnostic studies include the PET (positron emission tomography) scan and electrophysiological studies. The electrophysiological

studies are invasive procedures that involves the introduction of an electrode catheter percutaneously from the femoral vein through the inferior vena cava so the catheter tip is near the tricuspid valve. Graphic readings are taken to record bundle of His activities, including intra-atrial conduction, and conduction across the AV node (Rahimtoola et al., 1987).

NURSING DIAGNOSIS

Nursing diagnosis and intervention of the MI patient include the following.

Alteration in Comfort: Pain Related to Myocardial Ischemia or Necrosis. It is essential that pain be relieved.

1. Administer drug therapy as ordered and note response. Usually morphine sulfate (IV), NTG (IV), and O_2 are given.
2. Monitor BP, hemodynamics, and heart sounds as pain occurs.
3. Use nonpharmacological pain relief techniques and promote a relaxed, quiet, restful environment.
4. Maintain bed rest during episodes of pain, and allow the patient to assume a position of comfort.
5. Record the patient's description of the pain and determine aggravating factors, including breathing patterns.
6. Administer O_2 as needed to relieve pain.

Potential Alteration in Cardiac Output Related to Loss of Myocardial Contractility

1. Plan all activities to minimize oxygen demands.
2. Identify, report, and assist in the correction of signs and symptoms of decreased cardiac output.
3. Monitor BP, TPR, and apical pulse every 2 to 4 hours.
4. Monitor cardiac rhythm.
5. Administer O_2 as ordered.
6. Monitor breath sounds at least every 4 to 6 hours.
7. Monitor heart sounds at least every 4 to 6 hours.
8. Monitor ABGs, electrolytes, cardiac enzymes.
9. Monitor PAP, PCWP, CVP.
10. 12-Lead ECG.
11. Intake and output every 2 to 4 hours.
12. Monitor IV fluids.
13. Administer medications as ordered and monitor response.
14. Encourage appropriate diet—avoid ice.
15. Instruct patient to avoid activities that increase cardiac workload, such as Valsalva maneuver. Provide stool softeners or laxatives.

Anxiety Related to Perceived or Actual Threat of Loss of Biological Integrity

1. Use comfort measures, maintain quiet environment, and promote relaxation.
2. Facilitate contact with family members and significant others who will comfort and support the patient.
3. Use a calm voice and reassuring actions during care.
4. Explain procedures and tests to patient and family; orient to critical care area.
5. Administer sedative as needed to lessen anxiety.
6. Explain care and procedures.
7. Encourage expression of feelings.

Knowledge Deficit Regarding Disease Process

1. Begin patient and family teaching as soon as the patient is stable. Refer to a formal cardiac rehabilitation program when available.
2. Review explanation of heart condition: extent of infarct; associated complications—dysrhythmias, angina, CHF, pulmonary edema, cardiogenic shock, post-MI syndrome; nature of disease process—risk factors and precipitating factors.
3. Explain the importance of rest balanced with limits of exercise and activity as he/she progresses through the rehabilitation program.
4. Explain the importance of controlling existing conditions that aggravate recovery; e.g., hyperlipidemia, diabetes, hypertension.
5. Explain the importance of weight control.
6. Explain the importance of stress management.
7. Explain the importance of avoiding or modifying activity following heavy meals, alcohol consumption, emotional stress, and extreme temperatures.
8. Explain the importance of independence and responsibility of self-care.
9. Explain the importance of modifying activity during sexual intercourse including: approaching sex gradually, having sex when well rested, avoid sex when physically or emotionally stressed, avoid sex after heavy meal or alcohol

consumption, provide comfortable atmosphere, choose comfortable position, and recognize warning signs of heart strain (Boykoff, 1989).

10. Encourage the patient to communicate feelings and concerns with family or support group.

11. Discuss signs and symptoms of extending MI vs angina.

12. Explain the importance of seeking emergency care if chest pain is unrelieved with rest and nitroglycerin.

13. Explain the importance of diet—avoid caffeine, high-fat, high-cholesterol, high-sodium foods.

14. Explain the importance of avoiding tobacco.

15. Explain the importance of resting after meals.

16. Explain medications, including name, dosage (amount and time), purpose, and side effects.

17. Explain why over-the-counter (OTC) medications should be avoided until they are checked with a physician.

18. Explain why constipation and straining should be avoided.

19. Explain why physician should be consulted before resuming sex, travel, driving.

20. Explain why isometric-type exercises and heavy lifting and pushing should be avoided.

21. Explain monitoring daily activities; to space activities throughout the day to avoid fatigue (Carpenito, 1989; Holloway, 1989).

INTERVENTIONS

Nursing Management of Complications

Management of the patient with an acute MI centers around maintaining adequate myocardial oxygenation and decreasing myocardial workload, relieving pain and anxiety, managing dysrhythmias, and observing for and intervening promptly to prevent or minimize complications. Complications include congestive heart failure (CHF), which can lead to pulmonary edema (PE); cardiogenic shock (see Chap. 7); papillary muscle dysfunction (which is indicated by the development of a new murmur and must be treated with afterload reduction and emergency mitral valve replacement); ventricular aneurysm (an outward pouching of the ventricle and rupture); pulmonary embolism (from deep vein thrombosis).

Three additional complications of MI are pericarditis, endocarditis, and Dressler's syndrome.

Pericarditis. Inflammation of the pericardium may occur as a complication of MI in about 15% of affected patients. The patient usually presents with precardial pain, pericardial friction rub, dyspnea, weakness, fatigues, low-grade fever, and increased anxiety level. Precardial pain is usually sharp and stabbing in nature and is often aggravated by inspiration or coughing. Precardial pain must be distinguished from the pain of an acute MI.

Pericardial friction rubs are the most common method of diagnosing pericarditis. The friction rub is usually heard best on inspiration with the diaphragm of the stethoscope placed over the second, third, or fourth intercostal space at the sternal border. Friction rubs have been described as grating, scraping, squeaking, or scratching sounds. This rubbing sound results from an increase in fibrous exudate between the two irritated pericardial layers, causing increased friction as the heart beats within the pericardial sac. The pericardial friction rub may be the hallmark of a transmural MI, in which damage to the entire myocardial wall has occurred.

The treatment of patients with pericarditis involves relief of pain, usually through medication (antibiotics if the causative agent is bacterial in origin), corticosteroids for relief of inflammation process, and treatment of other systemic symptoms. In some extreme cases where relief is not obtained or the inflammation is of a lasting nature, a pericardiectomy may be indicated. Complications of untreated pericarditis include pericardial effusion, cardiac tamponade, chronic pericarditis, and constrictive pericarditis.

Endocarditis. Infective endocarditis, formerly termed bacterial endocarditis, is an infection of the endocardial tissue. It is caused by a variety of microbes, and frequently involves the heart valves. Bacteria of the genus *Streptococcus* are the organisms most commonly responsible for subacute infective endocarditis. Endocarditis can also be caused by staphylococci, gram-negative bacilli (such as *Escherichia coli* and Klebsiella), and fungi (such as *Candida* and *Histoplasma*).

The reason for developing endocarditis is poorly understood, but several notions appear to be consistent. The infecting agent is a highly virulent organism. Over 50% of the infections occur in individuals with valvular disease. Also, the particular species of bacteria involved develops properties that allow the organisms to adhere to the endothelial surface of the heart (Guzzetta and Dossey, 1984).

Infectious lesions or vegetations form on the

heart valves. These lesions have irregular edges and have been known to have a cauliflowerlike appearance. The mitral valve is the most common area to be affected, followed by the aortic valve. The vegetative process can grow to involve the chordae tendineae, papillary muscles, and conduction system. Therefore, the patient may develop dysrhythmias or die of heart failure.

Clinical manifestations of endocarditis can include fever, chills, cough, weight loss, fatigue, new murmur, congestive heart failure, pericardial friction rub, myocardial infarction, clubbing of the fingers, positive blood cultures, anemia, and ECG changes. The presenting symptoms will be determined by the valve involved, the organism present, and the length of time and extent of growth of the vegetative process. Treatment involves diagnosing the infective agent, treating with appropriate antibiotics or antifungal agents, and ultimately valve replacement surgery.

Dressler's syndrome (Post-Myocardial Infarction Syndrome). This is thought to be an autoimmune response to the AMI. On the third to fifth day of a post-transmural infarct, a pericardial rub may be heard in approximately 25% of patients. In about 2 to 5% of these patients, pericarditis with effusion develops 1 to 4 weeks postinfarct. It is usually treated symptomatically with aspirin, indomethacin (Indocin), and steroids; anticoagulants are usually discontinued. The patient must be observed for pulsus paradoxus as an early sign of cardiac tamponade (Kinney et al., 1991).

Medical Intervention

Medical intervention in MI is usually divided into two types of treatment: the medical approach and the surgical interventions.

Medical Approach

The medical approach to the treatment of MI generally includes oxygenation, rest, hemodynamic monitoring, and the use of pharmacological agents.

Oxygen is important to assist the myocardial tissue to continue its pumping activity and to repair the damaged tissue around the site of the infarct. Rest is imperative, and assistance with activities is required until the patient has stabilized. Then, progressive return to daily activity can begin in order to reduce the feelings of fear, anxiety, frustration, and loss of control. Hemodynamic monitoring is used to determine fluid balance and the overall functioning of the left ventricle (Braunwald et al., 1988; Hurst and Logue, 1990).

Pharmacological agents used in the treatment of MI can be divided into several groups.

Analgesics. These are used for pain; usually morphine IV or meperidine (Demerol) IV.

Nitroglycerin. Nitroglycerin IV is often used to decrease cardiac pain and limit complications (CHF) of an acute MI. It is usually given 5 to 10 μg/min in titrated doses every 5 to 10 minutes for a total of 100 to 200 μg/min until PCWP is below 20 mm Hg and/or the systolic blood pressure falls to below 90 to 100 mm Hg or side effects occur (Gunnar et al., 1988; Underhill et al., 1990).

Antiarrhythmics (Table 8-4)

Type IA. These are local anesthetics agents with anticholinergic effects; e.g., quinidine, disopyramide (Norpace), procainamide (Pronestyl), encainide, and flecainide

Type IB. These are local anesthetics without anticholinergic effects: e.g., phenytoin (Dilantin), lidocaine, (Xylocaine), aprindine, tocainide, and mexiletine.

- Side effects can vary but particular attention should be given to AV blocks, bradycardia, and hypotension.
- The most common antiarrhythmic agent used for acute and immediate post-MI is a lidocaine intravenous drip with a loading dose (bolus) of 1 to 2 mg/kg over 20 to 30 minutes followed by maintenance dose of 2 to 4 mg/min by IV drip.

Type II. These are cardiotonic medications, e.g., digoxin and other digitalis preparations (deslanoside [Cedilanid], digitoxin).

Type III. These are antiadrenergic drugs such as beta-adrenergic blockers; e.g., propranolol (Inderol).

Type IV. These are calcium channel blockers; e.g., nifedipine (Procardia) and diltiazem (Cardizem) (Govoni and Hayes, 1985).

Thrombolytic Therapy. Other medical interventions are also employed during the treatment phase of the acute MI. One fairly common therapy is thrombolytic therapy using streptokinase (SK), urokinase, or tissue plasminogen activator (t-PA). Research has shown that occlusion of the coronary vessel does not cause immediate myocardial cell death. Irreversible injury begins within 20 minutes of the vessel occluding. During a period of 5 to 6 hours the irreversible damage begins at the endocardial surface and progresses

Table 8–4. THE USE AND EFFECTS OF VARIOUS ANTIARRHYTHMIC AGENTS

Agent	Administration	Metabolized + Excretion	Side-Effects	Recommended Therapeutic Serum Level (*Trough*)
Quinidine	per 200–300 mg every 6 hours: same dosage (used rarely)	Liver–greatest Renal decrease in alkaline urine	Nausea, vomiting, diarrhea, cinchonism, thrombocytopenia, hypotension, ventricular tachycardia	2–6 mg/ml
Procainamide	hr 100 mg q3 min/lupus, up to 1 g; then infusion of 2 mg po: 3–6 g/day every 3–5 h	50% Liver 50% Renal	Positive ANA with lupus-like syndrome, fever, gastrointestinal distress, agranulocytosis, hypotension, psychosis, hallucinations	3–8 mg/ml
Disopyramide	per 150 mg q6 h	Kidney Liver	Hypotension, heart failure, vomiting, dry mouth, urinary hesitancy, constipation, blurred vision, hypoglycemia	2–3 mg/ml
Lidocaine	IV: loading dose 1–2 mg/kg; then infusion of 1–5 mg/min IM: 3–4 mg/kg	Liver	Tremor, agitation, disorientation, seizures, respiratory arrest, A-V block with conduction diseases	2-6 mg/ml
Phenytoin	IV: 100 mg q5 min, up to 700 mg po: 200 mg bid after loading dose	Liver	Nystagmus, dizziness, ataxia, gastrointestinal distress, skin rash, megaloblastic anemia, hyperglycemia	10–20 mg/ml
Propranolol	IV: 1 mg q3–5 min, up to 10 mg po: 10–120 mg q4–6h	Liver	Heart failure, hypotension, bradycardia, insomnia, bronchospasm, nausea, vomiting, lethargy, dizziness, nightmares, diarrhea	
Bretylium	IV: 5–10 mg/kg over 10–20 min; can repeat at 15–30 min intervals (not more than 30 mg/kg) Give q6–8h or 2 mg/min infusion	70%–80% unchanged in urine	Hypotension, nausea, vomiting, enlargement of parotid glands	
Verapamil	IV: 5–10 mg May repeat in 30 min po: 60–120 mg q6h	Liver	Headache, nausea, vomiting, hypotension, heart failure, bradycardia, A-V block	
Tocainide	po: 400–600 mg q8h	Urine—40% Unchanged	Similar to lidocaine, pulmonary fibrosis, worsening of arrhythmias, visual distrubances, nausea, vomiting, anorexia	4–10 μg/ml
Flecainide	po: 100–200 mg q12h	Urine–86%	Dizziness, visual disturbances, dyspnea, nausea, constipation, exacerbation of heart failures and arrhythmias, conduction disturbances, tremor	0.2–1.0 μg/ml
Amiodarone	po: 200–300 mg q24h	Liver	Pulmonary fibrosis, conduction disturbances, liver injury, exacerbation of arrhythmias, corneal deposits, photosensitivity, thyroid abnormalities, neurologic problems, nausea, vomiting, constipation, bradycardia	1–2.3 mg/l

From Shoemaker, W. C.: *Textbook of Critical Care.* 2nd ed. Philadelphia: W. B. Saunders, 1989.

to the epicardium. The extent and progression of the injury is determined by the completeness of the occlusion and the presence of collateral circulation (Niemyski and Hellstedt, 1989). The goals are to dissolve the lesion that is occluding the coronary artery and to increase blood flow to the myocardium. The patient must have been symptomatic for no more than 3 to 6 hours, had angina for 20 minutes unrelieved by NTG, and an ECG with an ST segment of 3 mm or greater.

Streptokinase. This is a synthetic protein derived from group C beta-hemolytic streptococci that lysis clots by acting on plasminogen. Therefore, SK may cause allergic reactions, especially in patients who have had streptococcal infections and retain high levels of antibodies. The most common reactions are fever and drug rash (Brewer-Senerchia, 1989). The Gruppo Italiano per lo Studio della Streptochinaes nel' Infarto Miocardio, or GISSI trial, was carried out in the mid 1980s at 176 hospitals in Italy. The 11,712 patients were randomly assigned to receive 1.5 million units of IV streptokinase or standard care. The GISSI trial provided evidence that treating the MI patient with SK can significantly decrease mortality, especially when administered within 3 hours of onset of symptoms. The trial also demonstrated that significant bleeding complications were not common (Brewer-Senerchia, 1989). Since SK is derived from streptococci, it is a foreign protein in the body. Once SK has been given, antibodies may form within 5 days and remain for 6 months, resulting in resistance or reaction to a subsequent dose (Niemyski and Hellstedt, 1989).

The patient undergoes coronary arteriography. Streptokinase can be infused into the coronary arteries with a bolus of 25,000 to 50,000 U followed by a 2000 to 4000 U/min infusion; it can also be given 1.5 million units over 45 to 60 minutes IV. The artery usually reopens in 30 to 40 minutes. As reperfusion occurs, dysrhythmias are common, and are an indication of effectiveness. Reocclusion of the coronary artery and the resulting pain are indicators for a PTCA or an emergency coronary artery bypass graft (CABG).

Urokinase. This is a naturally occurring human proteolytic enzyme derived from cultured kidney cells. Unlike streptokinase, urokinase does not need to combine with plasminogen to become activated. It acts directly by converting plasminogen to plasmin. Similarly to SK, urokinase does not react with fibrin or fibrin-bound plasminogen, but causes a widespread systemic lytic effect by converting plasminogen to plasmin. The usual dose is 2 to 3 million units given IV bolus over 30 minutes, or intracoronary infusion of 4000 to 8000 U/min as a maintenance dose. The success of urokinase has been reported at rates of 60 to 89% (Kleven, 1988).

Tissue Plasminogen Activator. Another medical treatment for the MI patient is tissue plasminogen activator (Alteplase), which is a serum protease that affects the lysis of a clot more directly than SK. It was developed from human DNA and is currently manufactured using animal tissue culture. Since t-PA is a human protein, there are no expected allergic reactions to the medication and, if necessary, retreatment is possible. Once t-PA binds to fibrin, it can convert clot-bound plasminogen to clot-bound plasmin, producing a clot-specific state rather than a systemic lytic state. Intravenous t-PA is given 100 mg total with 60 mg given over the first hour and 20 mg per hour for the next 2 hours (Brewer-Senerchia, 1989; Kleven, 1988).

Two separate research trials (the TIMI 1 trial and the European Cooperative SK, t-PA trial) demonstrated the superior thrombolytic effect of t-PA. Similar bleeding events were observed with both medications. The TIMI 1 trial (214 patients) reported an efficacy rate of 60% of those assigned to the t-PA group vs 37% of those assigned to the SK group (Chesebro et al., 1987). The European trial (64 patients) reported a patency rate of 70% with t-PA after 90 minutes compared to 55% with SK (Verstraete et al., 1985). Both research trials reviewed the outcomes of PTCA following tPA and concluded that there was no real benefit for the patient and its use carried risk of reocclusion (29%), ventricular fibrillation, severe bradycardia, and hypotension (Califf et al., 1988).

At the present time, t-PA costs about $2300, whereas SK costs about $100 per standard dose (Vogel, 1991). It is advantageous to use because it can be repeated if the first attempt fails, and SK cannot be repeated for at least 6 months (Andrien and Lemberg, 1990). Streptokinase is advantageous because it has been associated with significantly lower rates of intracranial hemorrhage than t-PA (Brooks-Brunn, 1988).

Several thrombolytic agents are currently being researched for possible treatment of acute MI. One is anisoylated plasminogen–streptokinase activator complex (ASPAC, Eminase), and is referred to as a second-generation streptokinase. Another experimental agent is single-chain urokinase plasminogen activator (scu-PA), and is referred to as prourokinase (Kleven, 1988). The patient must have experienced chest pain for less than 6 hours, have an ST segment elevation, and have had no relief of chest pain from NTG.

Thrombolytic therapy is absolutely contraindicated in patients with active internal bleeding, a history of CVA, recent intracranial/intraspinal surgery or trauma, intracranial neoplasm, AV malformation, aneurysm, or severe or uncontrolled hypertension (Niemyski and Hellstedt, 1989).

Nursing care of the patient first and foremost must include a complete initial assessment for potential bleeding risks and constant reevaluation to monitor for bleeding complications once therapy has begun. The second consideration must be patient and family education of the potential risk for bleeding postprocedure and the urgency with which any bleeding within the first 24 hours, regardless of how minor, must be reported. A third concern is the reperfusion phenomenon, which includes relief of pain, arrhythmias, physiological changes, ECG evolution, and CK release. Patients with RCA occlusion frequently experience sinus bradycardia, cardiac arrest or AV blocks during reperfusion. Those with LAD occlusions may experience ventricular arrhythmias; and those with transmural ischemia will show a resolution of the ST elevations. After successful thrombolysis, the CK will rise rapidly, peaking in 13 hours or less (Brewer-Senerchia, 1989).

The patient must be constantly monitored for signs and symptoms of reocclusion evidenced by renewal of chest pain, ECG changes, or additional CK release. The physician may have to evaluate the patient for retreatment with t-PA, or for percutaneous transluminal coronary angioplasty (PTCA) and coronary revascularization by coronary artery bypass and graft (CABG).

Anticoagulant therapy is also used in patients presenting with a MI and in coordination with thrombolysis. Heparin is usually the drug of choice for treatment in the acute phase, whereas aspirin may be prescribed for long-term, at-home therapy. Heparin can be administered 5000 U subcutaneously every 12 hours, by IV as a bolus of 5000 to 10,000 U every 4 to 6 hours, or as a continuous infusion of 20,000 to 40,000 U/day after a loading dose of 5000 U. The antiplatelet effects of aspirin prevent reinfarction, and is usually recommended for all MI patients whether or not they are receiving thrombolytic therapy (Peterson and Emmot, 1989).

Surgical Interventions

Surgical interventions for patients with MI resulting from CAD include PTCA and coronary revascularization by CABG.

Percutaneous Transluminal Coronary Angiography (PTCA). Even though a PTCA is not a "true" surgical procedure, and is usually done in the cardiac catheterization laboratory, the procedure is surgery-like in nature, the physical set-up is similar, and there is the seriousness of a true surgical procedure. The purpose of PTCA is to compress intracoronary lesions to increase blood flow to the myocardium. It is usually the treatment of choice for patients with uncompromised collateral flow, noncalcified lesions, lesions not present at bifurcations of vessels, and the patient must be a candidate for CABG surgery. The PTCA is done in the cardiac catheterization laboratory with the operating room on standby. A balloon catheter is inserted in the manner of doing coronary arteriography, but it is threaded into the occluded coronary artery and is advanced with the use of a guidewire across the lesion. The balloon is inflated under pressure one or several times to compress the lesion (Fig. 8–10). Complications from a PTCA are not dissimilar from those of a cardiac catheterization. They can include dissection of the coronary artery, coronary occlusion, MI, bleeding, decreased pulses distal to the procedure site, allergic reaction to the dye, and death (Canobbio, 1990; Tilkian, 1986).

Because PTCA is less invasive and less costly than CABG, its use has rapidly increased from 32,300 in 1983 to 200,000 in 1990 (Frankl, 1990a). There is an anticipated success rate of over 85% for the less complicated lesions, and 60 to 85% for the more complex occlusions (Frankl, 1990a). Multiple lesions (two or three) are successfully treated, but the single proximal lesions that are found in the vessels other than the left main CA are still the vessels of choice.

The use of PTCA in acute MI is currently being researched. Although reperfusion during the early hours of an evolving infarct have proved successful, many questions remain. There is promising evidence for PTCA along with thrombolytic therapy (Frankl, 1990a). In unstable angina, PTCA has been successful (Faxon et al., 1984; Frankl, 1990b); however, there may be a risk of increased complications from PTCA because of coronary spasms associated with unstable angina.

Complications. Restenosis may occur within 8 months following PTCA. This complication has been seen in 25 to 35% of the patients, and may go as high as 40%, particularly for lesions of the LAD coronary artery.

Absolute contraindications for the PTCA include:

1. Absence of flow-limiting lesion
2. Multivessel disease with severe atherosclerosis for which CABG would be more appropriate
3. Significant obstruction of more than 50% of the left main coronary artery
4. Absence of cardiac surgical program available at the hospital.

Coronary Artery Bypass Graft (CABG). This is a surgical procedure in which the ischemic

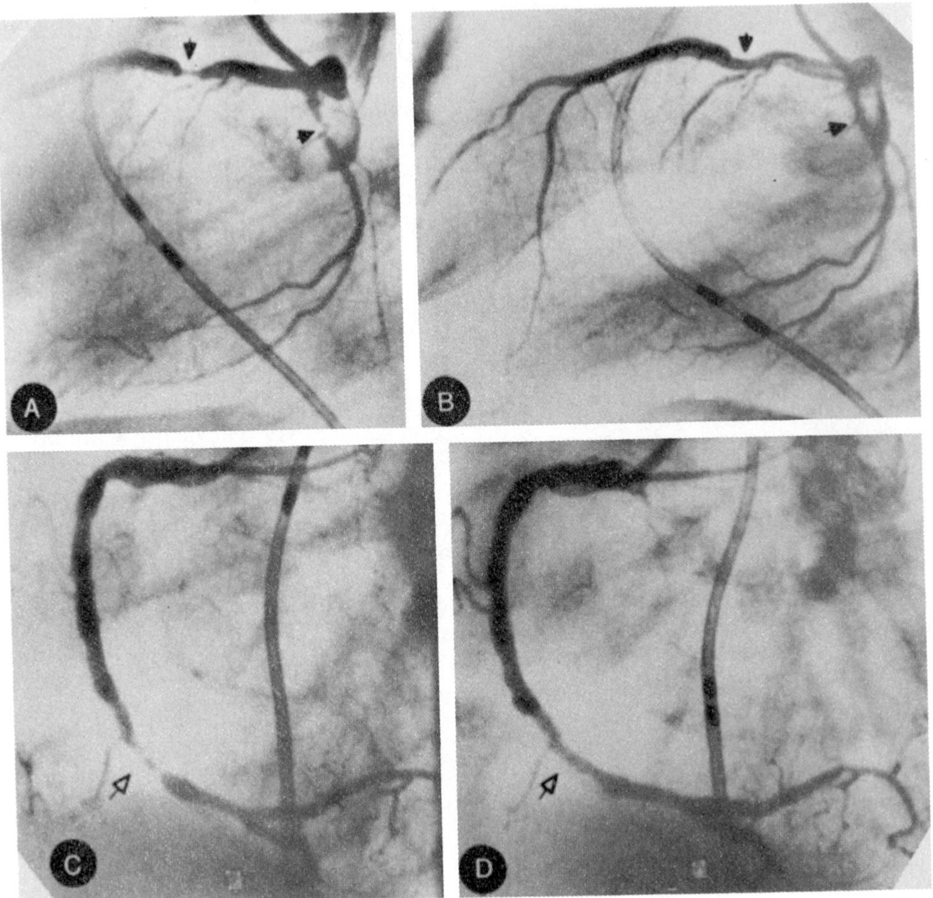

Figure 8-10. Radiographics of patients with triple vessel disease with images before and after angioplasty. (From Stertzer, S. H., et al. (1989): The setting of coronary angioplasty in multivessel disease: Current status and future directions *Cardiology Clinics*, 7(4):773.

area(s) of the myocardium are revascularized by implanting the mammary artery (IMA) or bypassing the coronary occlusion with a saphenous vein graft. The patient usually has a 75 to 80% flow occlusion in the coronary artery in question. There is a very low mortality rate (2 to 4%) with CABG, and the heart demonstrates a functional improvement of 90%.

Currently, CABG surgery is being performed for primary intervention of evolving AMIs, as therapy combined with thrombolytic therapy, and as emergency treatment after failed PTCA (Lynn-McHale, 1989). Indications for CABG include unresponsive chronic angina and preinfarction angina and triple-vessel disease. Indications for emergency CABG include unresponsive unstable angina, multivessel evolving AMI less than 6 hours after onset of symptoms, and evolving AMI when thrombolytic therapy or PTCA (or both) are unsuccessful (Lynn-McHale, 1989).

High-risk patients often benefit most from CABG. The degree of LV dysfunction is most likely to predict perioperative mortality. The procedure prolongs survival in high-risk patients when compared with medical therapy alone (Frankl, 1990b).

Differences between PTCA and CABG include successful PTCA is less traumatic, less costly initially, and requires a shorter hospital stay than CABG (Frankl, 1990b). However, CABG is more often indicated for a larger population of patients. In some instances, PTCA is difficult if not impossible for long-standing occlusions, multivessel disease, and incomplete revascularization. Patients who require CABG are those with stable angina, unstable angina, acute MI, and failed PTCA (Frankl, 1990b).

Coronary artery bypass graft surgery is performed in the operating room with the patient under general anesthesia and intubated. A midsternal, longitudinal incision is made into the chest cavity. The patient is put on cardiopulmonary bypass (CPB) during the procedure. The coronary arteries are visualized and a segment of the saphenous vein is grafted or anastomosed to the distal end of the vessel with the proximal end of the graft vessel anastomosed to the aorta. The internal mammary artery can also be used to create an artery-to-artery graft. The CPB is progressively discontinued, chest and mediastinal tubes inserted, and the chest is closed (Fig. 8–11).

When the chest is opened for heart surgery, the pleural space may be disrupted. If disruption occurs, the accumulation of air or fluid prevents the development of negative pressure necessary for normal respiration. Chest tubes are inserted to remove the air or fluid and to restore the normal negative pressure of the pleural space. The tube is connected to an underwater seal drainage apparatus that prevents backflow into the pleural space. The tube placed underwater creates a negative pressure. The air or fluid in the chest will drain into the apparatus or bottle in an attempt to equalize the negative pressure in the bottle. Air escapes through an air vent in the chest bottle, preventing pressure buildup. Fluid or blood draining from the chest cavity drains into the bottle and, if in large amounts, may necessitate a second collection bottle. Suction may be added to the system to facilitate air removal. The system must remain patent, open, and functioning at all times. Therefore, the chest tube is not to be clamped or a tension pneumothorax could result. The chest is radiographed to determine correctness of placement. Once the lungs have adequately reexpanded and negative pressure has been reestablished in the pleural cavity, the chest is radiographed again for final verification of expansion and the chest tube is removed. An occlusive pressure dressing is applied to the tube insertion site.

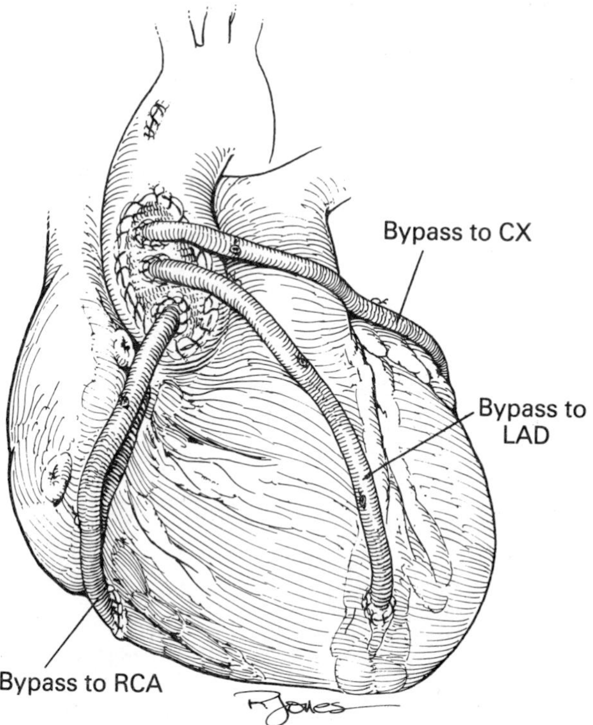

Figure 8–11. Triple coronary artery bypass graft with aortic patch. (From Cooley, D. A.: *Techniques in Cardiac Surgery*. 2nd ed. Philadelphia, W. B. Saunders, 1984.)

Complication. Cardiac tamponade is a complication that must be considered post-CABG. Cardiac tamponade is the collection of fluid in the posterior pericardial sac or mediastinal space. The blood returning from the great vessels to the heart and the ejection of blood from the ventricles is obstructed by the fluid collecting in the sac, which compromises cardiac filling. Signs of cardiac tamponade include decreased cardiac output, rising filling pressures, decreased arterial pressures, marked decrease in mediastinal tube drainage, mediastinal widening on chest x-ray, distant heart sounds, narrowing pulse pressure, and decrease in ECG voltage (Kinney et al., 1991). This is a life-threatening emergency and requires immediate surgical intervention.

Autotransfusion. This is a procedure that can be used during thoracic and cardiovascular surgery. The patient's own blood is collected, filtered, and reinfused back to the patient to minimize usage of blood from the blood bank and its potential complications. Regional anticoagulants such as citrate-phosphate-dextrose (CPD), acid-phosphate-dextrose (APD), or heparin are added to the autotransfusion collection system. The blood may be reinfused to the patient as whole blood or packed red blood cells (RBCs). Complications can include coagulation problems, hemolysis, air embolus, and sepsis. Autotransfusion can also be done following open heart surgery through collection of the blood from the mediastinal tubes. Anticoagulation in this instance is not warranted or necessary. It is imperative that the reinfusion apparatus remove all the air and filter out all clots before being returned to the patient.

Intra-Aortic Balloon Pump (IABP). The use of IABP counterpulsation may be seen in the post-MI patient with severe dysrhythmias or cardiogenic shock usually awaiting surgery, and acute left ventriculary power failure following heart surgery (Fig. 8-12). Refer to Chapter 7 for information relating to the use of the IAPB for cardiogenic shock.

Permanent Pacemakers

When a patient is admitted with an acute MI with the potential for developing serious bradydysrhythmias due to a block in the conducting system of the heart, temporary pacing is instituted. If a block persists beyond the acute phase, a permanent pacemaker is usually implanted.

The first implantable pacemakers were developed during the late 1950s and have gone through many changes in size, shape, power source, function, and encasing material. It is estimated there are 1 million persons worldwide with implantable pacemakers. In the United States, over 300 types of pacemakers are manufactured by numerous companies. Most pacemakers are multiprogrammable for rates, voltage, sensitivities, stimulus duration, and refractory periods.

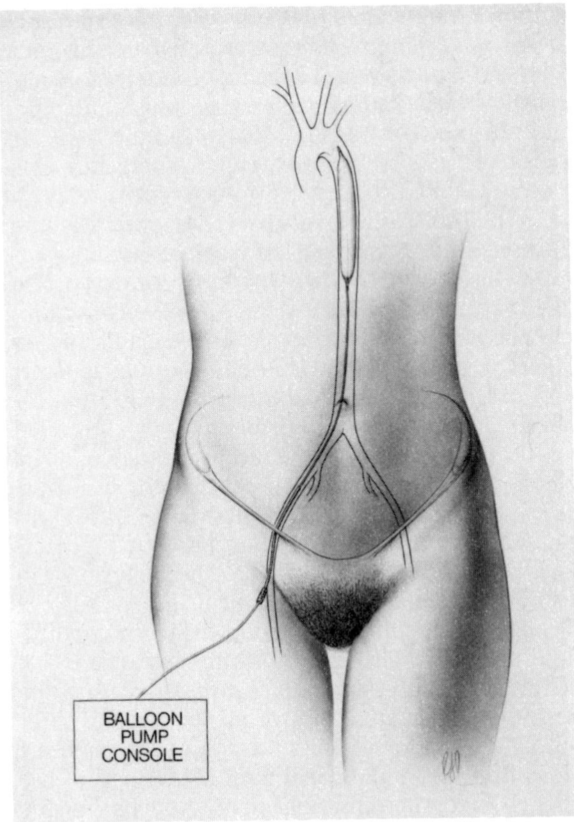

Figure 8-12. Correct positioning of percutaneous IABP in descending thoracic aorta. (From Shoemaker, W. C.: *Textbook of Critical Care.* 2nd ed. Philadelphia, W. B. Saunders, 1989.)

Eighty-six percent of implanted pacemakers are ventricular demand but have the variability to coincide with the patient's changing needs (Lasche, 1983).

Pacemaker functions are described in a code developed by the Inter-Society Commission for Heart Disease (ISCHD) in 1974, revised in 1980, and redescribed by the North American Society for Pacing and Electro-physiology (NASPE) in 1987 (Bernstein et al., 1987; Teplitz, 1991). The code is used to denote the capabilities of the pacemaker as programmed for an individual patient. The code originally had three letters, was updated to five in 1980, but is more commonly seen with the original three letters denoting the chambers paced, the chamber sensed, and the mode of response (Table 8-5).

The type of pacemaker that stimulates the heart at a constant rate regardless of any present cardiac rhythm is termed asynchronous. If attached to the atrium, the pacemaker is coded AOO, and if applied to the ventricles is VOO (see Table 8-5 for explanation of codes). Pacing devices that have the ability to sense as well as respond are classified as atrial and ventricular demand pacemakers, and are coded AAI, AAT, VVI, and VVT depending on their placement and inhibiting or triggering activity.

For patients with an acute MI resulting in an AV conduction disturbance, type II AV block, or complete heart block, a pacemaker labeled as an atrial synchronous ventricular pacemaker may be implanted. These are coded VAT and VDD. For patients with bradycardia in addition to an AV conduction disturbance, the AV sequential pacemaker (coded DVI) senses ventricular activity but paces both atria and ventricles. One of the most current and popular pacing devices used is classified as the universal pacemaker, and is coded DDD. It has multiple functions within one device. The universal, or fully automatic, pacemaker senses and paces both atria and ventricles

Table 8–5. THREE-POSITION PACEMAKER CODE (ICHD)

Chamber Paced	Chamber Sensed	Mode of Response
V—Ventrical	V—Ventrical	I—Inhibited
A—Atrium	A—Atrium	T—Triggered
D—Double (Dual)	D—Double (Dual)	D—Double (Dual) (Atrial triggered and ventricle inhibited)
	O—None	O—None

and varies the ventricular rate according to the atrial rate. The DDD pacemaker is indicated in patients with complete AV block with or without the sick sinus syndrome (Bernstein et al., 1987).

Most permanent pacemakers use lithium batteries as their power source. These models provide a longevity of 8 to 10 years in a system that can be sealed to prevent erosion by body fluids and leakage of battery materials. A permanent pacemaker can be inserted in a transvenous mode under local anesthesia with the lead wires traversing through the cephalic vein and the implant of the device on the right side of the chest. This procedure may be done in the operating room, but it is commonly done in the cardiac catheterization laboratory or special procedures area of the radiology department.

Patient and family education concerns about pacemakers include:

- Pulse checks
- Expected initial fatigue
- Keeping follow-up appointments
- Signs and symptoms of malfunctioning pacemaker
- Wound infection
- Permanent and temporary activity restrictions
- Electromagnetic interference
- Avoiding old wives tales and myths and concentrating on documented literature and physician's advice
- Use of electrical devices
- Leisure time and work-related activities, problems, and concerns
- Referral to pacemaker support groups
- The importance of carrying at all times the identification card concerning the manufacturer and other pertinent medical information
- The need for patient and family to review the information that the manufacturer provides with each device and to ask questions to allay misinformation and anxiety (Guzzetta and Dossey, 1984; Lasche, 1983; Teplitz, 1991).

Automatic Implantable Cardioverter Defibrillator

The automatic implantable cardioverter-defibrillator (AICD) is an implantable device for detecting and treating ventricular tachycardia (VT) or ventricular fibrillation (VF). Research has shown that 20 to 50% of such patients do not respond to antiarrhythmic agents (Manolis et al., 1989) and for which surgery is inappropriate. The AICD was approved by the U.S. Food and Drug Administration in October 1985. It consists of a pulse generator, one or two sensing electrode leads, and an anode and a cathode for cardioversion or defibrillation. The rate-sensing lead consists of a transvenous bipolar lead placed in the right ventricular apex or two myocardial leads screwed onto the left ventricle. The defibrillating lead consists of two patches, one usually placed at the junction of the superior vena cava and the right atrium, the other placed on the left ventricle (Manolis et al., 1989; Mirowski, 1985).

The AICD has about 3 years of monitoring life and is capable of delivering 100 to 150 shocks. A ventricular rate of around 155 beats per minute (adjustable range is 126 to 208 beats per minute) will be interpreted as VT or VF and will trigger the device. The AICD requires 5 to 10 seconds to sense VT or VF and another 5 to 7 seconds to charge the device and deliver a 28- to 32-J shock. If the arrhythmia persists, the device can recycle up to three times. After the fourth shock, there is a 30-second pause to recycle and to allow for detection of dysrhythmias for which shock would not be appropriate such as atrial fibrillation or sinus tachycardia. The AICD is activated or deactivated by using a doughnut-shaped magnet placed at the upper third of the device for 30 seconds (Manolis et al., 1989).

The AICD is surgically implanted by one of four thoracotomy approaches: left anterolateral thoracotomy, median sternotomy, subxiphoid, or subcostal. The leads are channeled under the skin and connected to the pulse generator placed in an abdominal pocket (Furst, 1988; Mirowski, 1985).

Nursing care of the patient with an AICD includes postoperative care, treatment of arrhythmias, psychosocial concerns, and discharge teaching. Postoperative care will be determined by the surgical approach used and other surgical procedures done at the same time. The nurse needs to monitor the patient for location and differentiation of pain, pulmonary status, altered mobility, and potential for infection.

Dysrhythmias will be treated according to ACLS policy if the device fails to correct the VT or VF. It is important to note that the AICD is placed in the inactive mode immediately postoperative to avoid inappropriate discharge for supraventricular tachycardias that are common postoperative problems.

Psychosocial concerns include stress, anxieties, and depression over quality of life and dependency on technology. Discharge teaching involves the patient and family and should include understanding of the function and activity of the device, how the AICD feels when activated, keeping track of the number of shocks delivered, maintenance of the device, testing and precautions procedure, review of CPR, and when to seek emergency assistance (McCrum and Tyndal, 1989; Miller, 1990; Thompson and Olash, 1990).

OUTCOMES

Patient outcomes or goals are generalized to encompass the wide spectrum of the patient who has experienced a MI, uncomplicated or complicated, requiring medical and/or surgical intervention. The patient will

1. Verbalize an absence of chest pain through hemodynamic stability
2. Demonstrate stable or improved cardiac output and cardiac index
3. Demonstrate reduced anxiety levels
4. Along with family and/or support system demonstrate increased understanding of disease process and health management through education and interactive discussion.

A suggested Nursing Care Plan for the Patient with Myocardial Infarction follows.

Congestive Heart Failure

Congestive heart failure (CHF), specifically left-sided CHF, is second only to dysrhythmia as the most common mechanical complication following a myocardial infarction, occurring approximately 50% of the time (Gunnar et al., 1988). Congestive heart failure is most commonly a complication of AMI, but CHF can also be a complication of CAD or hypertension. Ischemia of the left ventricle can cause the LV not to empty during systole. Diastolic filling increases and eventually the volume in the LV is so full that the pressure elevation is reflected backward into the left atrium and pulmonary veins, causing pulmonary congestion. Congestive heart failure is a clinical state in which the heart is unable to maintain the cardiac output necessary to meet the body's metabolic demands (Price and Wilson, 1986).

PATHOPHYSIOLOGY

Left-sided heart failure (LHF) is the inability of the left ventricle to maintain an adequate cardiac output. It is a syndrome or symptom of a physiological abnormal left ventricle and not a disease process itself. The pathology occurs in a fairly sequential pattern. The LV cannot pump effectively or efficiently, usually due to loss of muscle tissue from ischemia (MI). The ineffective pumping action causes a decrease in the cardiac output. The volume of blood remaining in the LV increases after each beat. As this volume builds, it backs up into the left atrium and pulmonary veins and into the lungs. Eventually there is accumulation of fluid in the lungs and pleural spaces, causing increased pressure in the lungs. There is impaired gas (oxygen and carbon dioxide) exchange in the pulmonary system. The backflow can continue on into the right ventricle and right atrium and into the systemic circulation. This type of failure is known as right-sided failure (RHF). As a compensatory mechanism, with an increase in the CO_2 levels in the lungs, the respiratory rate will increase to help eliminate the excess CO_2. This causes the heart rate to increase, pumping more blood to the pulmonary tree for that CO_2–O_2 exchange. The increased heart rate results in more blood being pumped from the systemic circulation into the cardiopulmonary circulation, which is already dangerously overloaded (Wright, 1990).

ASSESSMENT

Patient assessment includes the etiology of both right- and left-sided failure, signs and symptoms, precipitating factors, and diagnostic studies.

Etiology

The etiology or general causes of CHF include:

1. Decreased inflow of blood to the heart; e.g., hemorrhage, dehydration
2. Increased inflow of blood to the heart; e.g., excessive IV fluids, Na + H_2O retention
3. Obstructed outflow of blood from heart; e.g., damaged valves, narrowed arteries, hypertension
4. Damaged heart muscle; e.g., myocardial infarction, inflammatory processes
5. Increased metabolic needs; e.g., fever, pregnancy, hyperthyroidism, chronic anemia (Bates and Hockelman, 1983).

Specific causes of LHF and RHF are the following.

LHF

1. Coronary artery disease
2. Myocardial infarction

NURSING CARE PLAN FOR THE PATIENT WITH MYOCARDIAL INFARCTION

Nursing Diagnosis	Outcome	Intervention
Alteration in comfort: pain, related to myocardial ischemia or necrosis	Verbalizes absence or relief of chest pain Displays reduced tension/relaxed manner	Bedrest; position of comfort Assess description of pain and factors that can aggravate pain (e.g., respiration) Supplemental O_2 Administer medications and note response: Analgesics—Morphine Nitrates—NTG Beta-Blockers—propranolol (Inderal) Calcium Channel Blockers—nifedipine (Procardia) Monitor BP Nonpharmacological pain relief techniques: Relaxation techniques Quiet, restful environment Encourage periods of rest and sleep Organize care to allow for rest periods
Potential alteration in cardiac output related to loss of myocardial contractility	Will demonstrate stable or improved CO Cardiac rate, rhythm and hemodynamic measurements are within normal limits Absence of dysrhythmias Absence of pain with activity	Bedrest Assess and report signs and symptoms of decreased CO; e.g., BP, HR, urine output, fatigue, weakness; cool, pale, clammy skin Monitor BP, apical pulse, temperature, respirations every 2–4 hours and PRN Monitor cardiac rhythm; check strips every 4–6 hours and PRN Supplemental O_2 Auscultate breath sounds every 4–6 hours Auscultate heart sounds every 4–6 hours; watch for development of S_3 and S_4 Monitor lab data: serum enzymes—LDH_1, CPK-MB, SGOT: ABGs; electrolytes Monitor PA pressure, PCWP, CVP Review 12-lead ECG Intake and output every 2–4 hours Monitor administration of IV fluids Administer medications and note response: Inotropic—dobutamine (Dobutrex) Nitrates—NTG Diuretics—furosemide (Lasix) Antidysrhythmics—disopyramide (Norpace), procainamide (Pronestyl), lidocaine, phenytoin (Dilantin), propranolol (Inderal), bretylium (Bretylol), verapamil, nifedipine (Procardia), diltiazem (Cardizem) Monitor diet—low fat, low sodium; small, frequent feedings; avoid ice and caffeine Encourage to avoid Valsalva maneuver—provide laxative or stool softener Promote rest by providing quiet environment, and balancing activity and rest periods
Anxiety, related to perceived or actual threat of biological integrity	Will demonstrate reduced anxiety level Will demonstrate effective coping mechanisms Will participate in treatment and rehabilitation regimen	Provide comfort and education measures; e.g., quiet environment, relaxation techniques; acknowledge feelings of fear, orient patient and support system to procedures and surroundings, answer questions factually, encourage communication Monitor and minimize contact of patient with anxious family members Administer sedatives—diazepam (Valium), flurazepam (Dalmane), lorazepam (Ativan)

continued

NURSING CARE PLAN FOR THE PATIENT WITH MYOCARDIAL INFARCTION *Continued*

Nursing Diagnosis	Outcome	Intervention
		Encourage expression of feelings and anxieties—reassure the patient as appropriate with a calm voice, repeat information frequently
Knowledge deficit regarding disease process	Patient and/or support group will demonstrate increased understanding of disease process and health management through interactive discussion Identify possible life-style changes in preparation for discharge	Review patient understanding of his/her cardiac condition. Explain extent of infarct; associated complications; dysrhythmias; angina; post-MI syndrome, CHF; nature of disease process, including risk factors and factors precipitating angina Explain the importance of rest and of balancing progressive activity with rest Review importance of controlling existing conditions that aggravate CAD and inhibit recovery; e.g., hyperlipidemia, HBP, diabetes Encourage patient to control weight; lose weight if necessary Explain importance of using techniques to manage stress Review importance of physical activity and where to place limitations and restrictions; e.g., walking, jogging, swimming Avoid or modify activity following heavy meals, alcohol consumption, emotional stress, extreme temperatures, or temperature change Encourage independence in self-care Encourage communication of patient with family and/or support group Review coping mechanisms for possibility of role change in family group Review allowances and limitations of sexual activity Discuss signs and symptoms of MI vs angina Explain importance of calling physician if chest pain lasts more than 20 minutes and is unrelieved by NTG Review principles of cardiac rehabilitation: Diet; avoid caffeine, tobacco, limit certain foods (eggs, cream, butter, foods high in animal fat), rest after meals Medication; name, dosage, time, purpose, side effects Avoid OTC medication until cleared by physician Avoid constipation and straining at stool Avoid sitting in same position for extended periods of time Exercise program; at regular intervals, follow prescribed program, incorporate home exercise program Check with physician regarding resumption of sexual activity, travel, driving Avoid isometric-type exercises; heavy lifting and pushing

Data from Carpenito, L. J.: *Handbook of Nursing Diagnosis 1989–90*. Philadelphia, J. B. Lippincott, 1989; Guzzetta, C. E., and Dossey, B. M.: *Cardiovascular Nursing: Bodymind Tapestry*. St. Louis, C. V. Mosby, 1984; Johanson, B. C., et al.: *Standards for Critical Care*. St. Louis, C. V. Mosby, 1988; Moorhouse, M. F., et al.: *Critical Care Plans: Guidelines for Patient Care*. Philadelphia, F. A. Davis, 1987.

3. Hypertension
4. Rheumatic heart disease
5. Aortic valve disease

RHF

1. End result of left-sided failure
2. Pulmonary hypertension
3. Results of right ventricular infarction

Signs and Symptoms

Signs and symptoms that are observed for include the ones listed previously under nursing assessment as well as those specific for left- and right-sided failure.

LHF

1. Anxiety
2. Air hunger

3. Dyspnea/orthopnea
4. Diaphoresis
5. Rales/wheezes
6. Cyanosis
7. Increased HR
8. Elevated PCWP pressures (18 to 25 mm Hg or higher)
9. S_3 (?S_4) gallop
10. Murmur at apex
11. Dysrhythmias

RHF

12. Dependent edema
13. Jugular venous distension
14. Bounding pulses
15. Oliguria
16. Dysrhythmias
17. Elevated CVP
18. Liver engorgement and tenderness
19. Enlarged spleen
20. Decreased appetite, nausea, vomiting

Note: In left-sided heart failure, the detection of an S_3 or gallop rhythm is an important early sign. Detection of the S_3 sound and observation of other occurring signs can precipitate early and aggressive management of impending CHF to prevent further problems and complications.

Precipitating Factors

Precipitating factors for congestive heart failure include myocardial infarction, dysrhythmias (especially severe tachycardia or bradycardia), severe overexertion, sudden increase in environmental heat or humidity, anemia, thyrotoxicosis, and pregnancy and childbirth.

Diagnostic studies that are paramount for the diagnosis and competent treatment of the patient suspected of having CHF include

1. A complete history and physical examination incorporating all of the aforementioned assessment measures, signs and symptoms, and precipitating factors.

2. Chest x-ray to view the heart size and configuration and to check the lung fields to determine if they are clear or opaque (fluid filled). The procedure can be done in the radiology department, or if the patient is too unstable, it may be a portable x-ray study.

3. Hemodynamic monitoring will show elevated pulmonary artery (PA)/CVP pressures. The PA pressure reflects LV function; CVP reflects RV function (see Chap. 4).

4. Laboratory studies are monitored, specifically arterial blood gases (ABGs), which may indicate respiratory acidosis, metabolic acidosis, or if the patient is hyperventilating, respiratory alkalosis.

5. Liver function tests (LFTs) should also be noted. The liver can become congested, may enlarge and become tender, with ascites and/or jaundice becoming noticeable. Liver function will be diminished (Johanson et al., 1988; Kinney et al., 1991; Moorhouse et al., 1987).

NURSING DIAGNOSIS

Nursing diagnosis and intervention of the patient with CHF include the following.

Alteration in Cardiac Output: Decreased, Related to Decreased Myocardial Contractility

1. Administer O_2.

2. Position patient with head of the bed (HOB) elevated if BP stable.

3. Administer medications: e.g., IV—dopamine, dobutamine, amrinone; PO—digoxin, digitalis.

4. Monitor VS and hemodynamic measurements every 15 minutes until stable then every hour.

5. Monitor urine output every hour.

6. Administer vasodilators if the patient is normovolemic; e.g., morphine, nitroprusside, NTG, captopril, hydralazine, isosorabide, (isordil).

7. Administer diuretics as ordered; e.g., furosemide (Lasix).

8. Monitor serum electrolytes and ABGs every 6 hours until stable.

9. Administer and monitor effect of IV fluids with particular attention to recurring signs of CHF.

10. Provide quiet environment.

11. Provide for periods of uninterrupted sleep.

Alteration in Cardiac Output: Decreased, Related to Increased Afterload

1. Administer vasodilators as ordered; e.g., nitrates, nitroprusside, hydralazine, minoxidil, and prazosin. Vasodilators are used in MI patients who do not respond to diuretics alone. They reduce preload and afterload, improve cardiac output, and relieve myocardial ischemia. Complications to be alert for include hypotension, tachycardia, reduced cardiac output, and compromised peripheral perfusion (Gunnar et al., 1988).

2. Monitor V/S and hemodynamic measure-

ments every 15 minutes until stable then every hour.

3. Administer pain medication as needed.
4. Provide relaxing environment and encourage sleep.
5. Provide sedation as needed.

Impaired Gas Exchange Related to Ventilation—Perfusion Imbalance

1. Administer O_2 as ordered.
2. Elevate HOB if BP stable.
3. Monitor ABGs every four hours until stable.
4. Assess breath sounds every 2 hours.
5. Instruct in deep-breathing techniques.
6. Monitor fluid balance; e.g., daily weights, hourly input and output (I&O).
7. Monitor hematocrit and hemoglobin (H&H) daily for anemia.
8. Monitor and treat hyperthermia.
9. Provide for rest and sleep.

Potential for Fluid Volume Deficit Related to Excessive Diureses

1. Monitor I&O every hour.
2. Monitor response to diuretic.
3. Monitor daily weights.
4. Instruct patient and family on importance of oral fluid restriction.

Potential for Injury: Dysrhythmias Related to Electrolyte Imbalance

1. Monitor electrolyte/acid-base balance.
2. Administer potassium as ordered.
3. Monitor I&O.
4. Monitor ECG for signs of hypo-/hyperkalemia and digitalis toxicity.

Activity Intolerance Related to Generalized Weakness and Imbalance Between Oxygen Supply and Demand

1. Maintain O_2 during activities as needed.
2. Balance activities with rest periods.
3. Encourage independence through assistive devices and energy conservation.
4. Monitor response to exercise and gradually increase activity.
5. Assist patient as needed while encouraging independence (Carpenito, 1989; Fukuda, 1990; Moorhouse et al., 1987).

Interventions

Medical and nursing interventions and management of the patient with CHF center around a threefold approach: treatment of the existing symptoms of the crisis situation, preventing further or expanding complications, and treating the underlying cause.

Treatment of existing symptoms include:

1. Improvement in pump function through positive inotropic medications (dopamine, dobutamine) and cardiotonics (digoxin).

Reduction of cardiac workload and oxygen consumption by

- Avoiding anxiety-provoking situations.
- Elevating HOB.
- Schedule rest periods.
- Modify activities of daily living (ADL).
- Order vasodilators; e.g., NTG, captopril, morphine.

2. Intra-aortic balloon pump is used in severe CHF and cardiogenic shock to augment diastole, decrease afterload, and improve perfusion to the coronary arteries and vital organs.
3. Optimize gas exchange through supplemental oxygen, diuresis, and monitoring ABG's.

Control of sodium and water retention

- Diuresis; diuretics; e.g., Lasix, Diuril, Bumex
- Fluid restriction-oral
- Careful IV fluid administration
- Low-sodium diet
- Removal of fluid through thoracentesis, paracentesis, dialysis

4. Adequate nutrition through low calorie, low residue, bland small feedings.
5. Monitor cardiac output and pump function through hemodynamic monitoring measurements (Fukuda, 1990; Gunnar et al., 1988).

Complications

Complications for the patient with CHF can be quite critical. Interventions must be provided to avoid extending the existing conditions or allowing expansion of the process to encompass new, life-threatening complications. Two specific complications for which to monitor the patient are pulmonary edema and cardiogenic shock.

Pulmonary Edema

Pulmonary edema is an acute, life-threatening form of CHF. The pulmonary vascular system becomes so full and engorged that fluid seeps out of the vessels into the lung spaces. In an acute

MI, when the primary injury is to the left ventricle, thereby decreasing the pumping ability of the LV without compromising the pumping action of the RV, a temporary imbalance results in the output of the two pumps. The right ventricle continues to pump blood into the pulmonary system and the left side of the heart, and the left ventricle has increasing difficulty pumping the blood volume into the systemic circulation. The result is increasing volume and pressure of blood in pulmonary vessels, increasing pressure in pulmonary capillaries, and fluid leaking into the interstitial spaces of lung tissue.

Pulmonary edema greatly reduces the amount of lung tissue space available for gas exchange and results in clinical symptoms of extreme dyspnea, cyanosis, severe anxiety, diaphoresis, pallor, and blood-tinged, frothy sputum (Kinney et al., 1991; Price and Wilson, 1986). The ABGs will indicate a severe respiratory acidosis with low blood pH levels, low PO_2 levels, and usually rising PCO_2 levels. Pulmonary edema is treated by improving gas exchange through morphine IV, low levels of oxygen, and aminophylline; decreasing intravascular volume by using diuretics or, in some rare instances, phlebotomy; and decreasing venous return with the patient in a high Fowler's position and rotating tourniquets.

Cardiogenic Shock

Cardiogenic shock is the most acute and ominous form of pump failure. It is the inability of the heart to act as a pump. Shock can be seen following a severe MI, dysrhythmias, CHF, pulmonary embolus, cardiac tamponade, and abdominal aortic aneurysm. Often the outcome of cardiogenic shock is death; it carries a 85 to 95% mortality rate (McCance and Huether, 1990). Signs and symptoms include increased PA pressures; PCWP above 18 to 25 mm Hg; decreased CO and CI; decreased BP, without evidence of hypovolemia; cyanosis; decreased urine output; decreased or absent pulses; and restlessness and confusion. These patients need to be treated aggressively with vasopressors such as, dopamine, dobutamine, norepinephrine (Levophed), amrinone (Inocor).

An intra-aortic balloon pump (IABP) may be used to assist with circulation by decreasing afterload and augmenting diastolic pressure (Fig. 8–13). It is not uncommon for the patient to remain on the pump until surgical intervention can be done. For further detail, see Chapter 7.

The third part of the medical management program for patients with CHF is to treat the underlying cause. Once the crisis has passed and the patient is stabilized, the underlying cause or precipitating factor(s) for the complications must be addressed and treated. Treatment may encompass surgical or pharmacological intervention of a MI secondary to CAD, e.g., a CABG, PTCA, and cardiotonic drugs; valve replacement surgery as treatment of long-standing problems such as valvular diseases secondary to rheumatic heart disease; treatment modalities for pulmonary disorders (COPD); and management of hypertension (Gunnar et al., 1988).

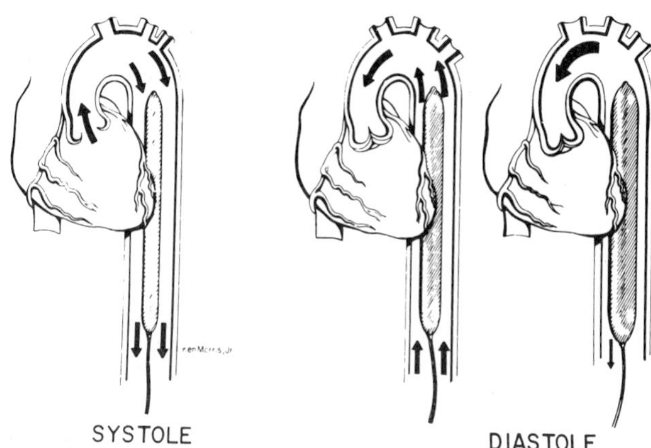

Figure 8–13. Mechanisms of action—intra-aortic balloon pump. Balloon deflates during systole, unloading ventricle; balloon inflates during diastole, increasing coronary perfusion pressure and myocardial oxygen supply. (From Shoemaker, W. C.: *Textbook of Critical Care*. 2nd ed. Philadelphia, W. B. Saunders, 1989.)

OUTCOMES

Outcomes for the patient with CHF include:

1. Cardiac output within normal limits
2. Absence of signs and symptoms of decreased cardiac output
3. Afterload is within normal limits
4. Normal ABGs
5. Absence of respiratory distress
6. Will be normovolemic and will not develop a fluid volume deficit
7. Absence of dysrhythmias
8. Increased level of activity without fatigue, weakness, discomfort, or other abnormal response.

Summary

This chapter has focused on the care of the patient with alterations in cardiac status. The normal anatomy and physiology of the heart have been reviewed and reasons for deviations from normal have been discussed. The pathophysiology of coronary artery disease has been described, including the potential complications of angina, myocardial infarction, and congestive heart failure. Nursing assessment, diagnosis, interventions and goals, and medical management specific to this population have been addressed. The purpose of this chapter has been to acquaint the critical care nurse with the problems and pathological conditions most commonly seen in the cardiovascular patient. It is hoped that this chapter will provide a beginning, basic understanding of the cardiovascular patient that will facilitate sound clinical judgment in planning care that is holistic and incorporates a cooperative, multidisciplinary approach.

■ References

American Heart Association (1989): *Heart Facts 1989.* American Heart Association.

Andrien, P., and Lemberg, L. (1990): Thrombolytic therapy in acute myocardial infarction. *Heart Lung* 19(1):102–104.

Bates, B., and Hockelman, R. A. (1983): *Physical Examination.* 3rd ed. Philadelphia: J. B. Lippincott.

Bernstein, A., et al. (1987): The NASPE/BPEG generic pacemaker code for antibradyarrhythmia & adaptive-rate pacing & antitachyarrhythmia devices. *PACE* 10(4):794.

Boykoff, S. L. (1989): Strategies for sexual counseling of patients following a myocardial infarction. *Dimensions of Critical Care Nursing* 8(6):368–373.

Braunwald, E., et al. (1988): *Heart Disease.* 3rd ed. Philadelphia: W. B. Saunders.

Brewer-Senerchia, C. (1989): Thrombolytic therapy: A review of the literature on streptokinase and tissue plasminogen activator with implications for practice. *Critical Care Nursing Clinics of North America* 1(2):359–371.

Brooks-Brunn, J. (1988): Thrombolytic intervention and its effect on mortality in acute myocardial infarction. Review of clinical trials. *Heart Lung* 17(6):756–760.

Califf, R. N., et al. (1988): Characteristics & outcomes of patients in whom reperfusion with intravenous tissue-type plasminogen activator fails: Results of the thrombolysis & angioplasty in myocardial infarction (TAMI) I trial. *Circulation* 77:1090.

Canobbio, M. (1990): *Cardiovascular Disorders.* St. Louis: C. V. Mosby.

Carpenito, L. J. (1989): *Handbook of Nursing Diagnosis 1989–90.* Philadelphia: J. B. Lippincott.

Castelli, W. P., et al. (1986): Incidence of coronary heart disease and lipoprotein cholesterol levels: The Framingham Study. *JAMA* 256(20):2835.

Chesebro, J. H., et al. (1987): Thrombolysis in myocardial infarction (TIMI) trial, phase I: A comparison between intravenous tissue plasminogen activator & intravenous streptokinase. *Circulation* 76:142.

Dossey, B., Guzzetta, C., and Kenner, C. (1990): *Essentials of Critical-Care Nursing. Body-Mind-Spirit.* Philadelphia: J. B. Lippincott.

Enger, E. L., and Schwertz, D. W. (1989): Mechanisms of myocardial ischemia. *Cardiovascular Nursing* 3(4):1–15.

Epstein, S. E., et al. (1982): Evaluation of patients after acute myocardial infarction: Indications for cardiac catherization & surgical intervention. *New England Journal of Medicine* (307)24:1487–1492.

Faxon, D. P., et al. (1984): Role of percutaneous transluminal coronary angioplasty is the treatment of unstable angina. *American Journal of Cardiology* 53(Suppl. C):131–135.

Frankl, W. S. (1990a): A comparison of coronary artery bypass surgery and percutaneous transluminal coronary angioplasty in the treatment of coronary artery disease, part I. *Modern Concepts of Cardiovascular Disease* 59(6):31–36.

Frankl, W. S. (1990b): A comparison of coronary artery bypass surgery and percutaneous transluminal coronary angioplasty in the treatment of coronary artery disease, part I. *Modern Concepts of Cardiovascular Disease* 59(7):37–42.

Fukuda, N. (1990): Outcome standards for the client with chronic congestive heart failure. *Journal of Cardiovascular Nursing* 4(3):59–70.

Furst, E. (1988): Cardiovascular technology. *Journal of Cardiovascular Nursing* 3(1):77–81.

Gardner, P. E. (1989): Cardiac output: Theory, technique, & troubleshooting. *Critical Care Nursing Clinics of North America* 1(3):577, 587.

Govoni, L. E., and Hayes, J. E. (1985): *Drugs and Nursing Implications.* 5th ed. New York: Appleton-Century-Crofts.

Greenspon, A. J., and Goldberg, S. (1983): Pathophysiology of angina pectoris due to coronary artery spasm. *Cardiovascular Clinics of North America* 14(1):17–29.

Gunnar, R. M., et al. (1988): Heart failure in acute MI. *Patient Care* 22(17):34–55.

Guzzetta, C. E., and Dossey, B. M. (1984): *Cardiovascular Nursing: Bodymind Tapestry.* St. Louis: C. V. Mosby.

Holloway, N. M., (1989): *Critical Care: Care Plans.* Springhouse, PA: Springhouse Corp.

Hudak, C. M., Gallo, B. M., and Lohr, T. (1986): *Critical Care Nursing: A Holistic Approach.* 4th ed. Philadelphia: J. B. Lippincott.

Hurst, J. W., and Logue, R. B. (eds.): (1990). *The Heart.* 7th ed. New York: McGraw-Hill.

Johanson, B. C., et al. (1988): *Standards for Critical Care.* St. Louis: C. V. Mosby.

Kannel, W., and Gordon, T. (1978): Evaluation of cardiovascular risk in the elderly: The Framingham Study. *Bulletin of New York Academy of Medicine* 54:573.

Kinney, M. R., Packa, D. R., Andreoli, K. G., and Zipes, D. P. (1991): *Comprehensive Cardiac Care.* 7th ed. St. Louis: C. V. Mosby.

Kleven, M. R. (1988): Comparison of thrombolytic agents: Mechanism of action, efficacy, & safety. *Heart Lung* 17(6):750–755.

LaRosa, J. (1991): An update from the national cholesterol education program: Implications for nurses. *Journal of Cardiovascular Nursing* 5(2):1–9.

Lasche, P. A. (1983): Permanent cardiac pacing: Technology & follow up. *Focus on Critical Care* 10(5):28–36.

Lynn-McHale, D. J. (1989): Interventions for acute myocardial infarction: PTCA and CABGS. *Critical Care Nursing Quarterly* 12(2):38–48.

Manolis, A. S., et al. (1989): Automatic implantable cardioverter defibrillator. *JAMA* 262(10):1362–1368.

Marriott, H., and Conover, M. (1989): *Advanced Concepts in Arrhythmias.* St. Louis: C. V. Mosby.

McCance, K., and Huether, S. (1990). *Pathophysiology.* St. Louis: C. V. Mosby.

McCrum, A. E., and Tyndal, A. (1989): Nursing care for

patients with implantable defibrillators. *Critical Care Nurse* 9(9):48–68.

McFarland, G. K., and McFarland, E. A. (1989). *Nursing Diagnostics and Intervention: Planning for Patient Care.* St. Louis: C. V. Mosby.

Miller, K. M. (1990): When your patient has an implanted defibrillator. *RN* 53(6):32–35.

Mirowski, M. (1985): The automatic implantable cardioverter-defibrillator: An overview. *Journal of the American College of Cardiology* 6(2):461–466.

Moorhouse, M. F., Geissler, A. C., and Doenges, M. E. (1987): *Critical Care Plans: Guidelines for Patient Care.* Philadelphia: F. A. Davis.

National Institutes of Health (1989): *Report of the Expert Panel on the Detection, Evaluation, and Treatment of High Blood Cholesterol in Adults.* NIP Publication, 89-2925. Bethesda, MD.

National Research Council, Committee on Diet and Health (1989). *Diet and Health: Implications for Reducing Chronic Disease Risk.* Washington, DC: National Academy Press.

Niemyski, P., and Hellstedt, L. F. (1989): Patient selection & management in thrombolytic therapy: Nursing implications. *Critical Care Nursing Quarterly* 12(2):8–24.

Ochsner, J. L. (1989): Early bypass operation after acute myocardial infarction. *Annals of Thoracic Surgery* (48):750–760.

Patterson, S., Piper, H., and Starling, E. (1914): The regulation of the heart beat. *Journal of Physiology* 48:465–513.

Peterson, J. E., and Emmot, W. W. (1989): Therapies to limit infarct size: Timing, dosage, & effectiveness. *Postgraduate Medicine* 86(3):54–63.

Price, S. A., and Wilson, L. M. (1986): *Pathophysiology: Clinical Concepts of Disease Process.* 3rd ed. New York: McGraw-Hill.

Rahimtoola, S., et al. (1987): Consensus statement of the conference in the state of the art of electrophysiology testing in the diagnosis & treatment of patients with cardiac arrhythmias. *Circulation* 75(4):3–11.

Subcommittee on Coronary Angiography (1987): Guidelines for coronary angiography. *Journal of the American College of Cardiology* 4(10):935–950.

Swan, H. J. C. (1975): The role of hemodynamic monitoring in the management of the critically ill. *Critical Care Medicine* 3(3):83–89.

Teplitz, L. (1991): Classification of cardiac pacemakers: The pacemaker code. *Journal of Cardiovascular Nursing* 5(3):1–8.

Thelan, L., Urden, L., and Davie, J. (1990): *Textbook of Critical Care Nursing: Diagnosis and Management.* St. Louis: C. V. Mosby.

Thibodeau, G. A. (1990): *Anatomy and Physiology.* 13th ed. St. Louis: C. V. Mosby.

Thompson, J., and Olash, J. (1990): Antitachycardia pacing with cardioverter-defibrillator backup for malignant ventricular dysrhythmias. *Journal of Cardiovascular Nursing* 4(2):33–43.

Tilkian, A. G., and Daily, E. K. (1986): *Cardiovascular Procedures: Diagnostic Techniques and Therapeutic Procedures.* St. Louis: C. V. Mosby.

Underhill, S. (1989): *Cardiac Nursing.* 2nd ed. Philadelphia: J. B. Lippincott.

Underhill, S., Woods, S., Froelicher, E., and Halpenny, C. (1990): *Cardiovascular Medications for Cardiac Nursing.* Philadephia: J. B. Lippincott.

Vander, A., Sherman, J., and Luciano, D. (1985): *Human Physiology: The Mechanism of Body Function.* New York: McGraw-Hill.

Verstraete, M., et al. (1985): Randomized trial of intravenous recombinant tissue-type plasminogen activator vs. intravenous streptokinase in acute myocardial infarction. *Lancet* 1, 842–847.

Vogel, J. (1991): Management of acute myocardial infarction: A perspective. *Clinical Cardiology* 14:5.

Von Rueden, K. T. (1989): Acute myocardial infarction. In: K. T. Von Rueden and C. A. Walleck (eds.). *Advanced Critical Care Nursing: A Case Study Approach.* Rockville, MD: Aspen Publishers.

Wenger, N. K. (1985): *Exercise and the Heart.* Philadelphia: F. A. Davis.

West, J. (1991): *Physiological Basis of Medical Practice.* Baltimore: Williams & Wilkins.

Wright, S. (1990): Pathophysiology of congestive heart failure. *Journal of Cardiovascular Nursing* 4(3):1–16.

Recommended Reading

Andrien, P., and Lemberg, L. (1990): Thrombolytic therapy in acute myocardial infarction. *Heart Lung* 19(1):102–104.

Enger, E. L., and Schwertz, D. W. (1989): Mechanisms of myocardial ischemia. *Cardiovascular Nursing* 3(4):1–15.

Gardner, P. E. (1989): Cardiac output: Theory, technique, & troubleshooting. *Critical Care Nursing Clinics of North America* 1(3):577–587.

Greenspon, A. J., and Goldberg, S. (1983): Pathophysiology of angina pectoris due to coronary artery spasm. *Cardiovascular Clinics of North America* 4(1):17–29.

Lynn-McHale, D. J. (1989): Interventions for acute myocardial infarction: PTCA and CABGS. *Critical Care Nursing Quarterly* 12(2):38–48.

Niemyski, P., and Hellstedt, L. F. (1989): Patient selection & management in thrombolytic therapy: Nursing implications. *Critical Care Nursing Quarterly* 12(2):8–24.

Chapter

9

Jeanette C. Hartshorn, R.N., Ph.D., FAAN,
Vicki L. Byers, R.N., Ph.D., and
Leslie Goddard, R.N., Ph.D.

Nervous System Injury

Objectives

- Describe the pathophysiology, nursing, and medical management of patients with increased intracranial pressure.
- Complete an assessment on a critically ill patient with nervous system injury.
- Describe the pathophysiology, nursing, and medical management of patients with head injury.
- Define current nursing and medical therapy for spinal cord injury.
- Discuss the nursing assessment and care of a critically ill patient with cerebrovascular disease.
- Define the pathophysiology and expected treatment for status epilepticus.

Neurological illness and trauma to the central nervous system are devastating and frequently life-threatening events. These patients have so many unique needs during the acute phase of their illness that caring for them is a challenge for the critical care nurse. Nursing care can make a significant difference for both the patient and family as they adjust to these events.

The brain is important in all aspects of our lives, for consciousness, thinking, problem solving, judgment, memory, language, perceptions, emotions, movements, and autonomic functions. The spinal cord is important because most sensory pathways go through the spinal cord on the way to the brain. Most motor pathways pass through the spinal cord on their journey to the rest of the body and most reflex activity is accomplished at the spinal cord level. When these structures are damaged, our activities are greatly altered. In this chapter, the pathophysiology, assessment, nursing diagnosis, interventions, and outcomes related to increased intracranial pressure, head injury, spinal cord injury, status epilepticus, and cerebrovascular disease are discussed.

Increased Intracranial Pressure

One of the most commonly encountered problems in the critical care setting is increased intracranial pressure (IICP). Planning for the care of these patients is based on the concepts of volume/pressure relationships, cerebral blood flow, cerebral edema, cerebrospinal fluid (CSF) changes, and herniation. Patients with IICP are dependent on astute and timely nursing assessment and interventions to limit the possible damage from the increased pressure. A plan of care must be developed for each individual patient as their responses to environmental changes are noted.

Under normal circumstances, intracranial pressure (0 to 15 mm Hg) fluctuates in response to changes in blood pressure, respiratory cycle, isometric contractions, coughing, and Valsalva maneuvers (i.e., holding breath, straining). With brain pathology (i.e., head injury, stroke, tumors, hydrocephalus, infections, cerebral edema, hematoma formation, anoxia), an increase in intracranial pressure is life threatening.

PATHOPHYSIOLOGY

Increased intracranial pressure (16 mm Hg and greater) is a life-threatening event occurring because the rigid cranial vault contains three types of noncompressible contents: semisolid brain, intravascular blood, and CSF. When the volume of any one of these three intracranial components increases, one or both of the other components must decrease proportionally or there is an increase in intracranial pressure (modified Monro-Kellie hypothesis).

As a way of compensating for an increased intracranial component, CSF is displaced into the spinal canal or undergoes an increased absorption into the venous system. In pathological conditions in which additional volume is added, like an increase in blood volume, cerebral edema, or hemorrhage, these compensatory mechanisms fail and additional intracranial volume is not tolerated. At this point, the patient begins to display symptoms of increased intracranial pressure. Physiologically, the brain is said to then lose its ability to compensate, which is demonstrated by an alteration in intracranial compliance.

Intracranial Compliance

Intracranial compliance is a measure of the brain's compensatory mechanisms and demonstrates the effects of volume on pressure. In Figure 9-1, the curve is flat until point A. Adding volume up to this point has very little effect on pressure; the ICP remains stable. This response is known as high compliance; the brain is able to adapt to changes in intracranial volume without a change in pressure (Nikas, 1987; Pacult and Gudeman, 1989; Rockoff and Kennedy, 1988). During normal compensation, CSF is displaced into the spinal subarachnoid space and blood is displaced into the venous sinuses. Nursing measures such as bathing, turning, and suctioning are safe to perform during this interval (Marshall et al., 1990; Miller, 1989a). Figure 9-1, point B on the steep portion of the curve demonstrates the time in which small changes in volume produce large changes in pressure. In Figure 9-1, point B demonstrates exhausted compensatory volume displacement mechanisms (low compliance) (Nikas, 1987; Rockoff and Kennedy, 1988). Patients on the steep portion of this curve can experience large and dangerous increases in ICP with ordinary activities of daily living or nursing care measures that were previously of little consequence (Marshall et al., 1990; Miller, 1989a). Patients in this situation must be monitored very closely.

Other causes of IICP include altered cerebral blood flow, loss of autoregulation, compression of the venous system, and herniation.

Altered Cerebral Blood Flow

Cerebral blood flow (CBF) brings oxygen and glucose to the brain for energy production. Waste products are also removed by the blood. When metabolism is increased, the CBF is increased to meet those demands (Marshall et al., 1990; Rockoff and Kennedy, 1988). Under pathological situations, CBF can increase to such an extent that it adds to brain bulk and consequently ICP (Marshall et al., 1990). On the other hand, a decrease in CBF while there is an increase in metabolic activity can render an area ischemic by increasing PCO_2 and causing cerebral edema, contributing to IICP (Marshall et al., 1990; Rockoff and Kennedy, 1988).

Cerebral perfusion pressure (CPP) is an estimate of the level of cellular perfusion. It is calculated by subtracting mean intracranial pressure (ICP) from mean systemic arterial blood pressure (MAP) (CPP = MAP − ICP). The acceptable range for CPP is 60 to 100 mm Hg. It is important to maintain CPP above 60 mm Hg in order to perfuse the brain with blood. A CPP of 60 mm Hg or lower is considered not only low, but potentially life-threatening (Nikas, 1987). When IICP approaches mean systemic arterial pressure, CPP decreases to a point where autoregulation is impaired and cerebral blood flow decreases. This decrease in flow will cause ischemia and eventually infarction of cerebral tissue if the situation is not corrected.

Autoregulation

Under normal limits, the cerebral vasculature exhibits pressure and chemical autoregulation. Pressure autoregulation provides a constant blood volume and CPP regardless of a wide range of

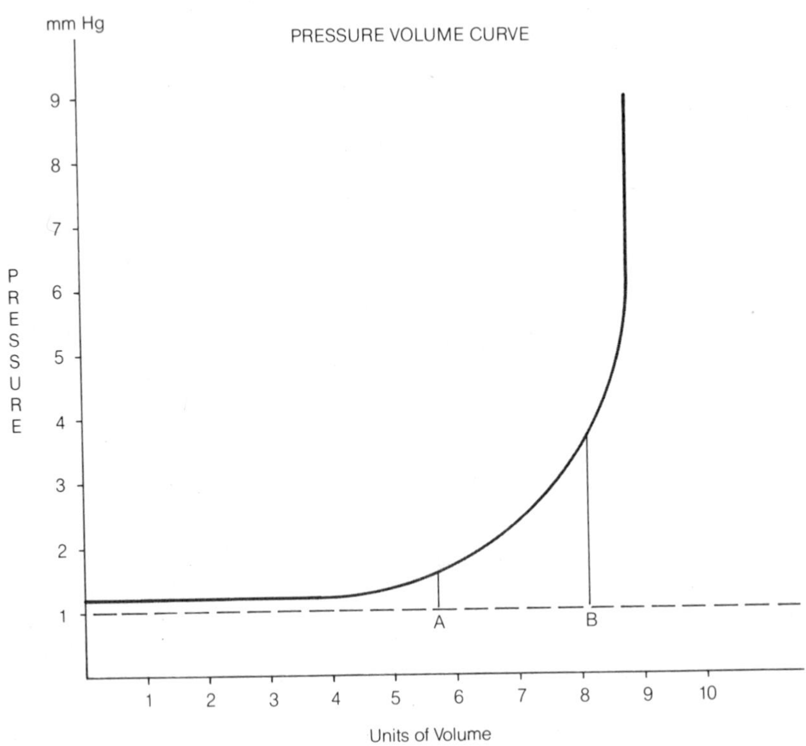

Figure 9-1. Pressure-volume curve. Up to point A, addition of volume had little effect on pressure; after that point, there is a *dramatic* increase in response to addition of volume, especially from point B onward. (From Hickey, J. V.: The Clinical Practice of Neurological Neurosurgical Nursing. 2nd ed. Philadelphia, J. B. Lippincott, 1986, p. 248.)

mean arterial pressure. Pathological states, like head injury, hemorrhage, or craniotomy lead to a loss of pressure autoregulation. When autoregulation is lost, hypertension increases CBF and hypotension causes ischemia. Both of these situations cause increased ICP. Cerebral perfusion pressure is a reflection of CBF, and it can be calculated at the bedside.

The cerebral vessels are also sensitive to chemical autoregulation. A $PaCO_2$ greater than 30 mm Hg and a PaO_2 of 50 mm Hg cause the cerebral arteries to vasodilate. $PaCO_2$ is the most potent vasodilator leading to an increase in CBF, cerebral blood volume, and ICP. Cerebral arteries are less sensitive to changes in PaO_2. The CBF is not affected until the PaO_2 is 50 mm Hg or less. A PaO_2 of 50 mm Hg will cause hypoxia and vasodilation of the cerebral vasculature, which will increase CBF and ICP (Marshall et al., 1990; Rockoff and Kennedy, 1988).

Obstructed Venous Outflow

Shunting CSF into the venous system is another way to compensate for an increase in intracranial volume. In pathological states, venous outflow can become obstructed in several ways. Different neck positions (hyperflexion, hyperextension, rotation) compress the jugular vein, inhibit venous return, cause central venous engorgement, and increase ICP (Nikas, 1989). A second mechanism for venous outflow obstruction is transmission of a high pressure that impairs venous return.

Mechanisms that increase intrathoracic or intra-abdominal pressure (i.e., coughing, vomiting, posturing, isometric exercise, Valsalva's maneuver, or positive end-expiratory pressure [PEEP]) produce increased pressure that impairs venous return. When the jugular vein is compressed, venous return is inhibited, resulting in venous engorgement. As venous outflow decreases, an increase in ICP occurs.

Cerebral Edema

Cerebral edema is an increase in the water content of the brain tissue. When cerebral edema occurs as a result of trauma, hemorrhage, tumor, abscess, or ischemia, an increase in ICP occurs. Experimental data suggest that as cerebral edema increases, there is a decrease in cerebral blood flow prior to IICP (Miller, 1989b). As cerebral blood flow decreases, cellular activity is impaired and signs and symptoms related to neurological dysfunction become apparent.

Cytotoxic and vasogenic edema are two categories of cerebral edema. Cytotoxic edema is characterized by intracellular swelling of neurons, which is most often due to hypoxia and hypo-osmolality. Hypoxia causes decreased adenosine triphosphate (ATP) production and leads to the failure of the sodium-potassium pump. As the activity of the pump ceases, sodium is not pumped outside the cell and potassium remains extracellular. In addition, water enters the cell and causes swelling. In cases of acute hypo-osmolality, water moves into the cell by osmosis. Thus, cytotoxic cerebral edema frequently accompanies states of diabetic ketoacidosis.

Vasogenic cerebral edema occurs as a breakdown of the blood-brain-barrier (BBB), leading to an increase in the extracellular fluid space. With the breakdown of the BBB, osmotically active substances (proteins) leak into the interstitium and draw the water from the vascular system. This results in an increase in extracellular fluid and a consequent increase in intracranial pressure. Head injury, brain tumors, and abscesses are common causes of vasogenic cerebral edema.

Herniation

When a mass effect occurs in the semisolid brain within a compartment, the pressure exerted by this mass is not equally divided, resulting in shifting or herniation of the brain from one compartment of high pressure to one of lower pressure. This causes pressure or traction on certain neurological structures, and an increase in neurological deficits or death can occur.

Herniation syndromes are classified as supratentorial (i.e., cingulate herniation, central herniation, and uncal herniation) or infratentorial (i.e., tonsillar herniation).

Cingulate Herniation. When a unilateral lesion creates a shift of brain tissue of one cerebral hemisphere under the falx cerebri to the other cerebral hemisphere, cingulate herniation occurs. This type of herniation compresses cerebral blood vessels and brain tissue, causing cerebral ischemia, cerebral edema, and increased intracranial pressure. Changes in arousal (level of consciousness) and mental status are associated with this type of herniation.

Central Herniation. A downward shift of the cerebral hemispheres, basal ganglia, and diencephalon through the tentorial notch causes central herniation (Morrison, 1990). The supratentorial contents compress vital centers of the brain stem. Early signs and symptoms include changes in arousal and mental status, increased muscle tone, motor weakness, change in the respiratory pattern (i.e., increased yawning, deep sighs, rate changes), small reactive pupils, and bilateral Babinski reflexes. Late signs and symptoms include decorticate posturing and Cheyne-Stokes respirations.

Uncal Herniation. When a unilateral lesion above the tentorium forces the uncus of the temporal lobe to displace through the tentorial notch, uncal herniation is the result. This displaced uncus compresses the midbrain, causing dysfunction of the parasympathetic fibers of the ipsilateral third nerve. Signs and symptoms include unilateral pupil dilation, ipsilateral third nerve palsy, and contralateral hemiplegia. Without treatment, the patient becomes unresponsive to the environment and progresses into full coma. In addition, brain stem dysfunction (loss of oculocephalic reflex, fixed midposition pupils, altered respirations), and decerebrate posturing is present.

Tonsillar Herniation. When the cerebellar tonsils are displaced through the foramen magnum, tonsillar herniation results. This displacement distorts the brain stem, compresses the medulla and causes fatal damage to the respiratory and cardiac centers.

Any change in intracranial compliance, cerebral blood flow, autoregulation, and cerebral edema can potentially cause IICP.

ASSESSMENT

Nursing Assessment

Nursing history and neurological assessment can provide needed information about the patient's current condition. Initial and ongoing assessment of the patient with IICP will provide an active picture of improvement or deterioration and will guide therapeutic efforts.

Ideally, the patient is the primary source of the historical data. If the patient is unable to give the history, then family or friends should supply information related to symptoms, onset, progression, and chronology of the event. If headache is a presenting symptom, then information must be obtained about the location, onset, type of pain associated with the headache, presence of other symptoms, duration, and what makes the headache better or worse. If the patient is admitted secondary to nervous system trauma, specific information concerning the mechanism of injury, immediate posttrauma care and emergency treatments are needed.

The Glasgow Coma Scale (GCS) is a standardized tool used as a guide in assessing the patient with head injury and IICP. The components of this assessment tool are eye opening, verbal response, and motor response (Fig. 9–2). A consistent stimulus is applied; either a verbal command or a painful stimulus. The responsiveness of the patient is expressed as a number according to the listed criteria. A high number (approaching 15) indicates normal functioning, whereas a low number (approaching 3) suggests impaired functioning. Generally, the actual numbers on the scale are less meaningful than the trend of scores. The GCS is a brief way of assessing consciousness. When more detail is needed related to the neurological status, assessment should be specific to the area of the brain that is involved. The advantages of using the GCS relates to its simplicity and universality (Ingersoll and Leyden, 1990). The major disadvantage is the GCS has limited applicability and does not replace neurological assessment.

When performing a neurological assessment, the critical care nurse focuses on mental status, cranial nerve functioning, and motor status. A neurological flow chart and narrative charting are frequently used to provide necessary information.

Glasgow Coma Scale

Eyes	Open	Spontaneously	4
		To verbal command	3
		To pain	2
	No Response		1
Best motor response	To verbal command	Obeys	6
	To painful stimulus*	Localizes pain	5
		Flexion-withdrawal	4
		Flexion-abnormal (Decorticate rigidity)	3
		Extension (Decerebrate rigidity)	2
		No response	1
Best verbal response**		Oriented and converses	5
		Disoriented and converses	4
		Inappropriate words	3
		Incomprehensible sounds	2
		No response	1
Total			3-15

Figure 9–2. The Glasgow coma scale, which is based on eye opening, verbal, and memory responses, is a practical means of monitoring changes in level of consciousness. If each response on the scale is given a number (high for normal and low for impaired responses), the responsiveness of the patient can be expressed by the summation of the figures. The lowest score is 3: the highest is 15. (Modified from Becker, D. P., and Gudeman, S. K.: Textbook of Head Injury. Philadelphia, W. B. Saunders, 1989, p. 388.)

Mental Status

When exploring mental status or consciousness, the critical care nurse assesses arousal and cognition.

Consciousness. The level of consciousness is evaluated by the patient's response to the environment. The highest level of response by the patient is an acknowledgment of the presence of the nurse (i.e., appropriate verbal response, gesture of greeting, eye contact). The lowest level of response by the patient is a lack of any response to the environment. Any change in the level of consciousness is an *early* sign of neurological deterioration and is one of the most important aspects of mental status assessment. Once consciousness is established, the nurse assesses the patient's orientation. Orientation is assessed in terms of person, place, and time.

Language Skills. The second component of mental status to be assessed is language skills. If the patient is not intubated, then it is important to assess his/her ability to talk. It is important to assess the patient's fluency of speech, word-finding difficulty, and whether the speech is spontaneous. An inability to talk is termed expressive aphasia (Dolan, 1991). If the patient is intubated, a similar format is possible by assessing his/her writing skills, which will provide information about expressive ability. The patient with expressive problems comprehends language and will follow command.

The other component of language to assess is the patient's ability to follow verbal commands. The patient may be presented with simple commands requesting that he/she do such simple things as pointing to the clock, pointing to the window, or raising the right arm. Upon successful completion of simple commands, the patient may be presented with a complex command such as raising the right arm and folding a piece of paper. The inability to follow commands is receptive aphasia (Dolan, 1991). The patient with receptive problems and not intubated can speak spontaneously. The verbal response does not follow the context of the conversation owing to the patient's lack of comprehension. The inability of the patient to talk or follow command is global aphasia. These simple tests assess the patient's ability to understand information presented to him/her.

Memory. The third component of mental status to assess is memory. Short-term memory is assessed by asking the patient to *recall* the names of three words or objects after a 3-minute interval. This simple test of recall can be used with the intubated patient. Instead of giving a verbal response to the nurse, the patient would write down the name of words or objects on a piece of paper (i.e., chair, clock, blue). Long-term memory is tested by asking questions about the patient's distant past (i.e., birth place, year of birth, year of graduation from school, year one was married). If the patient is intubated, the patient can write down on a piece of paper the answers to the long-term memory questions.

Cranial Nerve Functioning

Knowing the location of the each cranial nerve (Table 9–1) helps localize the lesion in the brain stem and assists the nurse in identifying specific patient problems related to the cranial nerve deficit. Ten of the twelve cranial nerves are located in the brain stem. On the initial baseline neurological assessment, all cranial nerves should be assessed. Subsequent neurological assessments focus on the cranial nerves II, III, IV, V, VI, VII, IX, and X. These particular cranial nerves regulate pupil response, eye movement, and protective mechanisms. Changes in the functioning of these cranial nerves will help to localize the level of brain stem involvement as well as identify significant changes in neurological status that require nursing intervention.

Cranial Nerve II. Tests for visual acuity, direct light response, and visual fields assess function of cranial nerve II. Testing all of these functions is important initially, but serial assessments can focus on direct light response and visual acuity only.

Cranial Nerves III, IV, and VI. The third cranial nerve is responsible for the consensual light response, elevation of the eyelids, and eye movement.

Cranial nerves III, IV, and VI affect extraocular movements of the eye (EOM's) (Fig. 9–3). When assessing EOM's, the nurse should check

Table 9–1. THE 12 CRANIAL NERVES

Cranial Nerve	Name	Major Functions
I	Olfactory	Smell
II	Optic	Vision
III	Oculomotor	Movements of eyes; pupillary constriction and accommodation
IV	Trochlear	Movements of eyes
V	Trigeminal	Muscles of mastication and eardrum tension; general sensations from anterior half of head, including face, nose, mouth, and meninges
VI	Abducens	Movements of eyes
VII	Facial	Muscles of facial expression and tension on ear bones (stapes); lacrimination and salivation; taste
VIII	Auditory	Hearing and equilibrium reception (vestibulocochlear)
IX	Glossopharyngeal	Swallowing; salivation; taste; visceral sensory
X	Vagus	Swallowing movements and laryngeal control; parasympathetics to thoracic and abdominal viscera
XI	Spinal acessory	Movements of head and shoulders
XII	Hypoglossal	Movements of tongue

From Marshall, S. B., et al.: Neuroscience Critical Care. Philadelphia, W. B. Saunders, 1990.

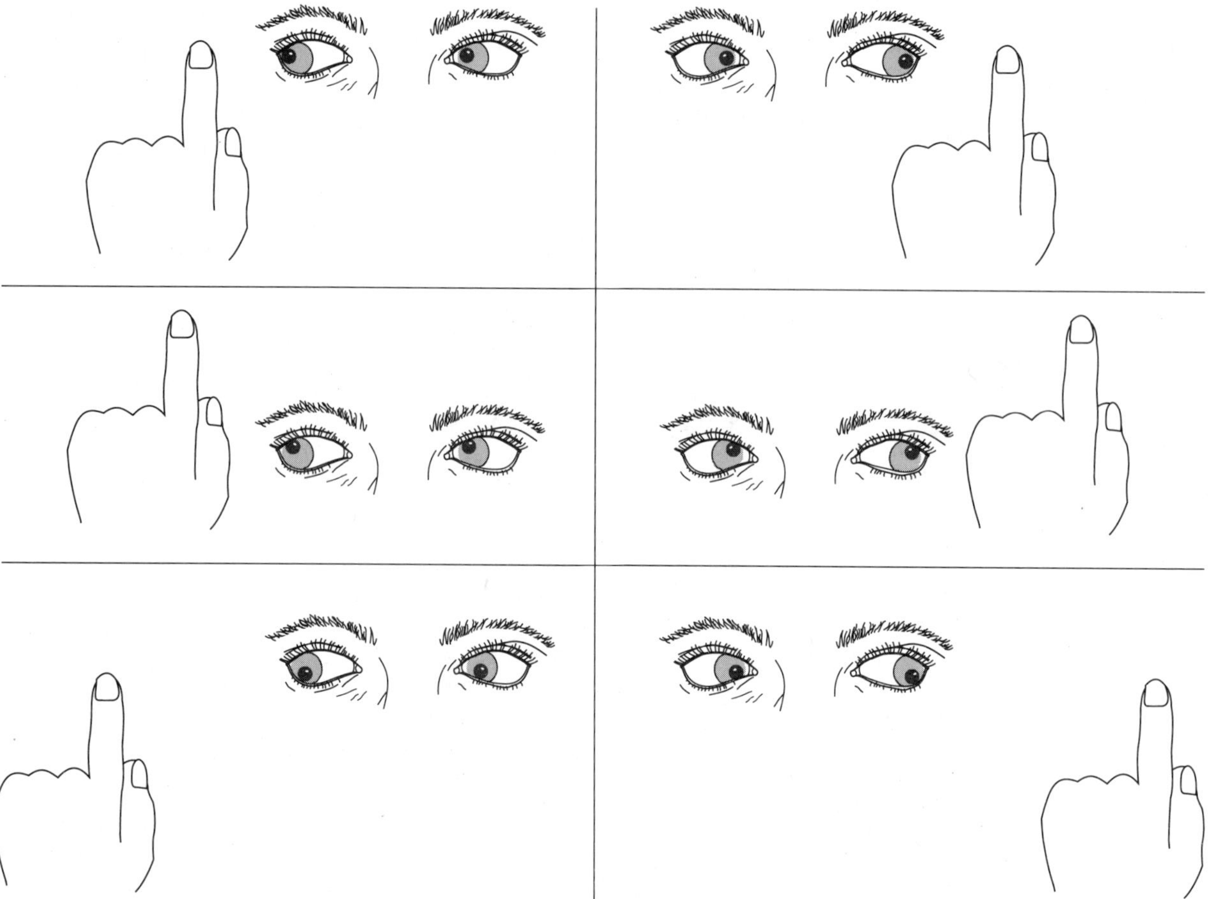

Figure 9-3. Extraocular movements. Patient is instructed to follow examiner's finger without moving the head from side to side or up and down. (From Simpson, J. F., and Magee, K. R.: Clinical Evaluation of the Nervous System. Boston, Little, Brown, 1973, Fig. 12.)

gaze and note the presence of nystagmus. In the unconscious patient, eye movements, as an indication of brain stem activity, are tested by the oculocephalic response (doll's eyes maneuver) (Fig. 9-4). When the doll's eyes maneuver is intact, the eyes move in the opposite direction when the head is turned. Abnormal responses include movement of the eye in same direction as the head or staying midline when the head is turned. An abnormal response indicates a disruption in the processing of information through the brain stem. Contraindications to performing oculocephalic testing include cervical cord injuries and severely increased ICP. An alternative test usually only performed by physicians is the oculovestibular response (ice water calorics). This also tests for brain stem function, but it is believed to be more reliable than the oculocephalic response. To test for the oculovestibular response, the head of the patient's bed is elevated 30 degrees and 30 to 50 ml of iced water is quickly injected into the ear. The normal response, indicating an intact brain stem, is that the eyes move in the direction of the ice water. Any other response is considered abnormal and indicates severe brain stem injury. An abnormal oculovestibular response is an ominous sign.

Examination of the pupils includes checking for size, shape, equality, and light reflex. Normal pupil size, which ranges from 1.5 to 6 mm in diameter, reflects a balance between the sympathetic and parasympathetic innervation. Exact measurement using a millimeter scale (Fig. 9-5) is the most reliable method of determining size and equality. Unequal pupils (anisocoria) normally occur in approximately 10% of the general population. Otherwise, inequality of pupils (greater than 1 mm) is a sign of pathology (i.e., IICP, ischemia, herniation, cervical cord trauma).

The light reflexes are tested with a bright

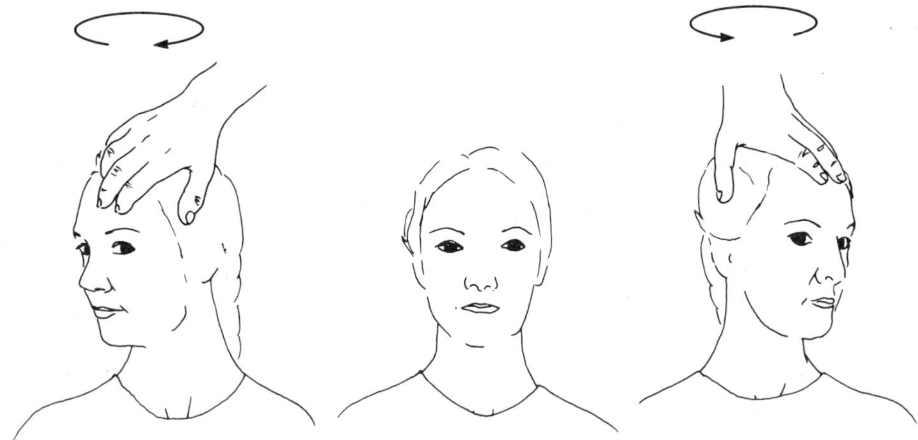

Figure 9–4. Doll's eyes. For doll's eyes to be present the eyes move in the opposite direction when the head is turned. Doll's eyes is absent when the eyes move in the same direction the head is turned or stay midline. (From Mitchell, P., Cammermeyer, M., Ozuna, J., and Woods, N. F.: Neurological Assessment for Nursing Practice. Reston, Virginia, Reston Publishing Co., 1984, Fig. 2–21.)

penlight in dim surrounding light. The direct light reflex is elicited by approaching the eye from the side with a penlight. The pupil should constrict as a response. The consensual light reflex occurs when the contralateral pupil constricts (Fig. 9–6). The rate of pupillary reaction is an important variable to assess. Reaction rates are generally described as brisk, sluggish, or nonreactive. A change from briskly to sluggishly reactive or sluggish to nonreactive is extremely important. These often subtle changes may be an indication of increasing intracranial pressure causing a deterioration in neurological status.

Differences between pupils are also important. For example, pressure on the pathway of the oculomotor nerve may cause the ipsilateral (same side as pressure) pupil to be dilated and sluggish or even nonreactive to light, whereas the contralateral (opposite side of pressure) remains normal in size and reactivity.

Cranial Nerves V, IX, and X. Testing cranial nerves V, IX, and X assesses the protective reflexes. Testing the cranial nerve V determines whether or not the corneal reflex is intact (Fig. 9–7). Observing for a bilateral blink is a way to test cranial nerve V. When there is an asymmetrical blink, a wisp of cotton is used to touch the cornea. The normal response is blinking in that eye. When this reflex is absent or diminished, the patient is at risk of developing a corneal abrasion.

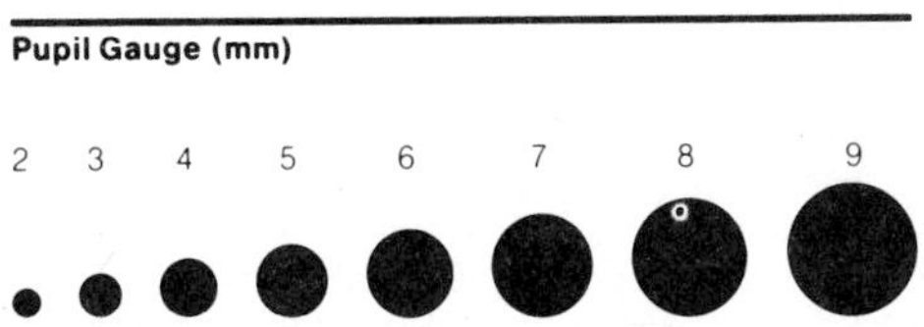

Pupil Gauge (mm)

2 3 4 5 6 7 8 9

Figure 9–5. Pupil gage in millimeters for measuring pupil size. (From Marshall, S. B., Marshall, L. F., Vos, H. R., and Chesnut, R. M.: Neuroscience Critical Care. Philadelphia, W. B. Saunders, 1990.)

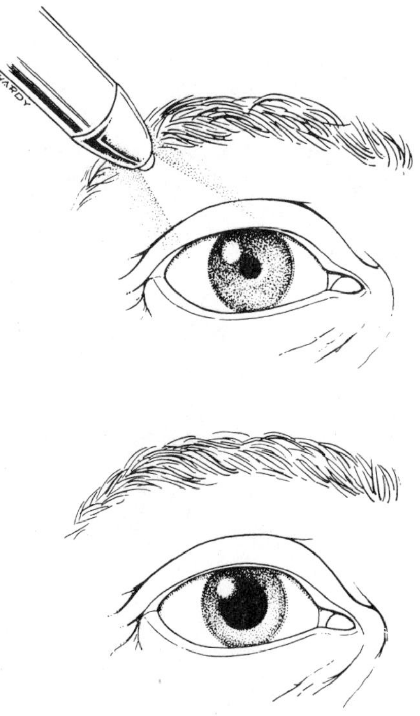

Figure 9–6. Light and accommodation reflexes. *Above,* pupil is constricted, as when exposed to light or near object. *Below,* the pupil is dilated, as when drawn or looking at a distant object. (From Chaffee, E. E., and Lytle, I. M.: Basic Physiology and Anatomy. Philadelphia, J. B. Lippincott, 1980, p. 275.)

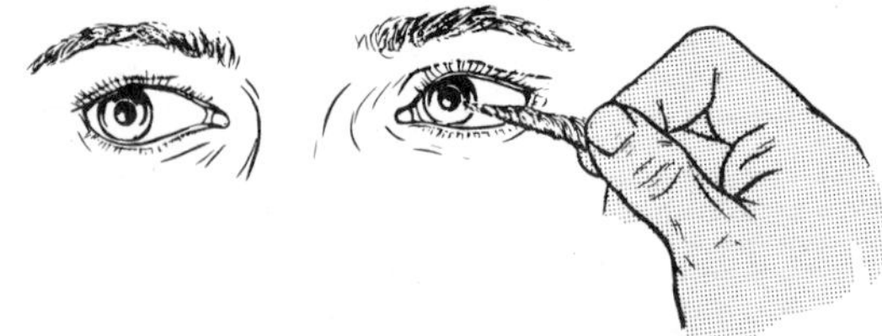

Figure 9-7. Corneal reflex. When spontaneous blinking is absent, the examiner touches a wisp of cotton to the cornea. A normal response is blinking and tearing of the eye stimulated. (From Van Allen, M. W., and Rodnitzky, R. L.: Pictorial Manual of Neurologic Tests. 2nd ed. Chicago, Year Book, 1984, Fig. 16c.)

Testing cranial nerves IX and X assesses the cough, gag, and swallowing reflexes. If the patient is able to follow commands, he/she should be instructed to cough and to swallow. To test the gag reflex, the patient must be asked to open his/her mouth and say "ah." During this maneuver, observe for symmetry, as the soft palate will rise on both sides while the uvula is midline. If the patient is unable to follow command or is unconscious, then stimulating the pharyngeal wall will elicit a "retching" response (Fig. 9-8). It is very important to have the head of the bed elevated 30 degrees with the patient lying on his/her side prior to testing the gag reflex. When these reflexes are diminished or absent, the patient experiences difficulty handling secretions and oral intake and is at risk of aspiration.

Cranial Nerves VII and XII. Testing the facial nerve (cranial nerve VII) requires the nurse to observe facial expression. Asking the patient to smile, frown, and puff out the cheeks accomplishes this goal of observing expression.

Cranial nerve XII moves the tongue and is assessed by asking the patient to stick out his/her tongue and move it from side to side. The nurse is observing for symmetry of movement. The nurse also inspects the surface of the tongue for atrophy.

Motor Status

Many centers of the brain are responsible for movement; therefore, motor assessment will detect the extent of damage to the motor system. In the assessment of the motor system, the nurse will focus on spontaneous movement of all extremities, muscle strength, muscle tone, coordination, and abnormal postures/reflexes, since muscle groups are assessed for symmetry.

Spontaneous Movement. This can be assessed by asking the patient to move the extremities on command or by observation while the patient moves around in bed. It is also important to notice and document changes in spontaneous movement.

Testing generalized muscle strength in the conscious patient consists of the performance of the drift test by the patient (Fig. 9-9). This test is very sensitive to the subtle changes in strength secondary to neurological deterioration. Lower extremity strength is tested by asking the patient to push his/her feet against the nurse's hands (Fig. 9-10). Patients with brain pathology are

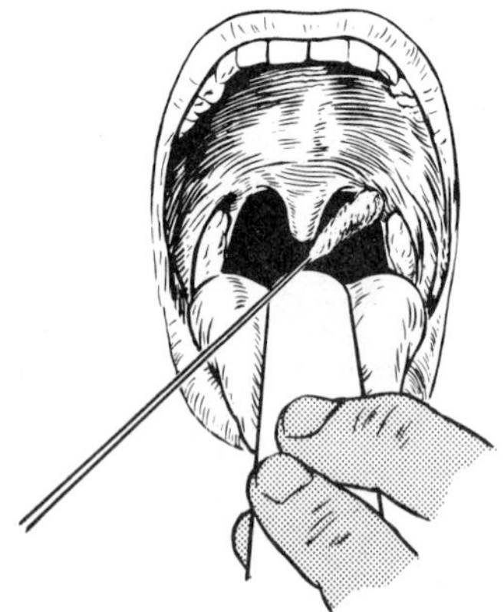

Figure 9-8. The gag reflex. In the conscious patient, ask the patient to say "ah." The examiner observes the rise of the soft palate and the midline uvula. In the unconscious patient, stimulate the posterior pharynx and observe the same response. (From Van Allen, M. W., and Rodnitzky, R. L.: Pictorial Manual of Neurologic Tests. 2nd ed. Chicago, Year Book, 1984, Fig. 20.)

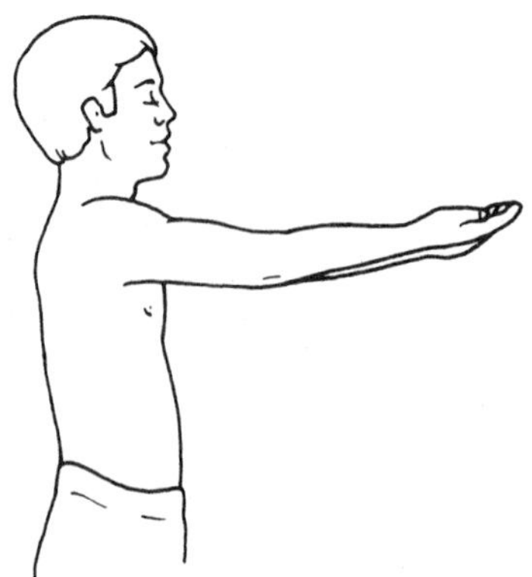

Figure 9-9. Drift test. With the eyes closed, the patient's arms are held straight out in front with the palms up for 20-30 sec. Watch how patient holds this position. Tendency to drift downward and pronating palms is a sign of muscle weakness. (From Hickey, J. V.: The Clinical Practice of Neurological Neurosurgical Nursing. 2nd ed. Philadelphia, J. B. Lippincott, 1986.)

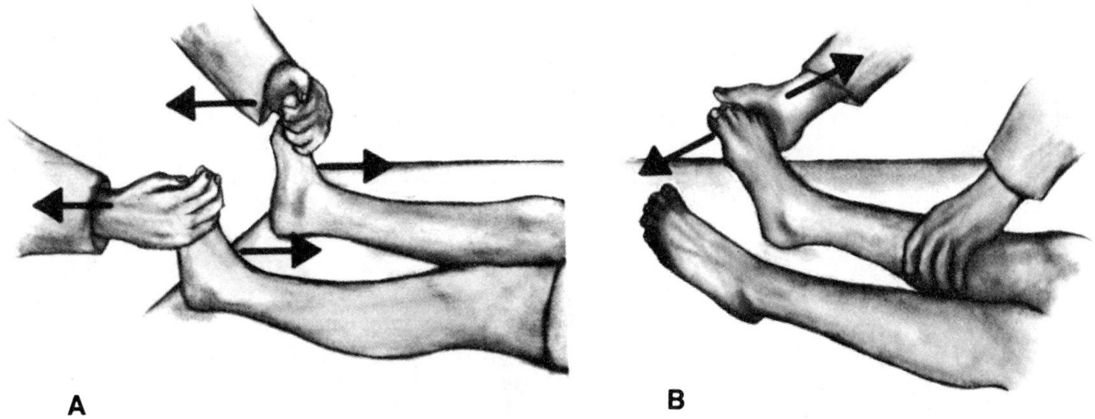

Figure 9-10. Testing lower extremity strength. *A*, Testing for dorsiflexion, and *B*, plantarflexion. (From Hickey, J. V.: The Clinical Practice of Neurological Neurosurgical Nursing. 2nd ed. Philadelphia, J. B. Lippincott, 1986, p. 80.)

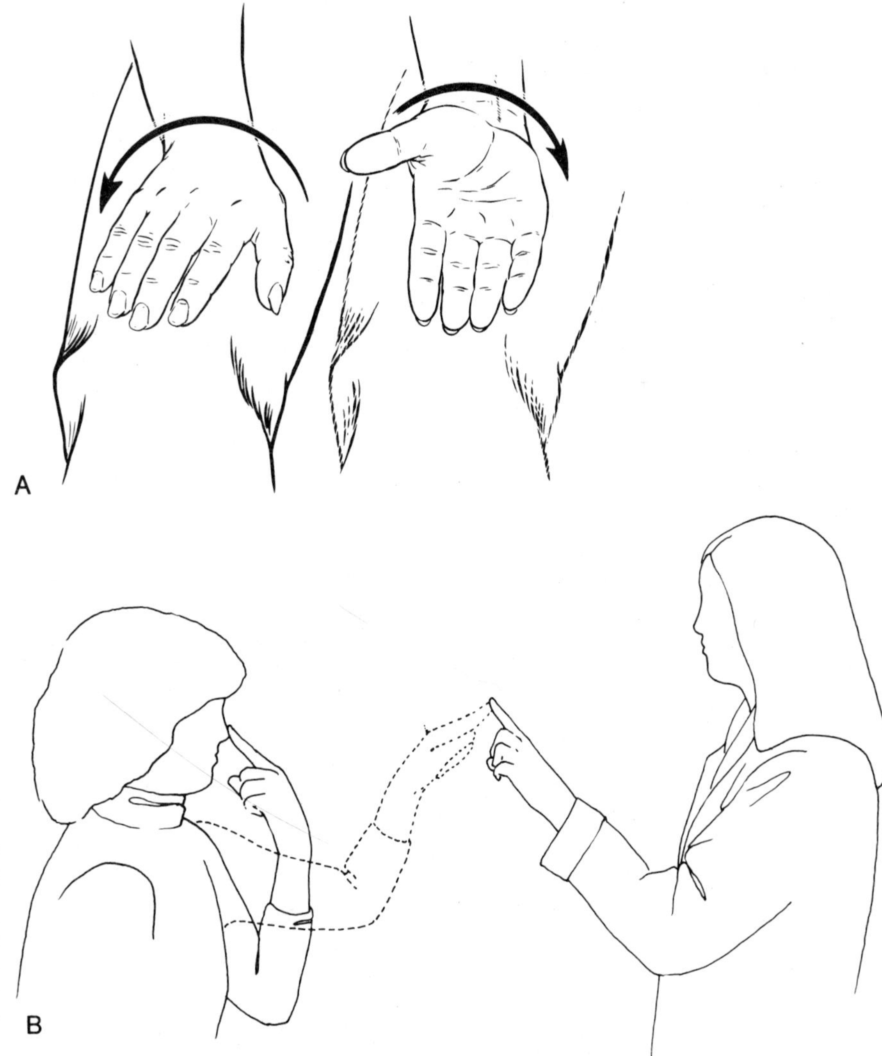

Figure 9-11. Tests for coordination. *A*, Alternating movements. *B*, Finger-to-nose test. A normal response is accurate, rapid, and coordinated. (*A* from Van Allen, M. W., Rodnitsky, R. L.: Pictorial Manual of Neurologic Tests. 2nd ed. Chicago, Year Book, 1984, Fig. 27a. *B* from Mitchell, P., Cammermeyer, M., Ozuna, J., and Woods, N. F.: Neurological Assessment for Nursing Practice. Reston, Virginia, Reston Publishing Co., 1984, Fig 2-10.)

told to exhale through the mouth during this test to avoid breath holding that could cause IICP. Specific muscle groups can be tested by exerting resistance ("push-pull") to the specific muscle group. It is possible to get an estimate of muscle strength in the patient who inconsistently follows commands or is restless. Attempts at pushing the patient's outstretched arms or legs down is one method of assessing strength informally. Unfortunately, it is not possible to test strength in the unconscious patient.

Muscle Tone. This is assessed by taking each extremity through a passive range of motion. Normal muscle tone shows slight resistance to the range of motion. Limp, flabby muscles are characterized by decreased or loss of tone, so there is no resistance to movement. Increased muscle tone is characterized by spasticity and rigidity, resulting in an increased resistance of muscle groups to range of motion.

Coordination of Movement. Coordination of movement is under cerebellar control. It can be assessed by asking the patient to perform rapid alternating movements or by placing the finger to the nose or have the patient run the heel down the shin bilaterally (Fig. 9-11). These tests require the patient to be able to follow verbal commands.

Abnormal Postures/Reflexes. Assessment for abnormal postures and reflexes is important in the brain-injured patient.

Hemiplegia. Early hemiplegia occurs when one side of the patient's body stops moving spontaneously and becomes paretic. This state indicates a cortical lesion and is a sign of further neurological deterioration secondary to a mass effect. The lesion (i.e., cerebral edema, hematoma, tumor) is compressing the motor fibers in the motor strip in the frontal lobe. Prolonged compression on motor fibers leads to paralysis.

Decorticate Rigidity. The second abnormal posture is decorticate rigidity (Fig. 9-12). This

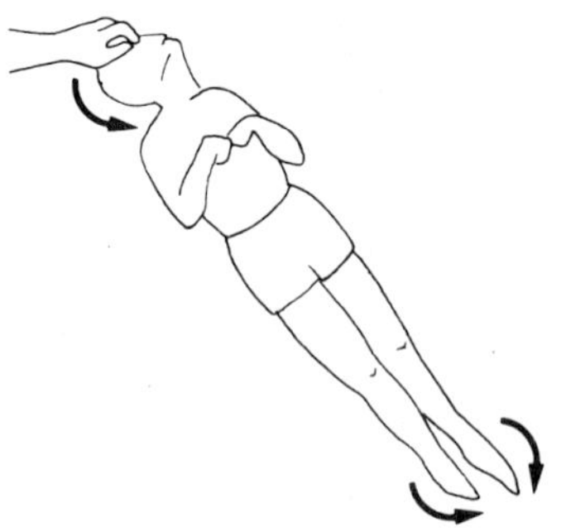

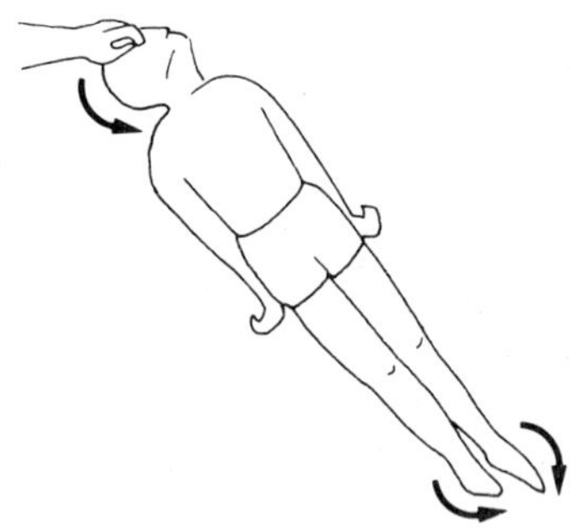

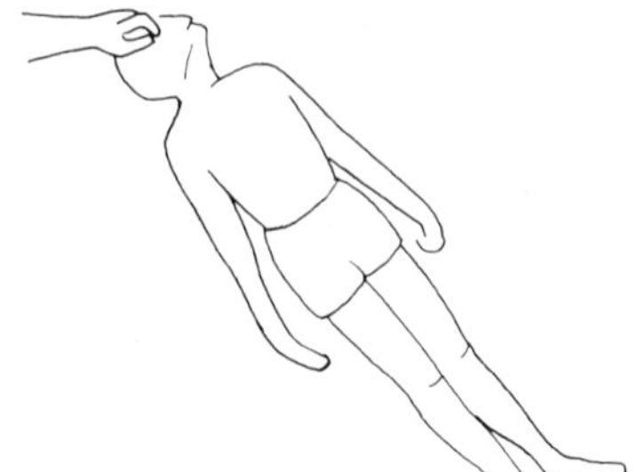

Figure 9-12. Abnormal postures. (From Marshall, S. B., Marshall, L. F., Vos, H. R., and Chesnut, R. M.: Neuroscience Critical Care. Philadelphia, W. B. Saunders, 1990.)

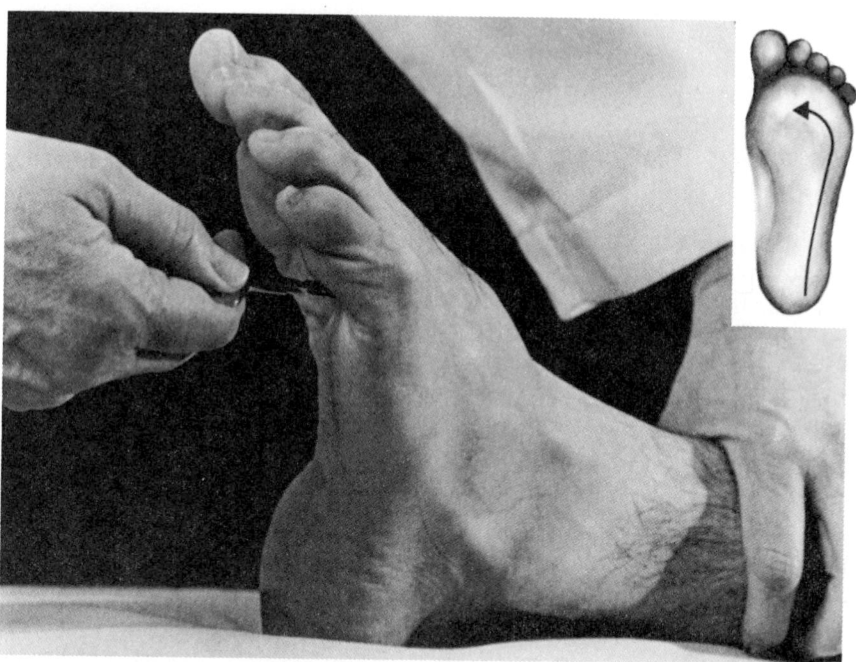

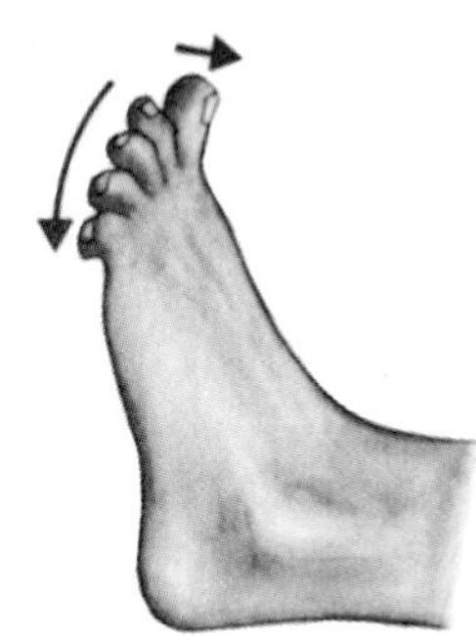

Figure 9-13. Babinski reflex. With a moderately sharp object, such as a key, stroke the lateral aspect of the sole from the heel to the ball of the foot, curving medially across the ball. Use the lightest stimulus that will provoke a response. Note movement of the toes, normally flexion. (Dorsiflexion of the great toe with fanning of the other toes indicates upper motor neuron disease.) (From Bates, B.: Guide to Physical Examination. Philadelphia, J. B. Lippincott, 1991, p. 537.)

posture can be the result of a cortical, subcortical, or diencephalon lesion. Characteristics of this posture are flexion of the upper extremities and extension with internal rotation of the lower extremities. Decerebrate posturing is the result of a midbrain or pons lesion. In this posture, the patient's jaws are clenched, extremities in full extension, feet in plantar extension, forearms pronated, and wrists and fingers flexed (Fig. 9-12).

In bilateral flaccidity there is no response to noxious stimuli (Fig. 9-12).

Both decerebrate and decorticate posturing can occur in response to noxious stimuli such as suctioning or pain.

Babinski Reflex. The major pathological deep tendon reflex is the Babinski reflex (Fig. 9-13). This reflex is assessed during the initial baseline assessment and periodically thereafter. The presence of a Babinski reflex is a sign of an upper motor neuron lesion and damage to the corticospinal tract in the adult. All of the assessments already discussed provide a complete neurological evaluation of the critically ill. In addition, the nurse also assesses the neurological parameters every 1 to 2 hours. Table 9-2 contains the components for hourly assessments for the patient with increased intracranial pressure, head injury, and CVA.

Table 9-2. COMPONENTS OF THE HOURLY NEUROLOGICAL ASSESSMENT FOR PATIENTS WITH IICP, HEAD INJURY, OR CVA

Mental Status	Focal Motor	Pupils	Brain Stem/Cranial Nerves
Glasgow Coma Scale Assesses level of consciousness, expressive language, ability to follow command	Move all extremities Strength all extremities (compares right and left side) Motor response (Glasgow Coma Scale)	Size Shape Reaction to light (direct and consensual) EOMs	Corneal reflex Present—immediate blinking bilaterally Diminished—blinking asymmetrically Absent—no blinking Doll's eyes (unconscious patient—no spinal fracture) Cough, gag, swallow reflex Observe for excessive drooling Observe for cough/swallow reflex

Vital Signs

Changes in vital signs appear late in the course of neurological dysfunction. Patients with neurological dysfunction are managed to limit extreme fluctuations in vital signs, since fluctuations can increase damage. Hyperthermia causes an increase in the metabolic demands of neurons, whereas extreme hypothermia leads to cardiac dysrhythmias. Respiratory changes correlate with lesions at various levels of injury; therefore, changes in respiratory rate, rhythm, and depth are important to note. Pulse and blood pressure changes are unreliable as part of the overall assessment. Both of these parameters are seen late in the course of IICP.

The Cushing reflex is a late sign of intracranial pressure and consists of a widening pulse pressure (systolic pressure rises faster than diastolic pressure) and bradycardia. It is essential that the nurse recognize that these changes occur late and, if they are the only assessment parameter used, the patient may have experienced severe damage by the time vital sign changes are seen.

Other Assessment Parameters

Other assessment parameters for the patient with IICP include ICP, arterial, and hemodynamic monitoring.

Intracranial Pressure Monitoring. The use of intracranial pressure monitoring is controversial; therefore, the benefits of ICP monitoring must outweigh the associated risk of morbidity.

Intracranial pressure can be measured continuously via the intraparenchymal, intraventricular, subarachnoid, and epidural catheters (Fig. 9–14). Intracranial pressure monitoring is indicated when ICP rises to 20 mm Hg. The mean ICP reading is taken at the end of the respiratory cycle and before inspiration. There are four types of ICP monitoring devices: intraparenchymal probe, intraventricular catheter, epidural probe, and subarachnoid bolt.

Intraparenchymal Fiberoptic Probe. The intraparenchymal fiberoptic probe (see Fig. 9–14a) is inserted into nondominant brain tissue. This device measures brain tissue pressure. The probe is connected to a monitor that has an analog reading and can interface with a monitor to visualize a waveform. The quality of the waveform and pressure readings are very similar to the intraventricular catheter. It is reported the intraparenchymal pressure readings are 3 to 5 mm Hg higher than the intraventricular readings (Ostrup et al., 1987). There are several advantages of this fiberoptic system: (1) its easy insertion; (2) it causes minimal trauma to tissue because of its small diameter (French); (3) the transducer is in the tip of the probe, so there is no concern related to the level of the transducer; and (4) it is associated with a lower incidence of infection because the intraparenchymal fiberoptic probe is not an air- or fluid-filled system (Ostrup et al., 1987). The major disadvantage of this system is that the fiberoptic probe is fragile and can break. If breakage occurs, then a new fiberoptic probe must be inserted. A second disadvantage of this new monitor device is the expense of the equipment.

Intraventricular Catheter. The intraventricular catheter is inserted into the lateral ventricle of the nondominant cerebral hemisphere. The catheter is connected by a stopcock to fluid-filled pressure tubing to a transducer (see Fig. 9–14b) that is positioned at the level of the foramen of Monro (middle of the ear as a reference point). The major advantages of this system includes accurate CSF pressure readings, therapeutic draining of CSF, and withdrawal of CSF for laboratory analysis (Franges and Beideman, 1988; German, 1988; Hudak et al., 1986). Disadvantages of this system include the risk of infection, unnecessary loss of CSF, and difficult insertion if the ventricles are small or displaced.

Epidural Probe. The epidural probe is placed between the skull and the dura mater in the epidural space (see Fig. 9–14c). Advantages of this monitoring system include the capability to monitor ICP without tearing the dura mater and reducing intracerebral infection. The major disadvantage is inaccurate pressure readings at high ICP levels.

Subarachnoid Bolt. The fourth intracranial pressure system is the subarachnoid bolt, placed in the subarachnoid space (see Fig. 9–14d). Advantages of this system include accuracy of CSF pressure measurement and ease of insertion. Major disadvantages of this system include frequent irrigations needed to maintain patency of the system and increased risk of infection.

Intraventricular and subarachnoid systems are maintained as closed systems to avoid contamination and infection. Another important consideration is maintaining the transducer at the level of the foramen of Monro (middle of the ear). In addition to leveling the transducer, zero balancing and keeping bubbles out of tubing will enhance the accuracy of the readings.

Hemodynamic Monitoring. All types of monitoring systems allow nurses to observe an ICP

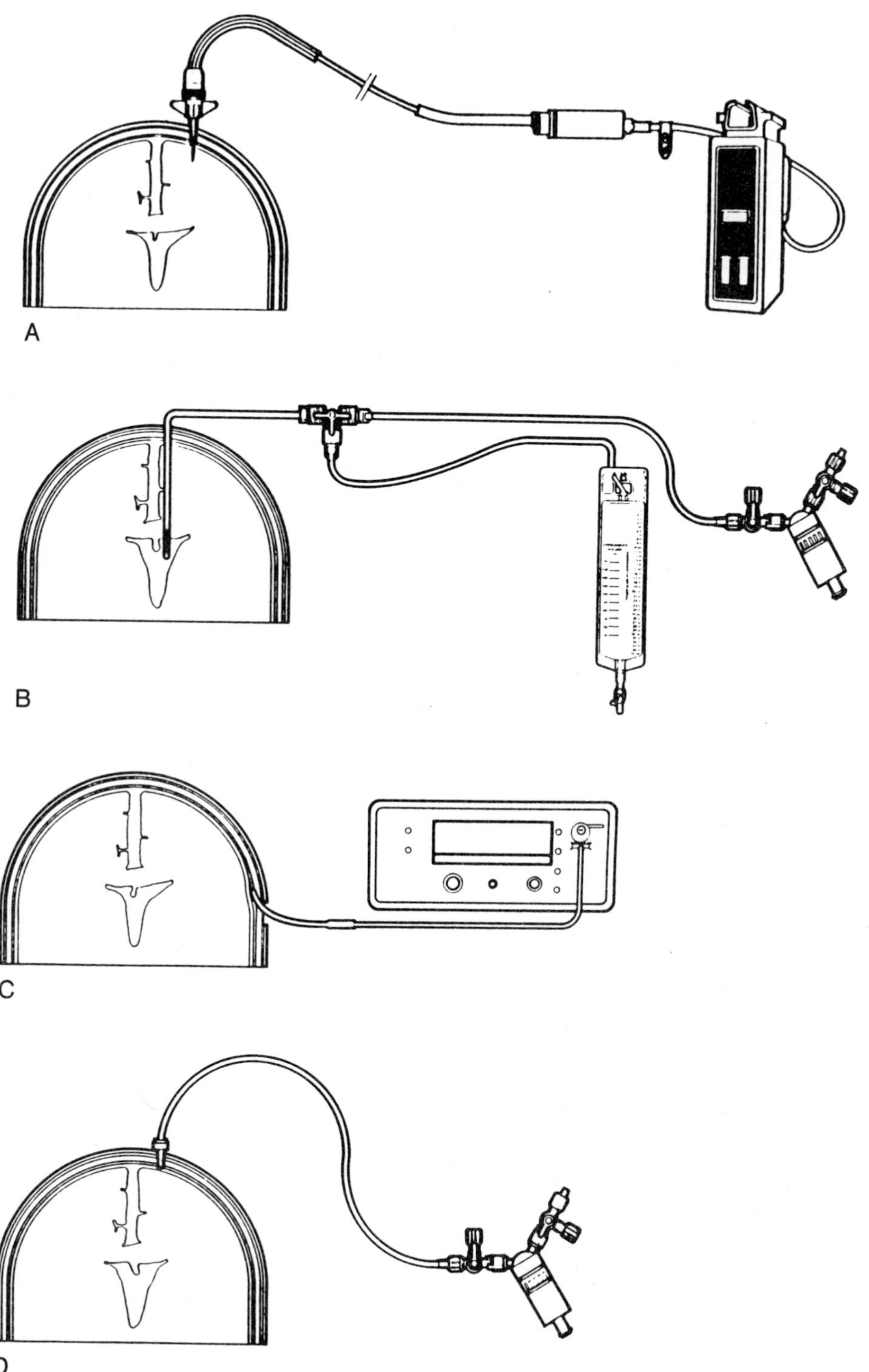

Figure 9-14. *A*, Intraparenchymal monitoring system. *B*, Intraventricular monitoring system. *C*, Epidural monitoring system. *D*, Subdural monitoring system. (Courtesy of Camino Laboratories, San Diego, California.)

waveform pattern. There are three types of waveforms (Fig. 9–15).

A waves (plateau waves) are waves between 50 and 100 mm Hg. These waves are associated with advanced intracranial hypertension. B waves less than 50 mm Hg correspond to respirations. B waves may serve as a warning to the nurse of the *potential* risk of intracranial pressure and impairment of intracranial compliance (Marshall et al., 1990). C waves are small waves (16 to 20 mm Hg) that correlate with changes in blood pressure and respirations. C waves lack clinical significance.

In assessing ICP, the nurse utilizes information about waveforms and potential changes to assure patient safety (see Fig. 9–15). Hemodynamic monitoring allows direct measurement of pulmonary artery and other pressures. These measurements are important for fluid management and overall management of the cardiovascular system. A potential problem common for the critically ill neurological patient receiving diuretic therapy and fluid restriction is dehydration. Monitoring pulmonary artery wedge (PAW) and pulmonary artery (PA) pressures allows the nurse to assess fluid status and prevent dehydration that could lead to hypotension and decreased cerebral blood flow. The PAW pressure is maintained in the range of 8 to 12 mm Hg (Marshall et al., 1990). The PA mean pressure range is 8 to 24 mm Hg (Marshall et al., 1990). The readings of PA and PAW should be taken at end expiration to minimize false readings affected by increased intrathoracic pressure (see Chap. 4).

Arterial Monitoring. Accurate assessment of arterial pressure is essential because it has a dramatic effect on ICP. Therefore, arterial pressure monitoring is frequently used for the patient with IICP. Arterial blood gas analysis to track the pH, PaO_2, $PaCO_2$, and O_2 saturation is also important because these substances have a significant effect on the cerebral vasculature.

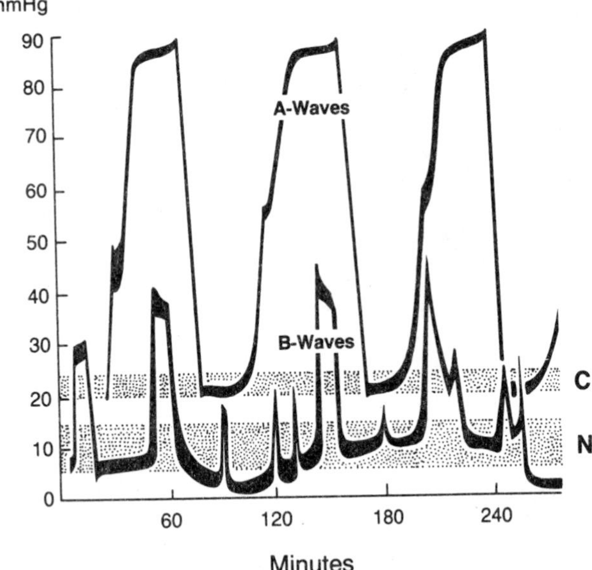

Figure 9–15. Intracranial pressure waveforms. Waveforms reflect pressure in mm Hg and time in minutes. Two abnormal waveforms are depicted, including A waves and B waves. A waves reflect intracranial pressure in the range of 50 to 100 mm Hg. They have a duration of 5–20 min or longer. Their waveforms have a distinctive plateau and they are referred to as "plateau" waves. B waves occur as sharp, peaked (saw-tooth pattern) rhythmic oscillations, which may reach a peak pressure of 50 mm Hg. They have a duration of 0.5–2.0 min. N refers to "normal" intracranial pressure waveforms and reflects a pressure within the range of 0 to 15 mm Hg. C refers to the pressure waveform for C waves. C waves are usually rapid, rhythmic waves with an amplitude of about 20 mm Hg. They occur every 4–8 min. (From Dolan, J. T. (ed.): Critical Care Nursing: Clinical Management Through the Nursing Process. Philadelphia, F. A. Davis, 1991, p. 93.)

Medical Assessment

The initial baseline laboratory tests obtained in the patient with IICP are the following:

* Arterial blood gases (ABGs)
* CBC (emphasis on RBC, Hct, Hgb)
* Coagulation profile (PT, PTT, platelet count)
* Electrolytes, BUN, creatinine, liver functions, serum osmolality
* Urinalysis, urine osmolality

The ongoing laboratory tests obtained in the patient with IICP are the following:

* ABGs
* Hct, Hgb
* Electrolytes, BUN, creatinine, serum osmolality

The x-rays and other diagnostic tests performed on the patient with IICP include the following:

* Computed tomography (CT scan)
* Skull x-rays
* EEG
* Cerebral blood flow studies
* Cerebral angiography

NURSING DIAGNOSIS

Nursing diagnoses appropriate for the patient experiencing increased intracranial pressure are:

* Decreased adaptive capacity: intracranial related to neurological illness/trauma
* Potential altered cerebral tissue perfusion related to IICP; decreased cerebral blood flow hypertension/hypotension
* Potential for ineffective breathing pattern/impaired gas exchange related to underlying neurological and respiratory problems
* Ineffective airway clearance related to cranial nerve impairment, obstruction in respiratory system, respiratory infections, and underlying neurological problem
* Fluid and electrolyte imbalance related to underlying neurological problem and treatment of IICP
* Altered nutritional status less than normal related to a hypermetabolic state following trauma/surgery
* Impaired mobility related to injury to the motor pathways in the brain
* Potential for infection related to invasive techniques and steroid therapy
* Altered thought processes related to IICP and structural damage ischemia
* Self-care deficit: activities of daily living related to the neurological deficits
* Potential for injury related to impaired mobility, memory/judgment, decreased attention span, and impulsiveness
* Ineffective family coping patterns related to the patient's neurological deficits

INTERVENTIONS

Nursing Interventions

Objectives of nursing management for the patient with increased intracranial pressure incorporate the following:

* Maintaining a normal intracranial pressure
* Maintaining adequate cerebral blood flow that is well oxygenated
* Maintenance of fluid and electrolyte balance
* Minimizing the hypermetabolic state, muscle wasting, and weight loss
* Prevention of the hazards of immobility
* Prevention of infections
* Minimization of impaired thought processes
* Protection from injury
* Promotion of self-care
* Promotion of effective family coping

Refer to the Nursing Care Plan for the Patient with Increased ICP, Head Injury, or CVA for a detailed description of specific nursing interventions.

General Nursing Care

For the last 20 years, nurse researchers have identified some nursing activities (i.e., suctioning, head positioning, repositioning, and hygiene measures) that are associated with increases in intracranial pressure (Boortz-Martz, 1985; Hulme and Cooper, 1976; Mitchell and Mauss, 1978; Mitchell et al., 1980; Snyder, 1983; Parsons and Shogan, 1984; Parsons et al., 1985). The ICP response to nursing activities is an individual patient response depending on the patient's position on the volume-pressure curve.

Head and body position is an important factor in minimizing IICP. Elevating the head of the bed 30 degrees and keeping the head in a neutral position in relation to the body facilitates venous drainage and decreases the risk for venous obstruction. When the head is turned 45 degrees, increases in ICP can occur. This is because the jugular vein becomes obstructed and venous drainage is impeded. Extreme hip flexion also causes elevation in ICP. Extreme hip flexion causes an increase in intra-abdominal and intrathoracic pressure and results in IICP.

Frequently, patients with IICP are fluid restricted. The goal of fluid restriction is to maintain intravascular volume without adding free water. An increase in free water (extracellular fluid excess) would increase cerebral edema and further increase ICP. Strict measurement of intake and output is required. When osmotic and loop diuretics are used, it is critical to monitor fluid and electrolyte status. Hypokalemia is common after mannitol therapy. This electrolyte imbalance is corrected with a potassium supplement. An elevation of serum osmolarity can occur with osmotic diuretic use. Hyperosmolarity can result in renal failure, neurological deterioration, and death if not corrected. Other factors leading to fluid and electrolyte imbalance are diabetes insipidus (DI) and the syndrome of inappropriate antidiuretic hormone (SIADH); either can occur with brain injury.

Hyperthermia increases the metabolic demand of brain cells, causing an increase in cerebral blood flow and IICP. Therefore, the body temperature should not exceed 38°C. Patients with neurological injury affecting the hypothalamus are particularly prone to temperature fluctuations. Often, they respond directly to environmental temperatures. Therefore, the envi-

NURSING CARE PLAN FOR THE PATIENT WITH INCREASED ICP, HEAD INJURY, OR CVA		
Nursing Diagnosis	**Outcome**	**Intervention**
Decreased adaptive capacity: Intracranial related to neurological illness/trauma	Intracranial pressure at rest will be within the range of 0-15 mm Hg Cerebral perfusion pressure (CPP) will be maintained at >60 mm Hg CPP = MAP − ICP Temperature 38°C Maintain head and body alignment Patient is awake and exhibits appropriate responses to the environment Absence of headaches ABGs WNL	Neurological assessments every hour Notify physician of changes Maintain airway Monitor ICP measurements continuously Record and report changes in readings Notify if CPP ≤ 60 mm Hg Elevate HOB 30-45° Monitor response to all nursing activities for increases in ICP Maintain head in neutral position Avoid extreme hip flexion, isometric exercises, straining with stool, breath-holding episodes IV fluids Fluid restriction as ordered (range 80-100 ml/hr) Do not suction for more than 15 sec at a time Hyperoxygenate with suctioning (pre and post) Maintain quiet environment Space nursing activities to avoid accumulative effect Monitor fluid and electrolyte status Monitor electrolytes, Hgb and Hct, BUN, creatinine Record I&O Administer medications as ordered (steroids, diuretics, anticonvulsants) Monitor side effects of medications Maintain temp at 38°C using hypothermia blanket, antipyretics Monitor ABGs—report if abnormal
Potential altered cerebral tissue perfusion related to IICP, decreased cerebral blood flow, hypertension/hypotension	Mean arterial pressure range 63-124 mm Hg Systolic BP 100-140 mm Hg Diastolic range 60-90 mm Hg Stable VS Urine output ≥30 ml/hr Hgb/Hct, WNL Normal sinus rhythm CVP 3-10 mm Hg PAWP 5-15 mm Hg Improved neurological status, especially LOC ABGs WNL No complications of therapy	Neurological assessment every hour Monitor BP and pulse every hour or as ordered Monitor correlation between BP and neurological status Monitor respiratory status Monitor ECG pattern continuously CVP and PAP as ordered Hourly urine outputs Specific gravity every 2 hr Check for hematuria Assess for signs of bleeding from chest, abdomen, pelvis, extremities Control scalp bleeding by compression Administer volume expanders (albumin, Plasmanate, blood products) Calm, quiet environment Administer medications as ordered Monitor effects of medications (antihypertensive agents, heparin, warfarin, antifibrinolytic agents) Administer medications for vasospasm (calcium channel blockers, steroid therapy, fibrinolytic agents [streptokinase]) Minimize restlessness and agitation Monitor electrolytes, Hgb/Hct, serum osmolality, ABGs Report if lab results are abnormal Monitor temperature, report if abnormal
Potential for ineffective breathing pattern/impaired gas exchange related to underlying neurological and respiratory problems	Maintain airway Vital capacity 60-75 ml/kg ABGs WNL O_2 saturation WNL 96% Breath sounds bilaterally	Monitor respiratory rate and rhythm Assess breath sounds every hour for 72 hr then prn Observe for anxiety, restlessness, trouble breathing Assist with clearing secretions with suctioning

NURSING CARE PLAN FOR THE PATIENT WITH INCREASED ICP, HEAD INJURY, OR CVA *Continued*		
Nursing Diagnosis	**Outcome**	**Intervention**
Ineffective airway clearance related to cranial nerve impairment, obstruction in respiratory system, and underlying neurological problem	CXR WNL No atelectasis/pneumonia Temp WNL No dyspnea, tachypnea No restlessness or anxiety Free from mucous plugs	Maintain patency of endotracheal tube or tracheostomy tube Observe for tolerance for turning on special beds Chest physiotherapy Administer antibodies as ordered Monitor O_2 saturation with arterial live or pulse oximeter Administer O_2 as needed Gradually decrease ventilatory assistance Assess for fatigue
Fluid volume deficit Electrolyte imbalance related to fluid restriction, diuretics, GI suction, DI, and SIADH	Urine output >30 ml/hr <200 ml/hr Good skin turgor Maintain admission weight Electrolytes, BUN, creatinine, Hct, WNL Serum osmolality <320 mOsm Normal sinus rhythm on rhythmic strip Normothermic Moist mucous membranes	Assess skin and mucous every 2 hr Foley catheter for strict I&O Report urine outputs <30 ml/hr or >200 ml/hr every 2 hr Weigh daily Monitor lab results: electrolytes, BUN, creatinine, Hct, Hgb, serum osmolality Monitor ECG Monitor temperature every 2 hr
Altered nutritional status < normal related to the hypermetabolic state	Maintenance of admission weight Absence of vomiting Absence of abdominal distention Bowel sounds present and active Absence of impaction Absorbing tube feeding Serum proteins and albumin WNL Positive nitrogen balance	Early nutritional support Auscultate bowel sounds prior to intermittent NG tube feeding or prn Palpate abdomen for distention Salem pump or NG tube for abdominal distention on low continuous suction Daily weights Monitor electrolytes, BUN, creatinine, Hct, Hgb, serum proteins Enteral nutrition Parenteral nutrition Check for NG tube residual when tube feedings are initiated Aseptic technique when manipulating central lines Don't infuse other fluids through line for nutritional support Monitor every hour Assess abdomen distention Record bowel evacuation Metamucil for diarrhea per order I&O
Impaired mobility related to increased ICP, head injury, CVA	Intact motor and sensory function on unaffected side Absence of edema Absence of thrombosis Absence of atelectasis Absence of skin breakdown	Neurological assessment Change positions every 2 hr (unless contraindicated by ICP) Skin assessment Range-of-motion of extremities prevent footdrop (i.e., high-top tennis shoes on 2 hr, off 2 hr, footboard) Monitor for local swelling, calf measurement Monitor color, temp, tenderness/pain over veins Antiembolism stockings Apply moist heat to area as ordered Anticoagulant therapy as ordered Monitor PT, PTT, Hct, Hgb, platelets Normal CXR Breath sounds present
Potential for infection related to invasive techniques and steroid therapy	Afebrile WBC WNL Negative cultures	Wash hands prior to contact with patient Aseptic technique when performing invasive procedures and working with patients, catheters, tubes

continued

NURSING CARE PLAN FOR THE PATIENT WITH INCREASED ICP, HEAD INJURY, OR CVA *Continued*

Nursing Diagnosis	Outcome	Intervention
		Discontinue invasive lines, catheters ASAP Use gloves when performing nursing activities Minimize patient exposure to infected staff/visitors Monitor results of CBC, report CBC abnormalities Obtain cultures and report abnormalities Monitor VS Assess VS, body fluids, skin for signs and symptoms of infection and report abnormalities Keep ICP and hemodynamic monitor devices a closed system Administer antibodies as ordered
Altered thought processes related to IICP	Appropriate behavior patterns Appropriate verbalizations Minimal memory impairments	Explain nursing activities prior to initiation Orient to person, place, time: Use clocks and calendars in patient room to help orient Avoid sensory overload Allow for frequent rest periods Provide a structured environment Continuity of staff taking care of patient Place call light, water, tissues within reach Identify objects by name Involve significant other in care and goal setting Identify behaviors occurring as a result of inaccurate thoughts and document these behaviors Teach patient, family, significant other in strategies to deal with altered behaviors Speak slowly, using concrete thoughts and allowing adequate response time from patient
Self-care deficit in activities of daily living (ADLs) related to the neurological problem	Perform self-care activities without a change in vital signs or ICP	Assist patient as necessary Monitor energy requirements and expenditure for self-care activity Assess activity tolerance (monitor heart rate) Assist in positioning patient for ADLs Keep objects within easy reach of patient Schedule frequent rest periods
Potential for injury related to impaired mobility, memory/judgment, decreased attention span, and impulsiveness	No falling No bruising from use of physical restraints Patient asks for assistance when needed	Identify certain behaviors that may increase risk for injury: restless, agitated, impulsive, short attention span Assess judgment and decision-making ability Remove clutter from environment Examine environment for potential risks
Ineffective family coping patterns related to the neurological problem	Verbalizes need for more information related to disease process or particular situation Discuss changes in patient/family as a result of neurological problem Demonstrates understanding of information given Decreased anxiety Significant other participates in care of patient Verbalizes feelings to nurses/other family members	Assess areas in which a knowledge deficit exists Provide adequate and correct information to patient/family Discuss usual reactions to neurological problem: stress, anxiety, inattention, depression, dependency Assess prior and coping skill and try to enhance those skills in dealing with current situation Provide information on routine care, hospital routines and services Assist family members to recognize roles to maintain family integrity Involve family members in care of patient Encourage the use of additional support systems—friends, clergy, professional health care providers

Data from Kim, M. J., et al.: Pocket Guide to Nursing Diagnoses. 2nd ed. St. Louis, C. V. Mosby, 1987; and Marshall, S. B., et al.: Neuroscience Critical Care. Philadelphia, W. B. Saunders, 1990.

ronmental temperature is kept cool for their safety.

Medical (Nonsurgical) Treatment

The first task of the physician is to decrease ICP and then identify the cause. Once the cause is discovered, treatment is centered on permanently decreasing the high intracranial pressure; maintaining the airway, providing ventilation and oxygenation; maintaining cerebral perfusion pressure; and decreasing the metabolic demands placed on the injured brain. Many of these medical interventions are used individually or in combination with each other.

Medical treatment of IICP usually includes hyperventilation, osmotic and loop diuretics, positioning, fluid restriction, corticosteroids, oxygenation, maintaining blood pressure, and decreasing the metabolic demand of injured brain cells.

Acute hyperventilation decreases PCO_2, causing vasoconstriction of the cerebral arteries, reducing cerebral blood flow, and decreasing IICP. Using hyperventilation over a long period of time is very controversial and may not reduce IICP significantly (Marshall et al., 1990; Ropper and Rockoff, 1988). However, physicians may utilize the technique by setting the ventilator at a rate that produces hyperventilation. In addition, the patient can be hyperventilated using the manual button on the ventilator or periodically hyperventilating by using the manual Ambu bag.

Osmotic diuretics (mannitol 20%) draw water from normal brain cells to the plasma, thereby decreasing ICP. The effects of decreasing ICP and increasing cerebral perfusion pressure occur within 20 minutes of infusion. The dosage range is 0.25 to 2.0 kg/dose (Ropper and Rockoff, 1988). Side effects of osmotic diuretics include hypotension, electrolyte disturbance, and rebound ICP. Osmotic diuretics are contraindicated in patients with renal disease. Since osmotic diuretics are not metabolized, the drug is excreted unchanged in the urine and will therefore affect specific gravity.

Loop diuretics (furosemide, ethacrynic acid) decrease IICP by removing sodium and water from injured brain cells. These agents also decrease CSF formation. The use of loop diuretics in the management of IICP remains controversial.

The use of corticosteroids for reducing ICP is controversial. Corticosteroids reduce cerebral edema associated with brain tumors, but studies are inconsistent in reporting the value of corticosteroids to reduce ICP in other intracranial conditions. Corticosteroids reduce CSF production as well as stabilize the blood-brain barrier and cell membranes, and these actions improve overall neuronal function. The most commonly prescribed corticosteroid is dexamethasone (Decadron). The initial dose of 6 to 20 mg IV is followed by 4 to 6 mg IV every 6 hours (Becker and Gudeman, 1989). The major side effects include muscle weakness, fluid retention, GI hemorrhage, nausea, abdominal distention, increased appetite, poor wound healing, and thrombocytopenia. The GI side effects may be prevented by using a H_2 receptor antagonist agent (cimetidine, nizatidine) and antacids (Marshall et al., 1990). Once the patient has been treated with corticosteroids, the drug must be carefully weaned. Abrupt withdrawal of steroids generally leads to a metabolic crisis (Cushing's crisis).

Patency of the airway is important for any patient, and the importance is no less for the patient with IICP. Without oxygen the brain cannot meet the metabolic demands, and the resultant hypoxia can lead to the death of neurons. For many patients with IICP, short-term management of the airway is accomplished by an endotracheal tube. Long-term management is by means of a tracheostomy tube.

Blood pressure must be carefully controlled in the patient with IICP since hypotension causes a decrease in CBF and this leads to cerebral ischemia. Hypertension (greater than 160 mm Hg systolic), on the other hand, worsens cerebral edema and leads to ischemia by compressing cerebral vessels. Mean systolic blood pressures greater than 160 mm Hg can be lowered by using labetalol or propranolol. These beta-blockers decrease the ongoing catecholamine release from sympathetic stimulation associated with neurological injury. The goal is to keep the patient with IICP normotensive and have a CPP in the range of 60 to 70 mm Hg (Ropper and Rockoff, 1988). These "high" systolic pressures are needed to achieve an adequate CPP when IICP is present. Some antihypertensive agents (nitroprusside, hydralazine) and some calcium channel blockers (verapamil, nifedipine) cause cerebral vasodilation. This vasodilation increases cerebral blood flow and causes IICP (Ropper and Rockoff, 1988). The use of these specific preferred vasodilators and calcium channel blockers are avoided in patients with poor intracranial compliance.

Seizure activity is another factor that raises

the metabolic rate, increases cerebral blood flow, expends oxygen, depletes energy stores, and causes IICP. Ischemia develops when flow can not meet metabolic demands. Seizures can be controlled with phenytoin (Dilantin), 15 to 18 mg/kg IV (loading dose). It is important not to exceed 50 mg/min in order to avoid the cardiotoxic effects of this drug. Diazepam (Valium), 5 to 10 mg IV bolus at a rate of 2 mg/min, can also be given to stop the seizures. If these measures fail and the patient is intubated, a neuromuscular blocker (pancuronium bromide, Pavulon) can be used.

Other pharmacological agents used to decrease the metabolic demand and to blunt environmental stimuli include morphine sulfate (small IV bolus or continuous dose 2 to 8 mg/hr), sedatives and muscle relaxants, and barbiturates. If barbiturates are used, the patient is intubated with mechanical ventilation, and has arterial pressure and intracranial pressure monitoring. Using either thiopental (short-term use) or pentobarbital (long-term use) is effective in reducing the metabolic demand on injured brain cells. Major side effects of barbiturate therapy are hypotension and myocardial instability. Table 9–9 outlines other nursing parameters associated with administering drugs.

Surgical Intervention

Surgical intervention may be required to remove the source of a mass or lesion causing the IICP. This involves the removal of infarcted areas and hematomas (epidural, subdural, or intracerebral). By removal of the clot, the mass lesion is gone, decreasing the brain component within the skull and also decreasing cerebral edema around the area of that clot. Such surgical measures then contribute to decreasing ICP.

Nursing Outcomes

Nursing outcomes for IICP are focused on maintaining ICP within the normal range (0 to 15 mm Hg), maintaining the airway, and promoting adequate oxygenation and cerebral perfusion pressure. Other patient outcomes are directed at maintaining fluid and electrolyte balance, preventing nutritional problems, preventing the hazards of immobility, and assisting the family with coping (see Nursing Care Plan for the Patient with Increased ICP, Head Injury, or CVA).

Head Injury

Head injury is a very common occurrence in the United States. Trauma is the leading cause of death between the ages of 1 and 44, with approximately 420,000 incidents of head injuries a year (Narayan, 1989). Severe head injury represents 10% of this figure, and mortality from head injury prior to hospitalization is considerable.

PATHOPHYSIOLOGY

When head injury occurs, it can damage the scalp, skull, brain and its pathways, meninges, cranial nerves, and intracranial vessels (Fig. 9–16). The head injury can be open or closed. An open head injury is when the scalp is torn or a fracture extends into the sinuses or middle ear. The meninges can also be penetrated. Closed head injury occurs when there is no break in the scalp. Acceleration-deceleration is a common mechanism for head injury. With this injury, the movement of the head follows a straight line and the moving head (acceleration) hits a stationary object (deceleration). Rotation or a twisting of the brain within the cranial vault adds to the insult, causing the extent of head injury to range from mild to severe.

Scalp Lacerations

Scalp lacerations are very common in head injury and can be associated with skull fracture. The scalp offers some resistance to compression and absorbs mild blows by distributing forces over the entire area of the scalp. Highly violent blows, however, do penetrate the scalp. In addition, the scalp is very vascular and can be the source of significant blood loss, which is difficult to stop. Once bleeding is stopped, it is important to clip the hair around the laceration. The wound is cleansed, debrided, inspected, and palpated for a depressed skull fracture. Inattention to these details can lead to infection.

Skull Fractures

The skull is composed of three layers that add stability and act as shock absorbers. The skull also has high compressive strength and is somewhat elastic. Following impact, the skull is compressed and there is an inbending of the skull at the point of impact and an outbending at the vertex. The area of outbending of tensile stresses

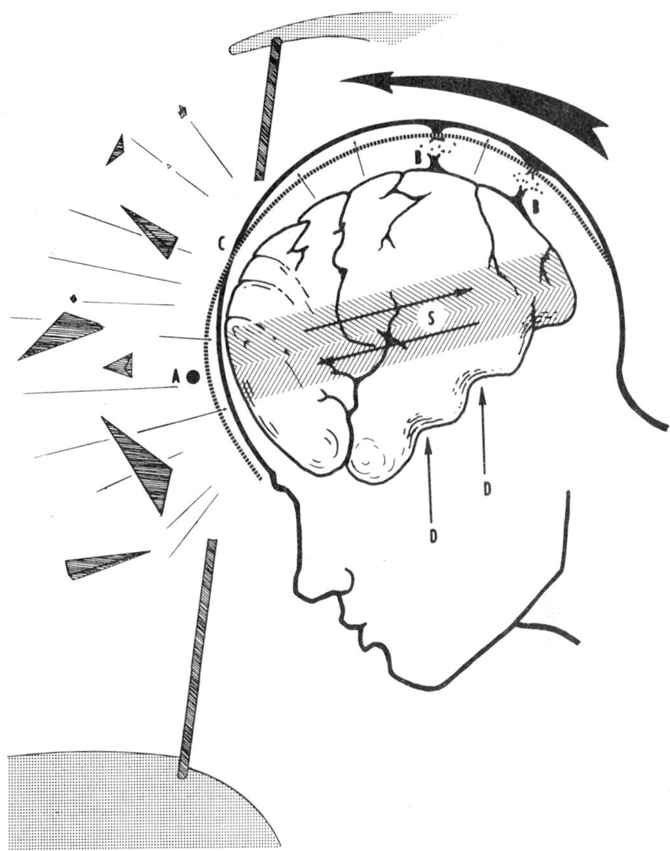

Figure 9-16. Closed blunt injury. Skull molding occurs at the site of impact. (A) Stippled line, preinjury contour; (C) solid line, contour moments after impact with inbending at (A), outbending at vertex. (B) Subdural veins torn as brain rotates forward. (S) Shearing strains throughout the brain. (D) Direct trauma to inferior temporal and frontal lobes over floors of middle and anterior fossae. (From Eliasson, S. G., Prensky, A. L., and Hardin, W. B.: Neurological Pathophysiology. 2nd ed. New York, Oxford University Press, 1978, Fig. 9-5.)

creates a fracture line that moves toward the base of the skull.

There are several types of skull fractures following head injury. These include linear, depressed, and basilar fractures.

Linear Skull Fracture

Linear skull fracture is the most common type. This fracture is uneventful unless there is an extension of the fracture to the orbit, sinus, or across a vessel. When there is extension of the fracture, the patient is admitted for observation of signs of intracranial bleeding.

Depressed Skull Fracture

A depressed skull fracture occurs when the outer table of the skull is depressed below the inner table of the surrounding intact skull. The dura may be intact, bruised, or torn. If the dura is torn, there is direct communication between the brain and environment, and meningitis can occur. In addition, the compressed and bruised brain beneath the depressed bone is the source of focal neurological deficit and may become an epileptogenic focal area. Mechanisms of closed head injury along with associated signs and symptoms are listed in Table 9-3.

Basilar Skull Fracture

A basilar skull fracture occurs at the base of the cranial vault and can extend into the anterior, middle, and posterior fossae. This type of fracture is difficult to confirm on a radiograph and is diagnosed by clinical presentation of the patient (Table 9-3). Dural tears are very common with a basilar skull fracture and may lead to meningitis. Drainage of CSF from the nose (rhinorrhea), postnasal drainage, and ear (otorrhea) may be indicative of a dural tear that allows a CSF leak. It is important to allow the CSF to flow freely. Nothing should be placed in the nose or ear although small bandages can be used to collect the drainage. The patient is also instructed not to blow his/her nose. If needed, suction catheters, nasogastric tubes, and endotracheal tubes should

Table 9–3. MECHANISMS OF CLOSED HEAD INJURY WITH ASSOCIATED SIGNS/SYMPTOMS—IMPACT BRAIN SET INTO MOTION INSIDE RIGID SKULL

Injury	Signs and Symptoms
Skull Fractures (Deformation of Skull, Secondary to Impact)	
Linear: Starts at outbended area, moves toward point of impact and to base of skull	Swelling, redness, bruising, tenderness on scalp, scalp laceration
Depressed: Outer table depressed below the inner table, associated with torn dura and brain beneath depressed bone is bruised	Palpation of depressed area in contour of skull; CSF leak from nose, ear, postnasal; scalp bruising, tenderness, laceration
Basilar: Fracture is the anterior, middle and/or posterior fossa along the floor of the cranial vault; dura is torn	
Anterior Fossa Fracture	Raccoon or panda eyes, periorbital edema, CSF leak nose, nasal congestion, cranial nerve deficits
Middle Fossa Fracture	CSF leak ear, hematympanum, battle sign, decreased hearing, cranial nerve deficits
Posterior Fossa Fracture	Bruising base of the neck, cranial nerve deficits
Cellular Injuries to Brain Cells (Interruption of Normal Connections Neurons, Pathways; Biochemical Changes Secondary to Stretching, Shearing, Rotational, and Hearing Forces Associated with Impact)	
Focal Injuries: Concussion, contusion, avulsion	
Concussion: Altered LOC, confusion, disorientation, retrograde amnesia	
Contusion: Injury can be the area directly beneath impact (coup) or injury can be to the brain's poles is bruised and swollen (countercoup), since these areas are prone to bleeding and swelling they act as an intracranial expanding mass	Altered level of consciousness, retrograde amnesia, motor deficits (weakness to paralysis) restlessness, combative, confusion, speech disturbances, cranial nerve dysfunction, decorticate and decerebrate posturing, abnormal breathing patterns, coma
Penetrating Injuries: Injury is caused by deep laceration of brain tissue, damage to the ventricular system	
Low Velocity: Stab wound—injury is caused by deep laceration of brain tissue, damage to the ventricular system	
High Velocity: Gun shot wound—extensive injury because of the entry of many bone fragments at the site, bullets spin irregularly creating many paths, increasing the brain damage, and shock waves cause brain disruption	
Diffuse Brain Injury: Tearing of axons and myelin sheaths secondary to generalized movement of brain from impact—prolonged coma, cranial nerve deficits, motor deficits	
Secondary Injury: Caused by IICP, cerebral edema, herniation, ischemia, hypoxia; these situations complicate intracerebral bleeds, focal and penetrating injuries	Prolonged coma, cranial nerve deficits, motor deficits
Intracerebral Bleeds (Cerebral Vessels Are Broken or Sheared Off Secondary to Impact)	
Epidural: Tearing of an artery from a skull fracture, brisk bleeding and rapid accumulation in the epidural space	Onset short period of LOC then lucid, then confusion, irritability, headache, deterioration LOC, motor, CN
Subdural: Tearing of bridging cortical veins—blood accumulates in the space between the dura and arachnoid	Acute and subacute—depressed LOC, pupil and EOM changes, motor changes; headache, *chronic* personality changes, gait problems
Subarachnoid: Bleeding into the subarachnoid space from the rupture of a traumatic aneurysm; altered LOC, headache, nuchal rigidity, photphobia	
Intraventricular: Bleeding to the ventricles; altered LOC, cranial nerve dysfunction, motor changes	
Intracerebral: Bleeding into brain tissue producing necrosis	Similar to focal injuries

be inserted through the mouth rather than the nose. If CSF is suspected to be present in drainage, a sample in a plain test tube is sent to the laboratory for analysis. Although used in the past, glucose test strips may not differentiate between CSF rhinorrhea and rhinorrhea from the respiratory tract (Nikas, 1987). Cranial nerves and the internal carotid artery passing through the skull floor can also be damaged in association with the injury.

Brain Injury

Brain injury from head injury is classified as primary and secondary brain injury.

Primary Brain Injury

Primary brain injury is the direct injury that occurs to the brain from an impact. With impact, the semisolid brain moves around inside the skull. The area under the direct impact is injured (coup injury). Injury to adjacent poles occurs from the movement of the brain inside the skull (contrecoup injury). The stretching, shearing, rotational, and tearing forces that result from impact cause an interruption of normal neuronal pathways.

On a cellular level following a direct injury, there is a series of biochemical events that contribute to the generation of free radicals (molecules or atoms that contain an unpaired electron in their outermost orbit, creating a lot of reactivity with other molecules) and the breakdown of the lipid neuronal cell membrane, which causes early neuronal deterioration (Hall, 1989). The patient shows signs/symptoms of neuronal deterioration and is unstable neurologically.

Concussion, contusion, penetrating injuries, hematomas, and intracerebral hemorrhage are all types of primary brain injury (Table 9–3). Concussion represents a mild form of head injury, whereas contusion, penetrating injuries, hematomas, and hemorrhage constitute severe head injuries.

Concussion. Concussion occurs when there is a mechanical force of short duration applied to the skull. This injury results in the temporary failure of impulse conduction. The neurological deficits are reversible and generally mild. Patients may lose consciousness for a few seconds at the time of injury, but lasting effects are not common.

Contusion. Contusion is the result of coup and contrecoup injuries, accompanied by bruising and generalized hemorrhage into brain tissue. Traumatic laceration of the cortical surface associated with contrecoup injuries may be greater than those seen directly under the point of impact. Signs and symptoms are variable (Table 9–3).

Penetrating Injuries

Penetrating injuries are the result of low or high-velocity forces such as gunshots, knives, or sharp objects. With this injury there is a deep laceration of brain tissue and possible damage to the ventricular system. A low-velocity (stabbing) injury is limited to the track of entry, and the greatest concern is bleeding and infection. A high-velocity (gunshot) injury causes extensive damage owing to the entry of bone fragments at the site, since bullets spin irregularly, creating many paths and shock waves that cause extensive brain damage.

A more global injury is a diffuse axonal involvement. With this injury there is widespread white matter axonal damage secondary to tearing and shearing forces. This type of injury is associated with disruption of axons in the cerebral hemispheres, diencephalon, and brain stem. Clinically, these patients show no, or only minimal, signs of recovery.

Hematomas

Epidural Hematoma. Collection of blood in the space between the inner table of the skull and the dura causes an epidural hematoma (Fig. 9–17). Many such hematomas are associated with a linear fracture of the temporal bone and result

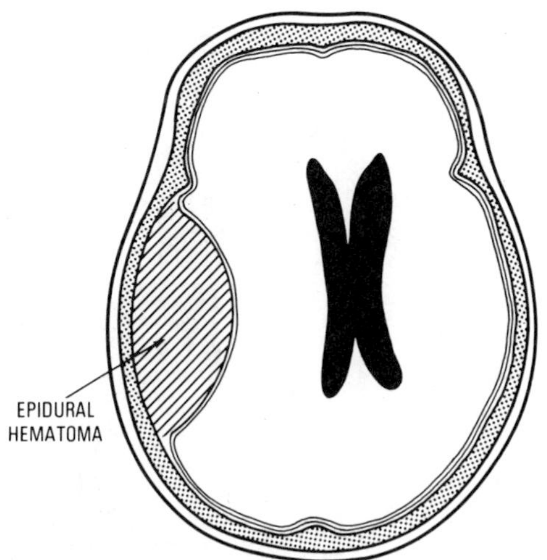

Figure 9–17. Epidural hematoma. (From Marshall, S. B., Marshall, L. F., Vos, H. R., and Chesnut, R. M.: Neuroscience Critical Care. Philadelphia, W. B. Saunders, 1990.)

from the tearing of the middle meningeal artery. Arterial blood accumulates rapidly in this space. The patient usually experiences a lucid period prior to neurological deterioration. Pupils are fixed and dilated on the side of the lesion.

Subdural Hematoma. Collection of blood in the subdural space causes a subdural hematoma (Fig. 9–18). It occurs when a surface vein is torn around the vertex. Subdural hematomas occur at all ages. In infants, they occur as a result of birth trauma; in the elderly, a subdural hematoma is most frequently the result of a fall. There are three kinds of subdural hematomas: acute, subacute, and chronic.

Acute subdural hematoma occurs within 24 hours of injury. This type of hematoma is seen in deceleration injuries and is associated with contusions. Subacute hematomas occurs after 24 hours and less than 1 week postinjury. Onset of symptoms is much slower and the symptoms are subtle. Prognosis is good for this kind of hematoma. Chronic subdural hematomas occur as a result of a low-velocity impact. They occur 1 week to several months after injury. In the elderly, these hematomas can be bilateral. The elderly are prone to subdural hematomas since they are prone to falling because of a decline in the motor system (balance and coordination deficits) due to normal aging. Signs and symptoms of subdural hematomas are discussed in Table 9–3.

Intracerebral Hemorrhage. An intracerebral hemorrhage is a large hemorrhage into brain tissue that creates a mass lesion. This lesion can occur anywhere in the brain. Signs and symptoms vary with this kind of lesion (Table 9–3).

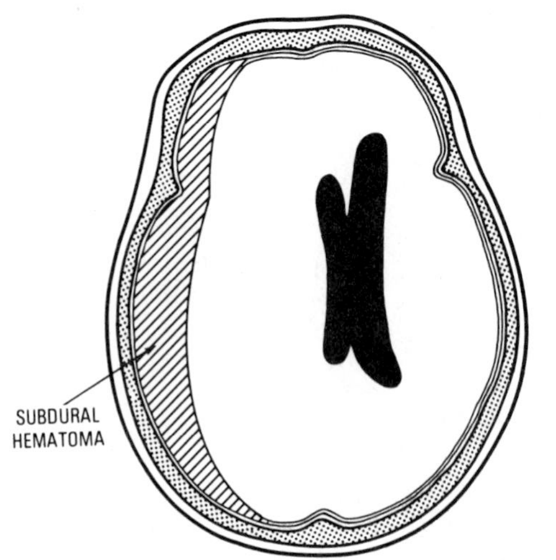

Figure 9–18. Subdural hematoma. (From Marshall, S. B., Marshall, L. F., Vos, H. R., and Chesnut, R. M.: Neuroscience Critical Care. Philadelphia, W. B. Saunders, 1990.)

Secondary Brain Injury

Secondary brain injury complicates the situation following the primary brain injury and is the result of hypoxia, hypotension, anemia, hypercarbia, uncontrolled IICP, cerebral edema, hypermetabolic state, infection, and fluid and electrolyte imbalance. All of these complications are caused by primary head injury and involve uncontrolled IICP and altered cerebral blood flow. These insults further add to the degree and extent of cellular dysfunction following head injury. All of these insults can increase brain damage and affect functional recovery.

ASSESSMENT

Nursing Assessment

The Glasgow Coma Scale is used as a guide in assessing the head-injured patient. In addition, the assessment of a patient must be supplemented with the neurological examination discussed in the previous section. Assessment should be specific to the area of the brain involved. If a patient has a brain stem injury, in addition to the Glasgow Coma Scale, the nurse would assess cranial nerves and respiratory rate and rhythm. All findings are documented with a description of the patient's behavior.

Another area for assessment is the respiratory status. About 60% of severely head-injured patients arrive at the hospital hypoxic (Nikas, 1987). A PaO_2 below 50 mm Hg causes vasodilation of cerebral vessels, increased cerebral blood flow, and IICP. Thus, this hypoxia can further compromise the patient's progress.

MEDICAL TREATMENT

Prompt and aggressive medical treatment is very beneficial for the head-injured patient. Medical assessment is based on the neurological examination, which includes reflex testing, ICP and hemodynamic monitoring, and respiratory assessment. The head-injured patient requires the same laboratory studies and diagnostic studies as the patient with IICP.

NURSING DIAGNOSES

The same nursing diagnoses are necessary for the head-injured patient and the patient with IICP (see Nursing Care Plan for the Patient with Increased ICP, Head Injury, or CVA). These diagnoses cover both primary and secondary head injuries.

INTERVENTIONS

Nursing Interventions

The nursing interventions are the same as those for the patient with IICP (see Nursing Care Plan for the Patient with Increased ICP, Head Injury, or CVA). An important consideration for nursing intervention is the sequence and timing of these activities. When the patient is having episodes of IICP, it is important to control the patient's environment and activities to minimize stimuli that contribute to the IICP. A thorough assessment will assist the nurse in determining how to proceed with nursing care without jeopardizing the patient's status. For example, a patient with a severe head injury and excessively high ICP will require careful control of all activities. Thus, they will require rest periods after each nursing intervention to allow the ICP to return to normal.

Medical (Nonsurgical) Treatment

The nonsurgical treatment of the patient with a head injury is the same as for IICP. The emphasis is on reducing IICP, maintaining the airway, providing oxygenation, maintaining cerebral perfusion, and preventing secondary head injury.

A variety of surgical procedures exist for head-injured patients. For patients with a depressed skull fracture, elevation of the fracture may be needed depending on the nature of the fracture. Surgical removal of an epidural, subdural, or intracerebral hematoma may be performed to prevent a mass lesion from causing a shift in brain tissue or herniation, thereby minimizing neurological deterioration of the patient. Penetrating wounds to the skull and brain may necessitate a craniotomy to explore the pathway of the missile, repair laceration of intracranial vessels and brain tissue, remove bone fragments, and, in the case of a gunshot wound, retrieve the bullet.

Postoperative care is directed at maintaining normal ICP, cerebral tissue perfusion, and airway; preventing fluid and electrolyte imbalance and complications from immobility; avoiding nutritional deficits; and reducing the incidence of infection. The postcraniotomy patient will need to have the craniotomy dressing assessed for drainage (color and amount) and fluid accumulation under the skin flap. Once the dressing is removed, the incision is assessed for swelling, redness, drainage, and tenderness. Individuals with penetrating wounds to the brain are at high risk for the development of not only infections, but brain abcesses.

OUTCOMES

With diligent nursing and medical care, the head-injured patient should have positive outcomes from injury. Outcomes for the head-injured patient are as favorable as they are for the patient with IICP (see Nursing Care Plan for the Patient with Increased ICP, Head Injury, or CVA).

Spinal Cord Injury

There are approximately 200,000 people in the United States with spinal cord injury (SCI). Each year there are 10,000 to 12,000 additional victims who sustain SCI. Most of these individuals are men under 40 years of age. The causes of spinal cord injury are motor vehicle accidents, falls, sports injuries, missile injuries, and diving accidents. It is not uncommon to see head injury in association with SCI; therefore, SCI should be considered as a possibility in all unconscious patients.

PATHOPHYSIOLOGY

A SCI occurs when there is some type of sudden force exerted on the vertebral column resulting in damage to the spinal cord. A series of responses result from this injury. There is altered autonomic function leading to cardiovascular instability. The loss of sympathetic input (spinal nerves T-1 to L-1) creates bradycardia, hypotension, venous stasis, and loss of temperature control (spinal shock). Spinal shock is the temporary loss of autonomic, sensory, and motor functions below the level of the lesion, and is secondary to the loss of facilitory input from the brain and inhibitory input below the level of the injury. A sign of the termination of spinal shock is the return of reflex activity below the level of the lesion. Another response to injury is an inflammatory reaction that creates cord edema. Cord edema compresses spinal cord tissue as well as cord blood vessels. Cord edema can ascend or descend from the level of injury.

The injury itself creates a series of biochemical changes. Potassium is lost from inside the cell

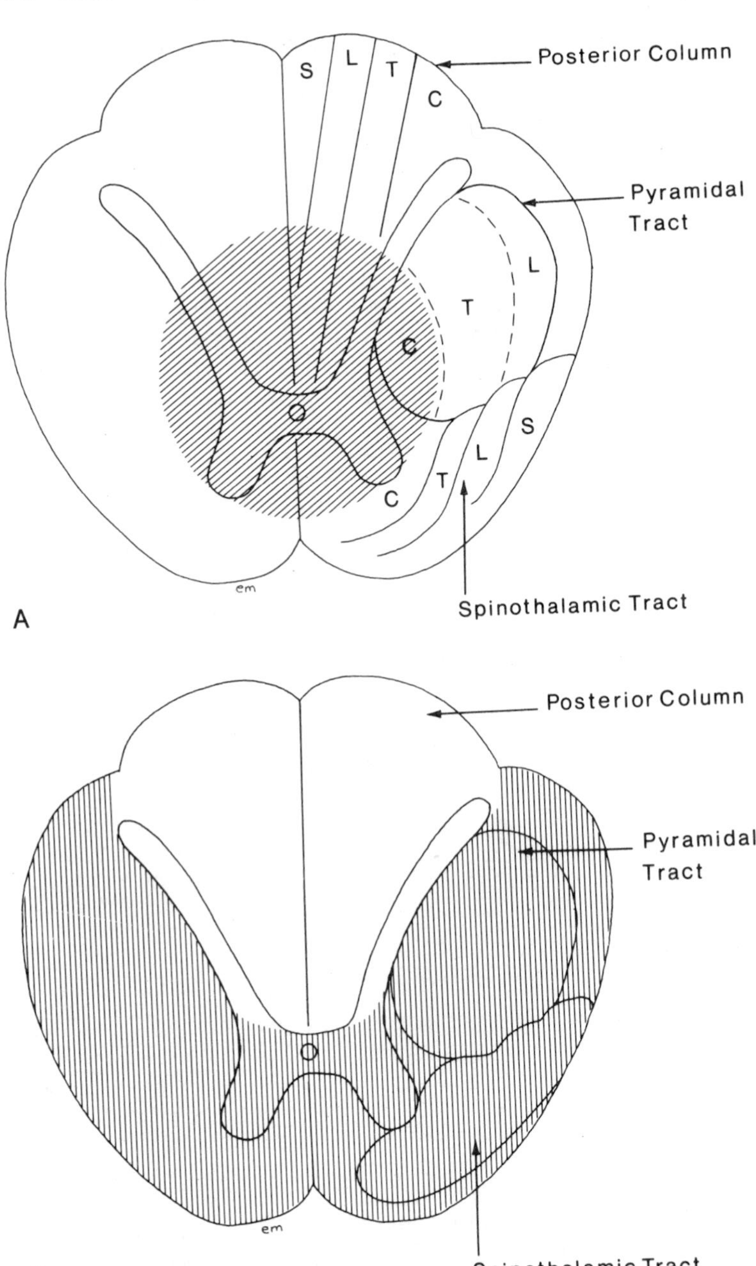

Figure 9–19. Incomplete spinal cord injuries. *A*, Central cord syndrome. Damage to the structures of the cervical cord gray matter and the pyramidal tract. More loss in the upper extremities. *B*, Anterior spinal cord syndrome. Damage to the anterior horn cells and the spinothalamic tract. Deficits are loss of motor function and pain and temperature below the level of the lesion.

to the extracellular compartment. It is postulated that this biochemical change causes spinal shock (Adelstein, 1989). There is also a calcium influx inside the cell that leads to the lipid membrane breakdown of neurons. Free oxygen radicals are also produced, which potentiate further breakdown of cell membranes. There is a release of vasoactive substances (norepinephrine, histamine, dopamine, prostaglandin) as a result of these biochemical changes. This event leads to vasoconstriction of the blood vessels, decrease in tissue O_2, a buildup of lactic acid, and ischemia. If the ischemia is not reversed, axonal degeneration and conduction failure of the neuron occur. Eventually there is cell death and permanent loss of function. This process also occurs with head injury.

The final response to spinal cord injury is vascular change. Instantly after injury, there are microscopic hemorrhages in the central gray matter of the spinal cord. After several hours, these hemorrhages invade the surrounding white mat-

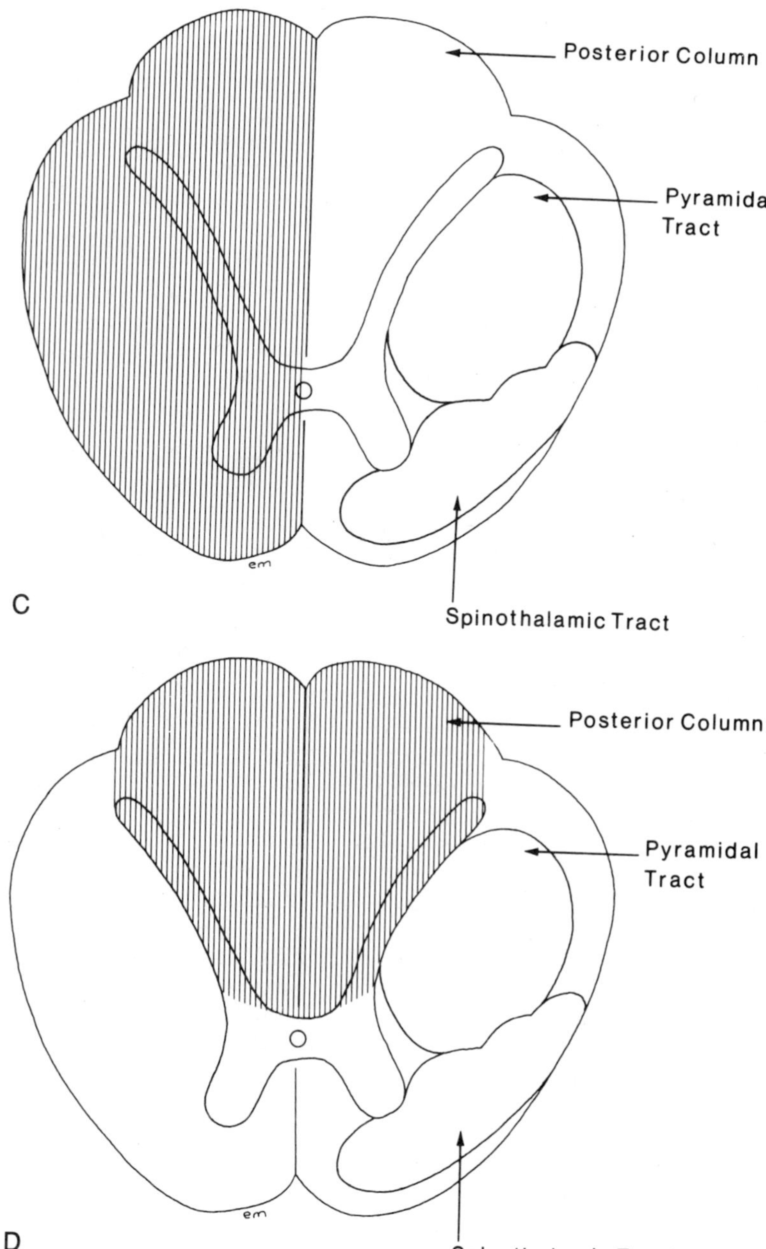

Figure 9–19. *Continued C,* Brown-Séquard syndrome. Hemisection of the spinal cord results in loss of motor function and touch, pressure, and position sense ipsilateral to the lesion and loss of pain and temperature sensation on the contralateral side of the body. This lateral disparity results because the spinothalamic tracts (pain and temperature) cross at the spinal level, whereas the dorsal columns and the corticospinal tracts decussate in the medulla. *D,* Dorsal column syndrome. Damage is to the dorsal column pathway. The deficit is loss of touch, vibration, and position sense below the level of injury. Motor function is preserved. (From Marshall, S. B., Marshall, L. F., Vos, H. R., and Chesnut, R. M.: Neuroscience Critical Care. Philadelphia, W. B. Saunders, 1990.)

ter, cord blood flow is decreased, and ischemia results.

A SCI can result in a complete or incomplete lesion. A complete lesion causes total loss of motor and sensory functions below the level of injury. An incomplete lesion results in the sparing of motor and sensory functions below the level of injury (Fig. 9–19). Most patients with an incomplete lesion show a mixed pattern of motor and sensory functions rather than a classic syndrome.

ASSESSMENT

Nursing Assessments

Airway and Respiratory Status

Assessment of the airway and respiratory status is the first assessment priority. The higher the level of spinal cord injury, the greater the functional impairment. Respiratory problems are frequently associated with spinal cord injury. Ineffective breathing patterns are commonly caused by paralysis of the diaphragm or intercostal muscles and from chest trauma. Therefore, the lungs must be auscultated for the presence of breath sounds in all areas as well as the presence of adventitious sound. Observing the respiratory rate, along with the rhythm and depth of respiration, is also important. Signs of respiratory distress may include excessive retraction of accessory neck muscles with respiratory effort, paradoxical expansion of the abdominal wall with inspiration, and cyanosis. Baseline ABGs collected when the patient arrives in the unit will provide important information about the actual exchange of gases within the lung.

Patients with high cervical fractures (vertebrae C-1 to C-5) with spinal cord involvement can experience hypoventilation with or without sleep apnea. This hypoventilation syndrome starts with vague complaints of the patient's experiencing air hunger and drowsiness with sighing respirations. When the patient is questioned, he/she is anxious, disoriented, or confused. Although the patient appears anxious and potentially responsive to a sedative, it is important not to sedate the patient since the drug will worsen hypoventilation and the patient may experience respiratory arrest as he drops off to sleep. If the patient is awakened prior to the respiratory arrest, normal breathing occurs. This hypoventilation syndrome occurs because of the decreased sensitivity of the respiratory drive to carbon dioxide and mechanical factors like immobilization. The hypoventilation syndrome usually lasts for the first 10 days after injury, and mechanical ventilation at night is the treatment of choice. Oxygen is administered cautiously in those patients dependent on the hypoxic drive for breathing.

Respiratory impairment varies with the level of injury and type of injury (complete or incomplete). Patients with a complete lesion at vertebral levels C-1 to C-4 usually experience total loss of respiratory function. Patients with complete lesions at vertebral levels C-1 to C-3 are ventilator dependent. Patients with complete lesions at vertebral levels C-4 to C-5 experience phrenic nerve damage and are candidates for phrenic nerve pacers. Individuals with complete SCI injuries below vertebra C-5 will have intact diaphragmatic breathing without intercostal and abdominal muscle function. Individuals with a complete lesion from vertebral levels T-1 to L-2 will experience varying amounts of intercostal and abdominal muscle loss. Respiratory impairment results from the dysfunction or loss of the diaphragm, intercostals, and abdominal muscles. Individuals with incomplete spinal cord lesions present with varying degrees of respiratory impairment depending on the level of the lesion and if the motor system is impaired.

Neurological Assessment

Once airway and respiratory assessment is complete, the neurological examination follows. If the patient also has a head injury, an assessment of all components of the neurological examination is done as described in the previous section. For the patient with a SCI, comprehensive motor, reflex, and sensory assessments are done.

Motor and Reflex Assessments

An assessment of the spinal nerve innervation of major muscle groups is important for determining the level of injury to the motor system (Table 9–4). A grading of muscle strength is also part of the motor assessment (Table 9–5) since it offers a basis for comparative assessment throughout the course of treatment. The grading of muscle strength is based on the ability to move muscle group(s), holding a position against gravity, and maintaining that position against the nurse's resistance to the muscle group(s). By observation or asking the patient to move his/her right arm establishes the patient's ability to move the right arm, and is rated a 1 on the scale. When the patient holds his/her right arm extended in front of him/her with palms up and maintains the position for 6 seconds, the patient is rated a 3 on the scale. The last step is to apply resistance to the muscles of the arm when the patient has his/her right arm extended in front of him/her ("I am going to push your right arm down, so try to prevent me from doing that"). If the patient has difficulty resisting the examiner, the rating is a 4 on the scale. If the patient maintains the position with resistance, the rating is a 5 on the scale.

Superficial and deep tendon reflexes should also be included in the motor assessment (Fig. 9–20). Reflex testing assists in establishing the level of spinal cord injury and the return of deep tendon reflexes below the level of injury signals the end of spinal shock.

Deep tendon reflexes are obtained by a brisk tapping of a reflex hammer on the tendons of a muscle group (Fig. 9–20). The response is contraction of the stimulated muscle group. Deep tendon reflexes are graded according to the response elicited (0 = no reflex; 1 = hypoactive; 2 = normal; 3 = hyperreactive).

Superficial reflexes are cutaneous sensations over the abdomen and groin area. They are elic-

Table 9–4. SPINAL NERVE INNERVATION OF MAJOR MUSCLE GROUPS

Spinal Nerve	Muscle Group Movement	Assessment Technique
C-4 to C-5	Shoulder abduction	Shrug shoulders against downward pressure of examiner's hands
C-5 to C-6	Elbow flexion (biceps)	Arm is pulled up from resting position against resistance
C-7	Elbow extension (triceps)	From the flexed position, arm is straightened out against resistance
C-7	Thumb-index pinch	Index finger is held firmly to thumb against resistance to pull apart
C-8	Hand grasp	Hand grasp strength is evaluated
L-2 to L-4	Hip flexion	Leg is lifted from bed against resistance
L-5 to S-1	Knee flexion	Knee is flexed against resistance
L-2 to L-4	Knee extension	From flexed position, knee is extended against resistance
L-5	Foot dorsiflexion	Foot pulled up toward nose against resistance
S-1	Foot plantar flexion	Foot pushed down (stepping on the gas) against resistance

From Marshall, S. B., et al.: Neuroscience Critical Care. Philadelphia, W. B. Saunders, 1990.

ited by scratching the surface of the abdomen or groin area.

Sensory Assessment

Sensory assessment is performed to determine superficial response to pinprick (sharp, dull, hyperesthesia, absent), position sense, and temperature. The sensory dermatomes are the segmental distribution of sensation (Fig. 9–21). This mapping of areas of sensation on the skin is supplied by one spinal segment. For example, when the nurse tests the superficial sensation to pinprick on the lateral forearm, thumb, and index finger, the skin area is innervated by dermatome C-6. While undergoing sensory testing, the patient is instructed to close his/her eyes. Position sense is determined by having the nurse grasp the patient's thumb or big toe and move the digit up or down, or by leaving it in a neutral position. The patient is asked to identify the pattern of movement. Temperature is assessed by filling up one test tube with hot water and another test tube with cold water. The patient is asked to identify the sensation when the test tube touches the skin. Table 9–6 outlines the components of hourly assessments for the SCI patient without a head injury. Table 9–7 lists the components of the hourly

Table 9–5. MOTOR STRENGTH GRADING SCALE

Score	Motor Function
0	None
1	Trace
2	Not greater than gravity
3	Greater than gravity
4	Slight weakness
5	Normal

From Marshall, S. B., et al.: Neuroscience Critical Care. Philadelphia, W. B. Saunders, 1990.

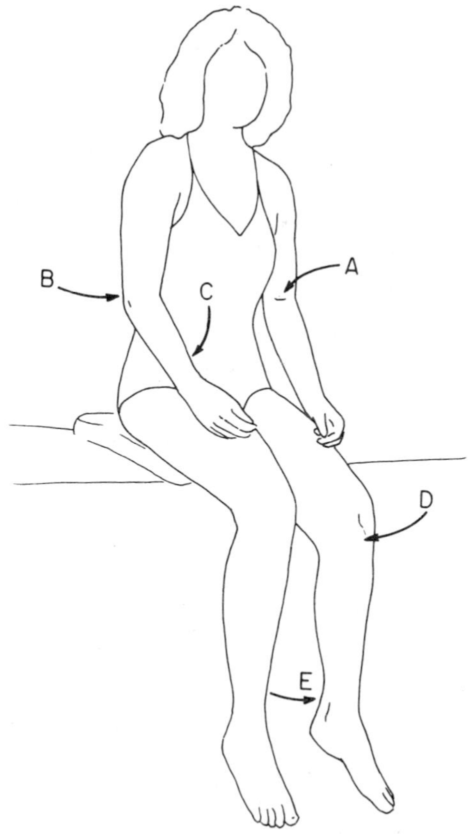

Figure 9–20. Deep tendon reflexes. (A) Biceps, (B) Triceps, (C) Brachioradialis, (D) Patellar, (E) Achilles. (From Mitchell, P., Cammermeyer, M., Ozuna, J., and Woods, N. F.: Neurological Assessment for Nursing Practice. Reston, Virginia: Reston Publishing Co., 1984, Fig. 2–16.)

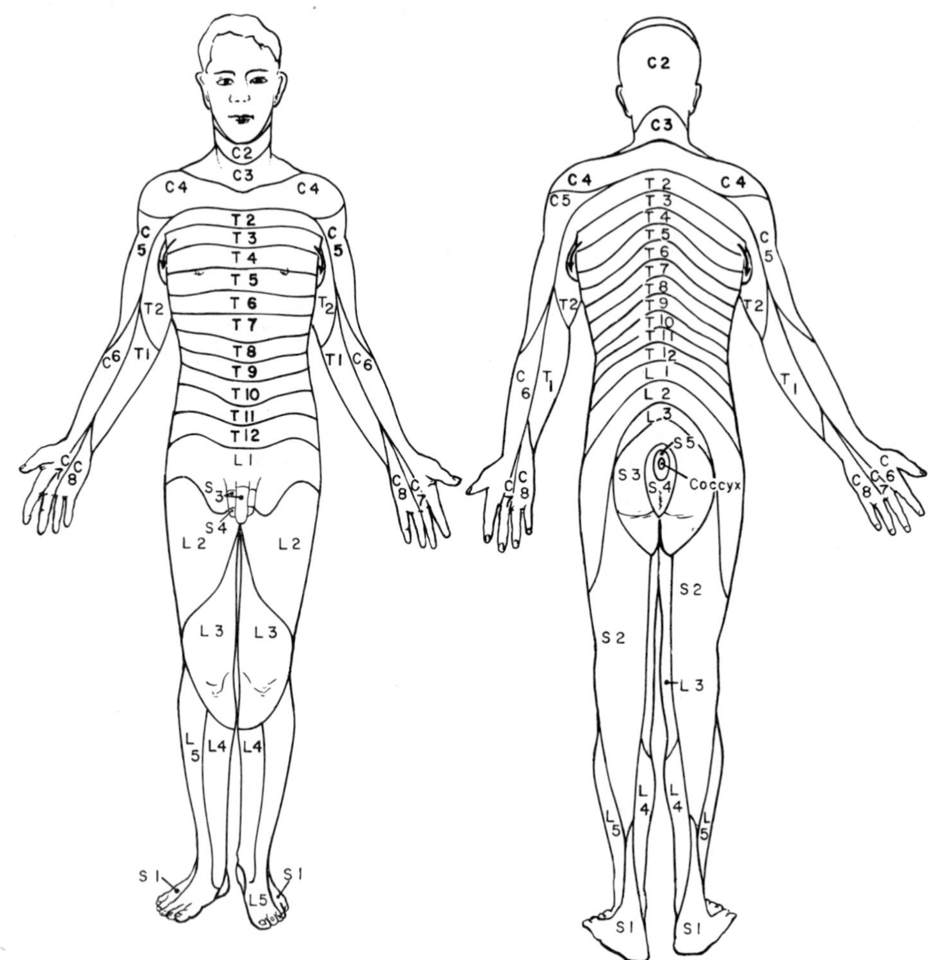

Figure 9–21. Sensory dermatomes. Cutaneous distribution of spinal nerves. (From Marshall, S. B., Marshall L. F., Vos, H. R., and Chesnut, R. M.: Neuroscience Critical Care. Philadelphia, W. B. Saunders, 1990.)

assessment for a patient with a spinal cord injury and head injury.

Hemodynamic Assessment

Another important assessment consideration is hemodynamic instability. The patient will need continuous hemodynamic monitoring during the acute period following the injury to assist in early recognition of hemodynamic instability. The usual hemodynamic response in injuries above the C-5 level is a decrease or loss of sympathetic innervation causing vasodilation, decreased venous return, and hypotension. The patient's vasomotor response returns over the course of a couple of months. Bradycardia is common and is due to the loss of sympathetic outflow and is aggravated by hypothermia and hypoxia. The patient, then, is at risk for vasovagal response when suctioned, which leads to hypoxia and vagal stimulation. This reflex is prevented by preoxygenating the patient prior to suctioning (Alspach, 1991).

Venous stasis occurs as a result of loss of vasomotor tone and paralysis. This stasis increases the risk of thrombosis in the legs and pelvis.

The high-level SCI patient (above C-5) also has trouble regulating body temperature. The level of injury interrupts the pathway between the hypothalamus and the blood vessels, causing body temperature to rise and fall according to the environmental temperature.

Gastrointestinal Tract Assessment

The gastrointestinal tract is another area to assess in the SCI patient. The loss of autonomic tone

Table 9–6. COMPONENTS OF THE HOURLY NEUROLOGICAL ASSESSMENT FOR PATIENTS WITH SCI WITHOUT HEAD INJURY

Motor	Sensation
Respirations Rate, rhythm, respiratory effort	Pinprick (sharp, dull) All surfaces of the body
Assess movement/strength bilaterally Shrug shoulders Elbow flexion Elbow extension Bending wrists Touching thumb to index finger Hand grasp Lift leg off the bed Bend knee Extend knee Pulls feet up Pushes feet down	Position sense Temperature All surfaces of the body

causes abdominal distention and paralytic ileus. A nasogastric tube for decompression is inserted until bowel sounds return. Gastric dilatation interferes with diaphragmatic functions, causing hypoventilation and fatigue while breathing. Stress ulcers can occur owing to vagus-stimulated gastric acid production. Steroid therapy is part of acute management, but also irritates the gastric mucosa, leading to the potential of additional GI problems. A thorough nutritional assessment is important since the injury leads to a hypermetabolic state.

Bowel and Bladder Assessment

Bowel/bladder atony occur during spinal shock. The bladder does not contract, and the detrusor muscle does not open secondarily to the paralysis. Urinary retention is a common problem and a Foley catheter during spinal shock is the treatment of choice. The bowel does not have peristaltic movement secondary to spinal cord injury. This loss of peristaltic movement places the patient at risk for a paralytic ileus. During the first 72 hours post-spinal cord injury, the placement of a nasogastric tube on low constant suction will decompress the bowel. Once bowel sounds return, flatus and a decrease in gastric output or a bowel movement removes the danger of an ileus. After this, a bowel program is initiated. This program consists of bisacodyl suppositories or enemas every other day, stool softeners, and digital stimulation to stimulate reflex colonic activity (Marshall et al., 1990).

Autonomic Dysreflexia

Autonomic dysreflexia (hyperreflexia) occurs after spinal shock has ceased and can be an ongoing problem for the SCI patient with a lesion above T-6. Autonomic dysreflexia is characterized by an exaggerated response of the sympathetic nervous

Table 9–7. COMPONENTS OF THE HOURLY NEUROLOGICAL ASSESSMENT FOR PATIENTS WITH SCI AND HEAD INJURY

Mental Status	Motor	Pupils	Brain-stem/Cranial Nerves	Sensation
Glasgow Coma Scale Assesses level of consciousness, expressive language, ability to follow command	Respirations Rate, rhythm, respiratory effort Assess movement/strength bilaterally Shrug shoulders Elbow flexion Elbow extension Bending wrists Touching thumb to index finger Hand grasp Lift leg off the bed Bend knee Extend knee Pulls feet up Pushes feet down	Size Shape Reaction to light (direct and consensual) EOMs	Corneal Reflex Present—immediate blinking bilaterally Diminished—blinking asymmetrically Absent—no blinking Doll's eyes (unconscious patient—no spinal fracture) Cough, gag, swallow reflex Observe for excessive drooling Observe for cough/swallow reflex	Pinprick (sharp, dull) All surfaces of the body Position Sense Temperature All surfaces of the body

system to a variety of stimuli (i.e., draft in the room, kinked Foley catheter, bladder distension, bowel impaction, routine bowel/bladder procedures). This exaggerated response by the sympathetic nervous system results from the lack of input from the brain owing to the blockage of the SCI. Common signs and symptoms are sudden, severe, pounding headache, elevated uncontrolled blood pressure, bradycardia, nasal congestion, profuse sweating above the level of the lesion, flushing of the face and neck, and anxiety. Blood pressure can rise to a dangerous or fatal level, making autonomic dysreflexia an emergency situation. The treatment is directed at finding and removing the cause (external or internal stimuli) of the exaggerated response. Once the cause has been located and removed, the symptoms will quickly disappear. Until that time, autonomic dysreflexia should be considered a severe medical emergency.

Skin Assessment

Inspection of the skin should be incorporated into the assessment. Owing to impaired circulation and immobility, the SCI patient is at risk for skin breakdown. The skin around the halo or tong pins should be inspected and pin care performed every 8 hours. Observing the site for redness, swelling, drainage, and pain should be incorporated into the plan. Inspection of areas under the Halo brace is important for the purpose of noting areas of skin breakdown.

Psychological Assessment

A psychological assessment is important during the acute period of injury. Initially the patient is concerned with surviving the injury and is incapable of realizing the extent of his/her injury or disability. The patient's perceptions are also impaired by medications and the physiological effects of injury. As the patient gains insight into the situation, it is important for the nurse to include the patient in planning his/her care and to give choices about that care. Family members also go through a similar experience as the patient. First there is shock related to the injury itself and the seriousness of the patient's condition. During this time, the family needs support and answers to their questions.

Medical Assessment

Common baseline laboratory studies include the following:

1. Chemical profile
2. Electrolytes
3. CBC
4. PT, PTT, platelet count
5. ABGs

Common diagnostic studies to confirm the extent of vertebral and spinal cord injury include:

1. Anteroposterior and lateral spine x-ray
2. Chest x-ray
3. CT scan
4. MRI
5. Myelography
6. Somatosensory-cortical evoked potentials (SEPs)

The SEPs are performed to see if sensory pathways between the site of stimulation and the site of recording are intact. This test requires tactile stimulation to elicit a response.

NURSING DIAGNOSIS

Nursing diagnoses appropriate for the patient with a SCI are:

1. Altered body alignment related to SCI
2. Ineffective breathing patterns/ineffective cough related to impaired diaphragm, poor chest excursion, diaphragm/intercostal muscle fatigue, ANS instability
3. Alteration in tissue perfusion related to cardiovascular instability (spinal shock)
4. Alteration in temperature (poikilothermia) related to loss of sympathetic innervation
5. Altered nutrition: less than body requirement related to paralytic ileus from SCI, stress ulcers from stress response and therapy, hypermetabolic state
6. Impaired mobility related to SCI
7. Fluid and electrolyte imbalance related to paralytic ileus, gastric suction, fluid overload
8. Alteration in bladder function related to atonic bladder, upper neuron lesion
9. Alteration in comfort related to spasticity, bladder spasms, dysesthesia from SCI
10. Self-care deficit related to impaired mobility
11. Powerlessness related to SCI and ineffective coping mechanism
12. Altered body image related to SCI

INTERVENTIONS

Nursing Interventions

The nursing interventions are focused on maintaining stabilization of the spinal alignment, maintaining the airway and respiratory status, and preventing complications associated with immobility and the spinal cord injury (see Nursing Care Plan for the Patient with Spinal Cord Injury).

Medical Interventions

Maintaining a patent airway and respiratory function is the first aspect of treatment. If the patient is having difficulty sustaining his/her own respiration, then mechanical ventilation is the treatment of choice.

Stabilization of the fracture/dislocation in order to bring about spinal alignment and prevent further neurological deterioration is accomplished by skeletal traction—halo brace/tongs (Fig. 9–22). If tongs are used initially to stabilize the spine, the amount of weight is very controversial. Usually 10 lb of traction is used initially, building up to 80 lb maximally. The halo brace offers many advantages such as easy access to the neck for diagnostic procedures and surgery, early mobilization, and ambulation. For both types of skeletal traction, pin care and skin assessment over pressure areas are important nursing interventions.

Maintaining perfusion pressure of the spinal

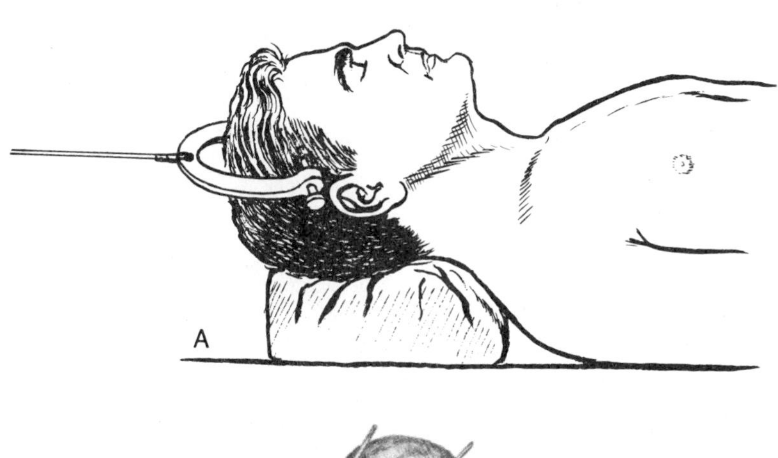

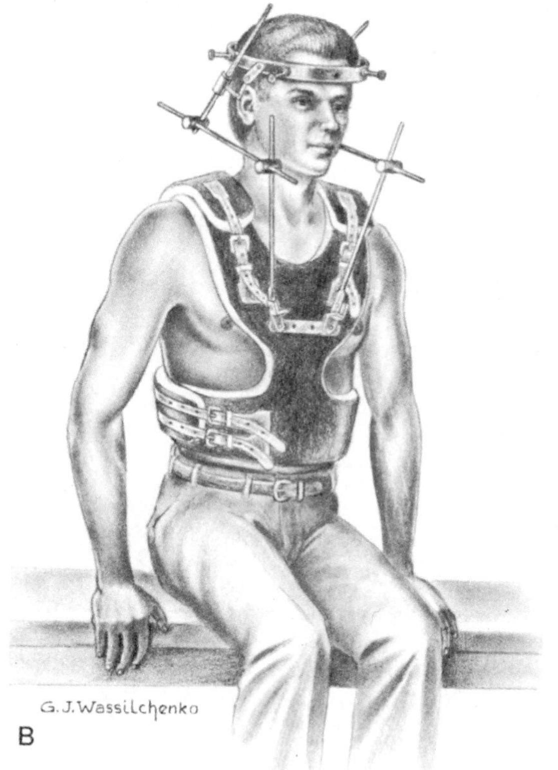

Figure 9–22. Skeletal traction with Crutchfield tongs. (From Hickey, J. C.: Clinical Practice of Neurological and Neurosurgical Nursing, Philadelphia, J. B. Lippincott, 1986, p. 400.)

NURSING CARE PLAN FOR THE PATIENT WITH SPINAL CORD INJURY

Nursing Diagnosis	Outcome	Intervention
Altered body alignment related to SCI	Vertebral alignment maintained Preservation of neurological function at initial SCI level	Maintain halo or tong traction or other device for immobilization Neurological assessments—motor, reflex, and sensory functions Report ascending lesion or progression of deficits from base line Safe use of special beds for turning Explain immobilization to patient and get his cooperation Pin care every 8 hr If skeletal traction slips or accidentally removed, maintain head in a neutral position Turning, lifting, transferring patient use 5 people with 1 person at head stabilizing neck, guiding traction Monitor temp, report if abnormal
Ineffective breathing pattern/ineffective cough related to impaired diaphragm, poor chest excursion, diaphragm/intercostal muscle fatigue, PE, ANS instability	Maintain airway Vital capacity 60–75 ml/kg ABG WNL O_2 saturation WNL 96% Breath sounds bilaterally CXR WNL No atelectasis/pneumonia Temp WNL No dyspnea, tachypnea No restlessness or anxiety	Monitor respiratory rate and rhythm Assess breath sounds every hour for 72 hr Observe for anxiety, restlessness, or statements related to "not getting enough air," "trouble breathing" Assist in cleaning secretions with suctioning or Quad coughing Encourage deep breathing and use of incentive inspirometer Maintain patency of endotracheal or tracheostomy tube (for intubation fiberoptic laryngoscopy or jaw thrust is used) Observe tolerance for turning on special frames or beds Chest physiotherapy Administer antibodies as ordered Monitor O_2 saturation with pulse oximeter Administer O_2 as needed Gradually decrease ventilatory assistance
Alteration in tissue perfusion related to cardiovascular instability (spinal shock)	Hemodynamic monitoring WNL Urine output ≥30 ml/hr VS stabile Normal sinus rhythm BP WNL	Monitor BP, pulse, respirations, temp every hour for 72 hr or as ordered Record I&O Urine output every hour Monitor fluid intake Use antiembolism stockings Administer medications to increase BP, bradycardia, dysrhythmias, volume expanders Monitor lab values CBC, Hgb, Hct, BUN, creatinine, electrolytes Report abnormal findings
Alteration in temperature (poikilothermia) related loss of sympathetic innervation	Maintain temperature at 37°C	Adjust environmental temperature to 75°F Correlate environmental temperature to body temperature Avoid the use of many blankets on patient For hyperthermia check environmental temperature, use cooling blanket and antipyretics when ordered
Alteration in nutrition < body requirements, related paralytic ileus from SCI, stress ulcers from stress response and therapy, hypermetabolic state	Bowel sounds present Absence of abdominal distention Absence of vomiting Potassium WNL Absence of T wave depression Gastric secretions and stool negative for occult blood Maintain gastric pH ≥3 Hct and Hgb WNL Maintain admission weight Return of bowel movements and flatus	Use of NG tube on low suction to prevent abdominal distention/possible aspiration Daily weights with bed scales Measure abdominal girths every 8 hr for 72 hr NPO until bowel sounds present Nutritional assessment Parenteral hyperalimentation if ordered When bowel sounds return, advance diet slowly, clear liquids in small amounts, and increase as tolerated Monitor serum albumin and proteins initially and every 3 days thereafter Monitor gastric pH of NG tube, aspirate; report if <3 Administer antacids, H_2 receptor blockers Monitor Hct and Hgb; report abnormal results Sudden unexplained shoulder pain can be referred pain from GI tract

NURSING CARE PLAN FOR THE PATIENT WITH SPINAL CORD INJURY *Continued*

Nursing Diagnosis	Outcome	Intervention
		Start bowel program when bowel sounds return Record bowel movement pattern
Impaired mobility related to SCI	Intact skin Calves and thighs symmetrical Absence of lower extremity (LE) edema No signs of pulmonary embolism Verbalizes importance of reposition Adequate nutritional status	Turn at least every 2 hr; use special bed, foam mattress, or air mattress Assess extremities for change in color, size, temperature Measure calf and thighs on admission and daily Report changes in circumference to physician Passive range of motion to LE qid Apply antiembolism stockings Remove antiembolism stockings every 8 hr for 30 min and assess legs Administer heparin 5000 U SC every 12 hr or as ordered Monitor PTT as long as heparin ordered; report abnormal results Inspect skin and give skin care every 2 hr Avoid skin wetness from perspiration, stool, urine Assess skin under halo brace or other braces Teach patient the importance of skin care and frequent repositioning
Fluid and electrolyte imbalance related to paralytic ileus, gastric suction, fluid overload	Electrolytes WNL Balanced I&O CXR WNL Maintain admission weight	Record I&O, specific gravity every 8 hr Monitor daily electrolytes; report abnormalities to physician Assess breath sounds Administer IV fluids Daily weights
Alteration in bladder function related to atonic bladder, upper motor neuron lesion	Output consistent with intake Absence of distention Normal temperature BUN, creatinine WNL No residual volume after catheter DC Negative urine cultures Clear urine No bladder spasms WBC WNL	Indwelling catheter initially during spinal shock Hourly urinary output Catheter case tid Avoid using a large-size Foley catheter Intermittent catheterization following spinal shock Acidify the urine—vitamin C, cranberry juice, apple juice Urinalysis daily for 72 hr then weekly Keep Foley bag off the floor and lower the abdomen Monitor urine pH; maintain < 5.8 Monitor WBC and report abnormalities
Alteration in comfort related to spasticity, bladder spasms, dysesthesia from SCI	Understands abnormal sensations/loss No skin breakdown No reports of bladder spasms No reports of spasticity Temperature WNL	Assess pain/discomfort Turn patient every hour Monitor temperature Report abnormal temperature to physician Protect anesthetic areas Utilize visual imagery/biofeedback, distraction Administer analgesics that will not cause respiratory depression
Self-care deficits related to impaired mobility	Performs self-care activities within ability of SCI	Help identify which activities patient can perform Offer encouragement throughout activity Involve family in care Allow patient to make decisions related to ADLs
Powerlessness related to SCI	Verbalizes increased control over activities	Encourage patient to talk about feelings about self and illness Include the patient in planning care Allow patient to make choices related to ADLs Display sensitivity toward events that could cause powerlessness Obtain patient views prior to providing information/directions Encourage patient to ask questions

Data from Kim, M. J., et al.: Pocket Guide to Nursing Diagnoses. 2nd ed. St. Louis, C. V. Mosby, 1987; and Marshall, S. B., et al.: Neuroscience Critical Care. Philadelphia, W. B. Saunders, 1990.

cord is the next focus of medical therapy. Since the goal is to maintain blood pressure within normal limits, using volume expanders is a preferred option in treatment. A Swan-Ganz catheter is used to determine the need for fluids.

Glucocorticoids have been used in the treatment of SCI for many years. The current controversy over the use of these drugs is in relation to the correct dosage needed to reverse the effects of SCI. A multicentered clinical trial to evaluate the efficacy of methylprednisolone is currently in progress. The dosing regimen is initiated with a bolus of 2000 mg, followed by a 24-hour infusion of methylprednisolone to maintain plasma levels to effect lipid peroxidation (Hall, 1989).

To prevent thrombus formation and pulmonary embolism, prophylactic anticoagulant therapy is initiated during the acute aspect of SCI as well as an antiembolic hose or a pulsatile hose.

OUTCOMES

During the past 20 years, functional outcomes for the SCI patient have been discouraging. With the advances in neuroscience research, and a better understanding of the pathophysiology of spinal cord injury, better treatment options, more skilled nursing care, and better rehabilitation opportunities the future for the SCI patient will be brighter. (See Nursing Care Plan for the Patient with Spinal Cord Injury.)

Acute Cerebrovascular Disease

Although cerebrovascular disease is the third leading cause of death (500,000 people/year) in the United States, over the last 20 years, there has been a decline in mortality resulting from cerebrovascular accident (CVA). Some factors responsible for this decline are improved control of blood pressure with antihypertensive medications, low-sodium and low-fat diets, and a decrease in cigarette smoking. Cerebrovascular accident is a broad term that covers a variety of intracranial vascular problems, which are usually found in the older population.

The critical care nurse encounters the patient with an intracranial hemorrhage more frequently than those with other kinds of cerebrovascular disorders. The patient with an occlusive stroke is seldom admitted to the critical care unit unless there is extensive neurological damage or decreased ventilatory ability.

PATHOPHYSIOLOGY

The mechanisms underlying CVA are due to atherosclerosis (thrombosis, embolism) or bleeding (hypertensive hemorrhage, aneurysms, arteriovenous malformation) of a cerebral vessel.

Blockage in a cerebral vessel results in a decrease in cerebral blood flow secondary to the blocked portion of the artery, and ischemia results. Along with ischemia there is inadequate oxygen delivery to brain cells, inadequate CO_2 removal, increased intracellular lactic acid production, decreased adenosine triphosphate (ATP), and disruption of the blood-brain barrier.

The underlying cause of a blocked artery is a thrombus or an embolus. Atherosclerosis, the most frequent cause of thrombotic disease, results in plaque present at bifurcations and curves in arteries. An embolus occurs when the plaque fragments, breaks off, and travels to the brain. When this plaque lodges in a cerebral artery, then cerebral blood flow is decreased. Cardiac sources of cerebral emboli (atrial fibrillation, rheumatic heart disease, acute MI, endocarditis, mitral valve prolapse, and valve prosthesis) are of paramount importance to be considered in treatment. In these cases, it is therefore important to treat the cardiac as well as neurological problem.

When a cerebral vessel ruptures, the result is a hemorrhagic CVA. The major types of hemorrhagic events are lacunar infarcts and bleeding into the subarachnoid space (i.e., ruptured aneurysm, arteriovenous malformation).

Chronic hypertension causes fibrinoid necrosis of the very small cerebral arteries, thereby causing reduction of the tensile strength in the vessel wall. This weakness causes the artery to leak, and blood escapes into brain tissue. The characteristic locations of lacunar infarcts are the basal ganglia, subcortical white matter, thalamus, cerebellum, and brain stem.

A ruptured cerebral aneurysm is a very common cause of subarachnoid hemorrhage (SAH). A portion of a cerebral artery that has an aneurysm presents as a bulging balloonlike area with a thin dome. Cerebral aneurysms occur at the bifurcation of large arteries at the base of the brain (circle of Willis) and rupture into the subarachnoid space of the basal cisterns. On occasion, cerebral aneurysms do rupture into the ventricular system or into brain tissue. When the aneurysm forms, a weakness in the arterial wall allows the development of the dome and neck of the aneurysm. Rupture usually takes place at the dome of the aneurysm. After rupture into the subarachnoid space, autoregulation is impaired. Subarachnoid hemorrhage secondary to a ruptured cerebral aneurysm is associated with a high morbidity and mortality. Most patients with a cerebral aneurysm are asymptomatic prior to the ruptured aneurysm. All patients with a ruptured cerebral aneurysm are at high risk for sudden death (Kirsch et al., 1989).

Prior to rupture, a cerebral aneurysm can mimick a mass lesion and compress brain tissue, cranial nerves, and blood vessels. Immediately following the rupture, there is bleeding into adjacent tissue, and increased intracranial pressure may be focal (near the aneurysm) or global. Cerebral blood flow is altered by increased intracranial pressure and impaired autoregulation. This altered cerebral blood flow causes a gradual ischemia. If the vessel does not seal off following the rupture, the intracranial pressure will equal the systemic arterial pressure and sudden death will follow (Kirsch et al., 1989).

Following the aneurysm rupture, the patient can also experience cardiac dysrhythmias, rebleeding, hydrocephalus, seizures, and vasospasm. The neurological injury can also be related to these events.

Cardiac dysrhythmia occurs as a result of stimulation of the sympathetic nervous system (Kirsch et al., 1989). Cardiac dysrhythmias can cause a transient loss of consciousness following acute aneurysm rupture. In addition to cardiac dysrhythmias, increased sympathetic tone also causes a high incidence of large T waves, prolonged QT intervals, and ST abnormalities (Kirsch et al., 1989).

Another problem following the initial aneurysm rupture is a rebleed prior to surgical clipping of the aneurysm. The mechanism causing a rebleed is an increased tension on the aneurysm wall (Kirsch et al., 1989). An increase in tension is due to hypertension and a sudden decrease in pressure around the aneurysm.

A subarachnoid hemorrhage can cause an impairment of cerebrospinal fluid circulation and reabsorption of CSF. A blood clot can destruct the flow in the ventricular system, causing an obstructive hydrocephalus. As blood enters the subarachnoid space, an inflammatory response is triggered. This inflammatory response can cause fibrosis and thickening of the arachnoid villi, which inhibits reabsorption. This inhibition of reabsorption of CSF causes communicating hydrocephalus. Both obstructive and communicating hydrocephalus cause increased intracranial pressure.

Another problem following a ruptured aneurysm is seizures. The incidence of seizures following an acute aneurysm rupture is as high as 26% (Kirsch et al., 1989). Seizures increase the metabolic demand and oxygen requirements of brain cells. Seizures occurring within the first 12 hours following rupture are attributed to increased intracranial pressure. After the initial 12 hours, but before surgical clipping of the aneurysm, seizures are associated with rebleeding of the aneurysm (Kirsch et al., 1989). Because of the potential danger of the effects of seizures, most patients are given phenytoin (Dilantin) to prevent seizures from occurring.

Cerebral vasospasm is a narrowing of arteries adjacent to the aneurysm, which results in ischemia and infarction of brain tissue if unresolved. The usual period of time for vasospasm to occur is 4 to 14 days after the rupture. The exact mechanism for vasospasm is unknown, but it is known that some factors contributing to vasospasm include structural changes in the adjacent cerebral arteries, denervation of adjacent arteries, generation of oxygen free radicals and release of vasoactive substances (serotonin, catecholamines, prostaglandins, oxyhemoglobin) that initiate vasospasm, an inflammatory response, and calcium influx.

Arteriovenous malformations (AVMs) of the brain are composed of tangled dilated vessels that form an abnormal communication network between the arterial and venous systems. Arterial blood is directly shunted into the venous system without a capillary network. The size and location of AVMs are varied, but they all cause varying degrees of ischemia, scarring of brain tissue, abnormal tissue development, compression, hemorrhage, hydrocephalus, and cardiac decompensation. Arteriovenous malformations are the leading cause of subarachnoid and ventricular hemorrhages in young people.

ASSESSMENT

Nursing Assessment

As with patients with IICP and head injury, nursing history and neurological assessment are very important. Mental status, cranial nerve functioning, and motor status are included in the assessment.

Since hemodynamic instability is common with acute CVA, the assessments of the airway, blood pressure, pulse, respirations, and fluid and electrolyte status are also priorities. The patient with a CVA will generally have intracranial pressure, hemodynamic status, and cardiac function monitored. Assessing functional status related to normal ranges of each of these parameters is also part of assessment skills.

Patients who undergo cerebral angiography need to have a baseline neurological assessment both prior to and after the procedure. The puncture site is inspected for hematoma or bleeding and is immobilized for 6 to 8 hours to prevent bleeding. When the femoral site is used, circulatory checks are performed bilaterally to include femoral and pedal pulses as well as color and temperature of the extremity.

Since there are a variety of medications used for occlusive and hemorrhagic CVA, assessing the patient for side effects of medications is incorporated in the nursing assessment.

Medical Assessment

The initial baseline laboratory tests obtained in the CVA patient are the following:

1. CBC (RBC, hemoglobin, hematocrit, platelet count)
2. Sedimentation rate
3. BUN, creatinine, electrolytes, serum osmolality
4. Fibrinogen levels (SAH)
5. Urinalysis and urine osmolality

Diagnostic tests that are performed to confirm the diagnosis of CVA include:

1. Chest x-ray (cardiac contour, pulmonary AVM)
2. CT scan of the brain (ischemia, hemorrhage)
3. MRI (sensitive to the presence and extent of ischemia)
4. Doppler carotid studies (middle cerebral artery stenosis/occlusion)
5. Transcranial doppler
6. Digital subtraction angiography (detects carotid occlusion and information about vertebral arteries)
7. Angiography (defines shallow ulcerated plaques, stenosis, mural thrombus, dissections, multiple lesions, aneurysms, AVMs; reveals poor blood flow, collateral flow)
8. Lumbar puncture (performed if CT scan does not demonstrate SAH, mass lesion, or obstructive hydrocephalus; diagnostic for SAH)

NURSING DIAGNOSIS

The patient with a CVA will have similar nursing diagnoses as the patient with increased intracranial pressure and head injury. Refer to the Nursing Care Plan for the Patient with Increased ICP, Head Injury, or CVA for the specific nursing diagnoses.

INTERVENTIONS

Nursing Interventions

For a patient with a CVA due to blockage, the nursing interventions are neurological assessment, administration of medications (i.e., anticoagulants, streptokinase, antihypertensive agents), observation for side effects of medications, and maintenance of hemodynamic stability. Since the risk of hemorrhage into an ischemic area is present in a hypertensive patient, blood pressure is reduced slowly, with the goal of preventing an intracerebral hemorrhage, but not low enough to cause ischemia. It is important to keep the CPP in the range of 60 to 70 mm Hg (Ropper and Kennedy, 1988). To prevent vasospasm, the blood pressure is maintained at an elevated level (systolic 160 to 170 mm Hg).

The patient with a hemorrhagic CVA presents the nurse with many challenges. When arterial blood enters the subarachnoid space, its presence is very irritating to the meninges. If conscious, the patient may complain of an extremely severe headache, experience photophobia, and have a stiff neck. These signs of meningeal irritation are very common following a subarachnoid bleed. This patient may also experience increased intracranial pressure, alteration in cerebral blood flow, hemodynamic instability, vasospasm, rebleeding, and hydrocephalus. A variety of medications are used with these patients depending on the cause of the bleeding. Possible medications are hypertensive agents, volume expanders, calcium channel blockers, steroids, mild sedatives, osmotic diuretics, and antifibrinolytic and anticonvulsant agents. Important interventions for the patient with a subarachnoid hemorrhage are a quiet environment, bed rest, and few visitors. Dimming the room lights and turning down the volume of the patient's monitors can be beneficial in reducing noxious stimuli. The interventions for the CVA patient are similar to those for the patient with increased intracranial pressure and head injury (see Nursing Care Plan for the Patient with Increased ICP, Head Injury, or CVA).

Medical (Nonsurgical) Treatment for Occlusive CVA

Quick, aggressive treatment of CVA is the current theme of medical treatment. The goal for management of CVA is maintaining cerebral blood flow to limit infarct size and to prevent ischemia that leads to cell death.

For a patient with an occlusive CVA, the medical treatment is to improve blood flow to impaired, perfused areas of the brain. This is done by increasing collateral flow, reducing viscosity, and removing the blockage. Hypervolemic hemodilution (dextran, albumin, plasma protein fraction [Plasmanate]) reduces viscosity and decreases hematocrit and platelet aggregation. These patients need to have a Swan-Ganz catheter in place to monitor cardiac reserve and pulmonary pressures.

Anticoagulation therapy is also used in occlusive CVA. Anticoagulation prevents or slows the progressive end-stage thrombosis. Heparin and then long-term use of warfarin maintain the patency of the arterial lumen. Anticoagulation prevents embolism from the heart. When anticoagulation is in use, however, there is danger of bleeding (see Nursing Care Plan for the Patient with Increased ICP, Head Injury, or CVA).

Randomized trials with thrombolytic therapy (tissue plasminogen activator [TPA], streptokinase, urokinase) are currently being used in several medical centers in the United States (Marshall et al., 1990; Wechsler, 1988). The goal of this therapy is to dissolve the clot and restore cerebral blood flow. Hemorrhagic complications are the major disadvantage of this therapy (Wechsler, 1988).

Other therapies for occlusive CVA are control of blood pressure, cerebral edema, and intracranial pressure. Control for these events was discussed in the previous section on increased intracranial pressure.

Surgical Treatment of Occlusive Stroke

Carotid endarterectomy is performed to remove plaque from the cervical internal carotid artery. During the first postoperative 24 hours, fluctuating blood pressure can occur. The most common fluctuation is hypotension with bradycardia, which might require treatment with a vasopressor agent. Hypertension has also been associated with cerebral hemorrhage. Other complications from this surgery are neck hematoma and myocardial infarction.

Another surgical procedure is the extracranial-intracranial bypass, which is very controversial. This procedure theoretically would increase cerebral blood flow to areas that were surgically inaccessible by bypassing occluded parts of the circulation. An external artery is grafted to an intracranial artery. In the randomized trials of this surgical procedure, the desired effects of increasing cerebral blood flow were not produced (Ropper and Kennedy, 1988).

Medical Management of Hemorrhagic CVA

Time is a critical factor in hemorrhagic CVA. Treatment is based on the size, extent, and location of the bleeding. The goal is to stop the bleeding and to prevent brain damage resulting from the bleeding. The level of consciousness is the single factor that guides treatment decisions. When the patient arrives at the hospital awake and responsive to the environment, and continues to maintain an intact mental status, medical treatment is the first choice. However, when the patient is admitted with, or develops, deterioration in mental status, the patient may be a surgical candidate, especially if there are large areas of hemorrhage or hemispheric bleeding.

Intracerebral hemorrhage caused by hypertension is treated by reducing the blood pressure gradually. Usually the goal is to maintain the systolic pressure at 160 mm Hg or the mean pressure below 110 mm Hg in the conscious patient. Examples of agents used for reducing the blood pressure are nitroglycerin, nitroprusside, and labetalol. Other therapies are directed toward minimizing increased intracranial pressure, cerebral edema, and hydrocephalus. For large hematomas and brain stem hematomas, surgical evacuation of the clot is necessary.

Subarachnoid hemorrhage secondary to a ruptured aneurysm or AVM requires medical and surgical interventions. Early medical treatment is aggressively aimed toward preventing a rebleed of the aneurysm and vasospasm as well as toward minimizing cerebral edema, hypertension, increased intracranial pressure, hydrocephalus, and seizures.

Aneurysm precautions directed at preventing a rebleed involve mainly control of the environment. It is necessary for the patient to be in an environment that is calm, quiet, and free from situations that would emotionally upset the patient. If the patient has photophobia, the room lights should also be dimmed to minimize the associated headache. Visitors are kept to a minimum during this acute period. A mild sedative and nonnarcotic analgesics for headache are given as needed. The other aspect of treatment is minimizing increased intracranial pressure to prevent rebleed. Head and body positions, prevention of strain, and isometric exercises become important components of therapy. A stool softener is ordered to prevent straining. The patient may be instructed not to assist in turning from side to side in bed.

A variety of techniques are used to treat vasospasm. The exact mechanism for vasospasm is unknown, so many treatments are used to minimize the condition. Volume expansion (albumin, plasma protein fraction [Plasmanate]) is one of these therapies. During the time hypervolemic hemodilution is used, the patient is monitored with a Swan-Ganz catheter. Volume expansion maintains intravascular volume and catecholamines are not released; therefore, preventing vasoconstriction of cerebral arteries. This therapy is directed at minimizing cerebral ischemia. Other modes of therapy include the administration of calcium channel blockers (nifedipine, nimodipine), hypertensive agents, steroids (methylprednisolone, dexamethasone [Decadron]), osmotic and loop diuretics (mannitol, furosemide [Lasix]), and anticonvulsants (phenytoin [Dilantin], phenobarbital, valproic acid).

Surgical Treatment of Hemorrhagic CVA

Surgical intervention for a intracerebral hematoma is dependent on the size, extent, and location of the hematoma. The surgical procedure is directed at removing the hematoma and necrotic tissue in the area.

Surgery for a cerebral aneurysm consists of occluding the neck of the aneurysm (use of a ligature/metal clip), reinforcing the sac (wrapping the sac with muscle, fibrin foam, solidifying polymer), and proximal ligation of a feeding vessel. If the neck of the aneurysm is narrow, then using a ligature or metal clip is desirable. When the neck of the aneurysm is too broad, then reinforcing the aneurysmal sac is then the goal of the surgery. Proximal ligation may be preferred when the aneurysm is of the internal carotid artery. The disadvantage of this procedure is decreased cerebral blood flow to certain parts of the brain. The trend is to stabilize the patient early and to take this patient to surgery early (within hours of the rupture). The timing of the surgery is important for acceptable neurological outcomes. The goal is to take the patient to surgery when there is minimal neurological dysfunction and prior to episodes of rebleeding or vasospasm.

Hemorrhage from an AVM is a low-pressure bleed, and the mortality from such a hemorrhage is lower than that of a ruptured aneurysm. The rebleed rate is also much lower than that of an aneurysm. Surgery for removal of the AVM is done either as a single step or in multiple stages. Postoperatively, the major problem is breakthrough bleeding from cauterized vessels. Rapid increases in blood pressure during recovery from anesthesia are to be avoided.

OUTCOMES

Patient outcomes for CVA include maintaining cerebral blood flow and minimizing complications associated with ischemia, cerebral edema, increased intracranial pressure, hydrocephalus, rebleeding, vasospasm, and seizures. The outcomes of the patient with a CVA are identical to the outcomes of the patient with increased intracranial pressure and head injury (see Nursing Care Plan for the Patient with Increased ICP, Head Injury, and CVA).

■ Status Epilepticus

A seizure is a sequela of a wide variety of neurological disorders and systemic diseases. A seizure is an abnormal electrical discharge in the brain that is a symptom of central nervous system irritability. Abnormalities may occur in the motor, sensory, or autonomic nervous system. Seizures consist of repetitive depolarization of hyperactive, hypersensitive cells at a rate of 300 to 1000 per second. When seizures occur in close proximity to each other, they have the potential to lead to a life-threatening situation, referred to as status epilepticus (SE).

PATHOPHYSIOLOGY

Status epilepticus can occur with any seizure type. The international classification of seizures is presented in Table 9–8. Status epilepticus is said to exist when seizures repeat frequently enough so that return of the normal state of brain function does not occur between the attacks. Specifically, status epilepticus is present when seizure activity lasts for 30 minutes (Riela, 1989). Status epilepticus is present in the case of partial seizures when the episode lasts 30 minutes or longer. It has been estimated that over 10,000 episodes of status epilepticus occur in the United States each year (Solomon et al., 1983; Treiman, 1983). Status epilepticus is more likely to occur

Table 9–8. INTERNATIONAL CLASSIFICATION OF EPILEPTIC SEIZURES

I. Partial or focal seizures
  A. Elementary
    1. Motor symptoms
    2. Sensory symptoms
    3. Autonomic symptoms
    4. Mixed symptoms
  B. Complex (temporal lobe or psychomotor)
    1. Impaired consciousness only
    2. Cognitive symptoms
    3. Affective symptoms
    4. Psychosensory symptoms
    5. Psychomotor symptoms
  C. Partial seizure that secondarily generalizes
II. Generalized seizures (without focal onset)
  A. Tonic-clonic (grand mal)
  B. Status epilepticus
  C. Absence attacks (petit mal)
  D. Tonic
  E. Clonic
  F. Myoclonic
  G. Atonic
  H. Akinetic
III. Unclassified (incomplete data)

Reproduced by permission from Rudy, E. B.: Advanced Neurological and Neurosurgical Nursing. St. Louis, C. V. Mosby, 1984; adapted from Gastaut, H.: Epilepsia 11:102, 1970.

with tonic-clonic seizures that have a specific causative factor than with seizures of an idiopathic nature. Brain tumors and brain trauma account for approximately 40% of the causes of SE (Janz, 1983).

The most frequent precipitating factor of status epilepticus is irregular intake of anticonvulsants, withdrawal from habitual use of alcohol or sedative drugs, electrolyte imbalances, or azotemia.

During status epilepticus metabolism and brain energy requirements may be five times greater than normal. When seizures are prolonged, calcium, prostaglandins, and various diglycerides accumulate in the nerve cells. This leads to cerebral edema and eventually nerve cell death (Solomon, et al., 1983). The pathological changes occurring from SE follow the pattern of cerebral hypoxia or severe hypoglycemia, although the precise mechanism to explain this is not known (Treiman, 1983).

In the tonic phase of SE, adequate oxygenation may be precluded by the tonic fixation of the chest wall and the obstruction of the airway by the glottis. In addition to these mechanical causes of inadequate ventilation, there are two additional deterrents to adequate ventilation. First, neurogenic pulmonary edema may be triggered by the massive autonomic discharges that occur. This may be associated with excessive bronchial secretions and bronchial constrictions. Additionally, respiratory centers in the brain stem may be effected by the abnormal neuronal discharge (Solomon, et al., 1983; Treiman, 1983).

The sympathetic nervous system effects of a seizure can lead to increases in serum epinephrine and norepinephrine to levels high enough to cause cardiac arrhythmias (Burnstine, et al., 1990; Treiman, 1983). Hypoxia and acidosis may also contribute to arrhythmias. In the initial stages, cerebral blood flow is increased along with the elevation of systemic blood pressure.

The autonomic dysfunction also causes hyperpyrexia, excessive sweating, and vomiting that leads to dehydration and electrolyte loss. Initial hyperglycemia is probably a result of the increased release of epinephrine and activation of hepatic gluconeogenesis (Glaser, 1983). With continuation of the seizure, energy stores are depleted, leading to hypoglycemia, an increase in the metabolism of lactic acid, and eventually to cytotoxic cerebral edema.

Mirskl (1990) notes that status epilepticus carries a mortality rate of approximately 2 to 10%. Death is more likely to occur when there is an underlying neurological disease responsible for the condition, and may result from the seizure or from the acute illness that precipitated the seizure (Celesia, 1983; Hauser, 1983). Generalized seizures that last for as little as 30 to 45 minutes result in neuronal necrosis in the areas of the basal ganglia, hippocampus, and neocortex even in the face of adequate oxygenation. This may result in permanent neurological deficits. To avoid permanent neurological dysfunction such as hemiparesis or chronic impairment of recent memory, even focal status and nonconvulsive status require prompt treatment (Treiman, 1983).

Additionally, status epilepticus may lead to other systemic complications. Renal failure may result from rhabdomyolysis and acute myoglobinuria. These may also cause hyperkalemia and acute intravascular coagulation (Treiman, 1983; Glaser, 1983). Prolonged clonic-tonic seizure activity leads to many systemic effects. Changes occur in the cardiovascular system because of increased demands from repeated skeletal muscle activity. Initially, tachycardia is present to increase cardiac output. Hypertension occurs to increase CBF in order to meet the metabolic demands of O_2 and glucose for neurons. As the seizure activity continues more stimulation of the vagus nerve occurs resulting in bradycardia. Cardiac dysrhythmias result from hyperkalemia (increased muscle activity), metabolic acidosis, and decreased respirations during SE.

Owing to the excessive muscle activity from prolonged skeletal muscle contraction and traumatic injury during SE, a disintegration of striated muscle fibers occurs. Myoglobinuria results from this muscle damage and may lead to renal failure.

ASSESSMENT

Nursing Assessments

Nursing assessments during status epilepticus incorporates neurological, respiratory, and cardiovascular assessment. Characteristics of the seizure and the neurological state between seizures are important aspects for the nurse to monitor and record. Documentation of the length of time and pattern of the seizure are necessary. Automatisms and head and eye deviation need to be noted. Assessment of respirations and monitoring of arterial blood gases is needed to assure adequacy of oxygenation. Because autonomic changes can result in pulmonary edema, it is imperative to note the onset of fine basilar crackles. Since status epilepticus may precipitate arrhythmias, cardiac monitoring and assessment are required.

Medical Assessment

Laboratory studies for the patient with status epilepticus should include electrocardiogram, serum electrolytes, serum medication levels, and blood and urine toxicology screens. Cardiac enzymes and arterial blood gases will assist in assessing the effect of the seizure on other body systems. Continuous cardiac monitoring needs to be in place prior to the administration of intravenous medications (Burnstine et al., 1990).

Appropriate radiological studies are needed to rule out a space-occupying lesion that may be responsible for the episode of SE. These may include computed tomography and electromagnetic resonance. Additional studies may be appropriate to rule out injury.

NURSING DIAGNOSES

Nursing diagnoses appropriate for the patient experiencing status epilepticus are:

* Potential for altered cerebral tissue perfusion related to the seizure activity
* Potential for ineffective breathing patterns/impaired gas exchange related to the seizure activity
* Potential for ineffective airway clearance related to underlying neurological problem and seizure activity
* Potential for fluid and electrolyte imbalance related to underlying neurological problem, status epilepticus, and drug therapy
* Potential for injury related to underlying neurological problems and/or seizure activity
* Altered thought processes related to the postictal state
* Impaired communication related to postictal state
* Potential for altered self-concept related to seizure activity
* Potential ineffective family coping related to patient's seizure activity

INTERVENTIONS

Nursing Interventions

Objectives of nursing management during status epilepticus need to incorporate the following:

* Maintain a patent airway
* Provide adequate oxygenation
* Maintain vascular access for administration of medications
* Maintain seizure precautions

A patent airway is facilitated by the use of an airway such as an endotracheal tube or nasal airway. This will also assist with removal of secretions that collect in the oropharynx. Supplemental oxygen is used to improve oxygenation. Suction equipment needs to be readily available to assist with airway clearance. Poor gas exchange during status epilepticus or as a result of respiratory depression from medications may necessitate intubation to adequately provide oxygenation. A nasogastric tube with intermittent suction is needed to assure that the airway is not compromised by aspiration.

Vascular access must be maintained to assure a route for administration of medication. The specific medication given will depend on the physician's preference and type of seizure. Seizure precautions are continued during status epilepticus. This should include padding the siderails on the patients bed and assuring that full length siderails are on the bed. The bed needs to remain in a low position with siderails up except when direct nursing care is being given. Do not use pad-

Table 9–9. DRUG THERAPY IN PATIENTS WITH IICP, HEAD INJURY, CVA, SCI, OR SE

Drug	Actions/Uses	Dosage/Route	Side Effects	Nursing Implications
Mannitol (20%)	Draws water from normal brain cells into plasma; reduces ICP; increases CPP	1.5–2 g/kg initial IV over 0.5–1.0 hr then 0.25–0.5 g/kg IV every 3–5 hr depending on ICP, CPP, serum osmolarity	Hypotension, dehydration, electrolyte imbalance, tachycardia, rebound edema	1–2 hr neurological assessments; monitor ICP, CPP, serum osmolarity; hourly I&O; daily weights, monitor electrolytes, monitor ABGs, VS
Furosemide (Lasix)	Renal tubular duiretic; reduces cerebral edema by drawing sodium and water out of injured neurons; decreases CSF production	1 mg/kg IV bolus every 6–12 hr (Becker and Gudeman, 1989)	Ototoxicity, polyuria, electrolyte disturbances, gastric irritation, muscle cramps, hypotension	Same as above
Dexamethasone (Decadron)	Steroid that has a stabilizing effect on cell membrane and prevents destructive effect of free O_2 radicals; decreases inflammation by suppressing white cells	6–20 mg IV initial then 4–6 mg every 6 hr IV	Flushing, sweating, hypotension, tachycardia, thrombocytopenia, weakness, nausea, diarrhea, GI irritation/hemorrhage, fluid retention, poor wound healing, weight gain	Decreases effects of anticoagulants, anticonvulsants, antidiabetic agents; increases effects of digitalis; monitor glucose, potassium, daily weights; monitor VS; causes edema; taper drug prior to discontinuing
Cimetidine	Inhibits histamine at the H_2 receptor sites inhibiting gastric acid secretion; decreases GI irritation to stress response following neurological injury and steroid use	300 mg in 50 ml 0.9% NaCl every 6–8 hr	Diarrhea, increases BUN, creatinine, thrombocytopenia; increases prothrombin time, bradycardia	Increases toxicity of phenytoin, lidocaine, procainamide; antacids decrease action of cimetidine; give slowly IV—can cause bradycardia
Labetalol	Beta-blocker that is nonselecting; decreases blood pressure	200 mg in 200 ml 0.9% NS at 2 mg/min IV; repeat every 6–8 hr as needed or 20 mg/over 2 min IV bolus; may repeat 40–80 mg every 10 min not to exceed 300 mg (Skidmore-Roth, 1988)	Hypotension, bradycardia, CHF, ventricular dysrhythmias, drowsiness, lethargy, nausea, tinnitis, wheezing	Cimetidine increases hypotension; increases hypoglycemia; hourly I&O; daily weights; monitor BP, pulse; taper drug if long-term use
Phenytoin (Dilantin)	Inhibits the spread of seizures; SE	For status epilepticus 10–15 mg/kg loading dose IV not to exceed a rate of 50 mg/min; can be infused mixed with NS at doses of 20 mg/kg, rate not to exceed 50 mg/min	Bradycardia, hypotension nystagmus/ataxia—dose-related gingival hyperplasia, blood dyscrasias; rash	Slow rate down if bradycardia or cardiac arrhythmias occur; monitor ECG and BP; monitor lab; monitor respiratory status
Diazepam (Valium)	Depresses subcortical areas of CNS; SE	5–10 mg initially; may be repeated at 10 to 15 min intervals up to a maximum of 30 mg, rate of administration not to exceed 2 mg/min	Respiratory depression, hypotension, drowsiness, dry mouth	Monitor respiratory status; administer IV bolus in a large vein
Lorazepam (Ativan)	Same as diazepam	2–4 mg IV bolus	Respiratory depression, hypotension, drowsiness	Same as diazepam
Pentobarbitol	Sedation; barbiturate metabolism and energy requirements; may prevent peroxidation of lipid components of cell membrane; used for refractory ICP and refractory SE	For IICP: 3–5 mg/kg IV in boluses of 50–100 mg doses monitoring ICP—loading dose; hourly maintenance doses of 100–200 mg (1–2 mg/kg) For SE: 2–8 mg/kg IV loading dose; maintenance dose 1–3 mg/kg/hr IV	Hypotension (at time of bolus); myocardial depression; respiratory depression	Monitor ICP (goal is to decrease ICP 15–20 mm Hg), monitor CPP; monitor vital signs and hemodynamic status; response of individual patients is variable; each one must be monitored closely

ded tongue blades since it is virtually impossible to insert any object between the tonically clenched teeth of a patient undergoing a seizure. Patients have inadvertently been injured from aspirating teeth that were loosened during attempts to forcefully insert a padded tongue blade between their teeth. When a neuromuscular blocker is used, then an oral airway is inserted.

Medical Interventions

Status epilepticus needs to be stopped within 20 minutes. No consensus has been reached as to the drug of choice since no ideal drug exits (Treiman, 1983). For tonic-clonic status either diazepam (Valium) or lorazepam (Ativan) is given in an IV bolus for rapid control of status epilepticus (Kapil and D'Souza, 1985). Diazepam has a rapid onset and is given at a rate of 2 mg/min for a total dose of 30 mg. Diazepam does not mix with other solutions and is administered at the IV port closest to the catheter as possible. Lorazepam is given as an IV bolus of 2 to 4 mg (0.05 to 0.2 mg/kg) (Kapil and D'Souza, 1985). Lorazepam has a longer duration of action than diazepam.

Phenytoin is also given during SE and requires a loading dose that may require 20 minutes to administer. The drug is given no faster than 50 mg/min to a total of 15 mg/kg. Phenytoin mixes only with normal saline; however, it is stable in solution for only 20 minutes, making it impractical for intravenous piggyback administration. It may be given as a push after clearing the line with saline or slowly pushed with normal saline running.

Phenobarbital is also used intravenously in status epilepticus. It can be given intravenously at 5 to 8 mg as a slow intravenous push. Because of the potential for respiratory depression, it is not recommended for use with diazepam.

General anesthesia may be initiated with artificial respirations and cardiorespiratory monitoring if SE has not been terminated within 60 minutes. General anesthesia can be achieved in the critical care setting with low-dose continuous drip intravenous pentobarbital therapy. Patients should be assessed for evidence of hemodynamic instability. Treatment of this patient should incorporate control of metabolic disturbances (Mirskl, 1990; Swatz and Delgado-Escueta, 1987). Refer to Table 9–9 for drug therapy.

OUTCOMES

Patient outcomes for status epilepticus are focused on protection during this life-threatening episode and prevention of recurrence. The first outcome is that the patient will maintain an adequate breathing pattern. Second, the patient will not experience an injury related to the seizure activity. And finally, the patient will demonstrate knowledge of the disease process, including precipitating factors, medication routines, and side effects of medications.

SUMMARY

Status epilepticus is a life-threatening event. Astute nursing assessment, airway management, maintenance of cardiovascular and metabolic functions, and prevention of patient injury results in positive outcomes. Proper pharmacotherapeutic management is essential during the course of status epilepticus.

References

Adelstein, W. (1989): C-C fractures and dislocations. *Journal of Neuroscience Nursing* 21(3):149–159.

Alspach, J. G. (ed.) (1991): *AACN Core Curriculum for Critical Care Nursing.* 4th ed., p. 401. Philadelphia: W. B. Saunders.

Becker, D. P., and Gudeman, S. K. (1989): *Textbook of Head Injury.* Philadelphia: W. B. Saunders.

Boortz-Martz, R. (1985): Factors affecting intracranial pressure. A descriptive study. *Journal of Neuroscience Nursing* 17(2):89–94.

Burnstine, T. H., Lesser, R. P., and Hanley, D. F. (1990): Association of cardiorespiratory abnormalities. *Critical Care Report* 1(1):39–42.

Celesia, G. G. (1983): Prognosis in convulsive status epilepticus. *Advances in Neurology* 34:55–59.

Dolan, J. T. (ed.) (1991): *Critical Care Nursing: Clinical Management Through the Nursing Process.* Philadelphia: F. A. Davis, p. 93.

Franges, E. Z., and Beideman, M. E. (1988): Infections related to intracranial pressure monitoring. *Journal of Neuroscience Nursing* 20(2):94–103.

Germon, K. (1988): Interpretation of ICP pulse waves to determine intracerebral compliance. *Journal of Neuroscience Nursing* 20(6):344–351.

Glaser, G. H. (1983): Medical complications of status epilepticus. *Advances in Neurology* 34:395–398.

Hall, E. D. (1989): Free radicals and CNS injury. *Critical Care Clinics* 5(4):793–805.

Hauser, W. A. (1983): Status epilepticus: Frequency, etiology, and neurological sequelae. *Advances in Neurology* 34:3–14.

Hickey, J. V. (1986): *The Clinical Practice of Neurological Neurosurgical Nursing.* 2 ed. Philadelphia: J. B. Lippincott.

Hudak, C. M., Gallo, B. M., and Lohr, T. (1986): *Critical Care Nursing.* 4th ed. Philadelphia: J. B. Lippincott.

Hulme, A., and Cooper, R. (1976): The effects of head position & jugular vein compression on intracranial pressure in patients with severe head injury. In: J. Beks et al. (eds.). *Intracranial Pressure III.* Berlin: Springer-Verlag, pp. 259–263.

Ingersoll, G. L., and Leyden, D. B. (1990): The Glasgow Coma Scale for patients with head injuries. *Critical Care Nurse* 7(5):26–32.

Janz, D. (1983): Etiology of convulsive status epilepticus. *Advances in Neurology* 34:47–54.

Kapil, R., and D'Souza, B. (1985): Status epilepticus. *Critical Care Clinics* 1:339–353.

Kim, M. J., McFarland, G. K., and McLane, A. M. (1987): *Pocket Guide to Nursing Diagnoses.* 2nd ed. St. Louis: C. V. Mosby.

Kirsch, J. R., Diringer, M. N., Borel, C. O., and Hanley, D. F. (1989): Cerebral aneurysms: mechanism of injury and critical care interventions. *Critical Care Clinics* 5(4):755–772.

Marshall, S. B., Marshall, L. F., Vos, H. R., and Chesnut, R. M. (1990): *Neuroscience Critical Care.* Philadelphia: W. B. Saunders.

Miller, E. R. (1989a): Nursing care of the head-injured patient. In: D. P. Becker and S. K. Gudeman (eds.). *Textbook of Head Injury.* Philadelphia: W. B. Saunders, p. 405.

Miller, J. D. (1989b): Pathophysiology of human head injury. In D. P. Becker and S. K. Gudeman (eds.). *Textbook of Head Injury.* Philadelphia: W. B. Saunders, p. 517.

Mirskl, M. A. (1990): Status epilepticus: Rapid treatment with low-dose pentobarbital. *Critical Care Report* 1(1):150–156.

Mitchell, P., and Mauss, N. (1978): Relationships of patient/nurse activity to intracranial pressure variations: A pilot study. *Nursing Research* 27:4–12.

Mitchell, P., Ozuna, J., and Lipe, H. (1980): Moving the patient in bed: Effects on intracranial pressure. *Nursing Research* 30:212–218.

Morrison, C. A. M. (1990): Brain herniation syndrome. *Critical Care Nurse* 7(5):34–38.

Narayan, R. K. (1989): Emergency room management of the head-injured patient. In: D. P. Becker and S. K. Gudeman (eds.). *Textbook of Head Injury.* Philadelphia: W. B. Saunders, pp. 23–66.

Nikas, D. L. (1987): Critical aspects of head trauma. *Critical Care Quarterly* 10(1):19–44.

Ostrup, R. C., Luerssen, T. G., Marshall, L. F., and Zornow, M. H. (1987): Continuous monitoring of intracranial pressure with a miniaturized fiberoptic device. *Journal of Neurosurgery* 67:206–209.

Pacult, A., and Gudeman, S. K. (1989): Medical management of head injuries. In: D. P. Becker, and S. K. Gudeman (eds.). *Textbook of Head Injuries,* Philadelphia: W. B. Saunders, p. 209.

Parsons, L. C., and Shogan, J. S. (1984): The effects of the endotracheal tube suctioning/manual hyperventilation procedure on patients with severe closed head injuries. *Heart and Lung* 13:372–380.

Parsons, L. C., Peard, A. L., and Page, M. C. (1985): The effects of hygiene interventions on the cerebrovascular status of closed head injured persons. *Research in Nursing and Health* 8:173–181.

Riela, A. R. (1989): Management of seizures. *Critical Care Clinics* 5(4):863–879.

Rockoff, M. A., and Kennedy, S. F. (1988): Physiology & clinical aspects of raised intracranial pressure. In: A. H. Ropper and S. F. Kennedy (eds.). *Neurological & Neurosurgical Intensive Care.* 2nd ed. Rockville, MD: Aspen, pp. 9–21.

Ropper, A. H., and Rockoff, M. A. (1988): *Neurological and Neurosurgical Intensive Care.* Rockville, MD: Aspen, pp. 24–25.

Skidmore-Roth, L. (1988): *Mosby's Nursing Drug Reference.* St. Louis: C. V. Mosby.

Solomon, T. E., Kutt, H., and Plum, F. (1983): The management of status epilepticus. In: A. Hopkins (ed.). *Epilepsy.* New York: Demos, pp. 417–442.

Snyder, M. (1983): Relation of nursing activities to increases in intracranial pressure. *Journal of Advanced Nursing* 8:273–279.

Swatz, B. E., and Delgado-Escueta, A. V. (1987): The management of status epilepticus. In: A. Hopkins (ed.). *Epilepsy.* New York: Demos, pp. 417–442.

Treiman, D. M. (1983): General principles of treatment: Responsive and intractable status epilepticus in adults. *Advances in Neurology* 34:377–384.

Wechsler, L. R. (1988): Therapy for acute ischemic stroke. In: A. H. Ropper and S. F. Kennedy (eds.), *Neurological and Neurosurgical Intensive Care.* 2nd ed. Rockville, MD: Aspen, p. 203.

Recommended Reading

German, K. (1988): Interpretation of ICP pulse waves to determine intracerebral compliance. *Journal of Neuroscience Nursing* 20(6):344–351.

Hartshorn, J. C., and Hartshorn, E. A. (1986): Nursing interventions for anticonvulsant drug interactions. *Journal of Neuroscience Nursing* 18(5):250–255.

Hummel, S. K. (1989): Cerebral vasospasm: current concepts of pathogenesis and treatment. *Journal of Neuroscience Nursing* 21(4):216–225.

Leppik, I. E. (ed.) (1990): Status epilepticus in perspective. *Neurology* 40(5)(suppl. 2):1–51.

MacDonald, E. (1989): Aneurysmal subarachnoid hemorrhage. *Journal of Neuroscience Nursing* 21(5):313–321.

Mahon-Darby, J., Ketchik-Renshaw, B., Richmond, T. S., and Gates, E. M. (1988): Powerlessness in cervical spinal cord injury patients. *Dimensions of Critical Care Nursing* 7(6):346–355.

Manifold, S. L. (1990): Aneurysmal SAH: Cerebral vasospasm and early repair. *Critical Care Nurse* 10(8):62–69.

Palmer, M., and Wyness, M. A. (1988): Positioning and handling: Important considerations in the care of the severely head-injured patient. *Journal of Neuroscience Nursing* 20(1):42–49.

Pollack-Latham, C. L. (1990): Intracranial pressure monitoring: Part I. Physiological principles. *Critical Care Nurse* 7(5):40–51.

Pollack-Latham, C. L. (1990): Intracranial pressure monitoring: Part II. Patient care. *Critical Care Nurse* 7(6):53–72.

Ricci, M. M. (ed.) (1984): Core curriculum for neuroscience nursing. *Association of Neuroscience Nurses.* Chicago

Rutledge, B. (1989): Aneurysm wrapping: Principles application. *Journal of Neuroscience Nursing* 21(6):370–374.

Walleck, C. A. (1987): Intracranial hypertension: Interventions and outcomes. *Critical Care Nursing Quarterly* 10(1):45–57.

Chapter

10

Susan Zorb, R.N., M.S.N., CCRN
Phyllis A. Enfanto, R.N., M.S., CCRN

Acute Respiratory Failure

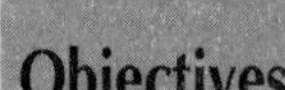

Objectives

- Describe the pathophysiology of acute respiratory failure.
- Compare the etiology, pathophysiology, assessment, nursing diagnoses, outcomes, and interventions for adult respiratory distress syndrome, acute respiratory failure in the patient with chronic obstructive pulmonary disease, and pulmonary embolus.
- Formulate a plan of care for the patient with adult respiratory distress syndrome.

Acute respiratory failure may occur in many settings. It may be the patient's primary problem, or it may be a complicating factor in other conditions. This chapter reviews the pathophysiology of acute respiratory failure as well as several common etiologies.

Definition

Respiratory failure is defined as an impairment of oxygen (O_2) uptake or carbon dioxide (CO_2) elimination, or a combination of the two (Luce et al., 1984). There are no absolute values for arterial PaO_2 or $PaCO_2$ that define respiratory failure. However, a PaO_2 of less than 60 mm Hg or a $PaCO_2$ of greater than 50 mm Hg is generally thought to be indicative of respiratory failure in the general population. Respiratory failure can be the result of failure of arterial oxygenation or failure of ventilation. It is divided into acute, which occurs rapidly with little time for bodily compensation, and chronic, which develops over time and allows the body's compensatory defenses to come into play.

Acute and chronic respiratory failure are not mutually exclusive. Acute respiratory failure, which is the subject of this chapter, may occur in a person who has chronic respiratory failure who develops a sudden respiratory infection or is exposed to other types of stressors.

Pathophysiology

FAILURE OF OXYGENATION

Failure of oxygenation is present when the partial pressure of oxygen (PaO_2) cannot be adequately maintained. There are five generally accepted mechanisms of reduced arterial oxygen concentrations (hypoxemia): (1) hypoventilation, (2) intrapulmonary shunting, (3) ventilation-perfusion mismatching, (4) diffusion defects, and (5) decreased barometric pressure (Ahrens, 1989a) (Fig. 10–1). All of these mechanisms may contribute

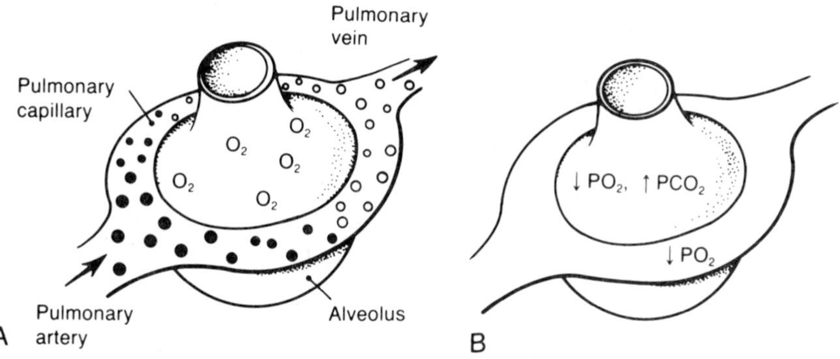

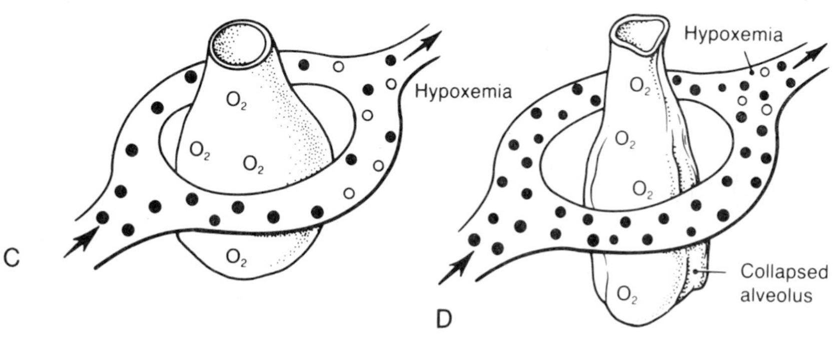

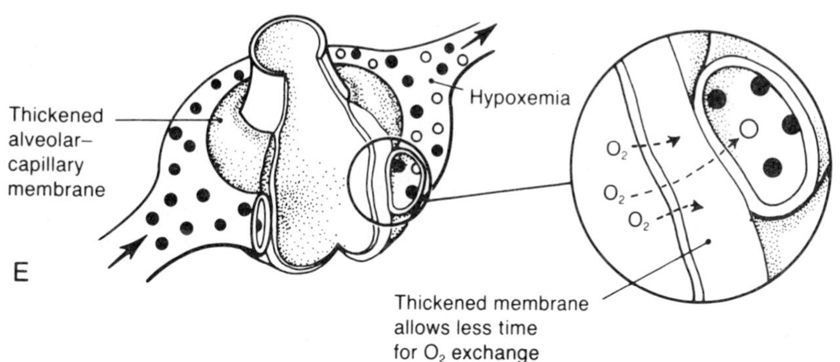

Figure 10–1. The four physiological causes of hypoxemia. *A*, A normal alveolar-capillary unit. Unoxygenated blood *(filled circles)* in the pulmonary capillary obtains O_2 from the alveolus. Oxygenated blood *(open circles)* leaves via the pulmonary veins. *B*, Hypoventilation results in an increased PCO_2 and decreased PO_2. *C*, Ventilation/perfusion mismatch resulting from poor alveolar ventilation; hypoxemia results. *D*, Right-to-left shunt. Hypoxemia results from many disorders, all of which lead to collapsed alveoli. *E*, Diffusion defect. The diffusion of O_2 across the alveolar-capillary membrane is decreased when the membrane is thickened or filled with fluid. (From Yee, B. H., and Zorb, S. L.: Cardiac Critical Care Nursing. Boston, Little, Brown, 1985, Fig. 5–4, p. 109.)

to the failure of oxygenation associated with acute respiratory failure. The least common mechanism, decreased barometric pressure, which occurs at high altitudes, is not addressed in this text. In addition, other conditions such as decreased cardiac output and low hemoglobin may result in tissue hypoxia.

Hypoventilation. In the normal lung, alveolar oxygen (PAO_2) is approximately equal to the PaO_2. Alveolar ventilation (VA) refers to the amount of gas entering the alveoli per minute. If the VA is reduced because of hypoventilation, the PAO_2 and the PaO_2 will be reduced. Factors that lead to hypoventilation include drugs such as morphine sulfate and other central nervous system depressants, as well as neurological disorders that cause a decrease in the rate or depth of respirations. The hypoxemia associated with hypoventilation can be successfully treated with supplemental oxygen administration (West, 1990). Hypoventilation also produces a rise in the alveolar carbon dioxide ($PACO_2$) level because the CO_2 that is produced in the tissues is delivered to the lungs but is not released from the body. This build-up of CO_2 in the alveoli further contributes to the reduced PaO_2 (West, 1990).

Intrapulmonary Shunting. In a perfectly functioning lung, the PaO_2 would exactly equal the PAO_2. However, this is not the case. Normally, a small amount of blood returns to the left side of the heart without engaging in alveolar gas exchange. This blood is referred to as the physiological shunt. If, in addition to the normal shunt, more blood returns to the left side of the heart without being oxygenated, it will cause a drop in the PaO_2. This condition exists when areas of the lung that are being inadequately ventilated are being adequately perfused (see Fig. 10-1). The blood, therefore, is shunted past the lung and returns to the left side of the heart unoxygenated. This intrapulmonary shunting is referred to as Q_s/Q_t disturbances. Q_s refers to the amount of shunted flow, whereas Q_t is the total amount of flow.

As the shunt increases, the PaO_2 continues to drop. This cause of hypoxemia cannot be effectively treated by increasing the inspired oxygen content (FIO_2) since the unventilated alveolar units will not receive any of the enriched air. Clinically, there are several methods to estimate the size of the shunt (Ahrens, 1989a). All of the methods are accurate about 70% of the time.

The most easily understood method for estimating a shunt is the calculation of the arterial/alveolar ratio (a/A ratio). In this method, the actual PaO_2 is compared to what it should be at a certain FIO_2. The alveolar oxygen tension is calculated using the following alveolar air equation.

$$PAO_2 = FIO_2\ (P_B - PH_2O) - PaCO_2/r$$

where

FIO_2 = fraction of inspired O_2

P_B = barometric pressure (760 mm Hg at sea level)

PH_2O = water vapor pressure (47 mm Hg at sea level)

$PaCO_2$ = pressure of arterial CO_2

r = respiratory quotient (usually 0.8)

$$PAO_2 = 0.21\ (760 - 47) - 45/0.8$$
$$PAO_2 = 93.5$$

$$a/A = 50/93.5$$
$$a/A = 0.53$$

If the patient is breathing room air ($FIO_2 = 0.21$) and has a PaO_2 of 50, and $PaCO_2$ of 45, the a/A ratio is 0.53. A normal a/A ratio should be 0.75, but any value greater than 0.60 may be clinically acceptable (Ahrens, 1989a). Use of the a/A ratio enables the clinician to assess the patient's response to therapy and to select the most appropriate FIO_2.

Ventilation/Perfusion Mismatching. The rate of ventilation ($\dot{V}$) usually equals the rate of perfusion ($\dot{Q}$) resulting in a ventilation/perfusion ($\dot{V}/\dot{Q}$) ratio of 1. If ventilation exceeds blood flow, the $\dot{V}/\dot{Q}$ ratio is greater than 1; if ventilation is less than blood flow, the $\dot{V}/\dot{Q}$ ratio is less than 1. In respiratory failure, $\dot{V}/\dot{Q}$ mismatching is the most common cause of hypoxemia. At any given moment, the lung will have various $\dot{V}/\dot{Q}$ ratios; one region may be better ventilated and another better perfused. In the failing lung, there may be a reduction in the ventilation to a region owing to increased secretions obstructing the airway or bronchospasms. If there is partial ventilation of the alveoli involved, the hypoxemia caused by this $\dot{V}/\dot{Q}$ mismatch will respond somewhat to an increase in FIO_2. If perfusion is reduced to an area with normal ventilation, as in pulmonary emboli, there will be an increase in dead space (V_{DS}) in relation to the tidal volume (V_T). The effect of this $\dot{V}/\dot{Q}$ mismatch will be discussed under failure of ventilation.

Diffusion Defects. The distance between the alveoli and the pulmonary capillary is usually only one or two cells thick. This facilitates efficient diffusion of O_2 and CO_2 across the cell membrane. In respiratory failure, the distance between the alveolus and capillary may be increased by the addition of fluid into the interstitial space (see Fig. 10-1). Changes in capillary perfusion pressure as well as leaking of plasma proteins into the interstitial space and destruction of the capillary membrane contribute to the build-up of fluids around the alveolus (Ahrens, 1989b). Fibrotic changes in the lung tissue itself may also contribute to a reduction in the diffusion capacity of the lung. As this capacity is reduced, PaO_2 is the first affected, and hypoxemia results. Because CO_2 is more readily diffusible than O_2, hypercapnea is a later occurring sign of diffusion defect.

Low Cardiac Output. Adequate oxygenation depends on a balance between O_2 supply and demand. Normal O_2 transport is between 600 and 1000 ml/min (Rutherford, 1989b). The major determinant of O_2 supply is the cardiac output (CO), as indicated by the formula for normal O_2 transport, $CaO_2 \times CO \times 10$ (CaO_2 = arterial O_2 content). As previously discussed in Chapter 4, CO is the product of heart rate times stroke volume. If the cardiac output drops, less blood is delivered to the tissues. In order to maintain aerobic metabolism, the tissues must extract increasing amounts of O_2 from the blood. When this increase in extraction can no longer compensate for the decreased cardiac output, anaerobic metabolism takes over. This results in a build-up of lactic acids, which will further depress the myocardium and result in an even lower cardiac output. The patient will exhibit low PaO_2 as well as low mixed venous oxygen saturation (SVO_2). This reduction in SVO_2 reflects the increased extraction of O_2 at the tissue level. This reduction in oxygenation is seen in patients with reduced cardiac output with or without concomitant pulmonary disease.

Low Hemoglobin. The majority of oxygen is transported to the tissues bound to hemoglobin. Each hemoglobin molecule can carry 1.34 g of O_2 when all of its O_2 bonding sites are completely filled. The term *oxygen saturation* refers to the percent of O_2 bonding sites on each hemoglobin molecule that are filled with O_2. For example, a hemoglobin molecule with one-half of its bonding sites filled is said to be 50% saturated. When breathing room air, a normal person's hemoglobin is about 95% saturated. Factors such as fever and acidosis reduce the hemoglobin affinity for oxygen and make it easier to unload the oxygen to the tissues. If a patient's hemoglobin level is below normal, O_2 supply to the tissues may be impaired and tissue hypoxia may occur.

Tissue Hypoxia. In acute respiratory failure, tissue hypoxia is what causes the damage. As previously mentioned, anaerobic metabolism occurs when the tissues can no longer obtain adequate O_2 to meet their metabolic needs. Anaerobic metabolism is inefficient and results in the build-up of lactic acids. The point at which anaerobic metabolism begins to occur is not known and may vary with differing organ systems. The effects of tissue hypoxia vary with the severity of the hypoxia.

Initially, mild central nervous system changes such as changes in visual acuity, impaired mental performance, and hyperventilation may be seen. As the hypoxia increases, changes may be seen in multiple organ systems. There may be a headache, change in the level of consciousness, convulsions, and permanent brain damage. Tachycardia and mild hypertension may be the initial signs in the cardiovascular system, followed by bradycardia, hypotension, and failure as the hypoxia worsens. Renal involvement will produce a decrease in urine output with sodium retention and proteinuria. Pulmonary hypertension is found owing to vasoconstriction in response to alveolar hypoxia. Treatment for respiratory failure will be discussed in each section.

FAILURE OF VENTILATION

Arterial carbon dioxide ($PaCO_2$) is the index used to evaluate ventilation. When $PaCO_2$ is increased (hypercapnia), ventilation is reduced. When $PaCO_2$ is reduced (hypocapnia), ventilation is increased. Hypoventilation and V/Q mismatching are the two mechanisms responsible for hypercapnia.

Hypoventilation. This is the cause of respiratory failure that occurs in patients with neuromuscular disorders, drug overdoses, and chest wall abnormalities (see Fig. 10–1). In hypoventilation, CO_2 accumulates in the alveoli and is not blown off. Respiratory acidosis occurs rapidly before renal compensation can occur. Mechanical ventilation may be necessary to support the patient until the initial cause of the hypoventilation can be corrected.

Ventilation/Perfusion Mismatching. Because the upper and lower airways do not play a part in gas exchange, the volume of inspired gas that fills these structures is referred to as dead space. This is normally 25 to 30% of the inspired volume.

A major mechanism for changes in $PaCO_2$ levels is an alteration in the amount of dead space in relation to the entire tidal volume (V_D/V_T). The amount of dead space in the lung increases when perfusion is reduced to an area that is ventilated because that area no longer participates in gas exchange. Changes in the V_D/V_T ratio must be accompanied by an increase in minute ventilation (V_E) in order for the $PaCO_2$ to remain normal. If the V_D/V_T increases without an accompanying change in V_E, then the $PaCO_2$ will increase.

Hypercapnia greatly increases cerebral blood flow and may result in headache, increased CSF pressure, and papilledema. The patient may appear restless and demonstrate slurred speech, mood swings, and a depressed level of consciousness.

Acute Respiratory Failure in Adult Respiratory Distress Syndrome

DEFINITION

Adult respiratory distress syndrome (ARDS) is a form of noncardiogenic pulmonary edema that can occur as a result of a variety of lung insults. It is a major cause of respiratory failure in patients with previously healthy lungs. Following a lung insult, there is an increase in the permeability of the alveolar capillary membrane. This is characterized by severe dyspnea, hypoxemia, and diffuse bilateral infiltrations on chest x-ray. The pathophysiological changes are similar to those that occur in the respiratory distress syndrome of the newborn.

The signs, symptoms, and pathophysiology that occur with ARDS were first described as a clinical syndrome in adults by Ashbaugh et al. in 1967. This term quickly replaced the many others that were previously used to describe patients with similar physical findings. These pseudonyms are presented in Table 10–1.

ETIOLOGY

Although the signs, symptoms, and pathophysiology are the same, there are many potential etiologies that have been implicated in the development or worsening of the ARDS (Table 10–2). The most frequently identified risk factors, or potential etiologies, are sepsis, aspiration of gastric contents, and massive trauma (Lillington and Redding, 1988).

The mortality rate for patients diagnosed with ARDS is greater than 50%, and increases to more than 85% when the etiology is sepsis or neoplastic disease (Raffin, 1987). Of those patients who recover, about 85% return to near-normal pulmonary function within 1 year.

The etiology of ARDS itself is most important when planning collaborative interventions to attain patient outcomes. Although treatment plans may be similar because of the overall problems with oxygenation and fluid balance, all of the possible underlying etiologies should be considered. This careful consideration may point the therapy in a direction that is different than originally anticipated, and improve the patient's chance of a successful outcome.

Table 10–1. PSEUDONYMS FOR ARDS

Adult hyaline membrane disease
Congestive atelectasis
Da Nang lung
High permeability pulmonary edema
Liver lung
Noncardiogenic pulmonary edema
Postperfusion lung
Posttraumatic pulmonary insufficiency
Posttraumatic wet lung
Pump lung
Respirator lung
Shock lung
White lung

Table 10–2. POSSIBLE ETIOLOGIES FOR ARDS

Anaphylaxis
Aspiration of gastric contents
Cardiopulmonary bypass
Diffuse pneumonia
Disseminated intravascular coagulation
Drug overdose
Eclampsia
Fat embolism
Fractures, especially of the pelvis or long bones
Goodpasture's syndrome
High altitude
Idiopathic
Idiosyncratic drug reaction
Increased intracranial pressure
Leukemia
Multiple transfusions
Multisystem trauma
Near-drowning
Neurogenic pulmonary edema
Oxygen toxicity
Pancreatitis
Paraquat toxicity
Prolonged mechanical ventilation
Pulmonary contusion
Radiation
Sepsis
Smoke or irritant gas inhalation
Surface burns
Thrombotic thrombocytopenic purpura
Uremia
Venous air embolism

PATHOPHYSIOLOGY

Regardless of the etiology of ARDS, the initial injury to the lung results in pulmonary hypoperfusion, which disrupts its normal function by damaging the alveolar or vascular epithelium (Fig. 10–2). The resulting tissue hypoxia then leads to a lactic acidosis and a release of vasoactive substances. Platelet and leukocyte aggregation also occur, serotonin is released, and there is embolization and occlusion of the pulmonary microcirculation due to intravascular clotting. There is also an increase in dead space. Each of

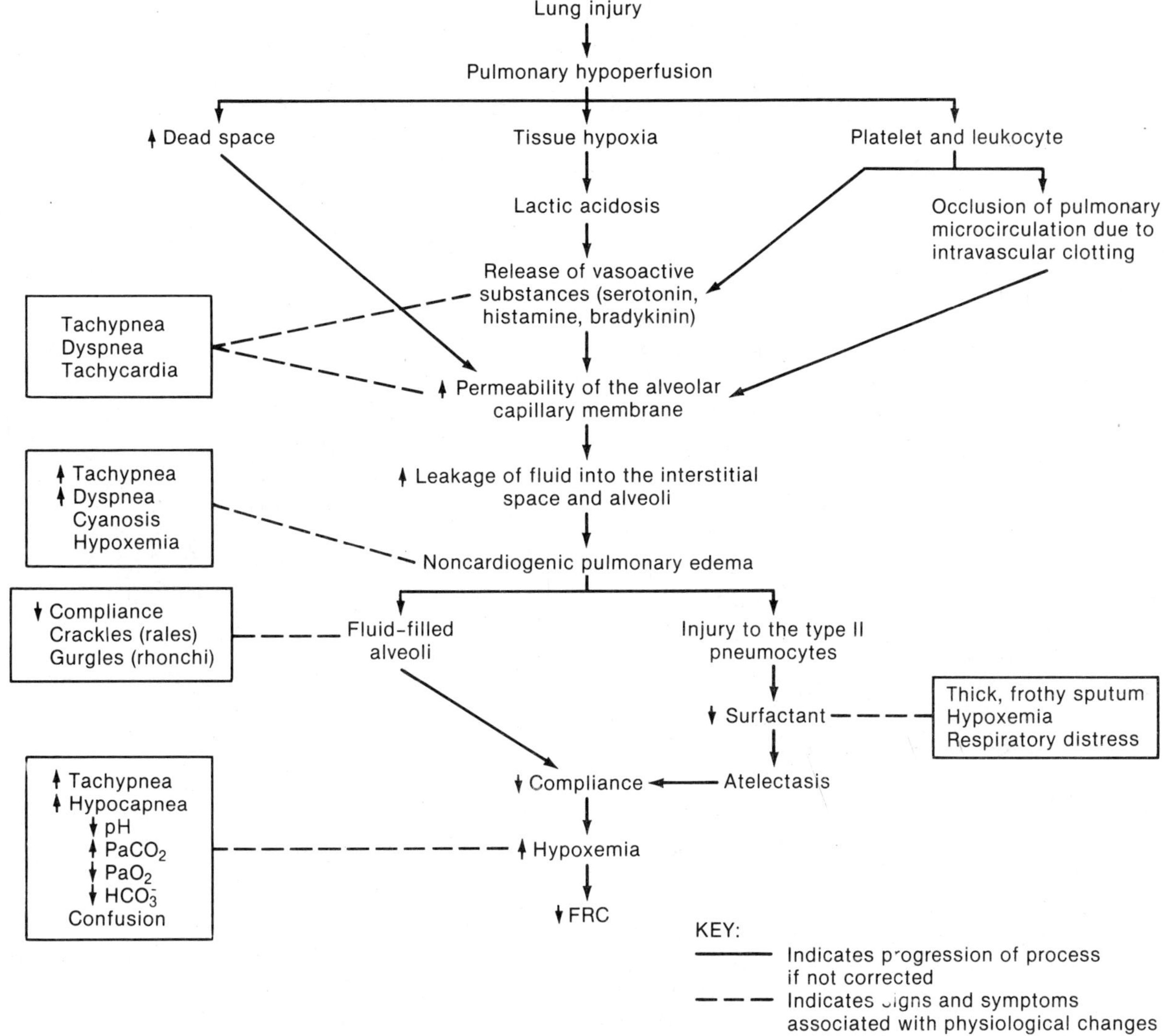

Figure 10-2. Pathophysiology of ARDS.

these three factors results in an increase in the permeability of the alveolar-capillary membrane. This allows fluid to gradually leak into the interstitial space and alveoli, causing pulmonary edema and alveolar collapse.

The edema, accompanied by a decrease in capillary perfusion, also results in a decrease in the production of surfactant owing to injury to the type II pneumocytes. The alveoli become more unstable and collapse unless filled with fluid. Gas exchange is impaired, and hypoxemia develops because the alveoli are either filled with fluid or collapsed.

Fluid continues to leak into the interstitial spaces, resulting in interstitial edema, compression, further collapse of alveoli, and an overall decrease in lung volume. This is exhibited by hypoxemia and a decrease in functional residual capacity (FRC). This along with the other changes results in an overall decrease in lung compliance. For the patient this means an increased work of breathing. The decrease in compliance is compounded by pulmonary vasoconstriction and bronchoconstriction due to the release of arachidonic acid metabolites (Raffin, 1987).

The alveoli will continue to receive blood flow even though they are not receiving adequate ventilation, causing intrapulmonary shunting. These changes along with the increase in wasted ventilation result in an overall $\dot{V}/\dot{Q}$ mismatch and hypoxemia. Clinically, the patient will hyperventilate in an attempt to increase the PaO_2. The result of the tachypnea is hypocapnia, increased airway resistance, increased oxygen consumption, and decreased compliance.

The resulting pulmonary dysfunction is compounded by a reflex increase in cardiac output and minute ventilation in an attempt to compensate for the hypoxemia. There is an increase in venous return due to the increased inspiratory effort needed to open the alveoli. Fluid continues to leak through the damaged capillary membranes into the interstitial spaces and compliance is further impaired (Matus and Glennon, 1988).

High levels of oxygen are often required to maintain adequate tissue perfusion despite the V/Q mismatch. When levels of oxygen greater than 50% are utilized for extended periods of time, the result may be oxygen toxicity. This will further compound matters because progression of oxygen toxicity leads to damage to the alveoli and an aggravation of the symptoms already present as a result of ARDS. Initial symptoms include tracheobronchitis, cough, inspiratory pain, and dyspnea (Matus and Glennon, 1988).

ASSESSMENT

Early assessment and diagnosis of ARDS will guide the caregivers to institute appropriate therapies, and decrease the chance that the initial changes will be compounded by the inappropriate use of oxygen, fluids, mechanical ventilation, and drugs. Symptoms of ARDS may not be present until 6 to 48 hours after the initial insult to the lung, and the critical care nurse is often the first to detect the early warning signs (Table 10–3).

One of the initial signs of ARDS is restlessness and a change in the patient's behavior. This can include mood swings, disorientation, and a change in the level of consciousness. Other early warning signs include dyspnea and hyperventilation with normal breath sounds. The dyspnea may not be evident in an otherwise young healthy patient, as he/she can easily double and triple minute ventilation at rest (Lake, 1984).

Patients may also exhibit a cough accompanied by respiratory alkalosis. If the patient is mechanically ventilated, the critical care nurse will see an increase in peak inspiratory pressures. This is an indication of the decrease in compliance. Pulse and temperature may be elevated, and chest x-rays are usually normal. These early warning signs should clue the health team members to search for potential causes of lung injury.

Table 10–3. EARLY WARNING SIGNS OF ARDS

Restlessness
Change in patient's behavior such as mood swings, disorientation, or a change in the level of consciousness
Dyspnea
Hyperventilation with normal breath sounds
Cough
Respiratory alkalosis
Increased peak inspiratory pressures
Normal chest x-ray
Tachycardia
Increased temperature

As the process progresses and PaO_2 drops, dyspnea will become severe, and there may be grunting with respirations (Table 10–4). The $PaCO_2$ will continue to drop, resulting in a respiratory alkalosis without improvement in oxygenation. On physical examination, there will be intercostal and suprasternal retractions. Hypocapnia and hypoxemia will not respond to increasing levels of oxygen. There will be tachycardia, pallor, and cyanosis.

The respiratory alkalosis will be accompanied by a metabolic acidosis due to lactic acid build-up. This can be confirmed by drawing serum lactate levels. As the ARDS progresses, the nurse will hear crackles, rhonchi, and bronchial breath sounds on auscultation. A chest x-ray will show bilateral patchy infiltrates, which progress to what is often referred to as white lung.

Table 10–4. LATE SIGNS OF ARDS

Decreased PaO_2
Severe dyspnea
Grunting with respirations
Decreased $PaCO_2$ with respiratory alkalosis
Intercostal and suprasternal retractions
Hypocapnia and hypoxemia
Tachycardia
Pallor
Cyanosis
Metabolic acidosis
Adventitious breath sounds—crackles, rhonchi, or bronchial breath sounds
Chest x-ray with bilateral patchy infiltrates
Decreased functional residual capacity
Increased peak inspiratory pressures

Pulmonary mechanics will show a decrease in lung volumes, especially FRC, and a decrease in static and dynamic compliance. As the patient's condition deteriorates, peak inspiratory pressures on the ventilator will continue to rise. Pulmonary artery pressure (PAP), pulmonary capillary wedge pressure (PCWP), and cardiac output (CO) can be normal, but if abnormal will help to guide treatment.

Assessment of a patient with ARDS should be collaborative. A key clinical finding that is often diagnostic of ARDS is a lung insult followed by respiratory distress with profound dyspnea, tachypnea, and hypoxemia that does not respond to oxygen therapy. Once diagnosed, important assessment data that will be used to guide treatment includes hemodynamic measurements, arterial blood gases, mixed venous blood gases, assessment of breath sounds, serial chest x-rays, fluid and electrolyte values, metabolic and nutritional needs, and psychosocial needs of the patient and family.

NURSING DIAGNOSIS

Several nursing diagnoses must be addressed when caring for a patient with ARDS. Addressing them will assist the nurse to meet the major goals of therapy. These goals include (1) increasing the delivery of oxygen to the tissues, (2) decreasing overall oxygen consumption, (3) supplying adequate nutrition to meet the metabolic demands of the patient, (4) maintaining fluid and electrolyte balance, and (5) providing support to the patient and family.

To meet these goals, the critical care nurse should devise a plan of care by addressing the following nursing diagnoses:

1. Ineffective breathing pattern related to increased alveolar capillary permeability and decreased lung compliance as indicated by dyspnea, cough, tachypnea, use of accessory muscles, and abnormal arterial blood gases
2. Impaired gas exchange related to increased alveolar capillary membrane changes, decreased surfactant, and embolization and occlusion of the pulmonary microcirculation as indicated by hypoxemia, restlessness, and increased $\dot{V}/\dot{Q}$ mismatch
3. Potential for infection related to illness and invasive procedures as indicated by elevated temperatures, warm, flushed skin, and increased white blood cell count
4. Potential fluid volume excess related to excess fluid intake as indicated by intake greater than output, elevated PCWP, and weight gain
5. Altered nutrition: less than body requirements related to increased metabolic demands and decreased ability to take in food due to infection, trauma, and mechanical ventilation as indicated by calorie counts that do not meet metabolic demands
6. Potential impaired skin integrity related to bed rest and inadequate nutrition
7. Alteration in tissue perfusion: cardiopulmonary related to microembolization of the pulmonary vasculature, decreased surfactant, and increased permeability of the alveolar-capillary membrane as indicated by atelectasis, pulmonary infiltrates, hypoxemia, and increased $\dot{V}/\dot{Q}$ mismatch
8. Potential alteration in tissue perfusion: peripheral related to vasoconstriction and hypoxemia as indicated by cold extremities, peripheral cyanosis, and abnormal mixed venous blood gases
9. Potential anxiety related to inability to speak, situational crises, uncertainty, and lack of control as indicated by elevated heart rate, blood pressure, and respiratory rate, increased muscle tension, and inappropriate behaviors
10. Potential ineffective family coping related to knowledge deficits of family members due to inadequate information and uncertain outcome as indicated by verbalization of fears.

Interventions

Interventions for a patient with ARDS should be collaborative and aimed toward common goals. Whether the consideration is oxygenation, nutrition, or family support, the outcomes are more easily reached when a collaborative approach is taken. The main factors to address when caring for a patient with ARDS include hypoxemia, fluid and electrolyte balance, nutrition, and psychosocial support.

OXYGENATION

The first intervention to attempt to relieve hypoxemia is to supply supplemental oxygen. These patients usually require intubation and mechanical ventilation. In order to achieve the desired PaO_2, the physician may initially use a high tidal volume. As the patient deteriorates and requires an FIO_2 greater than 50%, the physician will often add positive end-expiratory pressure (PEEP) in an attempt to improve oxygenation. This occurs by providing a positive airway pressure throughout the cycle that will reexpand collapsed alveoli and increase FRC. The anticipated result is greater oxygenation at a lower FIO_2.

Some patients remain hypoxic despite these interventions. The critical care nurse may observe that the patient continues to try to hyperventilate despite mechanical ventilation, often referred to as "bucking" the ventilator (Bradley, 1987). The patient tries to exhale during the inspiratory phase of the ventilator, and the result is a worsening of the hypoxemic state. The patient may be treated with sedatives (diazepam, lorazepam, morphine sulfate) to decrease anxiety and the work of breathing. If this is not effective, neuromuscular blocking agents (pancuronium bromide, vecuronium bromide) may be utilized to paralyze the skeletal muscles and allow the ventilator to completely control the work of breathing.

An arterial line and a pulmonary artery catheter will be needed to monitor the patient's hemodynamic status, blood pressure, and arterial blood gases. It is the critical care nurse's responsibility to collect these data, and the nurse and the physician analyze the data and make alterations in therapy.

Cardiac output, and subsequently blood pressure, are important parameters for the critical care nurse to monitor in a patient receiving ventilator support with PEEP. The increase in pleural pressure caused by the PEEP may result in a decrease in venous return, and a subsequent decrease in CO and blood pressure, causing a paradoxical decrease in oxygen delivery.

A decrease in CO may be critical in an already compromised patient with hypotension. Nursing interventions to promote venous return include elevating the foot of the bed 10 to 20 degrees and providing passive range-of-motion exercises. Urine output should also be monitored closely, and the physician should be notified if it drops to less than 30 ml/hr.

Peripheral circulation will need to be assessed and monitored closely, especially if the patient is on vasopressors. Signs of compromise include cold extremities, decreased or absent pulse, pallor, and cyanosis. The PEEP may need to be adjusted, along with tidal volume and FIO_2, to supply adequate tissue oxygenation. This is often determined by assessing samples of both arterial and mixed venous blood gases.

Frequent repositioning and good pulmonary hygiene are nursing interventions that will assist in decreasing the occurrence of atelectasis and pooling of secretions in the lungs. Repositioning will also decrease the occurrence of skin breakdown. Any increases in oxygenation that result from position changes should be analyzed and assessed. In the case in which lung disease is unilateral, improved gas exchange may be seen by placing the patient in the lateral position with the good lung down (Bradley, 1987). This allows greater blood flow to the better-functioning lung.

Along with maximizing oxygen delivery to the tissues, the critical care nurse must work collaboratively with the physician to decrease oxygen consumption. This includes measures to make the febrile patient normothermic, such as antipyretics, tepid baths, and a cooling blanket if necessary. Space activities out and provide substantial periods of rest. Another factor to consider is the comfort of the patient, and whether or not he/she is having any pain. Signs of pain or discomfort can include tachycardia, restlessness, guarding, and decreased attention span. Analgesics and comfort measures are indicated here.

FLUID AND ELECTROLYTE BALANCE

A second area of treatment that must be addressed is fluid and electrolyte balance. Careful assessment and treatment is paramount because the large volumes of fluid used to maintain intravascular volume and treat hypotension may worsen the pulmonary edema when it leaks through the alveolar capillary membrane. Intake and output, along with PCWP or PAD, must be monitored closely. Initially, PCWP and PAD may be normal or low. Intravenous fluid may be required, with the goal being to maintain the lowest PCWP and PAD needed to provide an adequate CO and tissue perfusion. Clinically, this is assessed by blood pressure, BUN, creatinine, mixed venous blood gases, and level of consciousness.

Controversy exists regarding the use of crystalloids or colloids in the treatment of patients with ARDS. Colloids have been used in an attempt to increase oncotic pressure within the vascular space, but because of the increased capillary permeability, the proteins can leak into the interstitial tissues and further compound the problem. Crystalloids are often chosen in the initial stages of treatment for ARDS when fluids are needed to maintain CO. It is important for the critical care nurse to inform the physician if the PCWP begins to rise, as this will probably be treated with fluid restriction and diuretics.

NUTRITION

The nutritional needs of the critically ill patient with ARDS must also be addressed, as the caloric requirements will increase 1.5 to 2.0 times normal (Lake, 1984). Many factors contribute to this increase in caloric requirements, such as stress, sepsis, trauma, and mechanical ventilation. If the nutritional requirements are not met, respiratory muscle function will be impaired owing to the negative nitrogen balance, and weaning will not be possible. Unless aspiration is a major risk, enteral nutrition is preferred because there are fewer overall complications than with the use of parenteral nutrition.

PSYCHOSOCIAL SUPPORT

As with all patients in a critical care setting, the health team members must always remember to provide a warm, nurturing environment in which the patient and family can feel safe. The onset of ARDS and its long recovery phase will result in stress and anxiety for both the patient and the family. The patient may also experience feelings of isolation on account of the long recovery phase.

All health care team members should take the time to sensitively explain procedures, equipment, changes in the patient's condition, and outcomes to patients and families. The patient should be allowed to participate in planning care as much as possible, and should feel comfortable verbalizing fears and questions to the staff. The isolation and accompanying depression can often be minimized by allowing frequent visits from families and friends while still providing adequate rest periods for the patient. Personal items from home, such as photographs of loved ones, may also assist the critical care nurse to meet the patient's psychosocial needs.

Other Therapies

Along with all of the therapies discussed, the physician may elect to provide other forms of treatment as well. In the presence of actual or presumed infection, many ARDS patients will be on antibiotics. Corticosteroids are sometimes used to assist the patient with the anti-inflammatory process during this period of stress. They also stabilize the capillary and cell membranes, enhance surfactant production, and decrease platelet aggregation (Lake, 1984). Although these properties are desired, they may also predispose the patient to an increased incidence of infection. The advantages of therapy must be weighed against the disadvantages in each case.

Outcomes

For each patient with ARDS, the therapies and interventions are chosen based on the clinical data for that individual. Therapies can be altered, changed, or discontinued depending on patient response. In each individual situation, health team members are working with patients and families to reach common goals and outcomes. The expected patient outcomes for a patient with ARDS include the following:

1. Stable blood pressure and cardiac output
2. Adequate oxygenation to the organs and peripheral tissues
3. Minimal damage to lung tissues
4. Decreased oxygen consumption
5. Adequate nutrition to effectively meet the metabolic demands
6. Optimal fluid balance
7. Effective breathing pattern and adequate gas exchange without mechanical ventilation
8. Normothermic (body temperature)
9. Absence of infection
10. Intact skin
11. Reduction or elimination of anxiety, fears, and social isolation

A review of the care of the patient with ARDS can be found in the nursing care plan.

Acute Respiratory Failure in Chronic Obstructive Pulmonary Disease

DEFINITION

Chronic obstructive pulmonary disease (COPD) refers to a group of disorders that result in obstruction of airflow in the lungs. These disorders include asthma, emphysema, and chronic bronchitis. Generally, COPD is marked by a gradual decline in the patient's lung function. However, acute respiratory failure can occur in the patient with COPD at any time. These patients normally have very little respiratory reserve, and any condition that causes increased work of breathing, worsened $\dot{V}/\dot{Q}$ mismatching, or increased secre-

NURSING CARE PLAN FOR A PATIENT WITH ACUTE RESPIRATORY FAILURE DUE TO ARDS		
Nursing Diagnosis	**Outcome**	**Intervention**
Ineffective breathing pattern related to increased alveolar-capillary permeability and decreased lung compliance as indicated by dyspnea, cough, tachypnea, use of accessory muscles, and abnormal arterial blood gases	Airflow maximized Absence of respiratory distress Unlabored respirations at rate of 12–18/min ABGs WNL	Assess and document respiratory status every 1 to 2 hr, including breathing pattern, rate, depth, and rhythm Assess chest expansion, use of accessory muscles, and breath sounds Position in semi–Fowler's, or that in which breathing pattern is most comfortable Medications to increase airflow as ordered; evaluate their effectiveness; may include drugs such as isoetharine hydrochloride (Bronkosol) and metaproterenol sulfate (Alupent) Anti-inflammatories as ordered; may include corticosteroids such as methylprednisolone Oxygen therapy or maintain mechanical ventilation as indicated Monitor for dyspnea and signs of increasing respiratory distress Assist with activities to conserve energy Provide patient with adequate periods of rest Monitor arterial blood gases If febrile, administer antipyretics as ordered to decrease temperature and, therefore, oxygen consumption
Impaired gas exchange related to increased alveolar-capillary membrane changes, decreased surfactant, and embolization and occlusion of the pulmonary microcirculation as indicated by hypoxemia, restlessness, and increased $\dot{V}/\dot{Q}$ mismatch	Adequate gas exchange ABGs WNL	Assess for hypoxemia and hypercapnea Assess for restlessness or change in the level of consciousness Position for maximal gas exchange; if only right lung affected, position with left lung down to improve gas exchange Provide supplemental oxygen as needed or maintain mechanical ventilation as indicated Encourage coughing and deep breathing Utilize paralysis and sedation as ordered to maintain optimal gas exchange Provide good pulmonary hygiene as needed Monitor ABGs Provide frequent periods of rest
Alteration in tissue perfusion: cardiopulmonary related to microembolization of the pulmonary vasculature, decreased surfactant, and increased permeability of the alveolar capillary membrane as indicated by atelectasis, pulmonary infiltrates, hypoxemia, and increased $\dot{V}/\dot{Q}$ mismatch	Adequate tissue perfusion to the cardiopulmonary system Unlabored respirations Heart rate and rhythm WNL Breath sounds normal Blood pressure and cardiac output WNL Absence of chest pain	Monitor and document vital signs Monitor CVP, PAP, PCWP, CO Monitor respiratory rate and pattern and breath sounds Maintain on a cardiac monitor and document any dysrhythmias Assess ECG for ischemia Monitor heart sounds Maintain oxygen therapy Institute measures to promote venous return such as raising the foot of the bed if patient becomes hypotensive Assess any chest pain and institute measures to relieve it Maintain vasopressors as ordered to maintain blood pressure
Altered nutrition: less than body requirements related to increased metabolic demands and decreased ability to take food in owing to infection, trauma, and mechanical ventilation as indicated by calorie counts that do not meet the metabolic demands	Metabolic demands decrease as condition improves Calorie counts will indicate that nutritional requirements are being met No weight loss Laboratory results WNL	If able to take food by mouth, provide frequent small meals that are high in proteins and calories Increase usual caloric intake by 1.5–2.0 times normal If mechanically ventilated, provide enteral or parenteral nutrition as ordered If utilizing enteral feedings, elevate the head of the bed and monitor gastric residual every 2 hr If utilizing parenteral nutrition, maintain strict aseptic technique when caring for the lines and administering TPN Monitor daily weights Maintain calorie counts

NURSING CARE PLAN FOR A PATIENT WITH ACUTE RESPIRATORY FAILURE DUE TO ARDS *Continued*

Nursing Diagnosis	Outcome	Intervention
Potential for infection related to illness and invasive procedures as indicated by elevated temperatures, warm, flushed skin, and increased white blood cell count	Temperature normothermic White blood cell count normal Absence of infection	Monitor temperature every 4 hr; more frequently if elevated Monitor WBCs; notify physician if elevated Reposition at least every 2 hr to assist with mobilization of secretions Provide good pulmonary hygiene Assess central line and intravenous site for signs of infection: redness, swelling, and drainage Use aseptic technique with all invasive procedures and dressing changes Change dressings per protocol, and prn if they become soiled
Potential fluid volume excess related to excess fluid intake as indicated by intake greater than output, elevated PCWP, crackles, and weight gain	Body weight WNL I&O balanced Electrolyte levels WNL PCWP in the range of 8–12 mm Hg Breath sounds clear	Weigh patient daily Monitor I&O Maintain fluid restriction if ordered Administer diuretics if ordered Assess for peripheral edema Monitor serum electrolytes; replace as ordered Monitor BUN and creatinine Measure urine specific gravity every shift and prn Monitor PCWP every hour and prn Administer inotropic and vasodilating medications as ordered Assess breath sounds every 2 hr and prn Maintain oxygen therapy as ordered Monitor ABGs
Potential impaired skin integrity related to bed rest and inadequate nutrition	Skin will remain intact Perfusion to all areas of the body maximized Nutritional status optimized	Assess every shift for areas of skin breakdown Keep skin clean and dry Apply protective creams Reposition patient every 1–2 hr If unable to turn patient owing to hemodynamic instability, place on specialized bed (e.g., air mattress, water mattress) Massage all bony prominences and around all reddened areas with each position change Assist with active and passive range-of-motion exercises Monitor lab values that may have an effect on skin, and report all abnormalities to physician: albumin, hematocrit and hemoglobin, uric acid, BUN, bilirubin, ABGs Collaborate with physician and dietitian in planning dietary intake, whether it be oral or parenteral Plan diet that has adequate intake of proteins, fluids, and calories Monitor and assess calorie counts
Potential alteration in tissue perfusion: peripheral related to vasoconstriction and hypoxemia as indicated by cold extremities, peripheral cyanosis, and abnormal mixed venous blood gases	Adequate tissue perfusion and cellular oxygenation of the peripheral system Oxygen consumption decreased Hypoxemia and vasoconstriction minimized Mixed venous blood gases have an O_2 saturation >70%	Monitor and document vital signs Assess quality of arterial pulses Assess skin temperature, color, and texture Assist with active and passive range-of-motion exercises Maintain oxygen therapy Reposition frequently and assess for increases in oxygenation; if only one lung is affected, oxygenation may improve if positioned laterally with good lung down Monitor temperature; if elevated institute measures to return it to normal Assess vasoconstrictive effects of medications Avoid long period of pressure to extremities Assess mixed venous blood gases

continued

NURSING CARE PLAN FOR A PATIENT WITH ACUTE RESPIRATORY FAILURE DUE TO ARDS *Continued*

Nursing Diagnosis	Outcome	Intervention
Potential anxiety related to inability to speak, situational crises, uncertainty, and lack of control as indicated by an elevated heart rate, blood pressure, and respiratory rate, increased muscle tension, and inappropriate behaviors	Vital signs WNL Muscle tension reduced; patient will remain relaxed Anxiety reduced, and patient will not exhibit inappropriate behaviors such as anger, fear, withdrawal, and regression	Monitor for signs of anxiety: increased heart rate, blood pressure, and respiratory rate, muscle tension, inappropriate behaviors Develop trusting relationship with the patient by utilizing calm, consistent, and reliable behaviors Always introduce yourself and all unfamiliar faces to the patient, and explain why they are there Thoroughly explain all procedures and happenings to the patient Avoid conflicts with the patient Provide nurturing environment and increase attention to the patient as indicated Allow the patient some control over decision making if possible Do not reinforce inappropriate behaviors Attempt to structure environment by providing consistent caregivers and decreased stimulation Teach relaxation techniques such as the utilization of slow rhythmic breathing during stressful periods Administer sedatives as ordered, if indicated Allow frequent family visits to decrease isolation
Potential ineffective family coping related to knowledge deficits of family members owing to inadequate information and uncertain outcome as indicated by verbalization of fears	Family integrity maintained Family members verbalize educational needs Family members verbalize fears and feel comfortable asking questions related to patient's prognosis Family members work together in making decisions for their loved one when necessary	Assess family unit and coping behaviors Establish healthy relationship with the family Assist family to identify roles to maintain family integrity Assist family members to verbalize distress Sensitively explain procedures, equipment, changes in the patient's condition, and outcomes to family members Always allow time for family members to ask questions and verbalize fears Inform family of resources available to them, such as chaplain and psychiatric liaison Assist family to prioritize their needs Provide conferences with family and health care providers to supply information, be supportive, and allow family to see that all members of health care team are working together to provide the best quality and continuity of care for their loved one

tions and bronchoconstriction may result in acute respiratory failure.

PATHOPHYSIOLOGY

The abnormality associated with COPD is obstruction to airflow. This obstruction may be caused by several factors, some of which are reversible and others of which are fixed.

Asthma

Asthma is a reversible airway obstruction caused by bronchospasm. This bronchospasm results in air trapping, prolonged expiration, $\dot{V}/\dot{Q}$ mismatching with an increased intrapulmonary shunt, and cough productive of thick, tenacious sputum. The bronchial airways are hyperactive and respond to both intrinsic stimuli such as emotions and sympathetic and parasympathetic balance and extrinsic stimuli such as various antigens and airway irritants (Matus and Glennon, 1988). In addition to the bronchospasm, bronchial wall edema and increased mucus secretion add to the amount of obstruction.

The lungs become overinflated and stiff, which increases the work of breathing and results in hyperventilation and a decreased $PaCO_2$. Status asthmaticus occurs when the bronchoconstriction is no longer responsive to bronchodilator therapy, and acute respiratory failure ensues. The patient experiences fatigue from the severe dyspnea, cough, and increased work of breathing. Hypercapnia and acidosis develop and cardiac output falls as a result of a decreased venous return that is related to the increased intrathoracic pressures. Dehydration due to hyperventilation and reduced oral intake may further impair cardiac output and contribute to circulatory collapse.

Emphysema

Emphysema is a nonreversible obstructive disease characterized by the destruction of the alveolar walls and connective tissue with the loss of elastic recoil. Owing to this tissue destruction, the terminal airways collapse during expiration and secretions are retained, leading to increased infections. V/Q mismatching occurs as a result of gas trapping and generalized pulmonary artery constriction. Diffusion is reduced because of the reduction of alveolar surface area. This results in chronic hypercapnia. Cor pulmonale may occur as the right ventricle dilates and hypertrophies in response to the elevated pulmonary artery pressure. Acute respiratory failure may occur when infection develops or when other bodily stressors such as surgery or shock place demands on the pulmonary system.

The emphysematous patient is often a man in his mid-50s who complains of increasing shortness of breath for the past several years with no cough or a nonproductive cough. He may have had recent weight loss. His chest is overexpanded and he appears to puff as he breathes, despite arterial blood gases which may be within normal limits. The normal appearance of the arterial blood (pink), coupled with the appearance of shortness of breath, leads to the name of "pink-puffers."

Chronic Bronchitis

Chronic bronchitis is defined as a productive cough for at least 3 consecutive months documented for over at least 2 consecutive years. Chronic bronchitis results from an increase in the number of mucus-secreting glands accompanied by swelling, inflammation, and hypertrophy of the mucosal layer of the bronchial tree. In addition, thick, tenacious mucus clogs the airway. Areas of cilia are also destroyed, which contributes to the patient's inability to clear increased mucus.

In the early stages, chronic bronchitis is reversible by reducing exposure to causative agents such as cigarette smoke or air pollutants. As the disease progresses, however, the changes in the airways become irreversible. As in other types of obstructive disorders, expiration is prolonged. Air trapping and hypercapnia will occur, and cor pulmonale is usually present. As in emphysema, anything that increases the work of breathing may result in acute respiratory failure. Owing to the constant presence of thick, tenacious sputum, these patients are especially prone to the development of a superimposed respiratory infection.

The patient with chronic bronchitis is often a man in his mid-40s with the cough history previously described. He may report increasing dyspnea on exertion and reduced exercise tolerance. He will often have cyanosis and signs of fluid retention, such as ankle edema and neck vein distention. His arterial blood gases may reveal hypoxia and CO_2 retention. The chronic bronchitic patient is often referred to as a "blue bloater," since the appearance of the arterial blood is poor and the patient appears bloated with edema.

Assessment

Regardless of the specific underlying pathophysiology, the patient with COPD is at risk for the development of respiratory failure and requires constant close assessment. Dyspnea and hyperventilation are early signs of respiratory failure in the patient with chronic pulmonary disease. However, these classic symptoms may be part of the patient's baseline respiratory status. It is important for the critical care nurse to obtain an accurate assessment of the patient's usual respiratory status so that subtle changes will not be missed.

Worsening cough, increased sputum production, or a change in the character of the sputum may signal the development of a respiratory infection that could produce profound respiratory failure. Wheezing indicates narrowing of the airways from bronchospasm. The patient will be more comfortable in the upright position, and may show retraction of the intercostal muscles with inspiration. Tachycardia and hypotension may result from reduced cardiac output.

Pulmonary function studies will show a marked reduction in expiratory flow. Functional residual capacity will be increased owing to air trapping. Crackles may be heard throughout the lung fields. The chest x-ray will show the flat low diaphragm characteristic of patients with COPD.

Arterial blood gases (ABGs) are a sensitive

monitor for the patient's status. It is extremely important to know the patient's baseline levels, as the person with COPD may have chronically abnormal ABGs. In the asthmatic patient, ABGs are often normal except during an acute attack when the $PaCO_2$ may drop because of hyperventilation. In this instance, a return to a normal $PaCO_2$ in the face of an ongoing episode may be an early sign of impending failure. Hypercapnia is a late-occurring, ominous sign. The COPD patient who chronically retains CO_2 may have baseline ABGs that show both the PaO_2 and $PaCO_2$ to be in the range of 50 to 59 mm Hg with a normal pH. When acute failure ensues, the $PaCO_2$ will rise and the PaO_2 may fall further, resulting in tissue hypoxia and acidosis.

Because ABGs are invasive and require frequent blood sampling, other methods are being developed for constant monitoring of the patient's oxygenation and ventilation. Pulse oximetry measures the oxygen saturation of the hemoglobin molecule and provides the clinician with a practical noninvasive method of assessing oxygenation (Rutherford, 1989b). In the ventilated patient, exhaled gas can be analyzed for CO_2 content, providing an assessment of ventilation (St. John, 1989). Both of these techniques may be used in the patient with COPD who has developed acute respiratory failure. Interpretation of the data, however, must take into account the patient's previously impaired respiratory function.

Nursing Diagnosis

The nursing diagnoses for the chronic pulmonary patient who develops acute respiratory failure include all of the diagnoses previously discussed in the section on ARDS. In addition, the following nursing diagnosis pertains to a patient with COPD.

Decisional Conflict: Personal health related to whether or not to be intubated during an acute event because of the uncertainty of the outcome of weaning.

Interventions

The goals of therapy in this group of patients are to sustain them during this episode of acute failure and to return them to their previous level of functioning. In many cases, this is not possible, and each episode of acute failure leaves the patient with chronically diminished function. The most important intervention is adequate body positioning. This intervention is aimed at both preventing and treating respiratory problems (Bushnell and Morrison, 1979). Frequent repositioning fosters the mobilization of secretions and prevents the development of atelectasis and pneumonia.

Postural drainage may be useful but is often contraindicated in patients with compromised cardiac output. Adequate hydration is important to loosen secretions and maintain adequate blood volume. Infections are treated with appropriate antibiotics. Bronchodilators, such as theophylline, are employed to counteract the bronchospastic component.

Oxygen therapy is judiciously prescribed, and its effects carefully monitored. Patients who normally retain CO_2 breathe as a result of their hypoxic drive. If the PaO_2 is rapidly increased, the hypoxic drive is eliminated and the patient will stop breathing. Therefore, low-flow oxygen therapy is initially tried. The patient's response to this is evaluated and changes are made accordingly. The goal of therapy is to achieve a PaO_2 that will provide adequate tissue oxygenation while enabling the patient to continue to breathe unassisted.

Intubation and mechanical ventilation in this patient population are the therapies of last resort. Every effort is made to avoid intubation in the patient with COPD because the risk of complications is high and the long-term prognosis is often poor. Menzies et al. (1989) found that out of 95 patients with COPD, complicated by acute respiratory failure requiring ventilation, 59 were dead within 1 year and 23 were never successfully weaned from the ventilator. However, intubation allows for optimal pulmonary toilet and clearing of secretions, and mechanical ventilation reduces the work of breathing. If the process that precipitated the acute respiratory failure can be successfully treated, the chances are good that the COPD patient will be weaned from the ventilator and return to previous activities.

Acute Respiratory Failure Due to a Pulmonary Embolism

DEFINITION

A pulmonary embolism (PE) is the blockage of a pulmonary artery from a thrombus that usually arises from the systemic veins and results in obstruction of blood flow to the lung tissue (Matus and Glennon, 1988; Levy and Stein, 1984). It is a fairly common complication of hospitalization today. The site of origin for these thrombi are usually the deep veins in the lower extremities of the body, mainly the calf, plantar, and femoral veins. They can also occur from the right side of the heart and the pelvis. The thrombi break off and travel through the venous system into the right heart and out to the lungs.

A PE can be acute or massive, and partial or complete. Acute thromboembolism is usually characterized by the presence of many small emboli lodged in the distal branches of the pulmonary artery, causing a partial occlusion. A massive PE is when the thrombus is lodged in a major branch of the pulmonary artery, causing a complete blockage of one or both of the major pulmonary arteries. The more massive the PE, the more grave the prognosis.

ETIOLOGY

The three main mechanisms that favor the development of a venous thrombi are (1) venous stasis, or a reduction in blood flow; (2) the presence of a disease state that may alter the coagulability of blood; and (3) damage to the vessel walls. Specific etiologies that fall into these three categories are listed in Table 10–5. Both a hypercoagulable state and venous wall damage contribute to the development of a thrombus, but may not cause a thromboembolism alone. They are seen in conjunction with other factors that result in stasis.

Table 10–5. ETIOLOGIES THAT CONTRIBUTE TO THE DEVELOPMENT OF PULMONARY THROMBOEMBOLISM

- Venous Stasis
  - Prolonged bedrest
  - Immobility
  - Obesity
  - Decreased cardiac output due to:
    - Prolonged surgical procedure
    - Atrial fibrillation
    - Congestive heart failure (CHF)
    - Myocardial infarction
  - Pregnancy
  - Chronic obstructive airway disease
  - Postoperative state
  - Advanced age
- Disease States and Altered Coagulability
  - Hip fractures
  - Malignancy
  - Hematologic disorders
  - Use of contraceptives (estrogens increase coagulability and platelet aggregation)
  - Postoperative period (due to abrupt discontinuation of anticoagulants)
  - Pregnancy
  - Antithrombin III deficiency
  - Chronic CHF or atrial fibrillation
  - Thromboembolism
  - Dehydration
- Vessel Wall Damage
  - Venostasis
  - Trauma
  - Sepsis
  - Burns
  - Venous punctures
  - Atherosclerosis

PATHOPHYSIOLOGY

Once a thrombus is formed in the venous system it can easily be dislodged with activities such as standing. Once dislodged, the thrombus travels up to the heart, through the right atrium and ventricle, and out into the pulmonary artery. Large clots may lodge in a major pulmonary vessel, and smaller ones often travel to the distal branches of the pulmonary artery vasculature. The result in either case is the obstruction of blood flow to the pulmonary system. The hemodynamic changes that occur will result in alterations in both the cardiac and pulmonary systems.

As emboli lodge in the distal vessels, and even the larger vessels, blood flow to the alveoli beyond that occlusion will be eliminated. The result is a lack of perfusion to ventilated alveoli, an increase in dead space, a V/Q mismatch, and a decrease in CO_2 tension in the embolized lung zone (Roberts, 1987). Gas exchange cannot occur and hypocarbia results. The hypocarbia affects the bronchial smooth muscle by causing bronchoconstriction, an increase in pulmonary resistance, and a decrease in compliance.

Pneumoconstriction in the terminal airways of the nonperfused lung zones results in alveolar shrinking and a decrease in the amount of wasted ventilation. Although this is a protective mechanism to shunt inspired air to the functioning alveoli, the result will be an increase in the work of breathing for the critically ill patient.

The reduction in blood flow to the alveoli also results in hypoxia for the type II pneumocytes, which are responsible for producing surfactant. Although the effects are not seen for 24 to 48 hours, the decrease in surfactant results in an unequal gas distribution, an increase in the work of breathing, and stiffened and collapsed alveoli. Ventilation is then shifted away from these units.

Atelectasis and shunting may also occur owing to the release of serotonin from the platelets that surround the clot. The result is peripheral airway constriction, which often involves functioning alveoli (Roberts, 1987; Matus and Glennon, 1988). In this situation, there is perfusion with inadequate ventilation. This along with the other causes of $\dot{V}/\dot{Q}$ mismatch is manifested by arterial hypoxemia.

Pulmonary hypertension also contributes to the increased shunting that occurs with a PE. Pulmonary hypertension usually occurs when there is occlusion of greater than 50% of the functional cross-sectional area of the pulmonary vascular bed (Roberts, 1987). Hemodynamically, the critical care nurse will observe an increase in pulmonary vascular resistance (PVR), pulmonary artery pressure (PAP), and right ventricular work. The PAP will continue to rise as the PVR rises. Pulmonary hypertension is often diagnosed as a mean PAP greater than 15 mm Hg (Levy and Stein, 1984).

As the PAP rises, the patient will exhibit signs of breathlessness. In order to maintain CO despite the increased resistance, the right ventricle will continue to increase its work until it reaches maximum function. A normal right ventricle will have the ability to increase its mean pressure approximately 35 to 40 mm Hg (Levy and Stein, 1984). If the pulmonary obstruction continues beyond the limits of the right ventricle, it will fail. Clinically, the patient will exhibit a decrease in CO, syncope, and a shock state. This may be compounded by the release of reflex humoral factors such as serotonin that constrict blood vessels and further increase the pulmonary pressure (Roberts, 1987).

Pulmonary hypertension along with the release of humoral agents stimulates the juxtapulmonary capillary receptors (J receptors) that are located in the alveolar wall (Falotico, 1981). The patient will exhibit dyspnea and tachypnea, or rapid shallow breathing. This is a classic sign in patients with a PE.

One potential outcome for a patient with a PE is pulmonary infarction. This complication is most likely to occur in a patient with some underlying cardiopulmonary abnormality that has already impaired pulmonary circulation (Matus and Glennon, 1988). This would include patients with lung disease and congestive heart failure. Clinically, there would be alveolar hemorrhage, consolidation, and tissue necrosis. It may be complicated by lung abscesses, a pleural effusion, or pleuritic-type pain.

The overall prognosis following a PE is dependent upon two main factors. The first is whether or not there was any underlying cardiopulmonary problem that preceded the PE, and the second is the extent of the pulmonary vascular circulation that is occluded by the thrombus.

ASSESSMENT

Most critically ill patients have several of the risk factors associated with a PE; therefore, the critical care nurse should be astutely aware of the signs and symptoms of a PE. Some of the chief complaints of a patient with a PE include dyspnea, cough, diaphoresis, hemoptysis, pleuritic pain, syncope, apprehension, fever, palpitations, and leg or calf pain. A patient can present with all or none of these symptoms. Most frequently, however, patients present with a sudden onset of dyspnea or breathlessness (Levy and Stein, 1984; Matus and Glennon, 1988; Roberts, 1987).

Along with the patient's chief complaint, the critical care nurse should question the patient about current symptoms and obtain an accurate past medical and surgical history. Dyspnea should be described, including type of onset, whether it is transient or prolonged, and whether it occurs with activity or at rest. Chest pain should also be described, including location and radiation, character, frequency, and influence of respiration, position, movement, activity, and cough.

Past medical and surgical history is particularly important, especially if it unveils the presence of any of the potential etiologies or a prior history of emboli. Other factors that may be of importance when obtaining a past medical history are included in Table 10–6.

Table 10–6. PAST MEDICAL HISTORY THAT IS IMPORTANT IN THE DIAGNOSIS OF PULMONARY EMBOLI

History of heart, lung, or blood disease
Recent surgery, trauma, or bedrest
Long car trip
Pregnancy or use of birth control pills
Varicose veins
Recent increase in weight
Use of constricting undergarments
Occupation that requires prolonged standing

The dyspnea along with other symptoms may be transient or prolonged and vary in severity depending upon the extent of the PE. It is often precipitated by physical exertion, such as walking. When there is obstruction of greater than 50 to 60% of the pulmonary vascular tree, the patient may have substernal chest pain due to the pulmonary hypertension (Levy and Stein, 1984). A pleuritic pain that is greatest with inspiration and decreases when the patient is upright may indicate pulmonary infarction. Lightheadedness and syncope occur with a massive PE owing to the failure of the right ventricle.

On physical examination, there may be signs of tachycardia, which can also be transient. In the presence of pulmonary hypertension, there may be an increased intensity of the pulmonary S_2 heart sound (Matus and Glennon, 1988). Other possible cardiovascular symptoms the critical care nurse should assess for include distended neck veins, murmur of the tricuspid and pulmonic regurgitations, and an atrial or ventricular gallop on inspiration. If right ventricular failure has occurred, the patient will have arterial hypotension along with peripheral vasoconstriction and central cyanosis. The 12-lead electrocardiogram (ECG) may show nonspecific ST changes.

When tachypnea is present, the critical care nurse should carefully assess the patient's breath sounds. Initially there may not be any changes in breath sounds, or they may be decreased. This may be accompanied by mild rales or wheezing if there is underlying bronchial disease. In the presence of a pulmonary infarction, the nurse's assessment might reveal a cough with hemoptysis along with a pleural effusion and a friction rub (Matus and Glennon, 1988). Such a patient often also complains of pleuritic pain and exhibits splinting on inspiration.

Along with a complete cardiopulmonary assessment, the critical care nurse should observe the affect of the patient. Signs of apprehension are indicative of a possible PE. The nurse should also assess and document any edema, peripheral or central cyanosis, and the patient's position in bed. If a PE is suspected, further assessment should include searching for the presence of phlebitis. This includes tenderness, warmth, erythema, a cordlike vein, and a positive Homan's sign.

Along with the patient's history and physical examination, the physician involved in the case will order several laboratory and diagnostic tests in order to make a differential diagnosis. Once clinical symptoms suggest a possible PE, the physician may order a CBC, electrolytes, enzymes, arterial blood gases, a chest x-ray, and an ECG (Levy and Stein, 1984). Leukocytosis with an increased sedimentation rate, LDH, and SGOT point toward a pulmonary infarction. Electrolytes may show signs of dehydration. Arterial blood gases may reveal hypoxemia, hypocarbia, and respiratory alkalosis (Matus and Glennon, 1988). All of these findings may be altered in a patient with underlying pulmonary disease.

A chest x-ray may be nondiagnostic or may have subtle changes, including an elevated hemidiaphragm on the side of the embolus, an enlarged pulmonary artery, an unexplained density, decreased visualization of lung fields, or a pleural effusion (Roberts, 1987). Changes in the ECG usually do not occur unless there is massive embolization. Possible ECG changes include enlarged P waves, ST segment depression, peaked or inverted T waves, and a right axis deviation. Dysrhythmias such as paroxysmal atrial tachycardia or atrial fibrillation may also be present.

The next diagnostic test is a lung scan, although an abnormality is not always a specific diagnostic finding. Any pulmonary or cardiac disease that affects lung function may also cause an abnormality. If the perfusion abnormality is more localized to a lobe or a segment, it increases the probability of a PE (Matus and Glennon, 1988). A negative perfusion scan does, however, rule out a PE.

A ventilation scan will be performed next to assess the distribution of gas in the alveoli (Matus and Glennon, 1988). If abnormalities of ventilation occur in the same areas as abnormalities of perfusion, and the chest x-ray is normal, then there is a $\dot{V}/\dot{Q}$ mismatch due to an underlying lung disorder. The likelihood of a PE increases if there is normal ventilation in areas where there is a perfusion defect. If the diagnosis continues to be questionable, then the physician will order a pulmonary angiogram.

A pulmonary angiogram is an invasive procedure in which a right heart catheterization must be performed. It is diagnostic for a PE (Levy and Stein, 1984; Matus and Glennon, 1988). A radiopaque dye is injected into the pulmonary artery, and flow will be disrupted in areas where a defect or embolism is present.

Nursing Diagnosis

Several nursing diagnoses can be identified by the critical care nurse when planning the nursing care for a patient with a PE. Addressing these will assist the health team members to meet the major goals of therapy. These goals include: (1) to prevent any further decrease in the delivery of oxygen to the tissues, (2) to provide cardiopulmonary support, (3) to maintain fluid balance, and (4) to provide support to the patient and family.

To meet these goals, the critical care nurse should develop the plan of care by addressing the following nursing diagnoses.

1. Potential activity intolerance related to hypoxia as indicated by tachypnea, dyspnea, and abnormal arterial blood gases
2. Anxiety related to uncertain outcome as indicated by apprehension and nervousness
3. Decreased cardiac output related to increased pulmonary vascular resistance and right ventricular failure as indicated by jugular vein distention, cyanosis, hypotension, cold, clammy skin, decreased urine output, and dyspnea
4. Potential ineffective family coping related to knowledge deficit of family members owing to inadequate information and uncertain outcome as indicated by verbalization of fears
5. Impaired gas exchanges related to decreased perfusion of alveoli and atelectasis as indicated by dyspnea, tachypnea, hypoxemia, V/Q mismatch, and abnormal arterial blood gases
6. Potential fluid volume excess related to increased pulmonary vascular resistance as indicated by jugular vein distention, the presence of an S_3 gallop, edema, liver enlargement, and atrial dysrhythmias
7. Potential for injury related to coagulopathy due to anticoagulant therapy as indicated by excessive bleeding, easy bruising, and abnormal hematocrit and hemoglobin
8. Potential for pain related to decreased blood flow to the area due to thrombophlebitis as indicated by splinting with inspiration, shallow breathing, tachycardia, and complaints of pain.
9. Alteration in tissue perfusion: cardiopulmonary related to the interruption in the arterial flow of the pulmonary system due to the thromboembolism as indicated by dyspnea, tachypnea, tachycardia, abnormal breath sounds, cyanosis, pain, hypotension, ECG changes, and dysrythmias

INTERVENTIONS

In the case of a PE, the best therapy is prevention. Several prophylactic nursing interventions can be instituted in the hospitalized patient that may decrease the chance of the patient developing a PE (Falotico, 1981; Levy and Stein, 1984). Early ambulation postoperatively, or in cases in which this is not possible, use of pneumatic boots that provide intermittent compression of the lower extremities will increase venous flow. Walking schedules along with active and passive range-of-motion exercises will also increase circulation in the critically ill.

Some other nursing interventions that may reduce the risk of PE include remembering not to adjust the knee section of the patient's bed and to avoid using pillows below the knees. Proper application of elastic bandages and elastic stockings is also key. The patient should be instructed not to cross his/her legs and to make frequent position changes when sitting for long periods to promote circulation.

The presence of atrial dysrhythmias as well as signs of a deep vein thrombosis is an important indicator of a potential PE that should be assessed by the critical care nurse on an ongoing basis. Signs of thrombophlebitis, such as pain upon dorsiflexion of the foot, redness, swelling, warmth, tenderness, and low-grade fevers, should be documented in the nurse's note and reported to the physician.

Most critically ill patients will fall into a high-risk category for a PE and are often treated prophylactically by the physician. Treatment can include the use of low-dose heparin, aspirin, dipyridamole, and dextran (Falotico, 1981; Levy and Stein, 1984).

Once a PE has occurred, the interventions will be collaborative and focus on the common goals of alleviating symptoms, supporting cardiopulmonary function, and preventing further spread of the clot. The main factors that will be addressed include hypoxemia, fluid balance, pain, nutrition, supporting cardiopulmonary function, and preventing further emboli. Regardless of the factor addressed, the actual treatment will be dependent upon the degree of dysfunction caused by the PE.

Assessment by the critical care nurse includes searching for signs and symptoms of hypoxia and hypoxemia. One of the earliest signs of hypoxemia is restlessness. The presence of this early indicator should clue the critical care nurse to perform a more detailed assessment prior to instituting nursing interventions. It should include assessing for a respiratory rate greater than 20/min, pallor, nasal flaring, retractions of intercostal spaces, splinting, asymmetrical lung expansion, and cyanosis. Auscultation may reveal a friction rub, diminished breath sounds, crackles, rhonchi, or wheezes.

The goals when planning treatment for a patient with hypoxemia include relieving breathlessness, improving oxygen delivery, and preserving respiratory function. Nursing interventions include monitoring arterial blood gases for hypoxia and hypocarbia, and administering oxygen therapy with a doctor's order as needed. The severity of the PE dictates the mode of oxygen delivery. This may include the use of a nasal cannula or a face mask. If secretions are also interfering with respiratory function, the critical care nurse should focus on providing good bronchial hygiene, which includes assisting the patient to cough and deep breathe at least every 2 hours (Roberts, 1987). Postural drainage and chest physical therapy may also be needed.

Other nursing interventions that will assist in supporting pulmonary function include placing the patient in semi–Fowler's position and administering narcotics as ordered that will alleviate any associated pain as well as decrease the vasospasms (Huffman, 1983). The end result is an overall decrease in PVR. In the more severe cases, intubation and mechanical ventilation with positive end-expiratory pressure (PEEP) may be necessary to maintain adequate tissue perfusion. Cardiac monitoring is also important, as patients are at increased risk of developing dysrhythmias that may need to be treated (Dickinson and Bury, 1989).

Accurate monitoring of intake and output is another important intervention performed by the critical care nurse (Roberts, 1987). Owing to the loss in surfactant and the resultant change in the permeability of the alveolar membrane, there is an increase in interstitial edema and pulmonary congestion. The increase in PVR also contributes to CHF because of the increase in the workload of the right ventricle. It is therefore imperative that the critical care nurse assess the patient for signs of CHF and pulmonary edema. Some of the indicators include jugular vein distention, peripheral edema, crackles, dysrhythmias, and increasing tachypnea.

Along with being aware of the potential for CHF, the critical care nurse should also assess the patient for signs of shock (Roberts, 1987). If the PE extends, it can result in obstruction of a major portion of the pulmonary vascular system. Clinically, the critical care nurse will see a severe tachycardia followed by a decrease in CO and blood pressure.

Accompanying signs and symptoms may include inferior wall ECG changes, a right bundle branch block pattern, atrial dysrhythmias, and flipped T waves in the precordial leads. The nurse will also monitor and document CVP, PAP, urine output, peripheral pulses, level of consciousness, and skin temperature, color, and moisture. In some cases, there will be right and left ventricular failure, a decrease in CO, and a decrease in renal tissue perfusion. If not corrected, the result will be organ failure and death.

Collaborative interventions should be directed at alleviating the pain associated with a PE. The pain is often pleuritic and is due to a decrease in the O_2 (Roberts, 1987). It becomes more severe with deep breathing and coughing. Since these are two important activities, the patient may require a narcotic analgesic. Decreasing the patient's activity will conserve oxygen. If the patient also complains of calf pain due to a concurrent DVT, the critical care nurse can apply heat to the area for added comfort.

The severe dyspnea exhibited by a patient with a PE may interfere with the ability to consume a regular diet (Roberts, 1987). The critical care nurse can be creative in providing more optimal conditions to improve the patient's nutritional status. Smaller, more frequent meals, including food brought from home, may be helpful. If the patient's respiratory function is significantly improved following respiratory treatments, it may be more optimal to provide meals following the treatments. Calorie counts should be maintained to document adequate nutrition. The nurse should consult a dietitian for meal planning as needed.

Along with working collaboratively to assess the patient with a PE, and provide some measures to alleviate symptoms, the physician will also choose to treat the patient either medically or surgically. Along with oxygen therapy to maintain PaO_2 greater than 60 mm Hg, analgesics will be ordered to relieve pain (Levy and Stein, 1984). In the presence of CHF and cardiac failure, the physician may elect to use diuretics, such as furosemide (Lasix) and digoxin. When CO is impaired, vasopressor and inotropic agents are used.

Heparin is often the drug of choice for anticoagulant therapy (Levy and Stein, 1984; Matus and Glennon, 1988). Prior to initiating the treatment, the physician will order a prothrombin time (PT) and a partial thromboplastin time (PTT). The intravenous loading dose of heparin varies from 2000 to 10,000 U followed by a continuous infusion that is usually begun at about 1000 U/hr. This hourly dose is increased or decreased depending upon the results of subsequent PTTs. Optimal anticoagulation is obtained with a PTT that is 2.0 to 2.5 times normal.

Heparin therapy is continued for 7 to 14 days (Levy and Stein, 1984; Matus and Glennon, 1988). Usually around day 4 or 5 of heparin therapy, warfarin (Coumadin) is begun. This oral anticoagulant often takes 4 to 6 days to reach therapeutic levels. Therapeutic levels are determined by drawing serum PT levels. Optimum therapy reveals a PT of 1.5 to 2.0 times normal.

Since adequate heparin therapy only prevents further spread of the clot, many physicians may elect to use a thrombolytic agent in the presence of a massive PE with severe hemodynamic compromise (Matus and Glennon, 1988). Thrombolytics can dissolve the clot and rapidly restore hemodynamic stability. Thrombolytics are begun during an acute event as soon as a diagnosis is made. The most frequently used thrombolytics are streptokinase and urokinase. When these drugs are discontinued, they are followed by heparin therapy. Two drawbacks of thrombolytic therapy are the cost and the increased risk of bleeding due to breakdown of beneficial thrombi and destruction of the clot that was repairing the break in a vascular membrane.

Surgical intervention may be necessary for some patients (Levy and Stein, 1984). This would include those in whom anticoagulants and thrombolytics are contraindicated, those who do not respond to medical treatment, those who are having life-threatening complications, and often those who have greater than 50% obstruction. Surgical procedures include an embolectomy, ligation of the inferior vena cava, or transvenous placement of a vena caval umbrella.

Outcomes

For each patient with a PE, the interventions chosen will be dependent upon the current clinical presentation as well as past medical and surgical histories. Treatments will also be adjusted based on patient response. Certainly, prevention is the best therapy. In each situation, health team members work together with the patient in order to meet common goals and outcomes and to return the patient to an optimal state of health. The expected outcomes for a patient with a PE include the following:

1. Adequate oxygen delivery to the tissues
2. Normal respiratory function, including no use of accessory muscles
3. Normal breath sounds
4. PaO_2 greater than 80%
5. No peripheral or sacral edema
6. Stable fluid balance with a urine output greater than 50 ml/hr
7. Stable blood pressure, CO, PAP, CVP
8. Stable cardiac rhythm; without signs of tachycardia, ECG changes, or dysrhythmias
9. Adequate caloric intake
10. Relief of pain
11. No further extension of clot
12. PT and PTT within therapeutic range

Summary

Acute respiratory failure is a disorder that can affect all segments of the population from young trauma victims to elderly people with long-standing pulmonary disease. Patients in the critical care areas are at high risk for acute respiratory failure related to ARDS and pulmonary emboli. The critical care nurse must be constantly alert to signs of impending failure. Changes in respiratory rate and character, breath sounds, and blood gases must be closely evaluated. Frequent position changes, good pulmonary toilet, and careful attention to the nutritional status all contribute to the successful maintenance of a patient's respiratory system and to the prevention of acute respiratory failure.

References

Ahrens, T. (1989a): Blood gas assessment of intrapulmonary shunting and deadspace. *Critical Care Nursing Clinics of North America* 1(4):641–648.

Ahrens, T. (1989b): Extravascular lung water concepts in clinical application. *Critical Care Nursing Clinics of North America* 1(4):681–688.

Ashbaugh, D. G., Bigelow, D. B., Petty, T. L., and Levine, B. E. (1967): Acute respiratory distress in adults. *Lancet* 2:319–323.

Bernard, G. R., and Bradley, R. B. (1986): Adult respiratory distress syndrome: Diagnosis and management. *Heart and Lung* 15(3):250–255.

Bradley, R. B. (1987): Adult respiratory distress syndrome. *Focus on Critical Care* 14(5):48–59.

Bushnell, S. S., and Morrison, M. L. (1979): Nursing care of the patient in respiratory failure. In M. L. Morrison (ed.). *Respiratory Intensive Care Nursing.* 2nd ed. Boston: Little Brown.

Dickinson, S. P., and Bury, G. M. (1989): Pulmonary embolism: Anatomy of a crisis. *Nursing '89* 19(4):34–41.

Falotico, J. B. (1981): Pulmonary embolism. *Critical Care Update* January: 5-8, 10-11, 14, 15, 38.

Huffman, M. H. (1983): Acute care of the patient with a pulmonary embolism due to venous thromboemboli. *Critical Care Nurse* 3(2):70-73.

Jacobs, E. R., and Bone, R. C. (1986): Clinical indicators in sepsis and septic adult respiratory distress syndrome. *Medical Clinics of North America* 70(4):921-932.

Lake, K. B. (1984): Adult respiratory distress syndrome (high permeability pulmonary edema). In G. C. Burton and J. E. Hodgkin (eds.). *Respiratory Care: A Guide to Clinical Practice.* 2nd ed. Philadelphia: J. B. Lippincott, pp. 854-875.

Levy, S. E., and Stein, M. (1984): Pulmonary embolism and infarction. In G. C. Burton and J. E. Hodgkin (eds.). *Respiratory Care: A Guide to Clinical Practice.* 2nd ed. Philadelphia: J. B. Lippincott, pp. 816-831.

Lillington, G. A., and Redding, G. J. (1988): What you need to know about ARDS. *Patient Care* March 15:67-78.

Luce, J. M., Tyler, M. L., and Pierson, D. J. (1984): *Intensive Respiratory Care.* Philadelphia: W. B. Saunders.

Matus, V. W., and Glennon, S. A. (1988): Respiratory disorders. In M. R. Kinney, D. R. Packa, and S. B. Dunbar (eds.). *AACN's Clinical Reference for Critical-Care Nursing.* 2nd ed. New York: McGraw-Hill, pp. 774-827.

Menzies, R., Gibbons, W., and Goldberg, P. (1989): Determinants of weaning and survival among patients with COPD who require mechanical ventilation for acute respiratory failure. *Chest* 95:398-405.

Raffin, T. A. (1987): ARDS: Mechanisms and management. *Hospital Practice* November 22(11):65-80.

Roberts, S. L. (1987): Pulmonary tissue perfusion altered: Emboli. *Heart and Lung* 16(20):128-139.

Rutherford, K. A. (1989a): Advances in the treatment of oxygenation disturbances. *Critical Care Nursing Clinics of North America* 1(4):659-668.

Rutherford, K. A. (1989b): Principles and application of oximetry. *Critical Care Nursing Clinics of North America* 1(4):649-657.

St. John, R. E. (1989): Exhaled gas analysis: technical and clinical aspects of capnography and oxygen consumption. *Critical Care Nursing Clinics of North America* 1(4):669-680.

West, J. B. (1990): *Respiratory Physiology—The Essentials.* 4th ed. Baltimore: Williams & Wilkins.

Recommended Readings

Ahrens, T. (ed.) (1989): Advances in Pulmonary Care. *Critical Care Nursing Clinics of North America* 1(4):641-722.

Burton, G. C., and Hodgkin, J. E. (eds.) (1984): *Respiratory Care: A Guide to Clinical Practice.* 2nd ed. Philadelphia: J. B. Lippincott.

Kersten, L. D. (1989). *Comprehensive Respiratory Nursing: A Decision Making Approach.* Philadelphia: W. B. Saunders.

Lillington, G. A., and Redding, G. J. (1988). What you need to know about ARDS. *Patient Care:* March 15:67-78.

Noll, M. L. (ed.). (1990): Respiratory Care in Adults. *AACN Clinical Issues in Critical Care Nursing* 1(2):237-326.

Zorb, S. L., and Stevens, J. B. (1990): Contemporary bioethical issues in critical care. *Critical Care Nursing Clinics of North America* 2(3):515-526.

Chapter 11

Charold L. Baer, Ph.D., R.N., FCCM, CCRN

Acute Renal Failure

Objectives

- Understand the definition and characterization of acute renal failure.
- Identify the phases of acute renal failure and the pathophysiology involved.
- Become familiar with the systemic manifestations of renal failure.
- Discuss the various nursing assessment activities, criteria, and procedures for determining care and treatment of the patient in renal failure.
- Develop a patient-centered plan of care based on diagnosis, goals, interventions, and outcome criteria.

Acute renal failure—Even the name of this pathophysiological condition suggests a major clinical challenge! The magnitude of the challenge, however, is difficult to ascertain because there are no precise tabulations of the current incidence of acute renal failure in the United States. Thus, one can only speculate that future occurrences will exceed the estimated 10,000 cases that now develop annually. In fact, it is likely that any number postulated at this time would be a drastic underestimation, particularly in view of the recent trends in health care. Such trends include the increasing numbers of acutely and complexly ill individuals who are cared for in tertiary care facilities; the rapidly changing demographics of the general population toward a more elderly segment; the continuing expansion of scientific and health care knowledge; and the addition of new technological apparatus. All of these trends support the speculation that the incidence of acute renal failure will indeed rise in the future.

The significance of the increasing incidence of acute renal failure is evident when one evaluates its impact on the individual and on society. From an individual perspective, the role of the renal system as the primary regulator of the internal environment means that it is essential to the continuing maintenance of life. Thus, for a critically ill individual who is already experiencing other major body system insults, the addition of a dysfunctional renal system will not only enhance the complexity of the patient's condition, but will also compromise the patient's ability to adapt to the other body system changes. The result is a severely compromised individual who requires numerous resources to sustain life and restore health. The impact on society relates to both the cost of the resources required to maintain the individual during a lengthy hospitalization, and to the individual's lost hours of productivity during the illness. In short, society experiences a double impact as a result of the dysfunctional adult.

Nursing's role in relation to the complex scenario of the critically ill patient and the renal system is to be sufficiently knowledgeable to assist in preventing acute renal failure, or in sustaining the individual during the acute renal failure episode. This chapter is designed to assist the clinician in meeting this challenge.

Definition

Acute renal failure can be technically defined as the abrupt cessation of renal function. Such a definition, however, is not very useful in the clinical setting. Instead, it is much more useful to define acute renal failure in terms of its onset, duration, and prognosis. This more specific definition provides clinical guidelines that describe what the patient is likely to experience during the acute renal failure episode.

Onset

The onset of acute renal failure is usually very sudden and is characterized by either anuria, oliguria, or polyuria. *Anuria* is the term used to designate a urine volume of less than 100 ml/24 hr, whereas *oliguria* refers to a urine volume of from 100 to 400 ml/24 hr, and *polyuria* describes a urine volume in excess of 400 ml/24 hr that accompanies a diagnosed state of acute renal failure. The oliguric state is the classic urine volume that accompanies acute renal failure, and thus it is the state most frequently encountered clinically. Polyuria, or nonoliguric acute renal failure, occurs much less frequently, but its incidence appears to be increasing. Individuals with nonoliguric acute renal failure may excrete 2 to 4 L of fluid per day, but the fluid is deficient in the solutes and waste products that compose normal urine. Anuria is the least frequently occurring of the urine volume states in acute renal failure, and total anuria is indeed rare.

Duration

Acute renal failure is a short-term, self-limiting pathology that usually lasts about 25 days or more. During that time frame, the individual progresses through four phases of the disease process, including onset, oliguria or anuria, diuresis, and convalescence. Table 11–1 summarizes these phases according to their definition, time span involved, renal blood flow and oxygen consumption, urine volume, and filtration clearance.

Onset Phase. The onset phase is the period of time that elapses from the occurrence of the precipitating event until the beginning of the change in urine output, usually either oliguria or anuria. This phase usually spans 0 to 2 days, during which time the normal renal processes begin to deteriorate. Renal blood flow and oxygen consumption decrease to about 25% of normal, urine volume decreases to 20% of normal,

Table 11–1. A SUMMARY OF THE PHASES OF ACUTE RENAL FAILURE

Phase	Definition	Time Span	Renal Blood Flow and O_2 Consumption (% of Normal)	Urine Volume (% of Normal)	Filtration Clearance (% of Normal)
Onset	The period of time from the precipitating event to the beginning of the oliguria or anuria	0–2 days	25	20	10
Oliguric-Anuric	The period of time during which the urine volume remains less than 400 ml/25 hr	8–14 days	25	5	10
Diuretic					
Early	The period of time when the urine output becomes greater than 400 ml/24 hr until the lab values stop rising	10 days	30	150	10
Late	The period of time from when the lab values begin to decrease until they stabilize		50	200	50
Convalescent	The period of time from the stabilization of lab values until totally normal renal function occurs	4–6 months	100	100	100

and filtration clearance decreases to 10% of normal. The individual experiencing the dysfunction cannot compensate for the diminished renal function and exhibits significant clinical signs and symptoms that are reflective of the chemical imbalances in the internal environment.

Oliguric-Anuric Phase. This phase encompasses the time during which the individual's urine volume remains less than 400 ml/day. It usually lasts 8 to 14 days, during which time renal blood flow and oxygen consumption remain at 25% of normal, urine volume decreases even further to 5% of normal, and filtration clearance remains at 10% of normal. The longer an individual remains in this phase, the poorer is the prognosis for recovery. The change in prognosis is directly related to the increased risks for fluid imbalances, electrolyte imbalances, and other complications that the individual encounters during this phase.

Diuretic Phase. The diuretic phase lasts about 10 days and comprises two stages, early and late.

Early Stage. This is the period of time when the urine output becomes greater than 400 ml/day and the laboratory values stop rising. During this stage, renal blood flow and oxygen consumption increase to about 30% of normal, urine volume increases to 150% of normal, and filtration clearance remains at 10% of normal. The improvement in renal blood flow and urine volume account for the stabilization of the laboratory values, while the lack of improvement in filtration clearance explains why those values do not begin to recede toward a more normal level.

Late Stage. This stage of the diuretic phase is the period of time that begins when the laboratory values begin to recede and lasts until they stabilize. In this stage, the stabilization of the laboratory values usually occurs at a level that is higher than the normal values for an individual. During this stage, the renal blood flow and oxygen consumption continue to increase to 50% of normal, urine volume peaks at about 200% of normal, and filtration clearance increases to 50% of normal. All of these improvements indicate that the individual's renal dysfunction is resolving, but there is still a significant risk for the occurrence of fluid imbalances, electrolyte imbalances, and other complications.

Convalescent Phase. The convalescent phase lasts 4 to 6 months and constitutes the remaining recovery time for the individual. This phase is initiated at the onset of the stabilization of the laboratory values and extends until they return to a totally normal level for the individual. The return to normal for an individual may indicate the return of 100% of normal renal function, or it may signal a return of only 97 to 99%. If the patient experiences such a 1 to 2% degree of residual impairment of renal function, it usually is not clinically significant. The elderly and patients with previously existing renal diseases are those most likely to experience such a degree of residual impairment.

■ Prognosis

The prognosis for patients who experience acute renal failure for returning to totally normal, or optimal, renal function is good in 50 to 60% of all cases. Of the remaining 40 to 50% of the patients, 25 to 30% will develop chronic renal failure and 15 to 20% will die as a result of not seeking health care soon enough, the complications secondary to the renal failure, or clinical mismanagement. A major component of the role of the nurse in caring for patients with acute renal failure is to be sufficiently knowledgeable and competent to be able to intervene with the latter group of patients to keep them alive. Unfortunately, the task is becoming more difficult because the technological advances are creating more opportunities for compromised patients to develop acute renal failure. Thus, even though the overall management therapies for patients with acute renal failure have improved, the statistical outcomes have not. The same mortality figures exist today that were documented nearly 25 years ago!

■ Etiology and Pathophysiology

There are numerous clinical conditions that can precipitate acute renal failure. In general, the causes of acute renal failure are usually classified into one of three categories, i.e., prerenal, postrenal, and parenchymal, depending upon where the precipitating factor exerts its pathophysiological effect upon the kidney. The three categories of etiologies and their correlating examples of clinical conditions are given in Table 11–2. Those conditions that can produce acute renal failure by interfering with renal perfusion are classified as prerenal. Those that can produce acute renal failure as a result of obstructing the flow of urine are classified as postrenal. Finally, those conditions that produce acute renal failure

Table 11–2. COMMON CAUSES OF ACUTE RENAL FAILURE

Classification	Examples of Clinical Conditions
Prerenal	
Hypovolemia	Vascular loss—hemorrhage
	Gastrointestinal loss—vomiting, diarrhea
	Renal loss—diuretic abuse, osmotic diuresis associated with diabetes
	Integumentary loss—burns, diaphoresis
Cardiovascular Failure	Myocardial infarction
	Tamponade
	Vascular pooling—sepsis
	Vascular occlusion—thrombosis, embolism
Postrenal	
Obstruction	Ureteral—fibrosis, calculi, crystals, clots, accidental ligation
	Bladder—neoplasms
	Urethral—stricture, prostatic hypertrophy
Parenchymal	
Glomerulonephritis	Acute poststreptococcal, systemic lupus erythematosus, Goodpasture's syndrome, bacterial endocarditis
Vasculitis	Periarteritis, hypersensitivity angiitis
Interstitial Nephritis	Acute pyelonephritis, allergic nephritis, hypercalcemia, uric acid nephropathy, myeloma of the kidney
Renal Vascular Disease	Renal artery occlusion, renal vein thrombosis
Acute Tubular Necrosis	
Postischemia	Hypovolemia, cardiogenic shock, endotoxic shock
Nephrotoxins	Heavy metals, organic solvents, glycols, antibiotics, anesthetics, radiographic contrast media
Pigments	
Hemoglobin	Intravascular hemolysis—transfusion reactions, toxic hemolysis
Myoglobin	Rhabdomyolysis—trauma, muscle disease, seizures, severe exercise, prolonged coma

by directly acting on functioning kidney tissue are classified as parenchymal. Overall, the disorders in the prerenal and postrenal categories (sometimes referred to as secondary renal problems) can often be reversed, and therefore will not result in acute renal failure if they are detected early and corrective interventions are instituted quickly. Parenchymal causes (sometimes referred to as primary renal problems), however, are more difficult to detect, are often not reversible, and thus often initiate the acute renal failure process.

PATHOPHYSIOLOGICAL MECHANISMS FOR MAINTAINING OLIGURIA

The pathophysiological mechanisms that maintain the oliguria that occurs during acute renal failure are interrelated entities. Five specific mechanisms have been identified: (1) increased renal vasoconstriction; (2) cellular edema; (3) decreased glomerular capillary permeability; (4) intratubular obstruction; and (5) the back leak of glomerular filtrate. However, the controversy continues regarding when and how many of these mechanisms actually operate in a patient experiencing acute renal failure. There appears to be some consensus that any or all of these mechanisms could be operative in any patient at any specific point in time to produce the oliguria.

The ischemic episode activates the renin-angiotensin system, which produces increased renal vasoconstriction and decreased glomerular capillary pressure, both of which decrease glomerular filtration rate. The decreased glomerular filtration rate and renal blood flow lead to tubular dysfunction, which not only produces the oliguria, but also results in further increases in renal vasoconstriction that continue to perpetuate the dysfunction.

The increased renal vasoconstriction also decreases renal blood flow, which can precipitate tubular damage. When the tubules are damaged, necrotic endothelial cells and other cellular debris accumulate and can obstruct the lumen of the tubule. This intratubular obstruction increases the intratubular pressure, which decreases the glomerular filtration rate and leads to tubular dysfunction and oliguria. In addition, the tubular damage usually produces alterations in the tubular structure that permit the glomerular filtrate to leak out of the tubular lumen and back into the plasma. This back leak of filtrate is a component of the tubular dysfunction that results in oliguria.

The ischemic episode also results in decreased energy supplies, such as adenosine triphosphate (ATP). Without ATP, the sodium-potassium adenosine triphosphatase (ATPase) of the cell membrane can no longer pump sodium out of the cell or accumulate potassium. Chloride enters the cell as depolarization occurs, and the result is an increase in cellular solutes that facilitate cellular edema. Cellular edema further decreases renal blood flow and glomerular filtration rate, damages the tubules, and ultimately leads to tubular dysfunction and oliguria. In addition, the ischemic episode decreases glomerular capillary permeability, which further decreases the glomerular filtration rate and leads to tubular dysfunction and oliguria.

The insult to the nephron that occurs as a result of nephrotoxic substances, such as heavy metals, contrast media, or pharmacological agents, is one of direct tubular damage. In other words, the nephrotoxic agent destroys component parts of the tubule, resulting in intratubular obstruction and the back leak of glomerular filtrate and all of the subsequent pathological alterations. The end result is tubular dysfunction and often oliguria.

In summary, the five pathophysiological mechanisms that are responsible for maintaining oliguria during acute renal failure all progress through tubular dysfunction. Thus, the individual with oliguric acute renal failure will have tubular dysfunction regardless of the cause or which of the five pathophysiological mechanisms are operative.

Systemic Manifestations

One of the facts about patients with acute renal failure that makes caring for them such a challenge is that every body system is affected by the dysfunctional renal system. Thus, the clinician must be knowledgeable about all of the potential ensuing problems and their pathophysiological mechanisms in order to deliver quality care. This knowledge base provides the foundation for formulating an appropriate plan of care for assisting the patient with acute renal failure in coping with the dysfunction. Table 11–3 summarizes the essential knowledge regarding the systemic manifestations of acute renal failure according to body system. Table 11–3 also lists the pathophysiological mechanisms that underlie a specific manifestation. There are, however, a few areas that should be clarified in relation to some of the body systems.

VASCULAR SYSTEM

When the electrolyte imbalances are considered, the clinician must know the specific types of alterations that are likely to occur during oliguric acute renal failure. The specific electrolyte imbalances that can be anticipated are summarized in Table 11–4. In addition, Table 11–5 summarizes the corresponding patterns of change that are likely to occur in the patient's urine laboratory values. It should be noted, however, that the specific underlying pathology for any specific condition could significantly alter the urinary laboratory values from those that are presented in Table 11–5.

The hypertension that accompanies acute renal failure is primarily due to fluid and sodium retention rather than an inappropriate activation of the renin-angiotensin system.

CARDIAC SYSTEM

The congestive heart failure that may occur as a manifestation of acute renal failure presents additional risks for the individual because it further compromises renal function by decreasing renal perfusion.

HEMATOPOIETIC SYSTEM

The increased susceptibility to infection presents a major problem for the already compromised patient with acute renal failure. Not only is the patient less able to combat infection, but he or she now requires numerous, repeated invasive procedures to maintain and sustain life, which will increase the risk of an infection occurring. The clinician must be ever vigilant regarding the potential for infection since sepsis has been documented as being the number one cause of death in patients with acute renal failure.

RESPIRATORY SYSTEM

The patient with acute renal failure is a prime candidate for respiratory system dysfunction. Therefore, the clinician must assist the patient in maintaining adequate ventilatory patterns. In addition, the magnitude of the acid-base imbalance

Table 11–3. THE SYSTEMIC MANIFESTATIONS OF RENAL FAILURE

System	Manifestation	Pathophysiological Mechanisms
Vascular	Fluid Overload	Decreased excretion
	Electrolyte Imbalances	Decreased excretion
	Metabolic Acidosis	Decreased hydrogen ion secretion Decreased sodium ion reabsorption Decreased bicarbonate ion reabsorption and generation Decreased excretion of phosphate salts or titratable acids Decreased ammonia synthesis and ammonium excretion
	Hypertension	Fluid overload Increased sodium retention Inappropriate activation of the renin-angiotensin system
Cardiac	Congestive Heart Failure	Fluid overload Hypertension
	Dysrhythmias	Electrolyte imbalances, especially hyperkalemia, hypocalcemia, and variations in sodium
	Pericarditis (seen more frequently in chronic renal failure patients)	Uremic toxins Increased pericardial membrane permeability
	Peripheral or Systemic Edema	Fluid overload and increased hydrostatic pressure (an associated decrease in osmotic pressure would increase the degree of edema) Right ventricular dysfunction
Hematopoietic	Anemia	Decreased erythropoietin secretion Loss of red blood cells through the GI tract, mucous membranes or dialysis Decreased red blood cell survival time due to uremic toxins Burr cells are produced by a hypertonic serum due to uremic toxins Uremic toxins interfere with folic acid action
	Alterations in Coagulation	Platelet dysfunction due to uremic toxins Hypocalcemia could contribute but rarely does because of the metabolic acidosis
	Increased Susceptibility to Infection	Decreased neutrophil phagocytosis and chemotaxis due to uremic toxins
Respiratory	Pulmonary Edema	Fluid overload Increased pulmonary capillary permeability Left ventricular dysfunction
	Pneumonia or Pneumonitis	Thick, tenacious oral secretions due to decreased fluid intake A weak, lethargic patient with a depressed cough reflex due to uremia Decreased pulmonary macrophage activity Fluid overload
	Kussmaul's Respirations	An increase in the rate and depth of respirations to decrease the carbon dioxide in the body to compensate for the metabolic acidosis
Gastrointestinal	Anorexia, Nausea, and Emesis	Uremic toxins Decomposition of urea in the GI tract releasing ammonia that irritates the mucosa
	Stomatitis and Uremic Halitosis	Uremic toxins Decomposition of urea in the oral cavity releasing ammonia
	Gastritis and Bleeding	Uremic toxins Decomposition of urea in the GI tract releasing ammonia that irritates the GI mucosa producing small ulcerations Increased capillary fragility
	Bowel Problems	Uremic toxins
	Diarrhea	Hypermotility due to electrolyte imbalances, especially hyperkalemia
	Constipation	Hypomotility due to electrolyte imbalances, decreased fluid intake, decreased activity, and decreased bulk in the diet

continued

Table 11-3. THE SYSTEMIC MANIFESTATIONS OF RENAL FAILURE *Continued*

System	Manifestation	Pathophysiological Mechanisms
Neuromuscular	Drowsiness, Confusion, Coma, and Irritability	Uremic toxins produce a uremic encephalopathy Metabolic acidosis Electrolyte imbalances
	Tremors, Twitching, and Convulsions	Uremic toxins produce a uremic encephalopathy
	Peripheral Neuropathy Stage 1—Restless leg syndrome and paresthesias Stage 2—Motor involvement leading to footdrop Stage 3—Paraplegia (Stages 2 and 3 are rare in acute renal failure patients)	Decreased nerve conduction, both motor and sensory, due to uremic toxins
Psychosocial	Decreased Mentation, Decreased Concentration, and Altered Perceptions (even to the point of frank psychoses)	Uremic toxins produce a uremic encephalopathy Electrolyte imbalances Metabolic acidosis Tendency to develop cerebral edema
Integumentary	Pallor	Uremic anemia
	Yellowness	Retained urochrome pigment is excreted through the skin
	Dryness	Decreased secretions from oil and sweat glands due to uremic toxins
	Pruritic	Dry skin Calcium and/or phosphate deposits in the skin Uremic toxins effect on nerve endings
	Purpura and Ecchymoses	Increased capillary fragility Platelet dysfunction
	Uremic Frost (seen only in terminal or severely critically ill patients)	Urea or urate crystals are excreted
Endocrine	Glucose Intolerance (usually not clinically significant)	Peripheral insensitivity to insulin due to uremia Prolonged insulin half-life due to decreased renal metabolism
Skeletal	Hypocalcemia	Hyperphosphatemia due to decreased renal excretion Decreased GI reabsorption due to decreased renal conversion of vitamin D
	Osteodystrophy	Increased osteoclastic activity in response to an increased secretion of parathormone
	Soft Tissue Calcification	Deposition of calcium phosphate crystals in soft tissue and other structures
Reproductive	Infertility	Decreased sperm production and decreased ovulation due to uremia
	Decreased Libido	A combination of the pathophysiological and psychological effects of uremia

that accompanies acute renal failure is usually so great that the individual cannot compensate, and thus will usually present with clinical signs and symptoms of metabolic acidosis.

GASTROINTESTINAL SYSTEM

The major clinical concern in relation to the anorexia, nausea, and emesis that occur in patients with acute renal failure relates more to the possibility of the individual becoming more catabolic owing to a lack of sufficient caloric intake than it does to the possibility of additional fluid and electrolyte abnormalities ensuing. This is because the more catabolic the individual becomes, the greater is the possibility that more body tissue will be broken down for energy. As more body tissue is broken down, more unexcretable waste products accumulate in the patient's serum; thus accelerating the uremic state.

The stomatitis associated with acute renal failure often contributes to increasing tissue catabolism by inhibiting the patient's ability to ingest food substances. The stomatitis is often so painful that the patient cannot tolerate the contact of liquids or solids against the oral mucosa.

Table 11–4. THE VARIATIONS IN SERUM LABORATORY VALUES ACCOMPANYING ACUTE RENAL FAILURE

Substance	Variation in Acute Renal Failure
Sodium	Increases or varies
Potassium	Increases
Chloride	Increases or varies
BUN	Increases
Creatinine	Increases
Calcium	Decreases
Phosphorus	Increases
Uric Acid	Increases
Carbon Dioxide-Combining Power	Decreases
Magnesium	Increases or normal
Osmolality	Increases or varies
Hematocrit	Decreases
Hemoglobin	Decreases

The gastrointestinal bleeding that occurs owing to uremia is an oozing of blood rather than a full blown hemorrhagic state. It certainly can progress to the hemorrhagic level, but in most patients it remains as a continuous small blood loss. Thus, the significance of gastrointestinal bleeding clinically is not so much in how it contributes to the patient's anemia but instead in how it participates in accelerating the uremic process. As the gastrointestinal bleeding continues, some of the blood is reabsorbed and metabolized by the body. Because blood is a protein, its metabolism further increases the amount of unexcretable nitrogenous waste products in the body and adds to the patient's already uremic state.

Table 11–5. THE VARIATIONS IN URINE LABORATORY VALUES ACCOMPANYING ACUTE RENAL FAILURE

Substance	Variation in Acute Renal Failure
Amount	Decreases
Specific gravity	Fixed at 1.010 (or less)
pH	Increases
Glucose	Normal
Protein	Normal (but can vary)
Creatinine	Decreases
Osmolaity	Decreases
Sodium	Decreases (but can vary)
Potassium	Decreases
Chloride	Decreases
Calcium	Decreases
Phosphorus	Decreases
Magnesium	Decreases
Urea	Decreases

NEUROMUSCULAR SYSTEM

The question of whether or not uremic toxins pass through the blood-brain barrier was once a major controversy among clinicians and scientists. Today, however, the issue appears to be somewhat clearer. There is definite evidence demonstrated by electroencephalography that uremic patients have altered brain wave patterns. The frequency and amplitude of the waveforms are altered from normal. Thus, at least some uremic toxins seem to pass through the blood-brain barrier.

PSYCHOSOCIAL SYSTEM

The clinician needs to remember that uremic patients have significant alterations in their mental processes. Therefore, they will often respond more slowly to questions and directives, tend not to remember as easily those instructional components of their care, and view the invasive procedures that they experience as being more threatening to them.

INTEGUMENTARY SYSTEM

The yellowness of the skin that uremic patients develop is due to the retention and excretion of urochrome pigment through the skin. Urochrome pigment is what normally gives urine its yellow coloration. When the patient is not excreting much urine, the pigment accumulates and seeks other excretory pathways. Uremic yellowness differs from the accompanying hepatic dysfunction in two ways: It is a duller yellow color, and it does not affect the sclerae of the eyes. Uremic yellowness is a definite yellow pigment—it is not golden, bronze, tan, or gray.

Clinical Assessment

The clinical assessment of the patient with acute renal failure follows the same format and includes the same components that are used in assessing any individual for whom care is planned and delivered. There are, however, some specific areas that should be noted and these are highlighted in this discussion. The clinician should incorporate these areas into the overall assessment process, without diminishing the importance of the areas that are not elaborated within this discussion.

PATIENT HISTORY

There are four aspects of the patient history that are significantly relevant to the renal system. Those aspects are renal-related symptoms, systemic diseases, family history, and medication history.

Renal-Related Symptoms. The renal-related symptoms that an individual reports can provide valuable clues that will assist the clinician in focusing the assessment to obtain essential data. Table 11–6 presents a list of the renal-related symptoms and their correlated potential pathologies. Most of the pathologies apply to both acute and chronic renal failure. The following pathologies are, however, more applicable to chronic renal failure: nephrotic syndrome, diabetes, and neoplasms.

Systemic Diseases. There are many systemic diseases that can have a direct effect on the renal system. Some of the most frequently encountered include cardiovascular diseases that result in hypotension, immunological diseases that result in sepsis, and hematopoietic diseases such as disseminated intravascular coagulation. Thus, when exploring the patient's history of systemic diseases, the clinician would certainly want to focus on those entities that are most likely also to affect the renal system.

Family History. Family history is an important assessment component for ascertaining not only those systemic diseases that an individual might be predisposed to develop, but also for delineating hereditary and other potential renal problems. Examples of such renal problems include hereditary disorders such as inherited glomerulonephritis, or Alport's syndrome; polycystic disease and medullary cystic disease; and metabolic entities such as calculi, amyloidosis, or hyperoxaluria. The hereditary renal diseases and other types of renal problems are of interest because they can assist in documenting a potential preexisting chronic renal condition.

Medication History. The clinician normally documents all prescribed and nonprescribed medications and their patterns and frequencies of ingestion by the patient. The significance of this information in relation to the renal system is in assessing the possibility of a nephrotoxic insult having occurred as the result of the chronic use or abuse of pharmacological agents, such as analgesics or antibiotics.

Vital Signs. When assessing the vital signs of a patient with acute renal failure, it is important for the clinician to remember that the blood pressure will probably be elevated; the pulse may also be elevated, and in some patients, irregular in rhythm; the respiratory pattern may be deep, rapid, and regular; and the body temperature may be either normal or in some patients elevated.

Table 11–6. THE RENAL RELATED SYMPTOMS AND THEIR CORRELATED POTENTIAL PATHOLOGIES

Symptom	Potential Pathology
Dysuria	Infection
Dribbling	Prostatic Enlargement
	Strictures
Edema	Failure
	Nephrotic Syndrome
Frequency	Infection
	Diabetes
Hematuria	Trauma
	Glomerular Membrane Diseases
	Neoplasms
Hesitancy	Prostatic Enlargement
Incontinence	Infection
	Neoplasms
	Prolapsed Uterus
Nocturia	Infection
Oliguria	Insufficiency
	Neoplasms
	Failure
Proteinuria	Glomerular Membrane Diseases
	Nephrotic Syndrome
Pyuria	Infection
Renal Colic	Calculi
Urgency	Infection
	Prostatic Disease

RENAL ASSESSMENT

Assessing the renal system includes performing the physical examination techniques of palpation and percussion, evaluating serum and urinary laboratory values, and consulting with the physicians regarding the noninvasive and invasive diagnostic procedure results. Overall, however, the clinician will not find the physical examination techniques of palpation and percussion to be particularly helpful in assessing the individual with acute renal failure.

Palpation. To palpate the kidneys, the clinician palpates the lower portion of the upper right and left quadrants of the abdomen. Usually only the lower pole of the right kidney is palpable. The purpose for palpating the kidneys anteriorly is to determine changes in kidney size. The clinician would also palpate the patient's flank area to try and elicit pain if an infection were thought to be present. The area palpated posteriorly is at the costovertebral angle.

Percussion. Percussion is performed in the same areas of the abdomen and flank that are used for palpation. The purpose of percussing the kidneys is to determine changes in size and to assess for surrounding areas of fluid accumulation.

Evaluating Laboratory Values. Because the renal system is the primary regulator of the internal environment of the body, any alteration in its function is rapidly evident in the serum and urine laboratory values. The clinician should evaluate the serum laboratory values of a patient with acute renal failure at least daily. The urinary laboratory values should also be monitored periodically, but much less frequently than serum values. The clinician assesses the laboratory values for deviations from normal and patterns of change that differ from those anticipated for an individual with acute renal failure. As previously noted, Tables 11–4 and 11–5 list the anticipated patterns of change for the laboratory values of an individual with acute renal failure.

When assessing a patient with acute renal failure and evaluating the laboratory values, the clinician must recall that the best measure of renal function is urinary creatinine clearance. Urinary creatinine clearance is calculated using the following formula: $U_c \times V/P_c = C_{cr}$. In this formula, U_c equals the concentration of creatinine in the urine, V equals the volume of urine per unit of time, P_c equals the concentration of creatinine in the plasma, and C_{cr} equals creatinine clearance. Creatinine clearance is an estimate of glomerular filtration rate and is measured in milliliters per minute. Thus, given the following set of patient data: $U_c = 175$ mg/100 ml; $V = 288$ ml/24 hr; $P_c = 17.5$ mg/100 ml; the patient's creatinine clearance would be calculated as

$$\frac{175 \text{ mg/100 ml} \times 288/1440 \text{ min/24 hr}}{17.5 \text{ mg/100 ml}} = 2 \text{ ml/min}$$

Because a normal creatinine clearance is about 120 ml/min, the clinician would recognize this creatinine clearance as being consistent with renal dysfunction.

Creatinine clearance is the best measure of renal function because creatinine is a metabolic byproduct of creatine and phosphocreatine in the muscles. Individuals do not usually alter muscle mass rapidly, so the levels of creatinine produced by the body remain relatively stable. Because the levels are usually so stable, they easily and rapidly reflect alterations in the system that normally excretes creatinine.

In lieu of using creatinine clearance to evaluate renal function, the next best measure to use would be serum creatinine, followed by serum blood urea nitrogen (BUN). Of these two values, BUN is the least reflective of renal function because the BUN can be influenced by other factors such as catabolism, bleeding, and dehydration. It should also be noted that the volume of urine output is not a good measure of renal function. Patients with nonoliguric or polyuric acute renal failure excrete large volumes of fluid with little solute. Thus, such patients still have renal dysfunction even though they are excreting large volumes of fluid. Patterns of urine output are more reflective of renal perfusion states than they are of renal function. Thus, the clinician should use patterns of urine output to assess renal perfusion rather than function.

Noninvasive Diagnostic Procedures. Paramount among the noninvasive diagnostic procedures for assessing patients with acute renal failure are measuring intake and output daily and obtaining daily weights. As simplistic as these assessment procedures are, there are still opportunities for errors. Because accuracy is so important, it is essential that appropriate measuring devices be used to obtain the amounts of urine rather than clinician "guesstimations." Likewise, since body weight is a measure that can be used to validate intake and output measurements, it is appropriate that the patient also have the body weight assessed daily. Certainly body weight and intake and output measurements may vary somewhat, but if the clinician recalls that there are about 500 ml in a pound, and factors the patient's insensible loss into the process, the two measurements should closely coincide.

Another noninvasive diagnostic procedure that is frequently used to assess the renal system is an x-ray of the kidneys, ureters, and bladder (KUB). This plain film of the abdomen is taken with the patient in a supine position and it reveals information regarding the size, shape, position, and possible areas of calcification of the kidneys. The KUB is usually performed prior to any invasive diagnostic procedures being conducted.

Table 11–7. INVASIVE DIAGNOSTIC PROCEDURES FOR ASSESSING THE RENAL SYSTEM

Procedure	Purpose	Technique	Potential Problems
Intravenous Pyelography	To visualize the renal parenchyma, calyces, pelves, ureters, and bladder to obtain information regarding size, shape, position, and function of the kidneys.	1. Have the patient void to empty the bladder. 2. Assist the patient in assuming a supine position. 3. Inject a contrast medium intravenously. 4. X-ray the kidneys and bladder at 5, 10, and 15 min.	Hypersensitivity reaction Acute renal failure Postinjection hematoma
Computed Tomography	To visualize the renal parenchyma to obtain data regarding the size, shape, and presence of lesions, cysts, masses, calculi, obstructions, congenital anomalies, and abnormal accumulations of fluid.	1. Assist the patient in assuming a supine position. 2. Remind the patient that at various times during the 40-min procedure, he/she will be asked to hold breath for a short time. 3. Inject a contrast medium intravenously. (This step may be omitted.) 4. X-ray the kidneys at 10-degree intervals and electronically transmit the information to a computer that creates an image of the kidneys and calculates their densities.	Hypersensitivity reactions if a contrast medium is used Postinjection hematoma
Nephrosonography	To visualize the renal parenchyma, calyces, pelves, ureters and bladder, to obtain data regarding the size, shape, position, and internal structure of the kidneys, as well as perirenal tissue. Also to assess and localize urinary obstructions and abnormal accumulations of fluid.	1. Assist the patient to assume either a sitting or prone position. 2. X-ray the kidneys and allow the inaudible, high-frequency sound waves to reflect off the kidneys and be transformed into an image that is projected onto an oscilloscope.	No potential problems currently identified
Nephrotomography	To visualize the renal parenchyma, calyces, and pelves in layers to obtain information regarding tumors, cysts, lacerations, or areas of nonperfusion.	1. Take plain x-rays of the kidneys. 2. Determine the arm to kidney circulation time of a substance. 3. Inject a loading dose of contrast medium intravenously. 4. Inject a second dose of contrast medium intravenously. 5. X-ray the kidneys at the predetermined circulation time. 6. Take tomograms of the kidneys at 1-cm intervals.	Hypersensitivity reaction Postinjection hematoma
Renal Angiography	To visualize the arterial tree, capillaries, and venous drainage of the kidneys to obtain data regarding the presence of tumors, cysts, stenosis, infarction, aneurysms, hematomas, lacerations, and abscesses.	1. Assist the patient to assume a supine position under the fluoroscope. 2. Administer a local anesthetic at the catheter insertion site. 3. Insert a catheter via the femoral artery to the aorta. 4. Inject a contrast medium via the catheter. 5. Take films of the kidneys during the arterial, nephrographic, and venous phases of filling. 6. Withdraw the catheter and apply a pressure dressing to the site. 7. Instruct the patient to remain on bed rest for 12 to 24 hr postangiography	Hypersensitivity reaction Hemorrhage at the catheter insertion site Acute renal failure

Table 11–7. INVASIVE DIAGNOSTIC PROCEDURES FOR ASSESSING THE RENAL SYSTEM *Continued*

Procedure	Purpose	Technique	Potential Problems
Renal Scan	To determine renal function by visualizing the appearance and disappearance of radioisotopes within the kidney. It also provides some anatomical information.	1. Assist the patient to assume a prone or other designated position. 2. Inject a radioisotope intravenously. 3. Take sequential films to illustrate the uptake and excretion of the radioisotopes by the kidneys.	Hypersensitivity reaction Postinjection hematoma
Renal Biopsy	To obtain data to make a histological diagnosis in order to determine the extent of the pathology, appropriate therapy, and the possible prognosis.	1. Assess the patient's clotting time, protime, and platelet count. 2. Check that all other appropriate prerequisite diagnostic tests have been completed. 3. Assist the patient to assume a prone position with the area to be biopsied slightly elevated using a support. 4. Cleanse and anesthetize the area. 5. Insert an exploratory needle while the patient holds breath to determine depth and position. 6. Reanesthetize the area if necessary. 7. Insert the biopsy needle and obturator while the patient holds breath. 8. Extract the obturator and replace it with the cutting prongs. 9. Obtain a tissue sample. 10. Remove the prongs, tissue, and needle and instruct the patient to breathe normally. 11. Apply gentle pressure to the site for 5 minutes, then apply a pressure dressing. 12. Instruct the patient to remain on bed rest for 24 hr.	Hemorrhage Postbiopsy hematoma

Invasive Diagnostic Procedures. The invasive diagnostic procedures that are used to assess the renal system include intravenous pyelography, computed tomography, nephrosonography, nephrotomography, renal angiography, renal scan, and renal biopsy. These procedures are summarized in Table 11–7, including their purposes, technique, and major potential problems. For any and all of these diagnostic procedures, the clinician would implement the following general interventions: (1) explain the procedure to the patient, emphasizing his/her responsibilities during the procedure; (2) reinforce the explanations that have been previously provided by other health care team personnel concerning the procedure; (3) carry out any preparatory activities required for the procedure; (4) provide appropriate fluids to assist the individual in maintaining an adequate hydration state prior to and after the procedure; (5) assist with the procedure whenever possible or necessary; (6) monitor the patient for any complications after the procedure; and (7) document the patient's response to the procedure.

Nursing Diagnoses and Interventions

The nursing care of the individual experiencing acute renal failure is based on three essential components: (1) knowledge of the systemic manifestations of renal failure; (2) an assessment of the individual's specific responses to the disease process; and (3) a comprehension of the general management goals for the individual. The first two components have previously been discussed, but the third component needs to be delineated. In general, there are eight management goals for an individual experiencing acute renal failure. Those goals are to (1) correct the primary disorder causing the renal dysfunction; (2) prevent infection; (3) treat the fluid imbalances; (4) treat the electrolyte imbalances; (5) treat the acid-base imbalances; (6) maintain the individual in an anabolic state; (7) treat the anemia; and (8) treat the uremic symptoms. Most of a clinician's interactions with a patient experiencing acute renal failure are aimed at meeting these goals and sustaining the individual during the time that is required for the condition to resolve.

The systematically derived plan of care for a patient with acute renal failure will be presented in the usual format, including the nursing diagnosis, goal statement, patient outcome criteria, and interventions (see also Nursing Care Plan for the Patient with Acute Renal Failure).

Table 11–8. A SUMMARY OF ECLECTIC NORMAL ADULT SERUM LABORATORY VALUES

Substance	Normal Value
Sodium	136–146 mEq/L
Potassium	3.5–5.5 mEq/L
Chloride	96–106 mEq/L
BUN	9–20 mg/100 ml
Creatinine	0.7–1.5 mg/100 ml
Calcium	8.5–10.5 mg/100 ml
	4.5–5.8 mEq/L
Phosphorus	2.0–4.5 mg/100 ml
	1.0–1.5 mEq/L
Uric Acid	2.5–6.0 mg%
Carbon Dioxide–Combining Power	24–28 mEq/L
Magnesium	1.6–2.2 mEq/L
Osmolality	280–295 mOsm/kg H_2O
Hematocrit	40–50%
Hemoglobin	12–16 g/100 ml

NURSING DIAGNOSIS: ALTERATIONS IN FLUID AND ELECTROLYTE AND ACID-BASE BALANCE

Goal. The general goal associated with this nursing diagnosis is to maintain, or reestablish, fluid electrolyte and acid-base balance. Certainly this and all other goal statements would be more specifically articulated as the goal was individualized to the specific patient.

Outcome Criteria. The outcome criteria that would demonstrate that the goal for this nursing diagnosis was met include a balanced fluid intake and output, minus insensible loss; a body weight within 2 lb of the individual's dry weight; stable vital signs within the normal range, or consistent with the patient's baseline values; a central venous pressure reading of between 5 and 8 cm; normal skin moisture, turgor, texture, and elasticity; normally hydrated oral mucous membranes; normal muscle strength; normal bowel sounds and fecal excretory patterns; negative Chvostek's and Trousseau's signs; an intact skeletal system; serum laboratory values within the ranges depicted in Table 11–8; and arterial blood gas values within the following normal ranges: pH 7.40 ± 0.03; $PCO_2 \pm 40 \pm 3$ mmHg; HCO_3 24 to 28 mEq/L; PO_2 90 ± 10 mmHg; and O_2 saturation $96 \pm 1\%$.

Interventions. The nursing interventions used in assisting individuals with acute renal failure in coping with the effects of the dysfunction can be independent, interdependent, or dependent in nature. This discussion encompasses all three types without differentiating one from the other. The rationale for the lack of differentiation is that the interventions are not clearly delineated and may alter category type depending on geographical area, nurse practice acts, and hospital policy. In addition, the discussion also includes both monitoring and intervening functions. Monitoring functions are those that assist the clinician in collecting additional data to use in the ongoing assessment process. Monitoring functions can assist in defining problems but they do not alter a patient's state. Intervening functions are those behaviors that will make a change in the patient's clinical state when implemented by the clinician.

The monitoring functions associated with this goal include (1) monitoring intake and output patterns at least every 4 hours; (2) monitoring the patient's weight daily; (3) monitoring serum laboratory values, especially BUN, creatinine, and potassium, at least daily; (4) monitoring arterial blood gas values as needed; (5) monitoring urinary laboratory values at least daily during the diuretic phase; (6) monitoring vital signs at least every 2 hours; (7) performing a complete cardiovascular assessment at least every 8 hours; (8) assessing apical and peripheral pulse differences to monitor for dysrhythmias at least every 2 hours; (9) performing a complete respiratory assessment at least every 8 hours; (10) performing a complete neurological assessment at least every 8 hr; (11) monitoring for clinical signs of cerebral edema at least every 4 hours; (12) monitoring Chvostek's and Trousseau's signs at least daily; and (13) monitoring the character-

NURSING CARE PLAN FOR THE PATIENT WITH ACUTE RENAL FAILURE

Nursing Diagnosis	Outcome	Intervention
Alteration in fluid and electrolyte and acid-base balance	Maintain or reestablish fluid and electrolyte and acid-base balance Balanced fluid intake and output A body weight within 2 lb of the individuals dry weight Stable vital signs consistent with the individual's baseline values CVP 5–8 cm Normal skin moisture, turgor, texture, and elasticity Normal hydrated oral mucosa Normal muscle strength Normal bowel sounds and elimination Negative Chvostek's and Trousseau's signs Intact skeletal system Serum lab values WNR Arterial blood gases WNR	Monitor I&O patterns every 4 hr Monitor daily weights Monitor laboratory values, especially BUN, creatinine, and potassium, daily Monitor arterial blood gases Monitor urinary lab values daily during diuretic phase Monitor V/S every 2 hr Cardiac respiratory and neurological assessment every 8 hr Assess apical and peripheral pulses every 2 hr Monitor for clinical signs of cerebral edema every 2 hr Monitor Chvostek's and Trousseau's signs daily Monitor characteristics of urine; e.g., color, odor, pH, specific gravity, protein, and glucose Catheterize patient with caution, only if necessary, and using strict aseptic technique Maintain prescribed fluid and electrolyte restrictions Administer all fluids and medication precisely Institute seizure precautions Administer blood prior to or during dialysis Prepare patient for dialysis or hemofiltration
Alterations in cardiac output	Maintain adequate cardiac output Stable vital signs Normal skin color, turgor, texture, and temperature Relaxed, sedate body posture and behavior Cardiac rhythm and rate that is consistent with fluid and electrolyte status	Assess apical and radial pulses every 4 hr Cardiovascular assessment every 8 hr Monitor fluid balance every 2 hr Monitor electrolyte balance daily Maintain all fluid and electrolyte restrictions Administer all fluids and medications precisely Prepare patient for dialysis or hemofiltration
Potential for infection	Prevent infection Stable vital signs; e.g., temperature Activity level consistent with patient's usual expenditure of energy Normal, intact skin; e.g., color, turgor, texture, temperature, and odor Decreasing size of any abrasions or cuts on skin Cognitive clarity and responsiveness Normal breath sounds Normal chest x-ray Urination pattern that is normal for individual Negative culture for all body fluids and wound areas WBC and differential consistent with normal for individual	Monitor environment, visitors, and personnel caring for patient for possible contamination Assess all abrasions or cuts in skin every 8 hr Monitor vital signs every 4 hr; e.g., temperature Assess cognitive clarity every 2 hr Monitor lab results and diagnostic tests daily Avoid abrasive and invasive equipment whenever possible Institute pulmonary preventive program; e.g., turning, coughing, deep breathing incentive inspirometry, every 2 hr Provide appropriate nutrients and calories consistent with restrictions Administer supplemental vitamins as prescribed *Note:* Patient will not usually receive antibiotics because of nephrotoxic potential to an already damaged renal system
Alterations in coagulation	Prevent abnormal or prolonged bleeding	Assess skin daily Monitor appropriate lab values daily

continued

NURSING CARE PLAN FOR THE PATIENT WITH ACUTE RENAL FAILURE *Continued*		
Nursing Diagnosis	**Outcome**	**Intervention**
	Presence of intact skin with no ecchymoses or petechiae Normal bleeding time of between 3 and 5 min Hemoglobin and hematocrit levels normal for patient	Assess patient's environment for items that may be hazardous to patient Avoid invasive procedures when possible Apply pressure to venipuncture and injection sites for 3–5 min Remove sharp objects from patient environment as possible Use electric razor Have patient wear hard-soled shoes when ambulating Prepare patient for dialysis
Alterations in breathing patterns	Normal, adequate respiratory pattern Respiratory rate, rhythm, and depth consistent with patient pathophysiological state Normal breath sounds Blood gases that are consistent with patient's state Serum CO_2 level between 24 and 28 mEq/L Activity pattern normal for patient. Cognitive clarity normal for patient	Monitor respiratory rate, rhythm, and depth every 2 hr Auscultating lung sounds every 4 hr Assess serum lab values and arterial blood gases daily, or as needed Assess cognitive clarity level hourly Monitor activity level every 8 hr Monitor patient environment for possible sources of respiratory contaminants Position patient in semi-Fowler's position Implement positive preventative pulmonary therapy every 2 hr Limit number and duration of interactions with individuals having upper respiratory infections—provide masks Administer medications prescribed Prepare patient for dialysis
Alterations in nutrition	Adequate nutritional intake. Body weight consistent with individual Appropriate caloric intake Anthropometric measurements Skin, nails, hair, and mucous membranes normal for patient's pathophysiological state Appropriate energy level Consistent cognitive clarity Serum lab values consistent with patient's pathophysiological state	Monitor body weight and caloric intake daily Anthropometric measurements weekly Monitoring skin, nails, hair, and mucous membranes daily Assess cognitive level every 4 hr Monitor serum lab values daily Provide diet with essential nutrients but within restrictions Oral hygiene before and after meals Remove noxious stimuli from patient's presence Provide rest periods prior to and immediately following meals Small, frequent feedings Encourage meal time to be social event to involve family, others Promote dietary goals with patient Administer medications, vitamins, and nutritional supplements as prescribed Administer hyperalimentation precisely as prescribed
Alterations in bowel elimination	Adequate bowel elimination—prevent constipation, avoid diarrhea Normal bowel habits for individual Character of stool is similar to patient's normal Comfortable elimination process Normal bowel sounds Abdominal and anal characteristics are normal Food and fluid intake consistent with restrictions Normal activity level Verbalizes comfort state of abdomen and lower GI tract	Assess bowel functions daily Monitor characteristics of stool after each evacuation Abdominal inspection every 4 hr Auscultate bowel sounds every 8 hr Inspect anal opening every other day Monitor fluid and food intake every 4 hr Monitor activity level every 4 hr Monitor serum lab values daily Assess all medication for potential detrimental effect on the GI tract Provide food and fluids within restrictions Assist patient in maintaining activity level Administer stool softeners as prescribed Administer gentle bulk-forming agents Occasional use of glycerin suppositories Provide privacy for patient during evacuation process
Impaired physical mobility	Promoting or increasing physical mobility Increase in functional ROM	Monitor patient's participation in ADL every 8 hr Assess degree and comfort of ROM every 8 hr Assess muscle tone and strength daily

NURSING CARE PLAN FOR THE PATIENT WITH ACUTE RENAL FAILURE *Continued*

Nursing Diagnosis	Outcome	Intervention
	Increased muscle tone and strength Increased patient participation in ADLs Stable patient gait on ambulation Full weight-bearing during ambulation Vital sign changes consistent with activity Verbalizes comfort during activities	Monitor gait and weight bearing ability when ambulating Assess vital signs and comfort level during activities Monitor serum lab values daily Assist patient in performing ROM exercises every 4 hr Assist patient in appropriate ambulation every 8 hr Have patient perform appropriate ADLs Provide for rest periods following activities Consult with occupational and physical therapist Establish an activity plan with patient Provide nutrition within restrictions Administer medications as prescribed Prepare patient for dialysis
Potential for Injury	Promote patient safety Maintain erect, stable posture during ambulation Sensorium free of vertigo and syncope Intact skin Neurological and neuromuscular functioning consistent with state Cognitive clarity Serum electrolyte and arterial blood gases consistent with patient's status	Assess posture and gait on ambulation Assess sensory, cognitive clarity, neurological, and neuromotor functions every 2 hr Assess patient's skin for intactness every 8 hr Assess for Chvostek's and Trousseau's sign daily Monitor serum lab values and arterial blood gases daily Provide hazard free environment Orient patient to surroundings daily or as needed Provide appropriate footwear for ambulation activities Encourage activities but avoid overstimulation Maintain seizure precautions Maintain nutritional and fluid restrictions Administer medications as prescribed Prepare for dialysis
Sensory-perception alterations	Decrease anxiety for patient Relaxed facial expression and body posture Appropriate eye contact Coherent logical communication patterns Normal affect and mannerisms Normal concentration and participation Participation in ADLs Appetite consistent with patient's pathophysiological state Consistent rest patterns Consistent personal hygiene Purposeful motor activity Consistent vital signs	Assess, e.g., patient's affect, facial expression, body posture, personal hygiene, eye contact, communication, activity, daily Monitor nutritional intake and appetite daily Monitor rest patterns daily Assess vital signs every 4 hr Monitor lab values every 4 hr Provide effective stimuli; avoid overstimulation Provide explanations of everything done Quality time with patient (10 min) four times a day Provide emotional support and reassurance Encourage expression of feelings Support patient's constructive coping mechanisms Assist patient to focus on concrete items Encourage family, clergy, and others to visit as appropriate Assist in identifying sources of anxiety Prepare for dialysis
Alterations in thought process	Promote effective communication Verbalizes orientation to person, place, and time Appropriate eye contact Clear, coherent communication Consistent affect and gestures Consistent concentration and participation Correct verbal responses to questions Appropriate activities Serum lab values consistent	Assess level of orientation every 4 hr Assess eye contact, communication, gestures, concentration, and participation during activities Assess verbal response to questions and resultant activity Monitor lab values daily Establish therapeutic rapport Structure interactions to be brief yet purposeful Assist in helping to differentiate stimuli Prepare patient for dialysis

continued

NURSING CARE PLAN FOR THE PATIENT WITH ACUTE RENAL FAILURE *Continued*		
Nursing Diagnosis	**Outcome**	**Intervention**
Potential for impaired skin integrity	Maintain intact integument Intact skin has color, odor, turgor, texture, temperature, elasticity, and degree of moisture consistent with patient's pathophysiological state Verbalizes a comfortable and intact integument	Assess skin daily Monitor fluid and food intake daily Assist with bathing activities using substance to prevent drying of skin daily Apply appropriate lotions or oils to skin every 4 hr Trim nails weekly Provide perineal care twice daily Turn or move patient hourly Assist with active or passive ROM exercises every 4 hr Institute adjunct therapies; e.g., bed padding, sheep-skin, massage Handle edematous tissue gently Administer medications as prescribed Provide fluid and food within restrictions Prepare patient for dialysis
Alterations in oral mucous membranes	Promote healing of the oral mucous membrances Maintain color, odor, intactness, turgor, texture, and moisture consistent with patient's pathophysiological state Verbalizes comfort of oral cavity and mucosa Verbalizes no change in oral temperature from food or fluids Verbalizes ability to taste food appropriately Adequate food and fluid intake to maintain desired weight consistent with patient's pathophysiological state Consistent lab values	Assess oral cavity and mucous membranes every 4 hr Assist with oral comfort level every 4 hr Monitor food and fluid intake daily Monitor patient weight daily Monitor serum lab values Assist patient with oral hygiene every 2 hr, prior to mealtime and at bedtime Adopt specific oral hygiene routine that produces cleanliness and comfort Rinse patient's mouth every hour Administer medications as prescribed Provide food and fluids at comfortable temperature Prepare patient for dialysis
Knowledge deficit	Provide patient with sufficient, accurate information to be an informed participant in own health care Verbalizes information known and asks questions about disease process and health care regimen Cooperates and participates in own health care	Assess content of patient's verbalizations and questions daily Monitor degree of cooperation and participation daily Provide specific, factual information about the disease process, its impact on the patient, and effect on care Reinforce information and update daily Include family in educational process If appropriate, arrange for former patient who has experienced renal failure to visit

istics and constituents of the urine, especially color, odor, pH, specific gravity, protein, and glucose at least daily.

Considering all of the concern that is generated regarding the volume of urine output excreted by a patient with acute renal failure, it is easy to understand why clinicians often automatically, but erroneously, insert indwelling urinary catheters into these patients. Certainly accuracy is to be strived for when assessing urine output, but never at the expense of jeopardizing the entire renal system. Indwelling catheters represent a major health hazard, i.e., infection, that could further compromise an already insulted kidney. In addition, the urinary output in 97% of all of the cases is going to remain oliguric for 8 to 14 days. Thus, the rules of thumb for the clinician regarding catheterization are (1) do not catheter-

Table 11-9. DAILY DIETARY REQUIREMENTS AND RESTRICTIONS IN ACUTE RENAL FAILURE

Dietary Component	Daily Amount in Acute Renal Failure
Water	400–600 ml plus the urine output
Calories	35–50 kcal/kg
Protein	0.5–1.5 g/kg
Sodium	500–1000 mg
Potassium	20–50 mEq
Phosphate	700 mg or less
Calcium	800–1200 mg
Carbohydrate	Unrestricted
Fats	Variable

Daily water-soluble vitamin supplements will also be required.

ize unless there is a physiological reason to do so; for example, the presence of a neurogenic bladder; and (2) if catheterization is necessary, intermittent catheterization using strict aseptic technique is preferable.

The intervening functions include (1) maintaining all prescribed fluid and electrolyte restrictions, usually very similarly to those displayed in Table 11–9; (2) administering all prescribed fluids and pharmacological agents precisely; (3) instituting seizure precautions; (4) administering any necessary blood transfusions prior to or during dialysis if possible; and (5) preparing the patient for dialysis as prescribed, or instituting hemofiltration as prescribed.

A major component of the above delineated intervening functions is that of assisting in treating the patient's hyperkalemic state. In general, there are three primary approaches to treating hyperkalemia: reducing the body potassium content; shifting the potassium intracellularly; and antagonizing the membrane effect of the hyperkalemia. These approaches, which may be used simultaneously or separately, are summarized in Table 11–10, including specific methods of treatment and the degree of effectiveness in decreasing plasma potassium and total body potassium content. As Table 11–10 indicates, there really are only two methods that are effective in reducing plasma potassium and total body potassium content in a patient with acute renal failure: dialysis and the use of cation exchange resins with sorbitol. Using other methods will only provide additional time for the clinician to implement the definitive therapy. In essence, the other methods can "protect" the patient for a short time until dialysis or the cation exchange resins are instituted and have had sufficient time to produce therapeutic results.

NURSING DIAGNOSIS: ALTERATIONS IN CARDIAC OUTPUT

Goal. The goal for this nursing diagnosis is to maintain an adequate cardiac output. Addi-

Table 11-10. TREATMENT APPROACHES FOR HYPERKALEMIA

Approach	Methods	Efficacy
Reduce the body potassium content	Decrease potassium intake	May decrease plasma and total body potassium content over time
	Increase the fecal excretion of potassium using cation-exchange resins such as Kayexalate	Takes hours to be effective but will eventually decrease both plasma and total body potassium content
	Increase the renal excretion of potassium by using mineralocorticoid agents, increasing salt intake, or using diuretic agents	Any of these would be effective in decreasing both plasma and total body potassium content if the individual has normal renal function
	Dialysis	Decreases both plasma and total body potassium content within a 4- to 6-hr time frame
Shift the potassium intracellularly	Administer glucose and insulin intravenously	Decreases plasma potassium for about 2 hr, but has no effect on total body potassium content
	Administer an alkali such as sodium bicarbonate	Decreases plasma potassium for a short time but has no effect on total body potassium content
Antagonize the cellular membrane effect	Administer calcium salts	Has no effect on either plasma or total body potassium content
	Administer hypertonic sodium salts	Has no effect on either plasma or total body potassium content

tional hypotensive episodes could exacerbate the existing renal insult.

Outcome Criteria. The outcome criteria that would indicate that this goal is being met include stable vital signs within the appropriate range for the individual; normal skin color, texture, turgor, and temperature; a relaxed, sedate body posture and behavior; and a cardiac rhythm and rate that is consistent with the patient's fluid and electrolyte status.

Interventions. The monitoring functions are a major component of the care that is delivered in relation to this nursing diagnosis. They include assessing apical-radial pulses at least every 4 hours to detect discrepancies between the two that might indicate a dysrhythmia; performing a total cardiovascular assessment at least every 8 hours; monitoring fluid balance at least every 2 hours; and monitoring electrolyte balance at least daily.

The intervening functions are relatively circumscribed and include maintaining all prescribed fluid and electrolyte restrictions, administering all prescribed fluids and pharmacological agents precisely, and preparing the patient for dialysis as prescribed, or instituting hemofiltration as prescribed.

NURSING DIAGNOSIS: POTENTIAL FOR INFECTION

Goal. Preventing infection is the primary goal associated with this nursing diagnosis. This goal is extremely important in caring for patients with acute renal failure because sepsis is the number one cause of death for this immunocompromised patient population.

Outcome Criteria. The clinician can determine that this goal is being met by noting the following about the patient: stable vital signs that are consistent with the baseline values for the patient, especially body temperature; an activity level that is consistent with the patient's usual expenditure of energy; either a normal, intact integumentary system or normal coloration, turgor, texture, temperature, and odor and decreasing size of any interruptions in the integument; cognitive clarity and responsiveness that is consistent with the patient's baseline; normal breath sounds upon auscultating the lungs; a chest x-ray that reveals no consolidation or infiltration; a micturition pattern that is consistent with the patient's baseline; negative culture results for all body secretions and wound areas; and a white blood cell count and differential that is consistent with the patient's baseline.

Interventions. The monitoring functions related to this goal include assessing the environment, visitors, and personnel who care for the patient in order to decrease the possible cross-contamination that can occur; assessing all interruptions in the integument at least every 8 hours; monitoring all vital signs at least every 4 hours; auscultating the patient's breath sounds at least every 4 hours; assessing the patient's cognitive clarity at least every 2 hours; and monitoring the results of all laboratory and diagnostic tests at least daily.

The intervening functions include avoiding invasive instrumentation and manipulation whenever possible; implementing positive preventative pulmonary maintenance therapies, such as turning, coughing, deep breathing, incentive inspirometry, and suctioning at least every 2 hours; maintaining the patient in an anabolic state by providing or administering the appropriate nutrients and calories consistent with the restrictions as prescribed; and administering nutritional supplements, such as vitamins, as prescribed. It is important to remember that in most cases, the patient will not receive a course of prophylactic antibiotic therapy because of the potential threat of nephrotoxicity to an already insulted renal system.

NURSING DIAGNOSIS: ALTERATIONS IN COAGULATION

Goal. The primary goal associated with this nursing diagnosis is to prevent abnormal or prolonged bleeding.

Outcome Criteria. The outcome criteria that will demonstrate that this goal is being met include the presence of an intact integument that evidences no ecchymoses or petechiae; a normal bleeding time of between 3 and 5 minutes; and hematocrit and hemoglobin levels that are stabilized within the baseline range for the individual. Other outcome criteria that could be used to evaluate whether this goal is being met do not seem to be useful because of the etiology of the coagulopathy and the presence of the uremic anemia. The existence of these pathophysiological entities will also alter other parameters that could be used to evaluate this goal.

Interventions. The monitoring functions that are appropriate for this goal include assessing the integument, especially in the areas of the extremities, at least daily; monitoring the appropriate laboratory values at least daily; and assessing the patient's environment for hazardous specific items, such as personal items or furniture, or their placement, that might cause injury to the patient.

The intervening functions include avoiding invasive instrumentation and manipulation whenever possible; applying pressure to all venipuncture and injection sites for at least 3 to 5 minutes postprocedure; structuring the patient's environment to minimize the hazards and maximize safety, such as placing frequently used items within easy reach, or positioning furniture with sharp edges away from the areas that the patient most frequently travels; instructing the patient on behaviors to implement that will maximize safety, such as using an electric shaver instead of a straight-edged razor, and wearing hard-soled slippers or shoes whenever traversing the halls or the confines of the room; and preparing the patient for dialysis as prescribed. In most patients, the coagulopathy that accompanies renal failure is a result of platelet dysfunction due to uremic toxins. Thus, instituting adequate dialysis is the best therapeutic measure to use in promoting normal coagulation processes.

NURSING DIAGNOSIS: ALTERATIONS IN BREATHING PATTERNS

Goal. The goal associated with this nursing diagnosis is to promote a normal, adequate respiratory pattern.

Outcome Criteria. To determine whether this goal is being met, the clinician would assess for the presence of the following outcome criteria: a respiratory rate, rhythm, and depth that is consistent with the patient's baseline and pathophysiological state; normal breath sounds that are free of adventitious sounds; blood gas values that are consistent with the patient's baseline and pathophysiological state; a serum CO_2 level between 24 and 28 mEq/L; an activity pattern that is consistent with the patient's baseline; and cognitive clarity that is consistent with the patient's baseline and pathophysiological state.

Interventions. The monitoring functions related to this goal include monitoring the patient's respiratory rate, rhythm, depth, and characteristics at least every 2 hours; auscultating the patient's lung sounds at least every 4 hours; assessing serum laboratory values and arterial blood gas values at least daily, or as appropriate; assessing the patient's level of cognitive clarity at least hourly; monitoring the patient's activity level at least every 8 hours; and monitoring the patient's environment for potential sources of upper respiratory tract bacterial contaminants.

The intervening functions include positioning the patient in a semi-Fowler's position to facilitate adequate respirations; implementing positive preventative pulmonary maintenance therapies, such as coughing, deep breathing, systematically altering position by turning, incentive inspirometry, and suctioning, at least every 2 hours; limiting the number and duration of interactions of individuals with upper respiratory tract infections who may come into contact with the patient; providing masks for frequent changing for individuals with upper respiratory tract infections who must be in contact with the patient; administering pharmacological agents, such as sodium bicarbonate, precisely as prescribed; and preparing the patient for dialysis as prescribed.

The clinician should recognize that Kussmaul's respirations are one type of altered respiratory pattern that is likely to be exhibited by the patient with acute renal failure. This pattern results from a respiratory attempt at compensating for the metabolic acidosis that the patient is experiencing. In such cases, the clinician should be prepared to support the altered pattern by proper positioning until more definitive therapy, such as dialysis or pharmacological agent administration, is instituted. Suppressing this altered respiratory pattern would only serve to counteract the patient's inherent compensatory mechanisms.

NURSING DIAGNOSIS: ALTERATIONS IN NUTRITION

Goal. Promoting adequate nutritional intake is the primary general goal associated with this nursing diagnosis.

Outcome Criteria. The outcome criteria that would demonstrate that this goal is being met include a dry body weight (clinically defined as that weight below which the signs and symptoms of hypotension occur) that is consistent with the patient's age, height, and body frame size; a caloric intake that is appropriate for the patient's age, height, weight, body frame size, energy expenditure, and pathophysiological state, usually in excess of 2500 calories to prevent additional catabolism; anthropometric measurements that are consistent with the patient's physical stature, such as a mid-arm circumference of greater than 26.3 cm, a mid-arm muscle circumference of greater than 22.8 cm, and a triceps skin fold of greater than 11.3 mm; integument, hair, nails, and mucous membranes that are consistent with the patient's pathophysiological state in terms of turgor, texture, intactness, and degree of hydration; an energy level that is consistent with the patient's pathophysiological state; cognitive clarity that is consistent with the patient's pathophysiological state; serum laboratory values that are either normal, as listed in Table 11–8, or consistent with the patient's pathophysiological state; and other serum laboratory values that are either consistent with the patient's pathophysiological state or are within the following ranges: total protein 6 to 8 g/100 ml; albumin 3.5 to 5.5 g/100 ml; transferrin 205 to 375 mg/100 ml; triglycerides 40 to 150 mg/100 ml; cholesterol 150 to 250 mg/100 ml; iron 75 to 175 mg/100 ml; vitamin B_{12} 180 to 1000 pg/ml; and folic acid 1.8 to 9.0 ng/ml.

Interventions. The monitoring functions related to this goal include monitoring body weight and caloric intake at least daily; obtaining anthropometric measurements at least weekly; monitoring the integument, hair, nails, and mucous membranes at least daily; assessing the patient's activity and energy level at least daily; assessing the patient's cognitive clarity at least every 4 hours; and monitoring the serum laboratory values at least daily.

The intervening functions include providing an oral or enteral diet that contains the essential nutrients but maintains the prescribed restrictions, as detailed in Table 11–9; assisting the patient with oral hygiene 10 minutes prior to the ingestion of food; removing all noxious stimuli from the patient's environment; providing at least 30 minutes of rest time prior to the ingestion of food; providing small, frequent feedings at times the patient has selected for ingestion; structuring the time of food ingestion to be a social event by inviting family members or other patients to join the patient; establishing competitive goals for the patient to achieve regarding the ingestion of food; administering pharmacological agents, vitamin supplements, and nutritional supplements as prescribed; and administering hyperalimentation precisely as prescribed, usually in a formulation similar to that given in Table 11–11.

The importance of the nutritional aspect of the care of the patient experiencing acute renal failure should not be underestimated. The research seems to indicate that individuals with acute renal failure who have a positive caloric balance have a much higher survival rate than those individuals with a negative balance. This outcome is predictable because an inadequate caloric intake would result in increased protein catabolism and accelerated formation and accumulation of uremic toxins. The catabolic processes are enhanced in these patients because their average metabolic rates while in acute renal failure are about 20% greater than normal. In addition, dialysis therapy also contributes to protein catabolism and further exacerbates the patient's nutritional needs. The loss of amino acids and water-soluble vitamins in the dialysate constitutes another drain on the patient's nutritional stores.

The pharmacological agents that are most likely to be administered to assist with meeting the goal of promoting adequate nutritional intake are antacid and phosphate-binding agents, such as aluminum hydroxide gels; gastric acid inhibitors, such as H_2-receptor blockers; and occasionally antiemetics. In addition, topical anesthetic agents may be prescribed for application to the oral mucosa if stomatitis is present to decrease the pain produced by the contact of food substances with the ulcerated mucosa.

NURSING DIAGNOSIS: ALTERATIONS IN BOWEL ELIMINATION

Goal. The general goal associated with this nursing diagnosis is to promote adequate bowel elimination. The patient with acute renal failure may fluctuate between having episodes of diarrhea and periods of constipation, depending upon the presence of electrolyte imbalances, especially hyperkalemia. Because the interventions for treating hyperkalemia have been previously discussed, and the fact that the patient is more likely to experience constipation as he/she progresses through the phases of acute renal failure, this discussion will focus on constipation as the primary alteration in bowel elimination.

Outcome Criteria. The clinician would assess for the presence of the following outcome criteria in order to determine whether the goal of promoting adequate bowel elimination related to constipation was being met: a pattern of bowel evacuation that approximates the patient's normal or baseline pattern, or is consistent with the patient's pathophysiological state; the evacuation of stool that is similar to the patient's baseline in terms of color, odor, consistency, size, and composition, or is consistent with the pathophysiological state; an evacuation process that the patient verbalizes as being comfortable; bowel sounds that are normal in terms of pitch and frequency of occurrence upon auscultation; abdominal and rectal orifice characteristics that are consistent with the patient's baseline upon inspection and palpation; fluid and dietary intake

Table 11–11. THE COMPONENTS OF HYPERALIMENTATION FOR PATIENTS WITH ACUTE RENAL FAILURE

Substance	Contents	Remarks
500 ml of 70% dextrose in water	Dextrose 350 g	Provides about 1400 kcal of energy
500 ml of 10% essential and nonessential amino acids	Amino acids 50 g	Provides about 200 kcal of energy The combination of these two substances, totaling 1000 ml, is usually infused at a rate of 80 to 100 ml/hr
500 ml 20% lipid emulsion	Lipids 100 g	Provides about 1000 kcal of energy Usually infused at a rate of 20 ml/h
Vitamins	Thiamine 10 mg Riboflavin 3 mg Niacin 40 mg Pantothenic acid 15 mg Pyridoxine 4 mg Ascorbic acid 100 mg Folic acid 400 μg Biotin 60 μg Vitamin B_{12} 5 μg Vitamin A 3300 IU Vitamin D 200 IU Vitamin E 10 IU	Patients may require additional amounts of these substances, especially of pyridoxine and ascorbic acid
Trace elements	Zinc 5 mg Copper 1 mg Manganese 0.5 μg Chromium 10 μg Selenium 40 μg	Patients may require additional amounts of specific trace elements
Electrolytes	Sodium 40 mEq/L Potassium 20 mEq/L Magnesium 8 mEq/L Calcium 5 mEq/L	These substances are usually added as combinations such as sodium chloride, potassium chloride, magnesium sulfate, and calcium gluconate
Other additives	Regular insulin Ranitidine Heparin	These substances would be added based on individual patient needs

that is consistent with the prescribed restrictions; an activity level that is consistent with the patient's pathophysiological state; and patient verbalizations regarding the degree of abdominal and lower gastrointestinal tract comfort at any specific time.

Interventions. The monitoring functions associated with this goal include assessing the patient's bowel evacuation pattern at least daily; monitoring the characteristics of the feces daily, or after each evacuation; performing a guaiac or other test to monitor for occult blood in the feces daily, or after each evacuation; inspecting the abdomen at least every 4 hours; auscultating bowel sounds at least every 8 hours; inspecting the rectal orifice at least every other day; monitoring the patient's fluid and dietary intake at least every 4 hours; monitoring the patient's activity level at least every 8 hours; assessing the patient's comfort level in terms of the abdomen and gastrointestinal tract at least every 8 hours; monitoring the patient's serum laboratory values at least daily; and assessing all pharmacological agents that the patient is ingesting in terms of their active or interactive effects on the gastrointestinal tract.

The interventions that the clinician would implement to assist the patient in promoting adequate bowel elimination related to constipation include providing fluids and foods that are consistent with the prescribed restrictions; assisting the patient in maintaining an activity level that is consistent with the pathophysiological state; administering stool softeners, such as docusate sodium as prescribed; administering bulk-forming, gentle cathartics, such as psyllium hydrophilic mucilloid, as prescribed; and occasionally, administering glycerin suppositories or non-magnesium-based laxatives as prescribed. In addition, it is important to create the appropriate environment for the evacuation process. Whenever possible, the patient should perform the evacuation process in an environment that closely approximates the normal. Thus, the clinician assists the patient by helping the patient assume the normal sitting posture, preferably in a bathroom or on a bedside commode, and providing privacy and as relaxed an environment as possible.

NURSING DIAGNOSIS: IMPAIRED PHYSICAL MOBILITY

Goal. Promoting or increasing physical mobility is the primary goal associated with this nursing diagnosis. In addition, the clinician must accomplish this goal within the constraints of the patient's pathophysiological state because increasing the patient's basal metabolic rate may lead to further catabolism. Goals for increasing mobility must be accomplished while maintaining adequate safety.

Outcome Criteria. The outcome criteria that would demonstrate that this goal is being met include patient verbalizations, or personnel documentation, reflecting an increase in passive, active, and functional range-of-motion of all joints and extremities; increased muscle tone and strength in all extremities; increased patient participation in the activities of daily living; a stable patient gait when transferring and ambulating; full weight bearing on all extremities during various types of activities; vital sign changes that are consistent with the amount of activity engaged in and the patient's pathophysiological state; and patient verbalizations of comfort during activities involving physical mobility.

Interventions. The monitoring functions that would be implemented in relation to this goal include monitoring the patient's participation in the activities of daily living at least every 8 hours; assessing the patient's verbal statements and staff documentation regarding the patient's degree of passive, active, or functional range-of-motion of all joint and extremities at least every 8 hours; assessing the muscle tone and strength of all of the patient's extremities at least daily; monitoring the patient's weight-bearing ability and gait each time he/she transfers or ambulates; assessing the patient's vital signs and response to activity during each activity; assessing the patient's comfort level during each activity; and monitoring the patient's serum laboratory values at least daily.

The intervening functions that would assist in meeting this goal are performing, or assisting the patient in performing, passive or active range-of-motion exercises of all joints and extremities at least every 4 hours; assisting the patient in ambulating a distance that is appropriate for the pathophysiological state at least every 8 hours; having the patient perform the appropriate activities of daily living within the constraints of the pathophysiological state; providing for at least 30 minutes of patient rest prior to engaging in any physical mobility activities; consulting with the occupational therapist for assistive devices that would facilitate the patient's participation in the activities of daily living; consulting with the physical therapist for other exercises or assistive devices that would assist the patient in increasing his/her physical mobility; establishing a plan with the patient for a series of daily activities that will progressively increase until the patient achieves a physical mobility level that is consistent with his/her baseline or pathophysiological state; providing a nutritional intake that is consistent with the prescribed restrictions; administering pharmacological agents, such as phosphate binders, vitamin D_3, and calcium supplements, as prescribed; and preparing the patient for dialysis as prescribed.

NURSING DIAGNOSIS: POTENTIAL FOR INJURY

Goal. The goal related to this nursing diagnosis is to promote patient safety. The patient with acute renal failure experiences so many systemic alterations that he/she is particularly susceptible to injury from both internal and external environmental hazards.

Outcome Criteria. To determine if this goal is being met, the clinician should assess for the presence of the following criteria: the maintenance of an erect stable patient posture upon arising and during ambulation; a sensorium that is consistent with the patient's pathophysiological state but free of vertigo and syncope; an intact integument that is consistent with the patient's baseline and/or pathophysiological state; neurological and neuromuscular functioning that is consistent with the patient's baseline and/or pathophysiological state; cognitive clarity that is consistent with the patient's baseline and pathophysiological state; arterial blood gas values that are consistent with the patient's baseline; and serum electrolyte levels that are consistent with the patient's baseline.

Interventions. The monitoring functions related to this goal include assessing the patient's posture and gait upon each arising and ambulation; assessing the patient's sensorium, cognitive clarity, neurological functioning, and neuromuscular functioning at least every 2 hours; assessing the patient's integumentary system, particularly for intactness, at least every 8 hours; assessing for Chvostek's and Trousseau's signs at least daily; monitoring the arterial blood gas values daily, or as available; and monitoring the serum electrolyte values at least daily.

The intervening functions aimed at assisting the patient in meeting this goal include structuring the patient's environment in order to minimize the hazards presented by the placement of furniture or personal items; orienting the patient to the surrounding environment at least daily and whenever items are moved or altered; assisting the patient in selecting the appropriate footwear for moving about the environment; maintaining an environment with sufficient stimuli to maintain orientation but not to excessively excite the patient; instituting seizure precautions by maintaining the bed in a low position, padding the side rails, maintaining the side rails in the up position while the patient is in bed, and including any other components of the institutional seizure precaution policy, such as an airway, a suction set up, or wall oxygen; maintaining all fluid and dietary restrictions as prescribed; administering pharmacological agents as prescribed; and preparing the patient for dialysis as prescribed.

The clinician should be alert to the need for additional safety precautions if the patient develops seizures due to the metabolic imbalances. The primary point to remember in such cases is that seizures are a warning sign and the clinician's primary role during their occurrence is one of observation. It is important to note where the seizure began and how it progressed, as well as its characteristics and duration. The patient's response during the episode should also be documented. Clearly, patient safety is an issue during the seizure, but the clinician should refrain from any type of physical restraint of the patient because this can often be deleterious to the patient. It is also important to remember that the patient who has experienced a seizure usually has difficulty handling secretions during the postseizure period, so the clinician needs to be prepared to assist the patient in order to prevent aspiration.

NURSING DIAGNOSIS: SENSORY-PERCEPTION ALTERATIONS

Goal. The goal associated with this nursing diagnosis is to decrease anxiety. Because of the pathophysiological alterations produced by acute renal failure, the patient tends to perceive stimuli differently than he/she did previously. Things may seem to assume a sense of exaggerated importance or personal threat. This perception is further exacerbated by sleep pattern disturbances, altered thought processes, and the fact that many of the therapeutic interventions implemented with these patients are invasive in nature.

Outcome Criteria. The outcome criteria that the clinician uses to assess whether this goal is being met include a relaxed facial expression and body posture; appropriate eye contact during interactions; coherent, logical, appropriately paced communication patterns; affect, mannerisms, and gestures that are consistent with the patient's baseline and/or pathophysiological state and appropriate for the interaction; levels of concentration and participation that are consistent with the patient's pathophysiological state; a level of participation in the activities of daily living that is consistent with the patient's pathophysiological state; an appetite and nutritional ingestion pattern that is consistent with the patient's pathophysiological state; rest patterns that are consistent with the patient's pathophysiological state; attention to personal hygiene that is consistent with the patient's pathophysiological state; purposeful motor activity; vital signs, autonomic responses, and serum laboratory values that are consistent with the patient's pathophysiological state; and the patient verbalizations.

Interventions. The monitoring functions related to this goal include assessing the patient's affect, facial expression, body posture, personal hygiene, eye contact, communication pattern, mannerisms, purposeful motor activity, gestures, concentration, level of participation, and verbalizations during each interaction; assessing the patient's level of participation in the activities of daily living at least daily; monitoring the patient's appetite and nutritional ingestion patterns at least daily; monitoring the patient's rest patterns at least daily; assessing the patient's vital signs and autonomic responses at least every 4 hours; and monitoring the patient's laboratory values at least daily.

The intervening functions include structuring the environment to decrease excessive stimuli, but including items that have personal meaning to the patient; briefly explaining to the patient everything that is done with him/her; spending 10-minute periods of time with the patient talking, listening, or in silence at least four times a day; providing emotional support, comfort, and reassurance; verbally and nonverbally encouraging the patient to express his/her feelings; supporting the patient's current coping mechanisms, but if they are maladaptive, assisting the patient in identifying more constructive behaviors; inviting the patient's family or clergyman to visit, as appropriate for the situation; selecting other patients for the patient to talk with, as appropriate for the situation; assisting the patient in identifying the sources of the anxiety whenever possible; and preparing the patient for dialysis as prescribed.

NURSING DIAGNOSIS: ALTERATIONS IN THOUGHT PROCESSES

Goal. Promoting effective communication is the goal associated with this nursing diagnosis. The pathophysiological alterations that accompany acute renal failure produce alterations in the patient's perception, cognition, attention span, and mental processes, such as information processing, reality orientation, problem solving, judgment, and comprehension.

Outcome Criteria. To determine whether this goal is being met, the clinician would assess for the presence of the following outcome criteria: verbal demonstration of the patient's orientation to person, place, and time; appropriate eye contact during interactions; clear, coherent, logical, appropriately paced communication patterns; affect, mannerisms, and gestures that are consistent with the patient's baseline and/or pathophysiological state and appropriate for the interaction; levels of concentration and participation that are consistent with the patient's pathophysiological state; the patient's verbal responses or questions that are indicative of an understanding of the content of the interaction; the patient's participation in activities that directly relate to the content of the interaction; and serum laboratory values that are consistent with the patient's pathophysiological state.

Interventions. The monitoring functions related to this goal include assessing the patient's level of orientation at least every 4 hours; assessing the patient's eye contact, communication patterns, gestures, mannerisms, level of concentration, and degree of participation during each interaction; assessing the patient's verbal responses and questions during each interaction; monitoring the patient's activities after each interaction; and monitoring the patient's serum laboratory values at least daily.

The intervening functions that are likely to help in meeting this goal include establishing a therapeutic rapport with the patient; structuring the interactions so that they are brief and focused; using various types of repetition to reinforce key points during the interaction; assisting the patient in differentiating the various types of stimuli that are encountered during the interaction; and preparing the patient for dialysis as prescribed.

NURSING DIAGNOSIS: POTENTIAL FOR IMPAIRED SKIN INTEGRITY

The integument is normally an excretory organ for specific secretions and some waste products. The skin of a patient with acute renal failure functions in the same way, only more so. In acute renal failure, the skin functions as a compensatory mechanism for excreting pigments and some substances that would normally be excreted in the urine. Thus, there is a primary potential that the integrity of the skin could be disrupted owing to scratching or other mechanisms that the patient uses to cope with the skin manifestations of acute renal failure.

Goal. The goal associated with this nursing diagnosis is to assist the patient in maintaining an intact integument.

Outcome Criteria. The outcome criteria that the clinician uses to determine whether this goal is being met include the presence of an intact integument that has the color, odor, texture, turgor, temperature, elasticity, and degree of moistness that is consistent with the patient's pathophysiological state; and the patient's verbalizations regarding the status of the integument.

Interventions. The primary monitoring functions related to this goal include assessing the patient's skin at least daily and monitoring the patient's fluid and nutritional intake at least daily.

The intervening functions include assisting the patient in bathing at least daily using a nonirritating, nondrying, non–lanolin-based substance, such as an oil- or oatmeal-based bath substance, or sodium bicarbonate bath water; applying non–lanolin-, light oil–based lubricating lotions at least every 4 hours to decrease the pruritus; trimming the patient's nails at least weekly to prevent abrasions or infection due to scratching; providing additional perineal care twice a day using a mild cleansing agent and water; implementing an hourly turning or movement schedule with the patient; performing active, or assisting the patient in performing passive, range-of-motion activities at least every 4 hours; implementing adjunct therapies such as a foam or another special type of mattress, protective padding, sheepskin pads, and massage to assist in decreasing pressure and friction at various points on the integument; handling and manipulating all edematous tissues gently and carefully; administering pharmacological agents as prescribed to assist in controlling the pruritus; providing fluids and nutritional substances that are consistent with the prescribed restrictions; and preparing the patient for dialysis as prescribed.

When the clinician is planning hygienic care for the patient with acute renal failure, there often is a tendency to strive to protect the already dry integument by scheduling bathing on an every other day or every 2 days regimen. Such an approach might assist in preventing additional skin drying, but it could alter the skin's compensatory ability to function as an organ of excretion. In order to facilitate the compensatory process, the patient needs clean skin and unclogged pores. Thus, a daily bathing schedule, or even more frequently for some patients, would be more appropriate.

NURSING DIAGNOSIS: ALTERATIONS IN ORAL MUCOUS MEMBRANES

The oral mucous membranes of the patient with acute renal failure often present a significant care challenge for the clinician. Not only does the patient experience uremic halitosis and stomatic ulcerations, but an altered taste sensation, dryness, crusting, occasional bleeding, and a whitish coating are also often present.

Goal. The goal related to this nursing diagnosis is to promote the healing of the oral mucous membranes in order to restore the integrity of the oral cavity.

Outcome Criteria. The clinician uses the following outcome criteria to determine whether this goal is being met: the color, odor, intactness, turgor, texture, presence of exudate, and degree of moistness of the oral mucous membranes; the patient's verbalizations regarding the degree of comfort related to the oral cavity; the patient's verbalizations regarding the effect of varying temperatures of fluids and food substances on the oral mucous membranes; the patient's verbalizations regarding the taste of various fluids and food substances; the amount and nutritional content of the fluids and food substances that the patient ingests daily; a pattern of daily weights that is consistent with the patient's baseline and pathophysiological state; and serum laboratory values that are consistent with the patient's baseline and pathophysiological state.

Interventions. The monitoring functions related to this goal include assessing the oral cavity and mucous membranes at least every 4 hours; assessing the patient's comfort level related to the oral mucous membranes at least every 4 hours; monitoring the patient's fluid and nutritional substance intake at least daily; monitoring the patient's weight at least daily; and monitoring the patient's serum laboratory values at least daily.

The intervening functions include assisting the patient in performing oral hygiene at least every 2 hours and prior to meals and at bedtime, using either a soft-bristled toothbrush or foam swab, a mild toothpaste, or a mixture of hydrogen peroxide diluted with two parts water and one part flavored mouthwash, floss, as appropriate, and a water-based lubricant for the lips; assisting the patient in rinsing the oral cavity at least hourly using a lemon or other flavored solution to mechanically cleanse and hydrate the tissues; administering pharmacological agents, such as antibiotic solutions or topical or anesthetic agents as prescribed; providing fluids and food substances at a temperature that is consistent with the patient's tolerance; and preparing the patient for dialysis as prescribed.

In providing, or assisting the patient with, oral hygiene, the clinician would not use lemon glycerin swabs because of their tendency to dehydrate the oral mucosa. In addition, the clinician assists the patient in rinsing the oral cavity thoroughly after using any cleansing solution containing hydrogen peroxide. If residual amounts of this oxidizing agent remain in the oral cavity, it can predispose the patient to developing an oral yeast infection.

NURSING DIAGNOSIS: KNOWLEDGE DEFICIT

The primary knowledge deficit that the patient with acute renal failure has is one of not comprehending all of the components and impacts of the disease process. The patient needs at least a rudimentary understanding of the following in order to be an informed participant in the health care that is delivered: the progression and prognosis of the disease state; the short- and long-term pathophysiological effects of the renal dysfunction; the impact of the dysfunction on the patient's daily pattern of functioning; the rationale for, and importance of, the daily invasive monitoring techniques; the rationale for the various fluid and dietary restrictions; the rationales underlying the use of the various pharmacological agents that are prescribed; the purpose, underlying principles, impact, frequency, and rationale for the prescribed dialysis therapy; and the patient's specific role in all of the various facets of the health care regimen. Certainly the clinician addresses these issues with the patient as they are appropriate and consistent with the patient's pathophysiological state. In addition, the clinician would utilize all of the appropriate teaching-learning principles when providing the patient with the appropriate information.

Goal. The goal related to this nursing diagnosis is to provide the patient with sufficient, accurate information to enable the patient to be an informed participant in the health care delivery regimen.

Outcome Criteria. The clinician uses the following outcome criteria to determine if this goal is being met: the patient's verbalizations and questions regarding the disease process and the health care regimen; and the patient's degree of cooperation with and participation in the health care regimen.

Interventions. The monitoring functions related to this nursing diagnosis include assessing the content of the patient's verbalizations and questions at least daily; and monitoring the degree of the patient's cooperation and participation in the health care regimen.

The intervening functions include providing the specific, factual information regarding the pathophysiological disease process, its impact on the patient, its progression and prognosis, and its prescribed therapeutic regimen of care; reinforcing verbally, or in writing, the information that is provided, either as appropriate or at least daily; including the family in the educational process so that they are also aware of the facts and can reinforce the information with the patient; and, if appropriate, arranging for a former patient who has experienced acute renal failure to talk with the patient.

As the clinician presents information to the patient, it is important to remember that the uremic state alters the reception, perception, interpretation, and retention of information. Thus, repetition and reinforcement are key components in the entire educational process. In addition, the patient's shortened attention span may require that the clinician divide the information into short 10- to 15-minute segments for presentation. Certainly the individualization of the educational process is mandatory when trying to meet this goal with the patient who has acute renal failure.

Medical Interventions

The medical interventions for the patient with acute renal failure are based on the general management goals that were previously discussed. The overall medical management plan involves a three "D's" approach to deal with the patient's renal dysfunction. This approach involves the three components of dietary management, diuretics, and dialysis. Each of these components is usually instituted early in the course of the disease process and the physician should be relatively aggressive in prescribing for their use.

DIETARY MANAGEMENT

Dietary management in patients with acute renal failure continues to be a major component of the therapeutic regimen. The overall goals of dietary management for these patients are to (1) minimize uremic toxicity; (2) minimize metabolic, fluid, and electrolyte imbalances; and (3) maintain adequate nutritional and anabolic states. The nutritional recommendations that have been established to assist in meeting these goals include a caloric intake of 35 to 50 kcal/kg of ideal body weight (IBW) per day; a protein intake of 0.5 to 1.5 g/kg of IBW per day, 75 to 80% of which is of high biological value and contains all of the required essential amino acids; a sodium intake of 0.5 to 1.0 g/day; a potassium intake of 20 to 50 mEq/day; a calcium intake of 800 to 1200 mg/day; and a fluid intake equal to the volume of the patient's urine output plus an additional 600 to 1000 ml/day. In addition, the physician would also prescribe multivitamins, folic acid, and occasionally an iron supplement to replace the water-soluble vitamins and other essential elements lost during dialysis.

If the patient is unable to ingest or tolerate an oral nutritional intake that is sufficiently adequate for sustenance, then hyperalimentation would be prescribed. Aggressive hyperalimentation therapy, similar to that which is detailed in Table 11–11 will supply the patient with sufficient nonprotein glucose calories, specific essential amino acids, fluids, specific electrolytes, and essential vitamins to create a more stable internal environment. Such an internal environment will not only prevent further catabolism, negative nitrogen balance, muscle wasting, and other uremic complications, but it will also enhance the patient's tubular regenerating capacity, resistance to infection, and ability to combat other multisystem dysfunctions. Of course, in order to facilitate the aggressive use of hyperalimentation, the physician must also prescribe aggressive, early dialysis therapy.

DIURETIC THERAPY

The use of diuretic therapy, especially the osmotic and loop diuretics, in managing patients with acute renal failure remains a controversial issue. The controversy is focused on the benefit to detriment ratio for the patient. It appears that both osmotic and loop diuretics may be effective in decreasing the insult to the kidney *if* they are administered promptly at the onset or within 4 to 8 hours of the onset of the oliguria. The hypothesis is that the diuretics will increase renal blood flow, glomerular filtration rate and intratubular pressure while decreasing tubular obstruction and dysfunction. The problem with using diuretics is that they may indeed only increase urine flow, without affecting glomerular filtration rate or tubular function, and thus would further compromise an already insulted renal system.

If diuretic therapy is implemented with a patient with acute renal failure, the physician would select either an osmotic agent or a loop-acting diuretic. This is because none of the other five categories of diuretic agents, including the mercurials, thiazides, carbonic anhydrase inhibitors, potassium sparers, and saluretics, will increase glomerular filtration rate and renal blood flow. In addition, only the loop-acting agents and the saluretics are effective for patients with renal dysfunction who have glomerular filtration rates of less than 20 ml/minute. Thus, most types of diuretic agents are ineffective for managing patients with acute renal failure.

DIALYSIS THERAPY

Dialysis therapy is the ultimate in supportive therapeutic measures for the patient with acute renal failure. Without some form of this mechanical substitute for renal function, the patient would not be able to sustain life during the dysfunctional episode. Thus, dialysis therapy is usually initiated early in the course of the renal failure in order to maintain the patient's serum creatinine below 10 mg/100 ml and the BUN below 100 mg%. Maintaining values below these levels creates an internal biochemical environment that facilitates the prevention of infection and the complications of uremia. Instituting dialysis early also increases the scope of other therapeutic interventions that can be implemented with the patient, including hyperalimentation.

The concept of dialysis therapy can be explored by first delineating its basic components. Following that delineation, the methods for vascular access and the two primary types of renal replacement therapy that are usually implemented with patients with acute renal failure, specifically hemodialysis and continuous arteriovenous hemofiltration (CAVH), will be detailed. In addition, intermittent peritoneal dialysis, which may also be used in some clinical settings, will also be discussed. The basic components of dialysis therapy include a definition, the purposes, the clinical indications, and the principles and mechanisms involved.

Definition

Dialysis is defined as the separation of solutes by differential diffusion through a porous membrane that is placed between two solutions. This general definition permits the clinician to distinguish among the various types of dialyses merely by identifying the porous membrane and describing the two solutions that are involved.

Purposes

The purposes of dialysis therapy are directly related to the functions of the renal system that it attempts to imitate. Those purposes are to (1) eliminate excess body fluids; (2) maintain or restore the electrolyte and acid-base balance of the circulating plasma; and (3) eliminate waste products and dialyzable toxins from the blood. Obviously, the kidneys perform several other functions that dialysis cannot imitate, such as secreting erythropoietin, activating the renin-angiotensin system, and converting vitamin D to its active metabolite vitamin D_3. Therefore, dialysis cannot ever totally replace the physiological functions of the renal system, but it can act as a sufficient substitute to sustain life during a crisis.

Clinical Indications

There are five broad categories of clinical conditions for which dialysis would be indicated: (1) acute and chronic renal failure; (2) severe water retention; (3) severe electrolyte disorders; (4) drug intoxication, assuming that the drug is dialyzable; and (5) in some instances, hepatic coma. Of these five categories, the first one, acute and chronic renal failure, is the most frequently encountered indication for dialysis therapy.

Principles and Mechanisms Involved

Dialysis therapy is based on the three physical principles that are related to the movement and transport of fluid and electrolytes within the body: osmosis, diffusion, and filtration. *Osmosis* is the movement of fluid, or water molecules, across a semipermeable membrane from an area of lesser solute concentration to an area of greater solute concentration. This movement continues until the concentrations of solute are equal on both sides of the membrane. *Diffusion* is the movement of solute molecules across a semipermeable membrane from an area of greater solute concentration to an area of lesser solute concentration. Diffusion continues until equilibrium is established across the membrane. *Filtration* is the movement of fluid across a semipermeable membrane from an area of greater pressure to an area of lesser pressure.

These three principles are influenced by many factors that determine the extent of their activity. Among those factors are the size of the pores of the semipermeable membrane, the size of the solute molecules, the osmotic concentrations and pressure gradients that are established, the temperature of the solution, and the rate of blood flow in the body. The size of the pores of the membrane and the size of the solute molecules determine which substances can participate in the transport processes. The gradients that are present determine the extent to which the various transport processes can occur. The gradients are sustained by the high rate of blood flow in the body. As the blood flows through the body, it continuously replaces the dialyzed blood with undialyzed blood. The undialyzed blood has very high concentrations of solutes, thus maintaining the established gradients. The temperature of the solution influences the velocity of the molecular movement, and thus affects the rate of the transport processes. An increase in the temperature of a solution will increase the rate of the transport processes that occur within the solution.

In addition to these principles, there are two other mechanisms that are used to support patients with acute renal failure. Those mechanisms are hemofiltration and ultrafiltration. *Hemofiltration* is a convective mode of blood cleansing wherein large fluid exchanges account for virtually all solute removal. As a convective mode it is not dependent on concentration or particle size. It may actually mimic the function of the kidney more closely than hemodialysis does, but it is much less efficient in removing small molecules. *Ultrafiltration* is the removal of plasma water and some small molecular weight particles using a pressure or osmotic gradient. Ultrafiltration is primarily aimed at controlling fluid volume, whereas dialysis and hemofiltration are designed to decrease waste products and fluid and electrolyte imbalances.

Vascular Access

An essential component for all of the renal replacement therapies that are used with patient's with acute renal failure is an adequate, easy access to the patient's blood stream. Without adequate access to the patient's blood stream, none of the renal replacement support therapies can be implemented. In addition, unless the access results in high rates of blood flow, such therapies will not be very effective. There are basically three mechanisms that are used to obtain access to the patient's vascular system for renal replacement therapy: temporary venous catheters, arteriovenous shunts, and arteriovenous fistulas. The temporary catheters and arteriovenous shunts are usually used with patients with acute renal failure because they can be used immediately and are less permanent than the arteriovenous fistulas.

Temporary Venous Catheters. Temporary venous catheters are usually inserted into either the subclavian, jugular, or femoral vein. The typical temporary access device has either a single or double lumen and is designed to be used only for short-term renal replacement therapy during acute or crisis situations. Examples of such devices are the Hickman, and Sheldon catheters.

Arteriovenous Shunt. An arteriovenous shunt consists of a surgically implanted extracorporeal apparatus that is used to connect an artery and a vein. Once the apparatus is in place, it can easily be opened, or in some cases, punctured to provide access to the blood stream. There are several types of shunts currently being used, but the most popular seems to be the Quinton-Scribner shunt, which is made of Silastic and Teflon and consists of two lengths of tubing joined by a connector. Each length of tubing has three portions, the first portion is implanted in the vessel and lies beneath the skin. The second portion is a steplike gradation that emerges from the plane of the vessel upward to exit onto the skin through a puncture wound. The third portion is external and lies flush with the skin. Access to the vascular system is obtained by removing the connector and attaching dialysis tubing directly to the arterial and venous lines of the shunt.

Arteriovenous Fistulas. An arteriovenous fistula is an internally, surgically created communication between an artery and a vein. The type of fistula most frequently created is the Brescia-Cimino fistula, which involves anastomosing the radial artery and cephalic vein in a side-to-side or end-to-side manner. The anastomosis permits blood to bypass the capillaries and flow directly from the artery into the vein. As a result, the vein is forced to dilate in order to accommodate the increased pressure that accompanies the arterial blood. This produces a vein that is much easier to cannulate for the renal replacement therapies. Table 11-12 summarizes the major advantages and disadvantages of the various vascular access devices.

Arteriovenous fistulas can also be created by using a variety of different types of grafts. The types of grafts most frequently used include the autogenous, or saphenous, vein graft; the human umbilical vein; the bovine carotid graft; the polytetrafluroethylene (PTFE), or Gor-Tex or Impra grafts; and the PTFE graft with a transcutaneous implant.

The clinician is always protective of the vascular access site and monitors it at least hourly. In addition, the clinician never uses an extremity that has an arteriovenous shunt or fistula in place for drawing blood specimens or obtaining blood pressure measurements. Such activities could produce pressure changes within the altered vessels that could result in either clotting or rupture. In either case, the loss of the vascular access site would be imminent.

Hemodialysis

This renal replacement therapy is the most frequently used in managing patients with acute renal failure. It can best be explored by examining the following aspects: a definition, clinical indications, the advantages, the disadvantages, the potential complications, and the contraindications.

Definition. Hemodialysis is the separation of solutes by differential diffusion through a celluloid membrane positioned between the patient's blood and the dialysate solution. An additional

Table 11-12. THE ADVANTAGES AND DISADVANTAGES OF VASCULAR ACCESS DEVICES

Type of Access	Advantages	Disadvantages
Temporary Access Devices	Easy insertion Available for immediate use No venipunctures are required for access Provides for easy access to the blood stream High flow rates are achieved Site can be reused at a later date	Insertion can be traumatic Located externally Creates alterations in body image Can be easily dislodged, resulting in hemorrhage Prone to infections and thrombosis Catheter may erode through the vessel or skin Requires very frequent monitoring and daily cleansing and care
Shunt	Can be placed in almost any vessel Availabe for immediate use No venipunctures are required for access Provides for easy access to the blood stream	Located externally Creates alterations in body image Can be easily dislodged, resulting in hemorrhage Prone to infections and thrombosis Restricts movement of the extremity Apparatus parts may erode through the skin Requires very frequent monitoring and daily cleaning and care
Fistula	Located internally Has increased longevity over other access methods Involves few complications Few limitations to movement Requires minimal monitoring and care	Needs 4-6 weeks to mature prior to being used Requires venipunctures for access May result in decreased circulation in the extremity May become occluded due to clotting Requires that constrictive clothing not be worn over the site

dimension of hemodialysis is that it is extracorporeal; meaning that it occurs in a receptacle that is located outside of the patient's body.

Clinical Indications. The clinical indications for hemodialysis are identical to those that were previously identified in conjunction with the discussion of the general concept of dialysis. Certainly acute and chronic renal failure continue to be the primary indications for hemodialysis.

Advantages. The two major advantages of hemodialysis are that (1) it requires only 4 to 6 hours per session, and (2) it is very efficient and corrects biochemical disturbances quickly.

Disadvantages. The disadvantages of hemodialysis include the following: (1) special staff education and training are required to implement the therapy; (2) acute fluid and electrolyte imbalances can occur rapidly; (3) a patient could easily hemorrhage or exsanguinate during the therapy; (4) there is a risk of contracting hepatitis as a result of the therapy; (5) the equipment is expensive; and (6) machine availability may be a problem at any specific time.

Potential Complications. The potential complications associated with hemodialysis therapy include (1) shunt, catheter, or fistula sepsis; (2) shunt, catheter, or fistula clotting; (3) hemorrhage; (4) hypovolemia; (5) acute electrolyte imbalances; (6) air emboli; and (7) disequilibrium syndrome. Disequilibrium syndrome is most likely to occur after the first, second, or third dialysis treatment, or in instances when there have been large decreases in BUN and creatinine levels in a short time frame as a result of dialysis. When BUN and creatinine levels are rapidly decreased during dialysis, the body makes compensatory adjustments. Because of the blood-brain barrier, dialysis will not deplete the concentrations of BUN, creatinine, and other uremic toxins in the brain as rapidly as it does those substances in the extracellular fluid. As a result, there is an osmotic concentration gradient established in the brain that allows fluid to enter until the concentration levels equal that of the extracellular fluid. The influx of extra fluid into the brain tissue to establish equilibrium creates a state of cerebral edema for the patient, resulting in severe headaches and occasionally seizures. Dialyzing the patient more frequently, but for shorter periods of time, to decrease the concentration differences more slowly usually decreases the incidence of disequilibrium syndrome.

Contraindications. The most frequently cited contraindications for hemodialysis therapy are hemodynamic instability, insufficient blood volume, or hypovolemia; an inadequate vascular access site; and the unavailability of the appropriate equipment. However, some physicians and dialysis centers contend that there are no contraindications to using hemodialysis therapy. The current trends appears to be one of using hemodialysis unless the patient's hemodynamic status is so compromised that flow rates would be insufficient for the therapy to be successful. In many intensive care units, however, the renal replacement therapy selected might temporarily be hemofiltration rather than hemodialysis. Hemodialysis would then be instituted when the patient had achieved a more stable state.

Hemofiltration

The process of hemofiltration can be examined using the same aspects that were discussed in relation to hemodialysis. Those aspects are a definition, the clinical indications, the advantages, the disadvantages, the potential complications, and the contraindications.

Definition. Hemofiltration is a convective mode of blood cleansing that is controlled by the patient's hydrostatic pressure. The process requires the infusion of large volumes of fluid in order to remove solutes.

Clinical Indications. The clinical indications for continuous arteriovenous hemofiltration (CAVH) include acute and chronic renal failure, persistent hypervolemia, cardiac failure, hepatic failure, cirrhosis, septicemia, septic shock, electrolyte imbalances, cerebral edema, adult respiratory distress syndrome (ARDS), acid-base imbalances, and to facilitate aggressive hyperalimentation therapy.

Advantages. The advantages of CAVH are that (1) it removes solutes gradually; (2) there is decreased risk of hemodynamic instability; (3) it provides increased flexibility in fluid administration plans; (4) it requires only minimal heparinization; (5) it can be used to maintain a metabolically stable state; (6) it is relatively inexpensive; (7) minimal staff education is required to implement the therapy; and (8) it seems to be ideal for physiologically unstable patients.

Disadvantages. The disadvantages of CAVH are that (1) it is not very efficient; (2) the patient must remain in bed during the entire therapy; (3) it requires at least mild anticoagulation; (4) and some type of vascular access site is necessary.

Potential Complications. There are numerous potential complications associated with CAVH.

Among those complications are (1) depletion syndrome, which results in the loss of vitamins, amino acids, and other substances; (2) acid-base imbalances; (3) fluid and electrolyte imbalances; (4) hemorrhage due to anticoagulation or disruption of the filter or tubing; (5) infection; (6) rupture or leakage of the filter; (7) clotting in the filter; and (8) loss of the vascular access site.

Contraindications. CAVH is contraindicated in patients with a systolic blood pressure lower than 60 mmHg, a hematocrit greater than 45%, or the inability to tolerate high volumes of fluid exchange. In addition, the patient must have an adequate vascular access site available.

Intermittent Peritoneal Dialysis

This renal replacement therapy is not as frequently employed for managing individuals with acute renal failure because of its comparatively slow ability to alter the biochemical imbalances. The process can be compared to the other renal replacement therapies by examining it according to the same parameters of a definition; the clinical indications; the advantages; the disadvantages; the potential complications; and the contraindications.

Definition. Peritoneal dialysis is the separation of solutes by differential diffusion through the peritoneal membrane that is positioned between an individual's blood and the dialysate solution that has been instilled into the peritoneal cavity. It is classified as intermittent when it is performed for a specified period of time, such as 36 hours, rather than as a continuous process.

Clinical Indications. The clinical indications for intermittent peritoneal dialysis include acute renal failure, severe water intoxication, electrolyte disorders, and drug intoxication resulting from overingestion of a peritoneally dialyzable drug.

Advantages. The advantages of intermittent peritoneal dialysis are that (1) the equipment is easily and rapidly assembled; (2) the equipment is relatively inexpensive; (3) minimal physical preparation of the individual is required; (4) there is minimal danger of acute electrolyte imbalances or hemorrhage occurring; (5) the dialysate can easily be individualized; and (6) the process can be implemented in either general care or specialty care areas.

Disadvantages. Intermittent peritoneal dialysis has several concomitant disadvantages, including the following: (1) the procedure is time intensive, usually requiring at least 36 hours for therapeutic effect; (2) biochemical disturbances are corrected slowly; (3) the individual will lose about 30 g of protein per a 36-hour dialysis session; (4) it may be difficult to gain or maintain access to the peritoneal cavity; and (5) there is always a risk that the complications that are delineated in the next section could occur.

Potential Complications. There are many complications that can result from the therapeutic use of intermittent peritoneal dialysis. Fortunately, most complications occur infrequently. The complications can be divided into three categories of etiologies: mechanical problems, metabolic difficulties, and inflammatory reactions.

The potential complications resulting from mechanical problems include the following: (1) perforation of abdominal viscera during insertion of the catheter; (2) hemorrhage from the catheter insertion; (3) preperitoneal placement of the catheter; (4) improper drainage due to blockage of the catheter; (5) leakage of fluid around the catheter; (6) pain during the catheter insertion; (7) discomfort due to the pressure of the fluid within the peritoneal cavity; and (8) pulmonary complications due to the pressure of the fluid in the peritoneal cavity.

Some of the potential complications that may result from metabolic difficulties are as follows: (1) hypovolemia due to too rapid removal of fluid; (2) hypervolemia due to impaired drainage of fluid; (3) hypernatremia due to too rapid removal of fluid; (4) hypokalemia due to using potassium-free dialysate; (5) alkalosis from using an alkaline dialysate; (6) disequilibrium syndrome due to too rapid removal of fluid and waste products; and (7) hyperglycemia due to the high glucose concentration of the dialysate.

The two potential complications that may result from inflammatory reactions are (1) peritoneal irritation produced by the catheter, and (2) peritonitis due to bacterial infection, which is the most common complication encountered in peritoneal dialysis therapy. The incidence of peritonitis appears to be related to the duration of the dialysis session. Some clinicians have found that peritonitis seems to occur more frequently when a session is prolonged beyond 36 hours.

Contraindications. There appear to be conflicting opinions as to what conditions might contraindicate the use of intermittent peritoneal dialysis therapy. The more liberal approach asserts that nothing contraindicates using peritoneal dialysis and that any obstacle can be overcome. The conservative approach contends that there are many conditions that would preclude using peritoneal dialysis because of the added risk to the patient's well-being. In response to this conflict, most physicians seem to accept a moderate approach concerning contraindications and tend to function somewhere between the two extremes. The moderate approach suggests that the following conditions at least be considered as contraindications to implementing peritoneal dialysis: (1) acute active peritonitis, (2) recent abdominal surgery, (3) known peritoneal adhesions, (4) severe abdominal trauma or burns, (5) a massive intraperitoneal hematoma; and (6) any major abdominally located vascular anastomosis.

Any or all of these therapies are likely to be prescribed by physicians as they attempt to select the best intervention plan for assisting the patient with acute renal failure in coping with the systemic alterations created by the disease state. The frequency and types of alternatives selected are, of course, based on each individual patient's response.

Preventative Measures

Considering the detrimental impact of acute renal failure on the critically ill patient's struggle for survival, it seems appropriate to briefly discuss how this devastating dysfunction might be prevented. The primary measures used to prevent acute renal failure are to: (1) maintain an adequate hydration state for the patient, especially preoperatively and prior to excretion urography studies; (2) maintain renal perfusion by administering as prescribed the following:

a. Vasoactive agents that are noted to increase renal blood flow, such as acetylcholine, low doses of dopamine, isoproterenol, kinins, prostaglandins, and calcium antagonists,

b. Volume expanders such as saline and mannitol,

c. Loop-acting diuretics

(3) continuously monitor the duration, dosage, and combinations of antibiotics administered to the patient; and (4) maintain an ongoing assessment of the patient's renal function.

Exploring the preventative measures that can be used to deter the onset of acute renal failure in critically ill patients seems like a perfect way to conclude this discussion. If such measures are aggressively pursued by the clinician, the patient may never have to experience the overwhelming impact of an insulted renal system. Unfortunately, all too frequently, such measures are overlooked or deferred as priorities within the context of the daily hustle and bustle of the intensive care unit. The result is that the patient then becomes much more vulnerable to the many physiological, pathophysiological, pharmacological, diagnostic, and therapeutic factors that could have a detrimental effect on the renal system. When that vulnerability is exploited and the patient experiences acute renal failure, the complexity of the patient care management increases. The clinician's skills, knowledge base, and other resources are taxed and the challenge begins! Hopefully the information presented in this discussion will assist the clinician in successfully meeting this patient care challenge.

Recommended Reading

Baer, C. L. (1990): Acute renal failure. *Nursing '90* 20(6):34–39.

Bergstrom, J. (1989): Toxicity of uremia: physiopathology and clinical signs. *Contributions to Nephrology* 71:1–9.

Brenner, B. M., Coe, F. L., and Rector, F. C. (1987): *Clinical Nephrology*. Philadelphia: W. B. Saunders.

Bremmer, B. M., and Lazarus, J. M. (1983): *Acute Renal Failure*. Philadelphia: W. B. Saunders.

Butt, K. M. H. (1983): Angioaccess. In: W. Drukker, F. M. Parsons, and J. F. Maher (eds.). *Replacement of Renal Function by Dialysis*. Boston: Martinus Nijhoff, pp. 171–185.

Collins, A. J., Keshaviah, P., Ilstrup, K. M., and Shapiro, F. (1985): Clinical comparison of hemodialysis and hemofiltration. *Kidney International* 28(Suppl. 17):S18–S22.

Drukker, W., Parsons, F. M., and Maher, J. F. (1983): *Replacement of Renal Function by Dialysis*. 2nd ed. Boston: Martinus Nijhoff.

Eknoyan, G., and Knochel, J. P. (1984): *The Systemic Consequences of Renal Failure*. Orlando, Florida: Grune & Stratton.

Finn, W. F. (1990): Diagnosis and management of acute tubular necrosis. *Medical Clinics of North America* 74(4):873–891.

Goldstein, M. S. (1983): Acute renal failure. *Medical Clinics of North America* 67(6):1325–1341.

Golper, T. A. (1985): Continuous arteriovenous hemofiltration in acute renal failure. *American Journal of Kidney Diseases* 6(6):373–386.

Harper, J. (1990): Rhabdomyolysis and myoglobinuric renal failure. *Critical Care Nurse* 10(3):32–34, 36.

Irwin, B. C. (1979): Hemodialysis means vascular access and the right kind of nursing care. *Nursing 79* 9(10):48–53.

Kramer, P. (1985): *Arteriovenous Hemofiltration*. Berlin: Springer-Verlag.

Lancaster, L. E. (1985): *The Patient with End Stage Renal Disease*. 2nd ed. New York: John Wiley & Sons.

Lancaster, L. E., and Baer, C. L. (1985): The pathophysiology of acute renal dysfunction. In: L. Schoengrund and P. Balzer (eds.). *Renal Problems in Critical Care*. New York: John Wiley & Sons, pp. 21–46.

Lawyer, L. A., and Velasco, A. (1989): Continuous arteriovenous hemodialysis in the ICU. *Critical Care Nurse* 9(1):29–32, 34–35, 38–41.

Mitch, W. E., and Klahr, S. (1988): *Nutrition and the Kidney.* Boston: Little, Brown.

Nahman, N. S., and Middendorf, D. F. (1990): Continuous arteriovenous hemofiltration. *Medical Clinics of North America* 74(4):975–983.

Norris, M. K. G. (1989): Acute tubular necrosis: preventing complications. *Dimensions of Critical Care Nursing* 8(1):16–26.

Porush, J. G. (1986, March): New concepts in acute renal failure. *American Family Physician* 33(3):109–118.

Price, C. A. (1989): Continuous arteriovenous ultrafiltration: A monitoring guide for ICU nurses. *Critical Care Nurse* 9(1):12–14, 17–19.

Ronco, C., Brendola, A., Bragantini, L., Chiaramonte, S., Feriani, M., Fabris, A., and LaGreca, G. (1985): Continuous arterio-venous hemofiltration. *Contributions to Nephrology* 48:70–88.

Schoengrund, L. (1985): Nursing management of the patient with acute renal failure. In: L. Schoengrund and P. Balzer (eds.). *Renal Problems in Critical Care.* New York: John Wiley & Sons, pp. 47–67.

Schrier, R. W. (1986): *Renal and Electrolyte Disorders.* 3rd ed. Boston: Little, Brown.

Strupp, T. W. (1988): Postshock resuscitation of the trauma victim: preventing and managing acute renal failure. *Critical Care Nursing Quarterly* 11(2):1–9.

Waltzer, W. C., and Rapaport, F. T. (1984): *Angioaccess—Principles and Practice.* Orlando, Florida: Grune & Stratton.

Whittaker, A. A. (1985, June): Acute renal dysfunction: Assessment of patient at risk. *Focus on Critical Care* 12(3):12–17.

Wilkins, R. G., and Faragher, E. B. (1983): Acute renal failure in an intensive care unit: Incidence, prediction, and outcome. *Anaesthesia* 38(7):628–624.

Wills, M. R. (1990): Effects of renal failure. *Clinical Biochemistry* 23:55–60.

Winkelman, C. (1985): Hemofiltration: a new technique in critical care nursing. *Heart and Lung* 14(3):265–271.

Wolfson, M. (1987): Nutritional support in acute renal failure. *Dialysis & Transplantation* 16(9):493, 496.

Chapter

12

Anne-Marie Jones, R.N., M.S.N., CCRN

Hematology/Immunology

Objectives

- Understand the basic anatomy and physiology, and normal functioning of the hematological and immune systems.
- Understand the pathophysiological processes that affect the hematological and immune systems.
- Discuss clinical manifestations, nursing and medical management of anemias, polycythemias, leukemia, disseminated intravascular coagulation (DIC), and thrombocytopenia.
- Discuss concepts of the immune system including organ and cell involvement, and immune mechanisms including defenses and responses.
- Discuss various disorders of and treatments for the immunocompromised patient including AIDS.
- Develop a plan of care for the patient with a bleeding disorder or who is immunocompromised.

Whenever a patient is critically ill, the hematological and immune systems become involved. Proper functioning of these systems is necessary for basic processes such as gas exchange, tissue perfusion, nutrition, acid-base balance, hemostasis, and protection against infection. Problems affecting these systems have been increasingly seen in critical care patients in recent years. Life-threatening disorders such as disseminated intravascular coagulation (DIC) and acquired immunodeficiency syndrome (AIDS) are two examples. The increased use of invasive monitoring and procedures has placed patients at risk for iatrogenic infections. Additionally, progress in the treatment of malignancies and immunotherapy related to organ transplant have introduced new problems for critical care patients and their caregivers.

Because critical care nurses are frequently challenged by the hematological and immunological systems, a basic understanding of the anatomy and physiology and the normal functioning of these two systems is necessary for comprehensive patient assessment. Knowledge of the pathological processes that affect these systems as well as subsequent medical and nursing interventions is necessary for the critical care nurse to provide the required standard of care. In this chapter, hematological/immunological anatomy and physiology is reviewed. Pathophysiology, medical treatment, and nursing management of selected disorders are then discussed.

Review of Hematological Anatomy and Physiology

The hematological system, through its various components, is involved in many cellular processes. In addition to transporting oxygen, carbon dioxide, nutrients, and wastes, the blood is vital in defense against infection, hemostasis, temperature regulation, and acid-base balance.

HEMATOLOGICAL FUNCTION OF ORGANS

Hematopoiesis is the formation and development of blood cells. Theoretically, all blood cells are derived from hematopoietic stem cells—these cells differentiate into erythrocytes (red blood cells, RBCs), leukocytes (white blood cells, WBCs), or thrombocytes (platelets) (Fig. 12-1). The hormone erythropoietin stimulates the formation and differentiation of red blood cells, whereas a substance known as thrombopoietin is thought to regulate the production and matura-

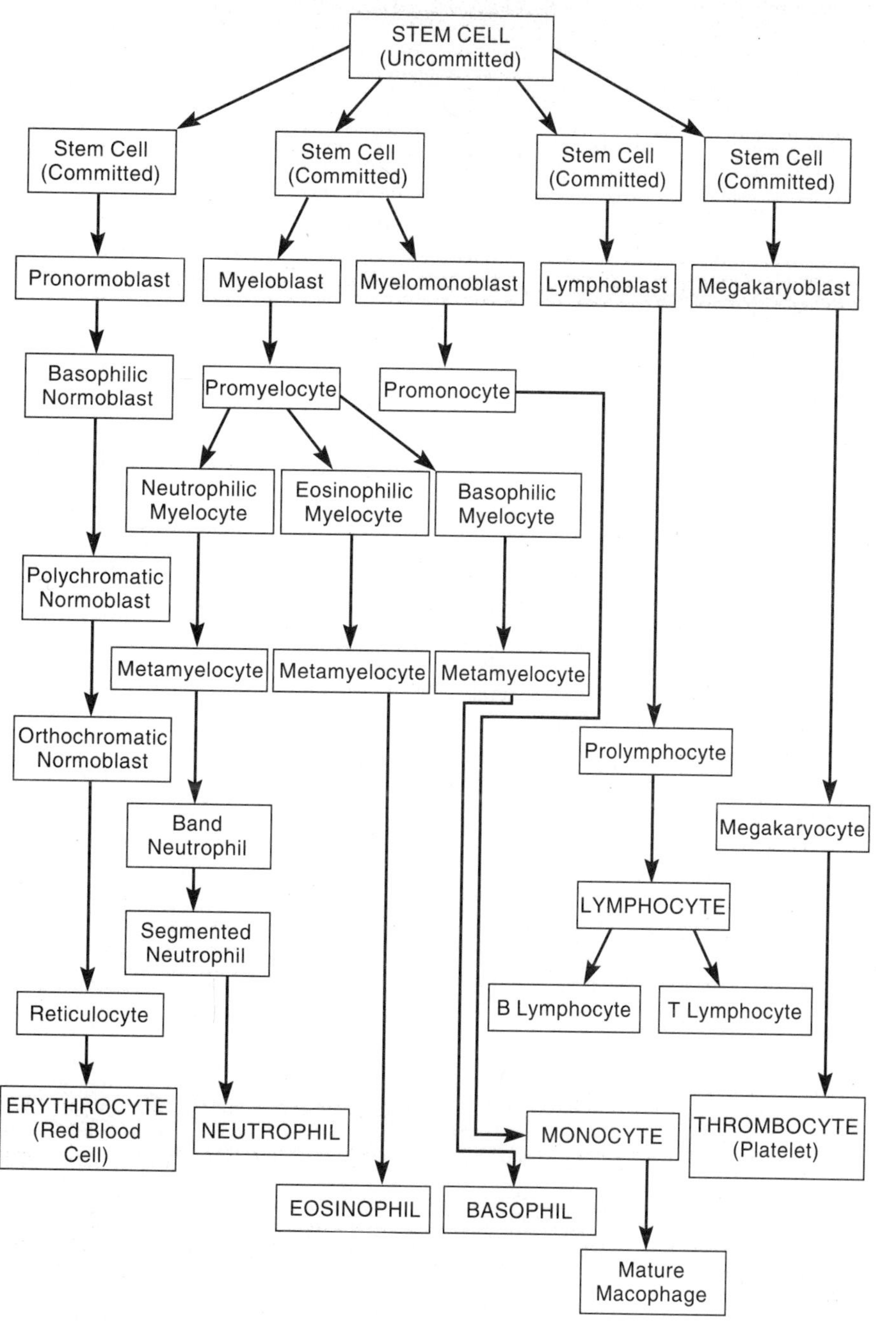

Figure 12-1. Blood cell differentiation from the stem cell.

tion of platelets. The bone marrow is the site of blood cell production. In early childhood, most bones are filled with blood-forming red marrow; in the adult, productive bone marrow is found in the vertebrae, skull, chest cage, ilium, and proximal long bones (Anderson and Bullock, 1988).

The spleen is a highly vascular organ that is involved in the production of lymphocytes, the filtering and destruction of erythrocytes, the filtering and trapping of foreign matter, including bacteria and viruses, and the storage of blood. Though it is not necessary for survival, the spleen plays an important part in protection against infection and hemostasis (Anderson and Bullock, 1988).

The liver produces clotting factors, utilizes bile from RBC breakdown, and detoxifies many substances in the blood; its proper functioning is essential for normal hemostasis and metabolism. The liver also filters and stores blood in addition to its many other metabolic functions (Dolan, 1991; Harvey, 1986).

The thymus gland and lymph nodes are also part of the hematopoietic system; they are primarily involved in immunological functions (Harvey, 1986).

CHARACTERISTICS OF BLOOD

The specific gravity of blood normally ranges from 1.048 to 1.066 and depends to a large extent on the number of circulating red blood cells. The higher the specific gravity, the more viscous the blood. The degree of viscosity will affect blood flow: the higher the viscosity, the slower the flow. Problems, such as abnormal clotting, are more likely to occur in the presence of sluggish blood flow.

In a normal state, arterial blood is bright red and venous blood is darker. This reflects the degree of hemoglobin oxygenation, and will vary. The osmotic pressure of blood, which is determined by the amount of salts, glucose, wastes, dissolved crystalloids, and plasma proteins, is maintained within normal limits by the kidneys. It averages 300 milliosmoles per kilogram (mOsm/kg) of water.

The pH, or hydrogen ion concentration, must remain within a narrow range for homeostasis to be maintained. The normal range is 7.35 to 7.45, which is slightly alkaline. Various buffering mechanisms in the body are involved in maintaining the pH within a normal range.

The volume of blood will vary depending on such factors as weight, sex, pregnancy, body position, age, nutritional status, temperature, and altitude. It represents approximately 8% of body weight. In the adult male, there is generally about 5 L of blood; in the female, about 3.5 to 4.5 L. In an adult with a 5-L blood volume, 4500 ml is in the systemic circuit. Of this, about 76% is in the veins and venules, 18% in the arteries, and 6% in the capillaries. The pulmonary circulation contains the remaining 500 ml of blood; 24% in the arteries, 50% in the capillaries, and 30% in the veins and venules (Jackson and Jones, 1988b).

COMPONENTS OF BLOOD

Plasma

The blood contains both circulating cells and plasma. Plasma, a pale yellow liquid, makes up about 55% of total blood volume, and is composed of serum and fibrinogen, a blood protein. Plasma contains a large number of substances, the highest percentage of weight being made up of the plasma proteins: albumin, serum globulins, fibrinogen, prothrombin, and plasminogen. These proteins participate in a variety of functions, including maintenance of intravascular blood volume through osmotic pressure, coagulation, blood clot dissolution, wound healing, and transport of various substances (Jackson and Jones, 1988b).

Cells

Cells constitute the remaining 45% of blood volume, and include erythrocytes, leukocytes, and platelets (Table 12–1; Fig. 12–2).

Erythrocytes

Also known as red blood cells (RBCs), erythrocytes are flexible biconcave discs without nuclei whose primary component is hemoglobin. Because of their unique configuration, RBCs can travel at high speeds, can bend, twist, and elongate themselves to facilitate passage through small areas and to expose more surface area for gas exchange. For each milliliter of blood there are approximately 5 million RBCs; they have a life span of about 120 days (Jackson, 1988a).

The RBCs are generated from precursor stem cells under the influence of a growth factor and the hormone erythropoietin. Erythropoietin is se-

Table 12–1. BLOOD CELLS—FUNCTIONS AND NORMAL VALUES

Cell	Functions	Normal Value	Alterations
Erythrocyte red blood cell (RBC)	Respiration Oxygen transport Acid-base balance	5 million/μl	Increased: polycythemia, dehydration Decreased: anemia, fluid overload, hemorrhage
Leukocyte white blood cell (WBC)	Immune response Defense against infection, foreign tissue	5000–10,000/mm^3	Increased: inflammation, tissue necrosis, leukemia Decreased: bone marrow depression (radiation, immune disorders)
Granular Leukocytes Neutrophils	(PMNs) Phagocytosis of invading organisms	50–70% of WBCs	Increased: inflammation, infection, surgery, MI Decreased: aplastic anemia, hepatitis, some pharmacological agents
Eosinophils	Defense against parasites; detox of foreign proteins Phagocytosis	1–5% of WBCs	Increased: allergic attacks, autoimmune diseases, parasitic infections Decreased: stress reactions
Basophils	Release heparin, serotonin, and histamine in allergic reactions; inflammatory response	0–1% of WBCs	Increased: postsplenectomy, hemolytic anemia, radiation
Nongranular Leukocytes Monocytes	Mature into macrophages; phagocytosis of necrotic tissue, debris, foreign particles	1–8% of WBCs	Increased: bacterial, parasitic, and some viral infections
Lymphocytes	Defense against microorganisms	20–40% of WBCs	Increased: bacterial and viral infections, lymphocytic leukemia Decreased: chemotherapy, immunodeficiencies
B lymphocyte	Humoral immunity and production of antibodies		
T lymphocytes	Cell-mediated immunity		
Thrombocytes (platelets)	Blood clotting; hemostasis	150,000–400,000/mm^3	Increased: polycythemia vera, postsplenectomy Decreased: leukemia, bone marrow failure, DIC, hemorrhage, hypersplenism

creted by the kidney in response to hypoxia and anemia (Jackson and Jones, 1988b).

Oxygen transport is the main function of erythrocytes. Hemoglobin binds with oxygen in the lungs and transports it to the tissues. The affinity of hemoglobin for oxygen depends on several factors, including blood pH, temperature, and the concentration of 2,3-diphosphoglycerate (2,3-DPG). Erythrocytes are also vital in maintaining acid-base balance in the body (Jackson and Jones, 1988b).

Reticulocytes are immature erythrocytes. Maturation of RBCs takes 4 to 5 days. When the demand for RBCs is great, as in hemorrhage or hemolysis, many of the cells released from the marrow are not mature, and an increase in reticulocytes is seen. Reticulocytes circulate about 24 hours before maturing (Dolan, 1991). If the demand for RBCs continues or increases, an increase in normoblasts may be seen; these cells are even more immature (Jackson and Jones, 1988b).

The hematocrit (Hct) is an expression of the ratio of RBCs to plasma. In males, a normal hematocrit is approximately 45%; in females, 40%. The normal hematocrit value, however, has a wide range and is affected by many factors, such as the level of hydration and altitude at which the patient lives. Hemoglobin values range between 14 and 18 g/100 ml in the male, and 12 to 16 g/100 ml in the female. In laboratory studies, the RBC count, hematocrit, and hemoglobin usually follow the same trends. For example, elevated values in all three will occur in dehydration, hemoconcentration due to blood loss, and polycythemia. Values will be decreased in anemia, fluid overload, and recent hemorrhage.

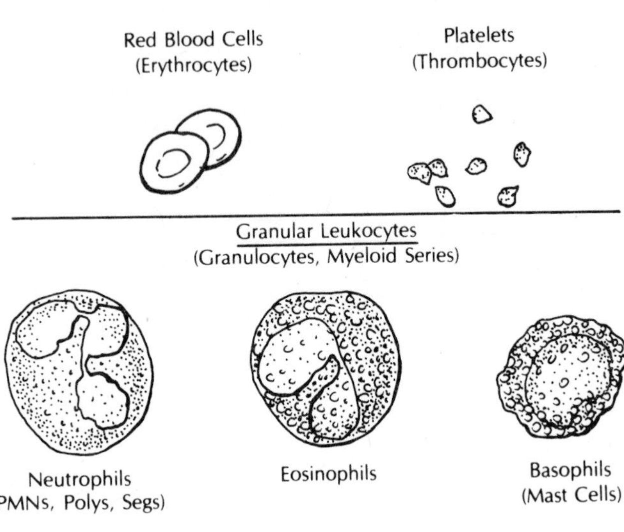

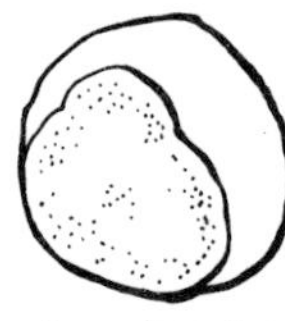

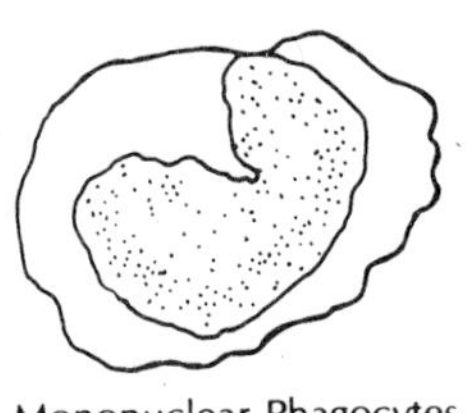

Figure 12-2. Differentiated blood cells. (Adapted from Harvey, M. A.: Study Guide to Core Curriculum for Critical Care Nursing. Philadelphia, W. B. Saunders, 1986, Fig. 6-1, p. 156.)

Leukocytes

Also known as white blood cells (WBCs), leukocytes are mobile cells that are larger, less numerous than RBCs, and have nuclei. There are a variety of leukocytes, specialized for different functions, and classified by their structure and affinity for certain dyes. The normal range of WBCs is 5,000 to 10,000/mm^3 of blood in the adult. Though WBCs are transported in the blood, many reside in the tissues. An increase in the total WBC count may be seen in inflammation, tissue necrosis, and leukemia. A decreased total WBC count reflects bone marrow depression, as may occur from radiation, viral infections, and immune disorders.

Primarily involved in the body's immune response, WBCs play a key role in the defense against infectious organisms and foreign antigens. They produce and transport factors such as antibodies that are vital in maintaining immunity (Bullock, 1988a). Though varied and with specialized functions, WBCs work in an integrated fashion to protect the body.

White blood cells are classified into two categories: granulocytes (polymorphonuclear leukocytes, polymorphonuclear neutrophils [PMNs or polys]), and nongranular leukocytes. The

PMNs include neutrophils, eosinophils, and basophils. Nongranular leukocytes include monocytes and lymphocytes.

Granulocytes

Neutrophils. Neutrophils, the most numerous of the granulocytes, constitute 50 to 70% of the total white cell count. They are further broken down into segmented neutrophils, in which filaments in the cell give the nuclei an appearance of having lobes, and band neutrophils, which are immature and have a thicker or U-shaped nucleus. Normally, segmented neutrophils make up approximately 56% of WBCs, whereas band neutrophils constitute only about 3% (Jackson and Jones, 1988b). The phrase "a shift to the left" refers to an increased number of "bands" as compared to mature neutrophils, and generally indicates an acute infectious process (Bullock, 1988a). Any inflammatory process will cause an increase in circulating neutrophils (Jackson and Jones, 1988b). Infection, surgical procedures, and myocardial infarction will also cause an increase in neutrophils. A decrease in neutrophils occurs with disorders such as hepatitis, aplastic anemia, various viral infections, and pharmacological agents such as sulfonamides and antihistamines (Holloway, 1988). The survival time of neutrophils is short—once released from the bone marrow, they circulate in the blood 4 to 8 hours before migrating to the tissues, where they live another 4 to 5 days (Guyton, 1986). When serious infection is present, neutrophils may live only a few hours as they phagocytize infectious organisms. Because of this short life span, drugs that affect rapidly multiplying cells (e.g., chemotherapeutics) will quickly decrease the neutrophil count, and thus alter the patient's ability to fight infection.

Neutrophils are attracted and migrate to areas of inflammation or bacterial invasion by the process of chemotaxis, which is mediated by substances released at the site of injury. There they ingest and kill invading microorganisms by phagocytosis.

Phagocytosis is the process by which antigens and damaged cells are removed from the tissues, and is carried out by granulocytes (especially neutrophils) and macrophages (matured monocytes). These phagocytes operate on a "search and destroy" principle. Once they have been attracted to an area by chemotaxis, a process called opsonization occurs, in which an antibody attaches to the phagocytic cells to enhance phagocytosis of bacteria (Fidler, 1988). Once the bacteria have been engulfed, they are killed and digested within the cell by lysosomal enzymes. It is by the process of phagocytosis that pus formation, or suppuration, occurs. Phagocytosis is a rapid process that is initiated within minutes of cellular injury (Fidler, 1988).

Phagocytosis also occurs in the lymphoreticular organs, which include the lymph nodes, thymus, spleen, and liver. When infectious organisms escape the local immune response, they enter the blood stream and lymphatic channels. In the blood stream, they are engulfed and destroyed by macrophages in the liver and spleen; in the lymph system, pathogenic substances are filtered by the lymph nodes and phagocytized by tissue macrophages. Here they may also stimulate the immune response by the lymphoid cells (Bullock, 1988a).

Eosinophils. Eosinophils are larger than neutrophils and make up 1 to 5% of the normal WBC count. They are important in the defense against parasites and are thought to be involved in the detoxification of foreign proteins (Jackson and Jones, 1988b). Eosinophils are found largely in tissues of the intestinal tract and lungs; they increase during an allergic reaction. Like neutrophils, eosinophils migrate to areas of infection and inflammation through chemotaxis where they participate in phagocytosis. Eosinophils contain bactericidal substances and lysosomal enzymes that aid in the destruction of invading organisms. Eosinophils also have a short survival time of 6 to 8 hours in the circulation, and 2 to 3 days in the tissues (Bullock, 1988a). An increase in circulating eosinophils is seen during allergic attacks, autoimmune diseases, and parasitic infections (Jackson, 1988a). A decrease in circulating eosinophils may occur in severe stress reactions because of the high levels of epinephrine and adrenocorticotropic hormone (Holloway, 1988).

Basophils. The third type of granulocyte is the basophil, which has large granules containing heparin, serotonin, and histamine. Basophils participate in the body's inflammatory and allergic responses by releasing these substances (Bullock, 1988a). Basophils, which constitute from 0 to 1% of the total WBC count, are not phagocytes but are important in acute systemic allergic reactions as well as the inflammatory response. They, like the other granulocytes, have a short life span. An increase in basophils may occur after splenectomy, with radiation therapy, and in hemolytic anemia (Holloway, 1988).

Nongranular Leukocytes

Monocytes. Monocytes are the largest of the leukocytes, though they constitute only 1 to 8% of the total WBC count. Once released into the blood stream, monocytes mature into macrophages, which are phagocytes. They function as "seek and destroy" scavengers. In addition to "eating" large foreign particles and cell fragments, macrophages are vital in the phagocytosis of necrotic tissue and debris. Like eosinophils, macrophages contain lysosomal enzymes and bactericidal substances. Macrophages also migrate to the tissues, where they become fixed, and are known as tissue macrophages. In the lung, these tissue macrophages are known as alveolar macrophages; in the liver, they are Kupffer cells; in connective tissue, they are histiocytes (Fidler, 1988; Bullock, 1988c). When activated by antigens, macrophages also secrete substances called monokines, which act as chemical communicators between the cells involved in the immune response. A monokine known as interleukin-1 influences the growth and cloning of lymphocytes, which enhances immunity (Fidler, 1988). Though monocytes may circulate only 36 hours, they can survive as tissue macrophages months or even years (Guyton, 1986; Bullock, 1988c). Monocyte values are increased in bacterial, parasitic, and some viral infections as well as collagen diseases and some malignancies (Jackson, 1988a).

Lymphocytes. Approximately 20 to 40% of the total WBC count is made up of lymphocytes in the adult. They are vital in the body's defense against bacteria, viruses, and other microorganisms; they also play a major role in tumor immunity, delayed hypersensitivity reactions, autoimmune diseases, and foreign tissue rejection. Lymphocytes are primarily concerned with the specific immune responses, and participate in two types of immunity: humoral immunity, mediated by B lymphocytes; and cellular immunity, mediated by T lymphocytes. B Lymphocytes, or B cells, originate in the bone marrow and are thought to mature there also. Their name is derived from the bursa of Fabricius, the site of B-cell maturation in birds. T Lymphocytes, or T cells, comprise the majority of circulating lymphocytes; they also live longer than B cells and participate in long-term immunity. T Cells are produced in the bone marrow, but migrate to the thymus for maturation. After maturation, T cells migrate to other lymphoid tissue or the blood stream, where they "patrol" for antigens. The life span of lymphocytes, which varies by type and whether they are circulating or in the tissues, ranges from a few days to years (Bullock, 1988c). Lymphocytes are increased in bacterial and viral infections, multiple myeloma, and lymphocytic leukemia. A decrease is seen with chemotherapeutic drugs, in immunodeficiency states such as AIDS, and with some forms of sepsis (Jackson, 1988a). Specific immunity is discussed more thoroughly later in the review of immunological anatomy and physiology section.

Thrombocytes

Known more commonly as platelets, thrombocytes are the smallest of the formed elements of the blood. A normal platelet count ranges from 150,000 to 400,000/mm^3 of blood. Platelets are necessary for blood clotting and hemostasis. They adhere to injured blood vessel walls and other surfaces, where they occlude rents and tears, preventing blood loss. Platelets also release mediators necessary for the clotting process. These substances include epinephrine and serotonin, which contribute to vasospasm; adenosine diphosphate (ADP), which is necessary for platelet adhesion and aggregation; and calcium and phospholipids necessary in various steps of the clotting process. *Adhesion* refers to the attachment of platelets to nonplatelet surfaces; *aggregation* is the adherence of platelets to each other to form plugs. Platelets have a life span of 7 to 14 days, and are continually being used to repair small vascular injuries that occur normally. Most are circulating throughout the blood, though the spleen normally stores up to 20% of platelets. *Thrombocytopenia* is a deficiency of platelets; *relative thrombocytopenia* refers to a functional abnormality of platelets though the count may be normal. Platelets are increased in compensation for hemorrhage, polycythemia vera, and leukemia, after splenectomy, and in some malignant diseases. A decrease in platelets is seen in bone marrow failure, hypersplenism, disseminated intravascular coagulation, hemorrhage, and with increased destruction of platelets (Jackson, 1988a).

Hemostasis

Hemostasis is the prevention of blood loss, or the process by which the body arrests bleeding. It involves several events and processes that are interrelated and occur simultaneously or sequentially. Research in this area continues to enhance our knowledge about exactly how hemostasis and blood coagulation occur.

When injury occurs to a blood vessel thereby allowing the escape of blood, the following physical events occur: (1) vascular spasm or vasoconstriction; (2) exposure of endothelial surfaces

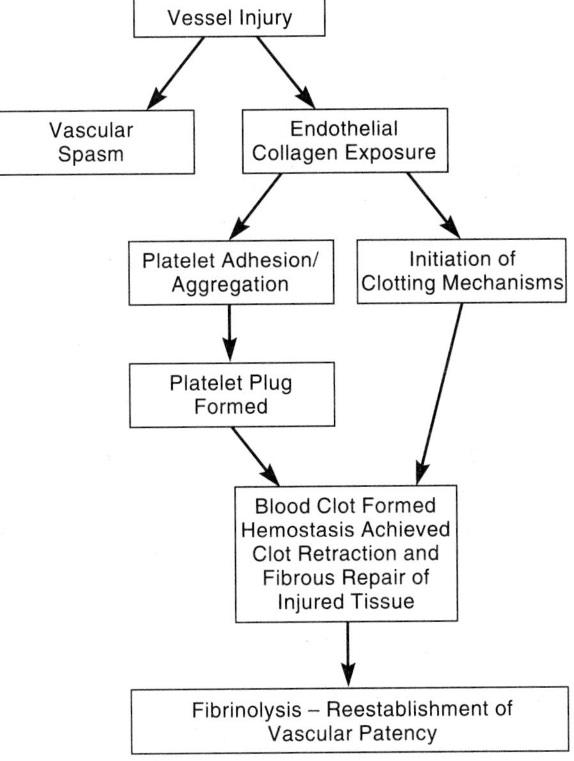

Figure 12-3. Hemostasis.

causes platelets to become sticky to enhance adhesion; (3) platelets aggregate to form plugs and release substances that facilitate the coagulation process; (4) a blood clot is formed through the activation of plasma coagulation factors; (5) clot retraction occurs to stabilize the clot; (6) fibrous repair of damaged tissue is initiated; and (7) the clot is eventually lysed (Jackson and Jones, 1988b) (Fig. 12-3).

Coagulation

The function of the body's blood coagulation system is to form a fibrin clot on the surface of the platelet plug. It involves a series of biochemical reactions that ultimately convert fibrinogen to fibrin, forming the fibrin clot. Fibrin threads trap platelets, RBCs, and plasma as the clot forms. The clot occludes the vessel lumen, then retracts, pulling the vessel edges together.

Coagulation occurs by two distinct pathways, the intrinsic and the extrinsic, which share a common "final" pathway resulting in a blood clot (Fig. 12-4). These separate pathways are basically alternate modes of activating a critical clotting factor, factor X. Both pathways begin with an initiating event, and have a "cascade" sequence of factor activation. Each factor must be activated by a preceding reaction.

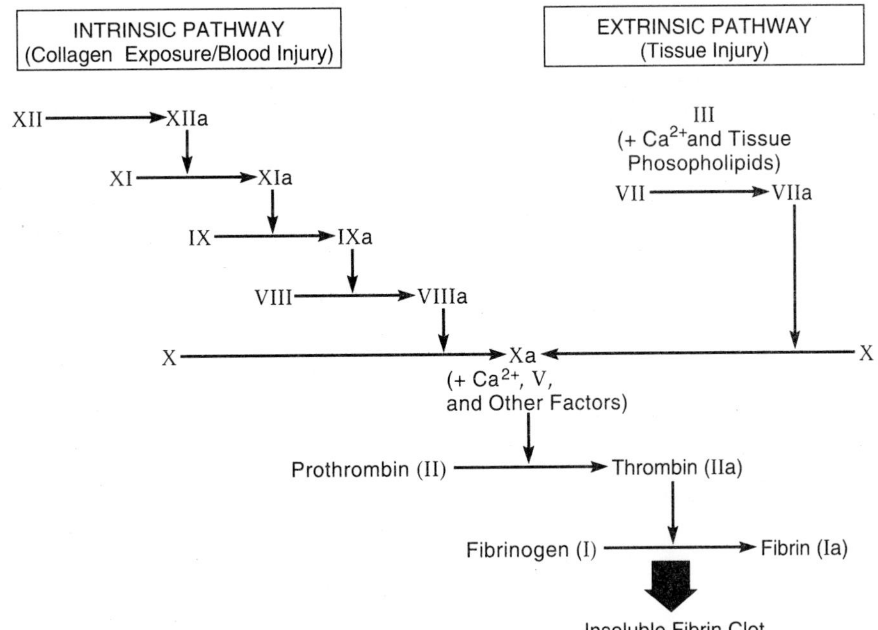

Figure 12-4. Coagulation pathways—intrinsic, extrinsic, and common.

The coagulation factors are mostly plasma proteins that are inactive enzymes (Table 12–2). With the exception of factors VIII and XIII, synthesis of these factors takes place in the liver. Hence, liver disease or injury can lead to problems with blood coagulation and bleeding. Several of the factors are vitamin K dependent, and thus a vitamin K deficiency can also lead to bleeding problems. Coagulation factors are designated by roman numerals according to their order of discovery, not their position in the clotting cascade.

Intrinsic Pathway

All factors needed for clot formation are contained in circulating blood. When blood is exposed to subendothelial collagen or is "injured," factor XII is activated to XIIa, which initiates coagulation via the intrinsic pathway. Factor XI is then converted to XIa, which in the presence of calcium activates factor IX. The sequence continues as factors IXa, VIII, calcium, and platelet phospholipids participate to activate factor X. The common pathway is thus triggered.

Extrinsic Pathway

When tissue injury occurs, a substance known as tissue factor, or thromboplastin (factor III), and phospholipids are released. In the presence of calcium, this activates factor VII, which converts factor X to Xa, thus entering the final common pathway for coagulation.

Common Pathway

In the common pathway, activated factor X (Xa) converts prothrombin (factor II) to thrombin in the presence of calcium and other cofactors. Thrombin, a powerful procoagulant, then converts fibrinogen (factor I) to fibrin, which forms a fibrin mesh and blood clot.

Thrombin also stimulates platelet aggregation, activates and enhances the activity of other clotting factors, and initiates the fibrinolytic system by converting plasminogen to plasmin.

Coagulation Antagonists and Clot Lysis

In order to maintain a balance between clot formation and bleeding, a system of checks and balances exists. Of the procoagulant forces, thrombin is the most powerful. Enough prothrombin is present in 10 ml of blood to clot 2500 ml of plasma in only 15 seconds (Jackson and Jones, 1988b). Thus, anticoagulant forces must be effective in preventing abnormal clotting.

Normal vascular endothelium is smooth and intact, preventing collagen exposure that initiates the intrinsic clotting pathway. In addition, negatively charged proteins are present on the endothelium that repel positively charged clotting factors. Rapid blood flow serves to dilute and disperse clotting factors. Clotting factors that are not contained within a formed clot are filtered and removed from the circulation by the liver. Several plasma proteins are present that localize clotting to the site of injury; they include antiplasmin and antithrombin III. However, the most potent anticoagulant forces are the fibrin threads, which absorb 85 to 90% of thrombin during clot formation, and antithrombin III, which inactivates thrombin not contained within the clot (Guyton, 1986). Heparin, produced in small quantities by basophils and tissue mast cells, acts as a potent anticoagulant. Heparin combines with antithrombin III to increase the effectiveness of

Table 12–2. BLOOD COAGULATION FACTORS

Factor	Common Names	Comments
I	Fibrinogen	Synthesized in liver
II	Prothrombin	Synthesized in liver; vitamin K dependent
III	Tissue thromboplastin Tissue factor	Extrinsic pathway's first factor
IV	Calcium	Necessary in several steps of coagulation
V	Labile factor	Synthesized in liver
VI	Not assigned	
VII	Proconvertin Stable factor	Synthesized in liver; extrinsic pathway
VIII	Antihemophilic factor A	Required in intrinsic pathway
IX	Plasma thromboplastin component (PTC) Christmas factor Antihemophilic factor B	Synthesized in liver; vitamin K dependent
X	Stuart-Prower factor	Synthesized in liver; vitamin K dependent; intrinsic and extrinsic pathways
XI	Plasma thromboplastin antecedent (PTA) Antihemophilic factor C	Required in intrinsic pathway
XII	Hageman factor	Intrinsic pathway's first factor
XIII	Fibrin-stabilizing factor	Stabilizes clot formation

the former; together this complex removes several of the activated coagulation factors from the blood (Bullock, 1988d).

Once hemostasis has been accomplished and blood vessel integrity restored, blood flow must be reestablished. This is accomplished by the fibrinolytic system, by which clots are broken down (lysed) and removed. Fibrinolysis is mediated by plasmin, an enzyme that digests fibrinogen and fibrin (Fig. 12–5). A plasma protein, plasminogen is the inactive form of plasmin; it is incorporated into the blood clot as it forms and cannot initiate clot lysis until activated. Many substances found in the body are capable of activating plasminogen, including thrombin and other activated clotting factors, lysosomal enzymes, urokinase (found in the urine), and streptokinase, which is released from streptococcal bacteria.

Fibrinolysis is very active within the microcirculation, where it maintains the patency of the capillary beds. Larger vessels contain less plasminogen activator; this may predispose them to clot formation (Jackson and Jones, 1988b).

When plasmin digests fibrinogen, fragments are produced that function as potent anticoagulants. These fragments are known as fibrin split products (FSPs) or fibrin degradation products (FDPs). In cases of excessive clotting and clot lysis, these FSPs contribute to the coagulopathy.

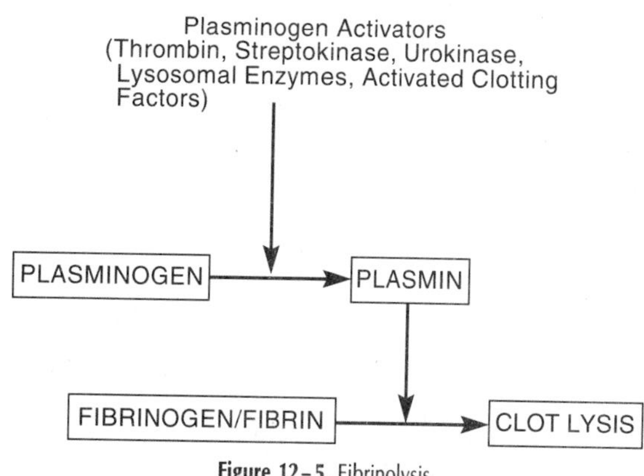

Figure 12–5. Fibrinolysis.

The FSPs are not normally present in the circulation but are seen in some hematological disorders as well as with thrombolytic therapy (e.g., the administration of streptokinase or tissue plasminogen activator [TPA]).

Laboratory studies that evaluate coagulation are listed in Table 12–3.

Selected Hematological Disorders

There are many pathological conditions that affect the hematological system, ranging from mild anemias to life-threatening bleeding disorders. In

Table 12–3. COAGULATION PROFILE STUDIES

Test	Normal Value	Comments
Lee White Clotting Time	6–12 min	Nonspecific for clotting abnormalities
Partial thromboplastin time (PTT)	60–90 sec	General indicator of blood's clotting ability— evaluates intrinsic pathway
		Used to monitor heparin therapy and detect bleeding tendencies, hemorrhagic disorders
		Increased in anticoagulation therapy, liver disease, vitamin K deficiency, DIC
Prothrombin time (PT)	11–16 sec	Evaluates extrinsic pathway; used to monitor oral anticoagulant therapy
		Increased with coumarin, liver disease, vitamin K deficiency, obstructive jaundice
Fibrinogen level	200–400 mg/100 ml	Decreased in DIC and fibrinolytic disorders
Fibrin split products (FSPs)	<10 μg/ml	Evaluates hematological disorders
		Increased in DIC, fibrinolysis, thrombolytic therapy
Platelet count	150,000–400,000/mm³	Measures number of circulating platelets
		Decreased in thrombocytopenia
Bleeding time	1–4 min	Evaluates platelet function
		Increased with thrombocytopenia and aspirin therapy
Calcium	9–11 mg/dl	Decreased in massive transfusions of stored blood

critical care, nurses see many of these disease states. The purpose of this section is to review those disorders that are most frequently seen in critical care, and pose the greatest risk to the patient.

RED BLOOD CELL DISORDERS

Anemias

Pathophysiology

The term *anemia* refers to a reduction in the number of circulating RBCs or hemoglobin, and is the most common form of hematopoietic disease (Jackson, 1988b). Simply put, there are too few RBCs and/or too little hemoglobin to fully oxygenate the tissues. When the blood's hemoglobin content is less than that needed to meet the body's demands, tissue hypoxia results (Dolan, 1991). Though symptoms may vary depending on the type, cause, or severity of anemia, basic clinical findings are the same.

As tissues become hypoxic, the substance 2,3-diphosphoglycerate (2,3-DPG) increases to cause hemoglobins to release oxygen. Blood flow is redistributed to those areas where oxygenation is most vital; i.e., the brain and heart.

There are many causes of anemia that are frequently seen in critical care. Posthemorrhagic anemia is caused by acute or chronic blood loss, such as from gastrointestinal bleeding or severe trauma. In aplastic anemia, bone marrow failure results in the inadequate production of all blood cells, including RBCs. Hemolytic anemia is an increase in the rate of destruction of RBCs. Causes of hemolytic anemia include autoimmune diseases, hereditary states such as sickle cell disease, trauma to cells from malfunctioning prosthetic heart valves or extracorporeal circulation, drug therapy, and certain infectious organisms (Jackson, 1988b).

Sickle cell disease, a form of hereditary hemolytic anemia, may occasionally be seen in critical care when the patient is in crisis. Because of an abnormal amount of hemoglobin S (HbS) in relation to hemoglobin A (HbA), red blood cells assume a sickle or crescent shape when there is a decrease in the oxygen concentration, decreased pH, or increased 2,3-DPG. This sickling alters the blood viscosity, impairing flow and leading to occlusion of the microvasculature. Though the sickling is reversible with the administration of supplemental oxygen, patients carry a varying number of irreversibly sickled cells that, when removed by the body, result in hemolysis and anemia. Sickle cell crisis is potentially life threatening as occlusion of the microvasculature leads to hypoxia, exacerbation of sickling, anoxia, infarction, and thrombosis in tissues and organs such as the brain, kidneys, spleen, and lungs (Belcher, 1989).

Clinical Manifestations

The generalized vasoconstriction that occurs and deoxygenated hemoglobin result in pallor of the skin seen in the anemias. The body tries to compensate for the lack of oxygen by increasing the heart rate, cardiac output, and respiratory rate. Laboratory findings include a decreased RBC count and hemoglobin and hematocrit levels. The reticulocyte count will usually be elevated, indicating increased RBC production. Hemolytic anemia patients will also have an increased bilirubin level. In aplastic anemia, the reticulocyte, platelet, and white blood cell counts will be decreased, as the marrow fails to produce any cells. In sickle cell disease, a stained blood smear reveals the sickled cells.

Symptoms of the various anemias are related to the tissue hypoxia and the body's resulting compensatory activities. General signs and symptoms include pallor, fatigue, weakness, and lethargy. The body shunts blood away from nonvital organs (such as the skin and kidneys) to perfuse the vital organs. More specific findings related to the body's attempt to compensate for the lack of oxygen in the tissues are tachycardia, palpitations, angina, systolic murmurs, dyspnea, and tachypnea.

Posthemorrhagic anemia will result in symptoms of hypovolemia, such as thirst, hypotension, and decreased urine output. Additionally, because of the altered perfusion and oxygenation of the brain, the patient may be restless and disoriented.

In aplastic anemia, patients may also present with bruising, nosebleeds, petechiae, and decreased ability to fight infections. These result from thrombocytopenia and decreased white blood cell counts, which occur when the bone marrow fails to produce blood cells.

Assessment of the patient with hemolytic anemia may reveal jaundice, abdominal pain, and enlargement of the spleen or liver; these findings result from the increased destruction of red blood cells, their sequestration (abnormal distribution in the spleen and liver), and accumulation of breakdown products.

Patients with sickle cell anemia may also have joint swelling or pain, and delayed physical and sexual development. In crisis, the sickle cell patient will often have decreased urine output and peripheral edema and signs of uremia because the renal tissue perfusion is impaired as a result of sluggish blood flow.

Medical/Nursing Management

Medical treatment of anemia includes identification and removal of any causative agents or conditions; improvement of tissue oxygenation with supplemental oxygen and blood component therapy; and cardiovascular system support as needed. For certain types of anemia, other interventions may be needed, such as a splenectomy in hemolytic anemia or bone marrow transplant for aplastic anemia. In sickle cell disease, oxygenation and correction of dehydration are important to reverse or prevent sickling of the erythrocytes.

Nursing management of anemia is based on the medical treatment and nursing assessment. Nursing diagnoses include altered tissue perfusion, impaired gas exchange, potential fluid volume excess/deficit, potential injury related to transfusions, and activity intolerance related to tissue hypoxia.

Physical assessment in anemia is vital; monitoring of vital signs, the ECG, hemodynamics, heart and lung sounds, and peripheral pulses will assist the nurse in assessment of tissue perfusion and gas exchange. Hypotension and orthostatic hypotension are particularly important signs indicating the patient is not tolerating the anemia. Additionally, mental status, urine output, and skin color and temperature are important indicators.

Laboratory results such as the CBC should be carefully followed. Other vital nursing interventions include promotion of rest, skin care, and careful administration of blood components, drug therapy, and intravenous fluids.

Polycythemia

Pathophysiology

The term *polycythemia* generally refers to an increased number of circulating RBCs and hemoglobin in the blood (Belcher, 1989). This causes the blood to be more viscous, and thus have sluggish flow. There are a number of disorders that can lead to hyperviscosity, but basic clinical findings and treatment related to altered blood flow and tissue perfusion are the same.

Polycythemia can be caused by overproductive bone marrow leading to an excess in all blood cells; a compensatory response to hypoxia, which stimulates the production of RBCs; or a state caused by the relative increase of cells to plasma, as in dehydration (Belcher, 1989).

Clinical Manifestations

Clinical findings of polycythemia are related to the increased resistance to blood flow and resulting compensatory activities. Patients may have neurological symptoms of dizziness, headache, blurred vision, or coma because the cerebral tissue perfusion is altered. The increased workload on the heart caused by the impaired flow and the body's attempted compensation may cause cardiovascular complications such as hypertension, congestive heart failure, and myocardial infarction. Altered tissue perfusion may lead to renal failure and neurological changes, such as headache and dizziness. The stagnant blood predisposes the patient to thrombus formation; thrombi may manifest as cerebrovascular accidents, myocardial infarctions, or gangrene of the feet. Bleeding disorders may also be seen as stagnant flow affects clotting factors. The liver and spleen may be enlarged as the cells are sequestered (Belcher, 1989). Laboratory reports will primarily reflect an increased erythrocyte count; depending on the exact disorder, the values of other formed elements will be elevated (Jackson, 1988b).

Medical/Nursing Management

Medical treatment includes treatment of the underlying disease process—for example, antineoplastic agents to suppress overproductive bone marrow, or correction of dehydration. Phlebotomy may be performed to relieve circulatory overload and reduce the hematocrit to 45% (Belcher, 1989).

Important nursing diagnoses in polycythemia are altered tissue perfusion, decreased cardiac output, potential for injury related to thrombus formation or hemorrhage, and potential fluid volume deficit related to phlebotomy/plasmapheresis.

Nursing assessment of the cardiovascular function in the patient with polycythemia should be carried out through monitoring of vital signs, the ECG, hemodynamics, heart and lung sounds, and peripheral pulses. Attention should also be given to mental status changes, renal function, skin color and temperature, and signs or symptoms of bleeding or blood clot formation.

As in other hematological disorders, laboratory results should be carefully followed. Administration of, and monitoring response to, chemotherapeutics, pharmacological therapy, and intravenous fluids are other nursing responsibilities. Patient weight and fluid intake and output should also be monitored.

WHITE BLOOD CELL DISORDERS

Many pathological disorders exist that can be classified as white blood cell disorders. Depending on the source, they may include neutropenia, various types of leukemias, lymphomas, and malignant myeloma (Bullock, 1988c; Jennings, 1985). Leukemia is briefly addressed here; lymphomas and malignant myeloma are not discussed in this text. The reader is referred to a more comprehensive reference on oncological disorders.

Neutropenia

Pathophysiology

Neutropenia is a neutrophil count of less than 2500/μl of blood resulting from the suppression of the bone marrow and its failure to produce adequate neutrophils (Bullock, 1988c). Patients with such low counts are predisposed to infections because of the body's reduced phagocytic ability. Neutropenia may be caused by acute or overwhelming infections, radiation, chemicals and drugs (benzenes, vinblastine, phenytoin, chloramphenicol), or other disease states (aplastic anemia, multiple myeloma, uremia).

Clinical Manifestations

Fever may be the only sign of infection in the neutropenic patient. Without phagocytosis, inflammation, heat, redness, and pain may be absent. Other clinical signs may include fatigue and weakness, chills, oral ulcers, sore throat, diarrhea, and tachycardia. Complications of neutropenia are most commonly septicemia and pneumonia as the body is not able to defend itself adequately against infection.

Medical/Nursing Management

The medical treatment of neutropenia is primarily aimed at preventing and treating infection. Anti-infectives and reverse isolation may be ordered; granulocyte transfusions may be necessary to replace deficient cells.

Potential for infection and altered oral mucous membrane are two important nursing diagnoses in neutropenia. Interventions to protect the patient from infection include close observation for signs of infection, being alert for any fever, good handwashing, maintaining skin integrity, promotion of adequate fluid and nutritional intake, perineal hygiene, reverse isolation as needed, and administration of antibiotics (see Nursing Care Plan for the Immunocompromised Patient). Scrupulous oral hygiene is necessary to promote integrity of mucous membranes and prevent infection.

Leukemia

Pathophysiology

Leukemia is a malignant disease that involves the blood-forming tissues and is characterized by a proliferation of abnormal or immature leukocytes. These cells accumulate in the lymphoid tissue and eventually infiltrate tissues throughout the body, involving all organs. The leukemias are classified by the type of cell and tissue involved as well as the course and duration of the disease. For instance, acute lymphocytic leukemia causes hyperplasia of lymphoid tissue and has a rapid onset and progression. Leukemia results in a loss of normal white blood cells, predisposing the patient to infection, as well as anemia and coagulation disorders because the bone marrow is unable to function properly to produce normal cells.

Clinical Manifestations

Clinically, the patient with leukemia may present with signs of recurrent infection or bleeding. The abnormal or immature white blood cells are not able to protect the body from infection, and the marrow fails to produce sufficient platelets. Mouth ulcers, pneumonia, gum bleeding, and epistaxis may be noted. Fatigue, lethargy, and weakness as well as pallor may result from anemia; the patient may also experience tachycardia and shortness of breath. Anorexia and weight loss may also be present. Other symptoms vary with organ involvement, and include decreased urine output, neurological changes, and enlargement of the liver, spleen, and lymph nodes.

Laboratory studies reveal an increased WBC count (15,000 to 500,000/mm^3 or higher) with a decrease in RBCs and platelets. Massive numbers of white blood cells are present on bone marrow biopsy (Belcher, 1989).

Medical/Nursing Management

Medical treatment of leukemia is aimed at stopping the proliferation of abnormal leukocytes and their infiltration into tissues. Medications depend on the classification of leukemia but may include antineoplastics such as methotrexate and corticosteroids. Radiation may be used to suppress bone marrow function. Bone marrow transplant is performed to provide normal productive tissue. Transfusions may be necessary to correct anemia or coagulation disorders. Infection is treated with antibiotics; reverse isolation techniques are instituted to protect the patient from infection. Additionally, intravenous hydration is maintained, and analgesics may be ordered to relieve pain.

Nursing diagnoses in leukemia include potential for infection and altered tissue perfusion, whose interventions have previously been discussed. Potential for bleeding, another nursing diagnosis, will be covered later.

BLEEDING DISORDERS

Patients with difficulty maintaining hemostasis are frequently seen in critical care. These bleeding disorders, referred to as coagulopathies, may be due to problems involving platelets, coagulation factors, or secondary to other pathological states. They may be inherited, such as hemophilia or von Willebrand's disease, or acquired, as in disseminated intravascular coagulation and vitamin K deficiency. See Table 12–4 for a list of terms associated with bleeding disorders.

Table 12–4. BLEEDING TERMINOLOGY

Term	Refers to
Ecchymosis	Blue or purplish hemorrhagic spot on skin or mucous membrane, round or irregular, nonelevated
Epistaxis	Bleeding from the nose
Hemarthrosis	Blood in a joint cavity
Hematochezia	Blood in stool; bright red
Hematoma	Collection of blood in tissue, space or organ; usually clotted
Hematemesis	Blood in emesis
Hematuria	Blood in urine
Hemoglobinuria	Hemoglobin in urine
Hemoptysis	Coughing of blood
Melena	Blood pigments in stool; dark or black
Menorrhagia	Excessive bleeding during menstruation
Petechia	Purplish red hemorrhagic spot, nonelevated, pinpoint, round

Disseminated Intravascular Coagulation

Pathophysiology

Disseminated intravascular coagulation (DIC) is a serious bleeding disorder that is characterized by an exaggeration of normal coagulation and profuse bleeding. Because clotting factors are used up in the abnormal coagulation process, it is also known as consumption coagulopathy. It is always secondary to another process, and can be triggered by a number of disease states. Mortality is greater than 50% in DIC, though the severity depends on the extent of the underlying disease process.

Disseminated intravascular coagulation can exist in chronic, acute, and subacute forms. The chronic form is most often caused by malignancy but may result from renal, liver, or metabolic disease. Acute DIC develops rapidly and is the most serious form of acquired coagulopathy. In subacute DIC, the patient has no clinical signs or symptoms, but laboratory findings indicate coagulation abnormalities (Holloway, 1988; Thelan et al., 1990).

The numerous conditions that can cause DIC include obstetrical emergencies such as amniotic fluid embolism and abruptio placentae; antigen-antibody reactions in anaphylaxis, incompatible blood transfusions, and transplant rejections; overwhelming infection, as in septic shock; prolonged hypotension from hemorrhage or cardiovascular failure; and acidosis (Dolan, 1991; Holloway, 1988) (Table 12–5).

Whatever the initiating event in DIC, procoagulants are released that cause diffuse uncontrolled clotting. The intrinsic and/or extrinsic

Table 12–5. CAUSES OF DIC

Infections	Bacterial (especially gram-negative), fungal, viral, mycobacterial, protozoan, rickettsial
Trauma	Burns, head, crush, or multiple injuries, snakebite
Obstetrical	Abruptio placentae, placenta previa, amniotic fluid embolism, retained dead fetus, missed abortion, eclampsia, hydatidiform mole
Hematological/Immunological Disorders	Transfusion reaction, transplant rejections, anaphylaxis, autoimmune disorders, sickle cell crisis
Oncological Disorders	Carcinomas, leukemias
Miscellaneous	Extracorporeal circulation, pulmonary or fat embolism, anoxia, acidosis, hyper- or hypothermia, hypovolemic or hemorrhagic shock, ARDS, sustained hypotension

pathways can be activated. Large amounts of thrombin are produced, which results in fibrin being deposited in the microvasculature, the consumption of available clotting factors, and the stimulation of fibrinolysis (Holloway, 1988).

Clotting in the microvasculature of the patient with DIC causes organ ischemia and necrosis. The skin, lungs, and kidneys are most often damaged. Thrombophlebitis, pulmonary embolism, cerebrovascular accident, gastrointestinal bleeding, and renal failure may result from thrombosis. Additionally, microvasculature thrombosis may result in acral cyanosis, purpura fulminans, or infarction and gangrene of the digits or tip of the nose (Thelan et al., 1990).

The fibrinolysis that follows results in the release of FSPs, which are potent anticoagulants that interfere with thrombin, fibrin, and platelet activity. Red blood cells are damaged as they try to pass through the blocked capillary beds; the damage to RBCs causes excess hemolysis. The lack of available clotting factors coupled with the

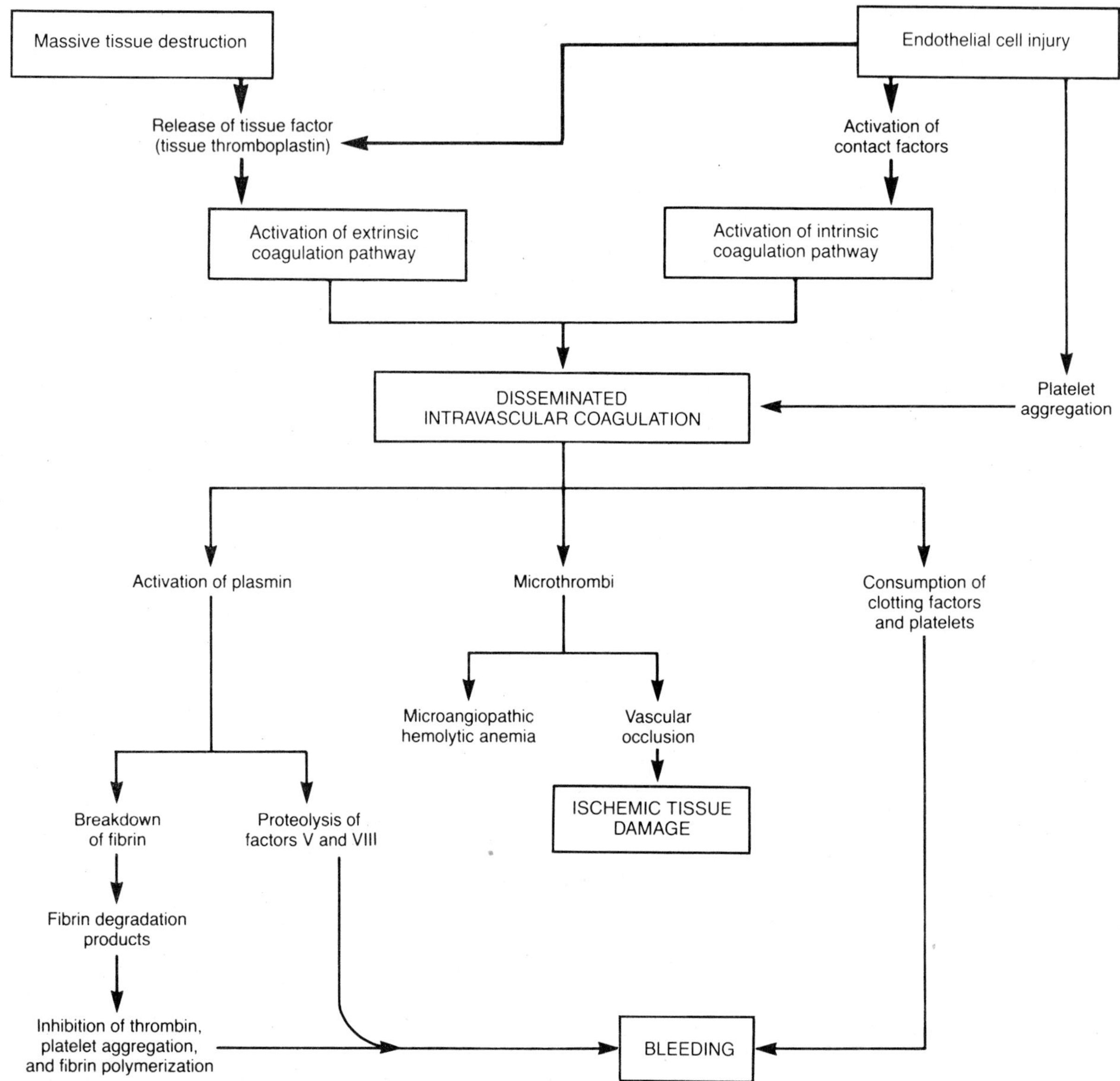

Figure 12–6. Pathophysiology of DIC. (From Cotran, R. S., Kumar, V., and Robbins, S. L.: Robbins Pathological Basis of Disease. 4th ed. Philadelphia, W. B. Saunders, Fig. 14–29, p. 700.)

anticoagulant forces results in the inability to form clots as needed, and predisposes the patient with DIC to hemorrhage (Fig. 12–6). Bleeding from venipuncture sites, catheters, incisions, body orifices, and into the skin occurs (Holloway, 1988).

Clinical Manifestations

Clinically, the patient with DIC presents with bleeding ranging from mild oozing from venipuncture sites to massive hemorrhage from all body orifices (Table 12–6). Petechiae, ecchymosis, and purpura may be present in the skin; gingival bleeding and epistaxis may be noted. Blood in the stool, emesis, and urine are common. Signs of organ ischemia and necrosis that result from microvasculature clotting may include angina, decreased urine output, gastrointestinal bleeding, dyspnea, and alterations in mental status. Acral cyanosis and infarction of digits and the tip of the nose may occur. Occult bleeding into body cavities such as the peritoneal and retroperitoneal spaces may be detected by vital sign changes or other classic signs of blood loss. Earlier signs of DIC may include more subtle changes. They include mental status changes, restlessness, confusion, dyspnea, and hypotension (Dolan, 1991).

Diagnosis of DIC may be difficult but is made on the basis of a combination of clinical symptoms, history, and a variety of laboratory studies. Lab findings in DIC include prolonged prothrombin time (PT), partial thromboplastin time (PTT), and thrombin time (TT); elevated levels of FSPs; and decreased levels of fibrinogen, plasminogen, platelets, and antithrombin III (Table 12–7).

Table 12–6. SYMPTOMS OF DIC

Oozing or bleeding from venipuncture sites, incisions, wounds
Bleeding around tubes: endotracheal, nasotracheal or nasogastric, urethral catheters
Bleeding from mucosal surfaces/body orifices: epistaxis, hematemesis, hemoptysis, melena, hematochezia, hematuria; gingival, scleral bleeding
Skin: ecchymoses, petechiae, pallor, mottling
Neurological: headache, altered level of consciousness, vertigo, lethargy, irritability, confusion, restlessness, focal deficits, seizures, coma
Cardiovascular: hypotension, tachycardia, ST-T wave changes
Renal: oliguria, hematuria
Gastrointestinal: abdominal pain, distention, hyperactive or absent bowel sounds
Other: anxiety, dyspnea, muscle weakness, fatigue, acral cyanosis, acidosis, hematomas, signs of thrombophlebitis

Table 12–7. LABORATORY FINDINGS IN DIC

Test	Alteration
Platelet count	Decreased
Prothrombin time (PT)	Prolonged
Partial thromboplastin time (PTT)	Prolonged
Thrombin time (TT)	Prolonged
Fibrinogen	Decreased
Plasminogen	Decreased
Fibrin split products (FSPs)	Increased
Antithrombin III	Decreased

Medical/Nursing Management

Medical treatment of DIC is aimed at treating the underlying cause, stopping the abnormal coagulation, and controlling bleeding (Table 12–8). Correction of hypotension, hypoxemia, and acidosis is vital, as is treatment of infection. Crystalloid intravenous fluids such as lactated Ringer's solution or normal saline are given to counteract hypovolemia from blood loss.

Heparin is sometimes given in DIC to interfere with the effects of thrombin, though its use is controversial (Dolan, 1991; Thelan et al., 1990; Young, 1990). The use of heparin is aimed at preventing further clotting and thrombosis that may lead to organ ischemia and necrosis. While

Table 12–8. MEDICAL TREATMENT OF DIC

Correct underlying problem
1. IV fluids, pharmacological therapy, respiratory and cardiovascular support to correct hypotension, infection, hypoxemia, acidosis, shock, electrolyte disturbances

Stop abnormal coagulation
1. Heparin to interfere with thrombin—bolus followed by continuous or intermittent infusion (controversial)
2. Antithrombin III to inhibit thrombin (investigational)

Control bleeding/restore hemostasis
1. Blood component therapy (platelets, FFP, cryoprecipitate) to replace platelets, clotting factors
2. Stabilize formed clots—aminocaproic acid used with caution to inhibit fibrinolysis

Treat/prevent complications
1. Blood components to correct anemia from hemorrhage
2. Cardiovascular and respiratory support to maintain cardiac output, optimal gas exchange, and tissue perfusion

Table 12–9. BLOOD AND BLOOD COMPONENT ADMINISTRATION GUIDE

Blood Component	Actions(s)	Administration/ Filter Set	Infusion Rate	Select Instructions
Whole Blood (WB)				
Stored WB	Increases blood volume and oxygen-carrying capacity of the blood.	Blood filter (170 μ)	2–4 hr	Gently but thoroughly mix WB by inverting bag several times to give a uniform suspension before administration. Infuse very slowly for first 15 min; observe patient for adverse reactions. Adjust infusion rate to infuse in 2 hr, unless patient's condition warrants slower infusion. Infusion should not take longer than 4 hr.
Fresh WB	Same as for stored WB; also provides platelets and clotting factors.	Component filter	2–4 hr	Same as for stored WB. If FWB is being used for viable platelets, use a component/platelet infusion administration set so that the platelets will be adequately maintained and transfused.
Red Blood Cells (RBCs)				
Packed RBCs	Increases oxygen-carrying capacity of the blood.	Blood filter	2–4 hr	Same as WB, except do not mix. When RBCs are prepared from a single plastic bag, they must be transfused within 24 hr. RBCs prepared in double plastic bags using a closed system have the same dating period as an original container of whole blood.
Fresh-Frozen RBCs	Same as for packed RBCs.	Blood filter	2–4 hr	Same as for packed RBCs.
Leukocyte-poor RBCs	Same as for packed RBCs.	Blood filter	2–4 hr	Same as for packed RBCs.
Platelet Concentrate	Increases platelet count; aids clot formation.	Component filter	Rapidly	Store at room temperature, and administer within 24 to 72 hr of preparation. Infuse concentrate rapidly, within 15 to 30 min. Check label on container, which specifies the number of units.
Fresh Frozen Plasma (FFP)	Raises clotting factor level.	Blood or component filter	Rapidly	Requires 30 min to thaw, notify blood bank early to facilitate preparation. Thus must be given within 6 hr of thawing.
Factor VIII				
Cryoprecipitated Antihemophilic Factor (cryo)	Raises factor VIII and XIII levels, prevents and controls bleeding in hemophilia A, hypofibrinogenemia.	Component filter	Rapidly	May not be refrozen. Administer rapidly, approximately 4 units (60 ml) in 15 min.
Antihemophilic Factor (AHF)	Same as for cryo.	Component filter	Rapidly	Refrigerate with diluent until used. Use within 60 min of preparation; administration should be completed 3 hr after mixing.
Granulocyte Transfusion (WBC)	Raises leukocyte level.	Platelet filter	2–6 hr (varies with each bag)	May be refrigerated for up to 24 hr without loss of effectiveness. Clear only with sodium chloride. Infuse over a 2- to 6-hr period; this depends upon the number of units in bag. Assess for infusion reaction; decrease infusion rate and call physician for orders. (Elevated temperature, rash, and chills are expected reactions.)

Table 12–9. BLOOD AND BLOOD COMPONENT ADMINISTRATION GUIDE *Continued*

Blood Component	Actions(s)	Administration/ Filter Set	Infusion Rate	Select Instructions
25% Normal Serum Albumin	Increases intravascular volume.	Special administration set with vial	Adjusted according to clinical response	Considered compatible with common IV solutions. Infuse carefully; adjust rate according to clinical response. This should be used cautiously in patients who are susceptible to volume overload. Because of the high osmotic power of this preparation, it can increase intravascular volume rapidly and result in congestive heart failure or pulmonary edema. Also, in patients with trauma or postoperative wounds bleeding may increase with the rise in intravascular pressure.
Plasma Protein Fraction	Increases intravascular volume and protein level.	Component filter	Adjusted according to clinical response	Compatible with most parenteral IV solutions. Infuse carefully, according to clinical response.

Microaggregate filters (20–40 μ) may be utilized in blood/blood component administration.
Potential Advantages:
1. Reduces febrile transfusion reactions.
2. Can be used for transfusion of multiple units (up to 10).
3. Can be used for transfusing all blood components.

Potential Disadvantages:
1. Increased cost for single unit transfusion.
2. Decreased flow rate with some types of microaggregate filters.

From Deloor, R.M., and Schreiber, M.J. The hematologic system. In: S. Millar, L.K. Sampson, and M. Soukop (eds.). *AACN Procedure Manual for Critical Care*. 2nd ed. Philadelphia, W.B. Saunders, 1985, pp. 410–430.

heparin's antithrombin activity prevents further clotting, it may increase the risk of bleeding, causing further problems.

Other pharmacological therapy in DIC may include the administration of aminocaproic acid (Amicar), which inhibits fibrinolysis by interfering with plasmin activity (Thelan et al., 1990). Aminocaproic acid is given in combination with heparin to prevent the lysis of existing clots, preventing the release of FSPs, and contributing to rapid cessation of hemorrhage. Another treatment being investigated for use in DIC is synthetic antithrombin III, which, like heparin, inhibits thrombin (Young, 1990).

Blood component therapy is used in DIC to replace deficient platelets and clotting factors as well as treat hemorrhage; and packed RBCs, whole blood, fresh frozen plasma, platelets, and cryoprecipitate may be given (Table 12–9). Transfusions of whole blood and packed RBCs are given to replace cells lost in hemorrhage. Fresh frozen plasma contains clotting factors V, VIII, XIII, and antithrombin III. Cryoprecipitate replaces fibrinogen and factor VIII.

Nursing care of the patient with DIC is aimed primarily toward the goals of prevention and recognition of thrombotic and hemorrhagic events. Continuous assessment for complications and aggressive interventions by the nurse will determine patient outcome. Psychosocial support of the patient and family, as in any critical illness, is of great importance.

Nursing diagnoses and interventions in DIC include altered tissue perfusion related to abnormal clotting and thrombosis (cerebral, peripheral, renal, and gastrointestinal), hypotension, or anemia; and decreased cardiac output related to fluid volume deficit and cardiac ischemia. Tissue perfusion and cardiac output can be assessed through monitoring vital signs, hemodynamic parameters, mental status, urine output, and cardiac rhythm. Peripheral pulses, capillary refill, and skin temperature and color should be assessed, as should bowel sounds.

Fluid Volume Deficit Related to Hemorrhage. The fluid volume deficit in patients with DIC should be assessed thoroughly and corrected by careful administration of fluids and blood components. Accurate intake and output measurements should be done hourly, including measurement of blood loss. Further bleeding should be prevented or promptly detected and controlled. To prevent further bleeding, skin integrity should be protected. Laboratory coagulation studies are to be carefully followed. Signs and symptoms of bleeding should be carefully monitored, including any oozing from venipunctures, catheters, incisions, mucous membranes, or body orifices. The nurse should assess urine, emesis, and stool for the presence of blood. Gastrointestinal function may be assessed through bowel sounds, the presence of nausea, vomiting, abdominal distention, or cramps. Skin should be assessed thoroughly for bruising or pressure areas. Careful cleaning and lubrication of the skin, frequent turning, and protection of pressure areas are necessary to keep skin intact. If possible, a flotation or air-fluidized mattress should be used. Suctioning should be performed only when necessary since even minimal pressure can cause trauma. Cuff blood pressures, including the use of noninvasive blood pressure machines, should be used as infrequently as possible. Rectal temperatures, suppositories, enemas, and douches should be avoided. Venipunctures and other needle sticks should also be avoided if possible; when necessary, only with small-gauge needles, and pressure should be held on sites for 10 minutes afterwards. Blood samples can be obtained through central lines, though placement of lines may also result in hemorrhage. Frequent oral hygiene with Toothettes or cotton swabs and normal saline rinses will help protect oral mucosa; toothbrushes and alcohol-containing solutions should not be used. An electric razor can be used if the patient must be shaved. Only paper tape should be used to avoid tissue trauma and bleeding on removal.

Impaired Gas Exchange Related to Pulmonary Ischemia (e.g., Pulmonary Embolism). Pulmonary function should be monitored to assess for impaired gas exchange. The patient's respiratory rate, depth, and pattern should be observed, and breath sounds auscultated to detect rales or rhonchi. Arterial blood gases should be monitored, and the patient should be assessed for restlessness, chest pain, or sputum production. Supplemental oxygen or ventilatory assistance should be administered as ordered, and the patient should be encouraged to turn, cough, and deep breathe and/or perform incentive spirometry as able.

Impaired Skin Integrity Related to Immobility, Trauma, and Invasive Procedures. As stated before, care should be taken to preserve integrity of the skin, and thorough assessment should be carried out frequently.

Anxiety Related to Fear of Dying, Procedures, and the Unknown. The patient with DIC and his/her family should be assessed for the level of anxiety and coping mechanisms available. Communication is to be encouraged, and feelings acknowledged. Involvement in the planning and implementation of care may return a sense of control. The nurse should be available to listen to, reassure, and support both patient and family. Information given should be accurate; false assurance is to be avoided. By maintaining an open, honest, and supportive environment, stress and anxiety may be lessened.

Alteration in Comfort: Pain Related to Tissue Ischemia, Bleeding into Tissues, and Therapeutic/Diagnostic Interventions. Pain relief and promotion of comfort may also diminish anxiety in the patient with DIC. The location, intensity, and quality of the patient's pain is to be assessed, along with the patient's response to discomfort. Pain medication should be offered as ordered, with attention to response to analgesics. Positioning with support and proper body alignment, with frequent changes, will also enhance the patient's level of comfort.

Thrombocytopenia

Pathophysiology

A quantitative deficiency of platelets is termed thrombocytopenia, and is a common cause of severe hemorrhage if not corrected. The pathophysiology may be related to decreased production of platelets by the bone marrow, increased destruction, or sequestration (abnormal distribution). Decreased production may result from bone marrow depression by toxic or chemotherapeutic agents, radiation, infection, or disorders such as aplastic anemia. Destruction of platelets is caused by their overconsumption, as occurs in DIC, or immune disorders. Prosthetic heart valves, extracorporeal circulation, and balloon counterpulsation may also damage platelets.

Clinical Manifestations

Clinically, the patient with thrombocytopenia presents with petechiae, purpura, and ecchymosis, with oozing from mucous membranes. Laboratory findings reveal a platelet count below 150,000. When the count is less than 50,000, bleeding may occur after injury or surgery. When the count drops below 20,000, spontaneous bleeding may occur. Fatal hemorrhage through the gastrointestinal tract or central nervous system is a great risk when the count is less than 5000 (Bullock, 1988d).

Medical/Nursing Management

Medical treatment of thrombocytopenia includes infusions of platelets to maintain hemostasis, steroids if the cause is an autoimmune disease, and splenectomy if refractory (Belcher, 1989). Nursing diagnoses, goals, and interventions are similar to those used for DIC.

White Clot Syndrome. This is a phenomenon also known as heparin-induced or heparin-associated thrombocytopenia (Kuhar and Hill, 1991). Though a rare complication of heparin therapy, the seriousness of the syndrome warrants suspicion when a patient on antiembolic drug therapy presents with multiple emboli. The disorder gets its name from the "white clot" aggregates of platelets and fibrin. It is thought to be an immune-mediated response, and is not dose related. Clinical signs of this disorder include symptoms of thrombosis (e.g., changes in extremity pulse, color, or temperature), a platelet count of less than 120,000, and a positive platelet aggregation test. Treatment is immediate cessation of heparin therapy. Other anticoagulants, such as warfarin sodium (Coumadin), aspirin, dipyridamole (Persantine), or dextran, may be substituted if necessary (Kuhar and Hill, 1991).

Other Coagulation Disorders

In addition to DIC and thrombocytopenia, several other disorders are seen in critical care areas that predispose patients to bleeding. They include vitamin K deficiency, liver disease, hemophilia, and von Willebrand's disease. Patients who receive massive transfusions of stored blood or packed cells also are at risk for developing coagulation problems.

Vitamin K Deficiency

Vitamin K is a fat-soluble vitamin that is not stored in the body, and thus is dependent on diet and absorption. It is essential in the formation of several of the clotting factors. Vitamin K deficiency may result from malabsorption, lack of intake, or liver disease. Laboratory studies reveal prolonged PT and PTT, though administration of vitamin K will correct abnormalities in 12 to 24 hours (Jackson and Jones, 1988a). The underlying cause of the deficiency should be treated, and supplements administered as necessary.

Liver Disease

One of the most common causes of bleeding disorders is liver disease (Jackson and Jones, 1988a). The patient with liver disease has an impaired ability to synthesize clotting factors, especially those that are vitamin K dependent. Portal hypertension may lead to enlargement of the spleen and sequestration of platelets, further contributing to bleeding tendency. A prolonged PT is found in laboratory studies; PTT may also be prolonged, and most clotting factors reduced. Treatment includes administration of fresh frozen plasma to replace clotting factors; platelets may also be necessary. Vitamin K may be given parenterally since malabsorption is common.

Massive Transfusions, Hemophilia, and von Willebrand's Disease

Hemorrhaging patients who receive only packed cells, stored whole blood, and crystalloid/colloid fluids lack replacement of labile clotting factors and platelets (Parrillo, 1991). Fresh frozen plasma and platelet infusions must also be given to maintain hemostasis (see Table 12–9). Hemophilia and von Willebrand's disease are hereditary disorders in which factor VIII is deficient. Treatment is based on local measures to control bleeding and factor replacement.

Nursing management is similar for any bleeding or coagulation disorder; see Nursing Care of the Patient with a Bleeding Disorder.

Review of Immunological Anatomy and Physiology

The body's ability to resist and fight infection is termed immunity. Our bodies are constantly exposed to bacteria, viruses, fungi, and parasites (some of which are normally present on the skin and many mucous membranes) that are capable of causing disease. In the healthy individual, an

NURSING CARE PLAN FOR THE PATIENT WITH A BLEEDING DISORDER		
Nursing Diagnosis	**Outcome**	**Intervention**
Altered tissue perfusion related to abnormal clotting, hypotension, and/or anemia	Maintain adequate perfusion and prevent damage to vital organs as evidenced by: Vital signs and hemodynamics stable and within normal limits Normal mental status ABGs within normal limits Urine output >30 ml/hr Absence of cardiac dysrhythmias Adequate peripheral pulses, skin warm with normal color	Monitor hemodynamics, vital signs, ECG, ABGs, I&O, and lab studies Provide good skin and oral care to promote circulation Assess for and report signs of altered perfusion: Cardiovascular: dysrhythmias, angina, hypotension, murmurs, tachycardia, dyspnea Cerebral: decreased level of consciousness, restlessness, confusion, irritability, pupillary changes, reflexes Pulmonary: dyspnea, tachypnea, rales/rhonchi, cyanosis, hemoptysis Renal: decreased urine output, hematuria GI: abdominal pain, distention, nausea/vomiting, hyperactive or absent bowel sounds, hematemesis, hematochezia/melena Peripheral: pallor, acral cyanosis, mottling, ecchymoses, petechiae, absence of or diminished pulses, edema Administer medical treatment per orders and observe response: Vasoactive, antiarrhythmic drugs Respiratory support; oxygen Antibiotics Heparin, aminocaproic acid Blood component therapy
Fluid volume deficit related to hemorrhage	Patient will be free of bleeding and normovolemic as evidenced by: Absence of oozing/bleeding Lab studies within normal limits Vital signs and hemodynamics stable and within normal limits	Monitor hemodynamics, vital signs, I&O, and lab studies Weigh dressings/linens to estimate blood loss Check body fluids for occult blood Assess for, note presence and degree, and report signs of bleeding: General: oozing or bleeding from venipunctures, intravenous access sites, incisions, wounds, mucous membranes and body orifices Cardiovascular: dysrhythmias, hypotension, murmurs, tachycardia, dyspnea Cerebral: decreased level of consciousness, restlessness, confusion, irritability, pupillary changes, reflexes abnormal Pulmonary: dyspnea, tachypnea, rales/rhonchi, cyanosis, hemoptysis Renal: decreased urine output, hematuria GI: abdominal pain, distention, nausea/vomiting, hyperactive or absent bowel sounds, hematemesis, hematochezia/melena Peripheral: hematomas, pallor, cyanosis, mottling, ecchymoses, petechiae, edema, bone and joint pain Control bleeding: Ice packs, pressure dressings or direct pressure over bleeding sites Leave existing clots undisturbed Topical hemostatic agents as ordered Prevent trauma Provide frequent, gentle skin and oral care Avoid venipunctures, injections, cuff BPs, rectal/vaginal exams, or medications Frequent position changes; air or flotation mattress; sheep skins Electric razor only Stool softeners, soft diet

NURSING CARE PLAN FOR THE PATIENT WITH A BLEEDING DISORDER *Continued*

Nursing Diagnosis	Outcome	Intervention
		Administer medical treatment per orders and observe response Aminocaproic acid Blood component therapy
Anxiety related to fear of death/procedure/unknown	Behavior reflects diminished level of anxiety Patient/family able to state verbal understanding of disease process and treatments; verbalize questions, fears, anxieties Patient/family participate in planning and implementation of care	Provide emotional support; develop rapport with patient and family; be available to patient and family; maintain open lines of communication; be honest, avoid false reassurance Assess level of anxiety, knowledge of disease process, and treatments Educate patient/family about disease process, treatments Explain procedures Involve patient/family in planning and implementation of care Use relaxation/imagery techniques; keep stressors to minimum Support positive coping mechanisms
Alteration in comfort: pain related to bleeding, altered tissue perfusion, procedures	Maintain optimum comfort; relieve pain as evidenced by verbal statements and behavioral clues of relief of pain	Assess location, intensity, duration, and quality of pain Administer analgesics as ordered/needed; observe response Position patient for comfort using proper body alignment, pillows for support, and padding pressure areas Use heat/cold treatments as warranted Provide quiet, calm, reassuring environment Remain with patient during procedures; allow family to as appropriate

intact and responsive immune system provides adequate protection. But the person whose immune system is not functioning properly is at risk for overwhelming, life-threatening infection. Such factors as disease, age, stress, and therapy can compromise an individual's immune system, providing an inadequate defense.

In critical care, patients' immune systems are often compromised by disease, procedures, and medications. Infectious disease processes can overwhelm the body's ability to "fight back." Diagnostic and therapeutic interventions such as invasive and surgical procedures put the patient at risk for infection. Additionally, many of the drugs and treatments administered can depress patients' immune systems. In the case of organ transplants, this immunosuppression is done purposely, but can result in the patient's inability to fight infection.

Critical care nurses' understanding of the normal immune system and its proper response to assault is paramount to good assessment skills and use of therapeutic interventions.

CONCEPTS IN IMMUNOLOGY

To understand immune physiology, the critical care nurse should have a working knowledge of a few key concepts. They include antigen, self versus nonself, tolerance, autoimmunity, and specificity.

An antigen is any substance that is capable of stimulating an immune response in the host. Under normal circumstances, an antigen is foreign to the host. Microorganisms (bacteria, viruses, fungi, and parasites), abnormal or mutated cells, foreign or transplanted cells, and foreign molecules (e.g., penicillin) can act as antigens (Miller and Habicht, 1991). An antigen is seen by the body as being foreign, or "nonself." The body normally protects cells or molecules that it senses as being "self," and attempts to destroy that that is nonself. The body distinguishes between self and nonself by the particular structure of proteins that are determined by chromosomes. Self can be recognized as nonself if it undergoes mutation, is in an abnormal location, or changes structure (Fidler, 1988).

The body's response to an antigen is determined by a number of factors, such as genetics, amount of antigen, and route of exposure (Miller and Habicht, 1991). Once a substance is recognized as an antigen, the body puts its natural and acquired defenses into action to destroy the invader and prevent disease.

Tolerance is the body's ability to recognize self as self, and therefore protect it. In autoimmunity, the body for some reason attacks self as nonself (i.e., has no tolerance), and an immune response is activated against body tissues. Autoimmunity can result from injury to tissues, infection, or malignancy. An example of an autoimmune disease is systemic lupus erythematosus (SLE).

Specificity refers to the fact that an immune response stimulates cells to develop immunity for a specific antigen (Fidler, 1988). B Lymphocytes are sensitized and produce antibodies that recognize, react with, and destroy only the specific antigens that they were synthesized in response to.

Whereas a *specific* immune response refers to the sensitization of lymphocytes and production of antibodies, *nonspecific* defenses include the processes of phagocytosis and inflammation. In *active* immunity, the body actively produces cells and mediators that result in the destruction of the antigen. *Passive* immunity is that which is transferred from another person (e.g., maternal antibodies transferred to the newborn through the placenta and breast milk).

ORGANS INVOLVED IN IMMUNOLOGICAL FUNCTION

The immune system is diffuse—it functions throughout the body and involves several different cells and organs. The lymphoreticular system consists of lymphoid tissue, lymphatic cells, and phagocytic cells in the body that engulf and process foreign materials to protect the body from invasion. The organs included in the lymphoreticular system are the bone marrow, thymus, lymph nodes, spleen, and liver (Fidler, 1988).

All blood cells are produced in the bone marrow, including those involved in immune defenses. The bone marrow is thought to be the site of maturation of B lymphocytes, which provide humoral immunity through antibody formation. The main function of the thymus is the maturation of T lymphocytes, which are involved in cellular immunity. It is located in the anterior mediastinum just beneath the sternum. The thymus is the central organ of the lymphatic system, and is largest during puberty, after which it begins to shrink. Lymph nodes are small, bean-shaped structures located in the head, neck, axillae, groin, and abdomen; they are connected by lymphatic vessels. Their function is to filter and cleanse interstitial fluid and circulate lymphocytes.

The blood is filtered in the spleen; foreign material, dead or abnormal cells, and debris are removed by phagocytes. The spleen also stimulates B and T lymphocytes to proliferate, differentiate, and produce antibodies in response to antigenic material that has been trapped, recognized, and processed. The liver also acts as a filter through phagocytosis—blood is cleansed of bacteria and foreign material absorbed from the gut (Fidler, 1988).

CELLS INVOLVED IN IMMUNOLOGICAL FUNCTION

Leukocytes, or white blood cells, are essential in the body's defense against invasion by foreign organisms. Both granulocytes and nongranulocytes are vital to immunity. The characteristics and functions of granulocytes (neutrophils, eosinophils, and basophils) and nongranulocytes (monocytes and lymphocytes) were discussed fully in the hematological anatomy and physiology review section.

IMMUNE MECHANISMS

An intact and healthy immune system consists of both natural, or nonspecific, defenses and acquired, or specific, defenses. The nonspecific defenses are the first line of protection; when they fail to protect the body from invasion, the specific defenses are put into action.

Nonspecific Defenses

The body's nonspecific defenses consist of physical and chemical barriers to invasion, the protective and repairing processes of inflammation and phagocytosis, and other substances that stimulate the body to fight back.

Epithelial Surfaces

The body's first line of defense against infection are physical and chemical barriers. The epithelial surfaces are those that are exposed to the environment and already colonized by a "normal" bacterial flora. These normal flora help to protect the body from pathogens; because they are attached to the epithelial surfaces, they prevent pathogens from doing so and gaining access to the body (Fidler, 1988).

Intact skin and mucous membranes provide a protective covering; they also secrete substances that have antimicrobial effects. For instance, sweat glands produce lysozyme, an antimicrobial enzyme, and sebaceous glands secrete sebum, which has antimicrobial and antifungal properties. The skin is also constantly exfoliating, which sloughs off bacterial and chemical hazards.

The pH of the skin and mucosae of the gastrointestinal and urinary tracts inhibits growth of many pathogens. Secretory immunoglobulin A (IgA) (an antibody) and phagocytic cells are present in respiratory and gastrointestinal secretions. In the respiratory tract, mucus and cilia work together to trap and remove harmful substances. Macrophages present in the alveoli engulf and destroy pathogens. The motility of the intestines maintains an even distribution of bacterial flora, preventing overgrowth and invasion, and promoting evacuation of pathogens (Fidler, 1988).

Inflammation and Phagocytosis

The second line of defense involves the processes of inflammation and phagocytosis. Inflammation is initiated by cellular injury, and is necessary for tissue repair, but can be harmful if uncontrolled. When cellular injury occurs, specific substances are released that act as mediators; they include histamine, serotonin, kinins, lysosomal enzymes, prostaglandin, clotting factors, and complement, which is a series of proteins that act in a cascade fashion to enhance the immune and inflammatory responses (Bullock, 1988a). These mediators increase blood flow, capillary permeability, and vasodilation, and promote chemotaxis and phagocytosis of neutrophils. The signs of inflammation, heat, pain, redness, and swelling are caused by these responses (Fidler, 1988). Antibody activity, phagocytosis, and inflammation are enhanced by complement (Fidler and Keen, 1988).

Other Nonspecific Defenses

Pyrogen is a substance that is released in inflammation, especially from neutrophils; it is thought to inhibit the growth of pathogens and enzymatic reactions by increasing body temperature. Another nonspecific defense involves the substance interferon. Interferon is an immunological agent produced in viral infections that acts to inhibit viral replication; it is also used in the treatment of malignant disorders (Fidler, 1988).

Specific (Acquired) Defenses—the Immune Response

The immune response protects the body from disease by recognizing, processing, and destroying foreign invaders. It also aids in the removal of damaged body tissues and cells, and defends the body against the proliferation of abnormal or malignant cells. It involves the interaction of macrophages and B and T lymphocytes.

There are two "arms" to the immune response—humoral immunity and cell-mediated immunity. These two forms are not mutually exclusive; they act together to provide immunity (Miller and Habicht, 1991).

Humoral Immunity

Humoral immunity is mediated by B lymphocytes and involves the formation of antibodies in response to specific antigens. Antigens bind to receptors on B lymphocytes. This activates B cells and causes the proliferation and differentiation of

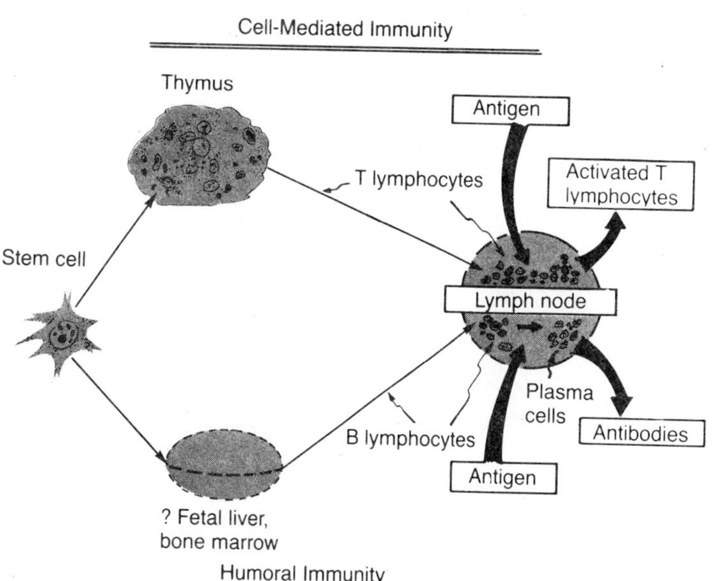

Figure 12–7. Formation of antibodies and sensitized lymphocytes in response to antigens. (From Guyton, A. C.: Textbook of Medical Physiology. 7th ed. Philadelphia, W. B. Saunders, Fig. 6-1, p. 61.)

plasma cells and the production of antibodies in response to specific antigens (Fig. 12–7). Once antibodies have been synthesized and released, they bind to their target antigen and form an antigen-antibody complex (Fig. 12–8). This complex is targeted for phagocytosis by neutrophils and macrophages. The antigen-antibody complex also activates complement. The humoral response and proliferation of B cells is regulated by the activity of T lymphocytes. Helper T cells promote B-lymphocyte activity and the production of antibodies, whereas suppressor T cells downgrade the humoral response (Fig. 12–9).

There are two phases in humoral immunity: the primary immune response and the secondary response. In the primary response, antigens that have evaded the nonspecific defenses are engulfed and processed by macrophages. The macrophages then present the processed antigens to the lymphocytes, which proliferate, differentiate, and produce antibodies. In this first exposure, antibodies appear in the serum after 7-10 days. Immunoglobulin M is the first antibody to appear, then IgG. The total antibody titer peaks around 21 days. It is in this primary response that the cells develop an immunological memory for antigens; this provides the basis for the secondary response on subsequent exposure (Bullock, 1988a; Fidler, 1988).

When a second or subsequent exposure to the antigen occurs, the secondary response occurs, which is much quicker, stronger, and longer lasting. Antibodies peak within 7 to 10 days and may be detectable in serum for years (Miller and Habicht, 1991).

Humoral immunity and antibodies can be passively transferred through serum. When an individual is deficient in B lymphocytes (such as in X-linked agammaglobulinemia and common variable immunodeficiency), sufficient antibodies cannot be produced, and the individual is at risk, especially for bacterial infections.

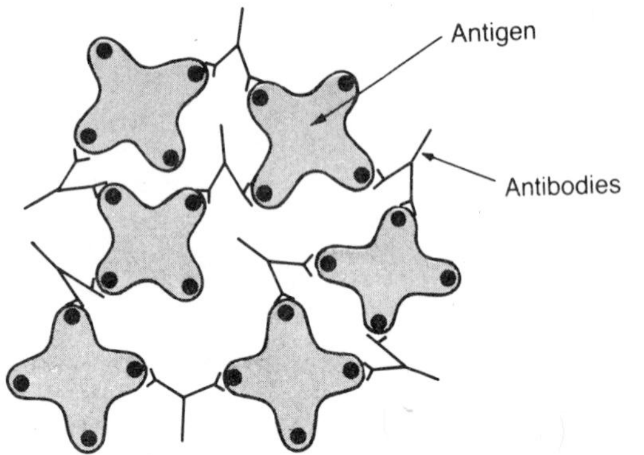

Figure 12–8. Binding of antigens and antibodies. (From Guyton, A. C.: Textbook of Medical Physiology. 7th ed. Philadelphia, W. B. Saunders, Fig. 6–4, p. 64.)

Immunoglobulins. Antibodies, also known as immunoglobulins (Ig), are produced in specific response to certain antigens. There are five classes of immunoglobulins: IgG, IgM, IgA, IgE, and IgD (Table 12–10).

The most abundant of the immunoglobulins is IgG, which is found in most body fluids. It is unique in that it crosses the placenta and provides passive immunity to the newborn through a variety of antibodies. Immunoglobulin G also activates and fixes complement, which enhances the effects of antibodies.

Immunoglobulin M is the first immunoglobulin synthesized in an immune response, with the titer rising before IgG. It is the largest antibody, and is present mostly in the blood stream. It causes agglutination, or the clumping together of antigenic particles, and also causes cell lysis.

Immunoglobulin A, also called secretory IgA, is an important part of the body's nonspecific first line of defense and prevention of disease. It is present in many secretions, such as saliva, sweat, tears, mucus, and breast milk. The breast-

Table 12–10. IMMUNOGLOBULINS

Immunoglobulin	Comments
G	Most abundant immunoglobulin (Ig) Present in intravascular and extravascular spaces Crosses placenta Coats microorganisms to enhance phagocytosis Activates complement system
M	First Ig produced in response to antigens Present mostly in intravascular space Activates complement system
A	Called secretory IgA—present in many body secretions: saliva, tears, sweat, mucus Protects epithelial surfaces Passes to newborn through colostrum and breast milk Activates complement system
E	Important in allergic and inflammatory responses; parasitic infections
D	Function/significance not well understood

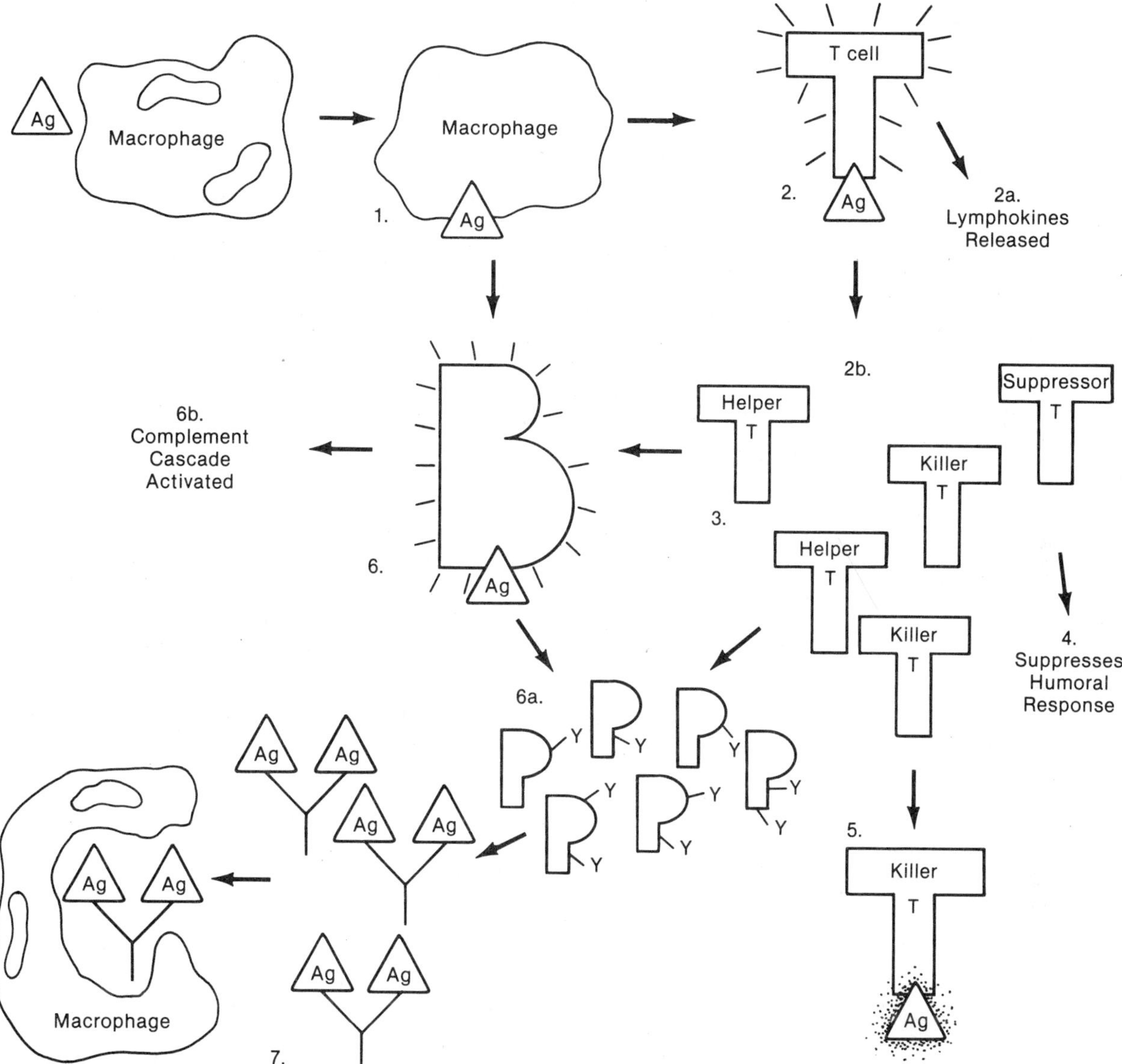

Figure 12–9. The immune response. *1,* Macrophages process antigen (Ag) and present to T lymphocytes. *2,* T Lymphocytes (T cells) recognize antigen—in response (*2a*) they release lymphokines (e.g., interleukin 2) and (*2b*) differentiate into helper T cells, suppressor T cells, and killer T cells. *3,* Helper T cells promote B-cell activity and antibody production. *4,* Suppressor T cells downgrade the humoral response. *5,* Killer T cells bind with and destroy antigens. *6,* B Lymphocytes (B cells) become activated after contact with antigen. *6a,* They proliferate and differentiate into antibody-producing plasma cells (P = plasma cells; Y = antibodies). *6b,* Activated B cells also activate complement. *7,* Antibodies bind with antigen, enhancing their phagocytosis and destruction by macrophages and neutrophils.

feeding infant receives protection from intestinal pathogens through ingestion of colostrum and breast milk. Immunoglobulin A inhibits the adherence of pathogens to epithelial cells by causing agglutination.

Immunoglobulin E is normally present in very low concentrations in the serum, but is important in allergic reactions. It binds with mast cells and basophils in epithelial surfaces effecting the release of histamine and vasoactive substances, resulting in allergic symptoms. Immunoglobulin E also plays an important role in the defense against parasitic infections.

The function of IgD is not understood, and has questionable significance in the immune response (Dolan, 1991).

Cell-Mediated Immunity

Cellular, or cell-mediated, immunity is more obscure than the humoral response. It is mediated by the T lymphocyte. When macrophages recognize foreign materials as being nonself, they trap, process, and present such materials to T lymphocytes. T Cells recognize these antigens processed by macrophages; they then proliferate, differentiate, and migrate to the site of the antigen, which is neutralized or destroyed. Differences between B and T lymphocytes are displayed in Table 12–11.

Once contact is made with a specific antigen, the T lymphocyte differentiates into T-helper (T_4) cells, T-suppressor (T_8) cells, and cytotoxic, or killer, cells (Bullock, 1988b). T-Helper cells enhance the humoral immune response by stimulating B cells to differentiate and produce antibodies. T-Suppressor cells downgrade and suppress the humoral response. In autoimmune diseases, there is a decreased activity of these suppressor cells, and an overactive immune response results in the attack on body tissues. The ratio of helper to suppressor T cells is normally 2:1; a normal immune response is dependent on the relationship between these two cells. An alteration in this ratio causes disease. For instance, a depressed ratio (a decrease of T-helper cells in relation to T-suppressor cells) is found in acquired immunodeficiency syndrome (AIDS), whereas a higher ratio (a decrease in T-suppressor cells) can be a feature of autoimmune disease (Miller and Habicht, 1991). Cytotoxic, or killer, T cells, participate directly in the destruction of antigens by binding to and altering the membrane surface, and disrupting the intracellular environment, which ultimately destroys the cell. Killer cells may also release a cytotoxic substance into the antigen cell that causes cell lysis (Bullock, 1988b). Another differentiated cell is known as the natural killer (NK) cell, and is thought to lyse virus-infected and neoplastic cells (Fidler, 1988).

T Lymphocytes also produce substances known as lymphokines, which, like the monokines secreted by macrophages, function as chemical communicators between cells involved in the immune response. Lymphokines cause chemotaxis and stimulate macrophage activity and the production of interferon (Fidler, 1988). An important lymphokine is interleukin-2, which bolsters the immune response (Fidler, 1988).

Additionally, T cells provide the body with immunosurveillance, in which they monitor blood, body fluids, and tissue for abnormal cells or tissue. It is this mechanism that is responsible for the rejection of transplanted tissue, which is recognized by T cells as nonself (Bullock, 1988b; Miller and Habicht, 1991).

Cell-mediated immunity cannot be transferred through serum; transfer takes place only through injection of sensitized T cells. Whereas humoral immunity is an immediate response, cell-mediated immunity is a more delayed reaction. It is important in viral, fungal, and intracellular infections, and is the mechanism involved in transplant rejection. Cell-mediated immunity is also important in the fight against neoplastic cells.

Table 12–11. COMPARISON OF B AND T LYMPHOCYTES

	B Lymphocyte	T Lymphocyte
Mediates	Humoral immunity	Cell-mediated immunity
Origin	Bone marrow	Bone marrow
Matures	Bursa of Fabricius in birds ? bone marrow	Thymus
Function	Immunoglobulin synthesis: IgG IgM IgA IgE IgD	Defense against viral, protozoan, and fungal infections Stimulates macrophages Regulates humoral response Transplant rejection Immunosurveillance for mutant or malignant cells
Transfer	By serum	Only through injection of cells

Selected Immunological Disorders

There are a number of pathological states that can alter the body's ability to fight disease. The immune system can fail to develop properly, lose its previous ability to react to invasion by pathogens, overreact to otherwise harmless antigens, or turn immune functions against self. Included in the long list of disorders of the immune system are hypersensitivity and anaphylaxis, autoimmune diseases, congenital immune disorders, acquired immune disorders, and malignant or neoplastic diseases of the lymphoid organs or tissues. However, in the intensive care unit, the predominant immune system problem seen is that of immunocompromise. This section will focus on the recognition and treatment of the immunocompromised patient.

IMMUNOCOMPROMISE

A nursing diagnosis seen frequently in critical care is "potential for infection" (see Nursing Care Plan for the Immunocompromised Patient).

Immunocompromise in the critically ill is caused by many factors. In addition to existing immunodeficiency diseases and life-threatening illness, immune defenses are altered by invasive monitoring, procedures, and the presence of opportunistic pathogens. These factors can worsen the patient's preexisting state or contribute to the development of new problems (Gurka, 1989).

Immune disorders can affect any or all of the various components of the immune system. Cell-mediated or humoral immune responses may be affected. The defect may be in the ability to phagocytize pathogens or in the complement cascade. Any defect in the immune system, whatever the component, will put the body at risk for disease.

Primary Immunodeficiency

Primary immune disorders or immunodeficiencies are those in which the primary dysfunction exists in the immune system (Golightly, 1991). Most primary immunodeficiencies are congenital; there is a failure of some part of the immune system to develop (Bullock, 1988b). Many disorders fall into this category (Table 12-12).

When the deficiency is in the stem cell, both humoral and cell-mediated immunity will be diminished or absent, as in severe combined immunodeficiency disease. A congenital humoral disorder results in a deficient production of immunoglobulin, and manifests itself through recurrent, severe, or unusual infections with extracellular bacteria (Fidler and Keen, 1988). X-Linked agammaglobulinemia and common variable immunodeficiency are examples of congenital humoral defects. When the defect is in cell-mediated immunity or the T cell, the patient has an impaired defense against fungi and intracellular microorganisms, as in DiGeorge's syndrome. Other primary disorders affect the function of complement or phagocytosis (Bullock, 1988b; Golightly, 1991). Complement defects diminish the activity of antibodies, phagocytes, and the process of inflammation. Phagocytic defects can result in an inadequate number or dysfunction of phagocytic cells (Fidler and Keen, 1988).

Table 12-12. PRIMARY AND SECONDARY IMMUNODEFICIENCIES

Primary	
B cell defects	X-Linked agammaglobulin of Bruton Common variable immunodeficiency IgA deficiency
T cell defects	DiGeorge's syndrome Nezelof's syndrome
Combined defects	Severe combined immunodeficiency disease (SCID) Ataxia-telangiectasia (AT)
Phagocytic defects	
Complement defects	
Secondary	
Infections	Measles, tuberculosis, acute viral, cytomegalovirus (CMV), HIV (AIDS)
Malignancies	Hodgkin's disease, acute and chronic leukemias, multiple myeloma
Autoimmune states	Systemic lupus erythematosus (SLE), rheumatoid arthritis (RA)
Diseases	Diabetes mellitus, renal disease, alcoholic cirrhosis
Drugs	Cytotoxic agents (chemotherapeutics, immunosuppressants), antibiotics, phenytoin
Other	Aging, stress, malnutrition, radiation, anesthesia

Secondary Immunodeficiency

In a secondary immunodeficiency, the immune disorder is the result of factors outside the immune system, and involves the loss of a previously functional immune defense. Also known as acquired immunodeficiency, secondary immunodeficiency causes include stress, aging, malnutrition, malignancies, chronic disease, pharmacological agents (e.g., chemotherapeutics, immunosuppressants), and infectious diseases such as AIDS (Bullock, 1988b; Dattwyler, 1991) (see Table 12-12).

Stress

When the body is under stress, physical or emotional, its ability to fight disease is affected. The mechanism is not well understood, but the increased release of adrenal hormones plays a part (Fidler and Keen, 1988). Serious illness, noise, lights, constant activity, procedures, and equipment are patient stressors in critical care units. Social factors such as bereavement, job loss, or divorce are stressors, as are pathological conditions such as tuberculosis, myocardial infarction, diabetes, and malignancy (Fidler and Keen, 1988). Surgery also causes stress, and many anes-

NURSING CARE PLAN FOR THE IMMUNOCOMPROMISED PATIENT

Nursing Diagnosis	Outcome	Intervention
Potential for infection related to immunocompromise or immunosuppression, invasive procedures, presence of opportunistic pathogens	Patient remains free of infection as evidenced by absence of fever, redness, swelling, pain, and heat; lab studies (WBC and differential, urinalysis, cultures) within normal limits; chest x-ray without infiltrates, absence of adventitious breath sounds	Establish baseline assessment with documented history, physical exam, and lab studies Assess patient for signs/symptoms of infection Vital signs with temperature at least every 4 hr—any elevation in temperature to be reported and investigated Monitor labs: WBC and differential, blood, urine, sputum, wound, and throat cultures; report abnormal results Note presence of chills, tachycardia, dysuria Pulmonary: observe for cough, sputum production, dyspnea; monitor ABGs for hypoxemia; assess breath sounds at least every 4 hr; monitor chest x-ray for infiltrates, changes; obtain sputum cultures as indicated Skin/mucous membranes/wound: observe mouth, skin, perineum, axillae, areas of pressure, breakdown, or excoriation, presence of lesions; note any pain, redness, swelling, pus formation, or heat at venipuncture, IV, wound, or incision sites; culture areas as indicated Prevent infection Strict handwashing before, during, and after any patient contact Promote optimal nutrition and hydration Pulmonary: encourage incentive spirometry every 1 hr; position changes and pulmonary toilet every 2 hr; chest physiotherapy and postural drainage; use strict aseptic technique for suctioning Skin/mucous membranes/wounds: avoid breaks in skin/mucous membrane integrity; provide meticulous skin care, keeping all areas clean, dry, and lubricated as appropriate; position changes every 2 hr; meticulous oral hygiene with nonirritating solutions and soft bristled brush; dressing changes as ordered to wound, incision, and invasive line sites, using strict aseptic technique Limit number of invasive devices/procedures as able (e.g., IV, central, Foley catheters); use strict aseptic technique when devices necessary Use private room and reverse isolation as necessary; limit number of visitors; restrict visitors/caregivers to those without infection; use gown, masks, gloves as needed Provide diet of well-cooked foods, avoid fresh fruits or vegetables if patient is neutropenic Keep room uncluttered and well cleaned; no standing water sources; discard any open containers or unused fluid solutions
Impaired skin/mucous membrane integrity related to immobility, invasive devices and procedures, dehydration, malnutrition, immunosuppression	Patient's skin and mucous membranes remain intact; will be absent of signs of pressure areas, breakdown, lesions, excoriation; skin turgor and moisture of mucous membranes will remain adequate; will remain free of signs of infection	Assess for alterations in integrity Skin and mucous membranes every shift for signs of pressure, breakdown, lesions, and excoriation Monitor incisions, IV and venipuncture sites, axillae, perineal areas, and so forth, for redness, swelling, pain, heat Prevent alterations in integrity Provide meticulous skin care; keep skin clean, dry, and lubricated Provide frequent mouth care with nonirritating solutions and soft bristled brush; maintain moisture of mucous membranes Turn/reposition the patient at least every 2 hr and PRN Use air-fluidized/alternating pressure mattresses, or eggcrate mattresses/pad bony prominences and pressure points

NURSING CARE PLAN FOR THE IMMUNOCOMPROMISED PATIENT *Continued*

Nursing Diagnosis	Outcome	Intervention
		Treat any pressure ulcers or areas of breakdown promptly; provide protection from further damage Maintain adequate hydration and optimal nutritional status Assist with mobility as able
Alteration in nutrition: less than body requirements related to NPO status (ET or NG tubes, surgery), anorexia, nausea/vomiting, painful oral mucosa	Patient will maintain optimal nutritional status as evidenced by adequate caloric and protein intake; ideal/stable body weight; laboratory values will remain within normal limits (total protein, serum albumin, electrolytes, hemoglobin, and hematocrit)	Assess baseline nutritional status Height and weight Laboratory values Presence of weakness, fatigue, infection, or other signs of malnutrition, food preferences, and deterrents to adequate intake of protein and calories Prevent alteration in nutrition Obtain dietary consult to determine nutrients/intake required Establish food preferences Determine deterrents to adequate intake: NPO status, presence of, e.g., anorexia, nausea, vomiting, stomatitis Monitor daily weight, lab values, protein and caloric intake, I&O Encourage small, frequent, high-calorie and high-protein meals Provide meticulous mouth care before and after meals Encourage meals from home/significant others and relaxed atmosphere/socialization during meals Administer antiemetics as needed, 30 min prior to meals Assess need for enteral/parenteral nutritional therapy; administer as ordered and observe response
Knowledge deficit related to disease process, critical routines/procedures/treatments, immunosuppressive therapy	Patient verbalizes understanding of disease process, treatments, medication regimens	Assess patient's level of understanding and ability to comprehend information, readiness to learn Orient patient to critical care unit, routines, procedures Instruct patient/significant others about diagnosis, treatments, medications, need for optimal nutrition and adherence to medication regimen Answer questions promptly and honestly; maintain atmosphere of mutual respect and approachability; be available to patient and family to answer questions Reinforce patient education and compliance with plan of care

thetics used in surgery further depress the immune response.

Age

The very young and very old are immunocompromised. The newborn is protected by maternal antibodies up to several weeks or months, but then becomes susceptible to infection until it develops a competent immune system of its own. Elderly patients have diminished immunity. With age, thymus involution results in a decreased cell-mediated immunity. Antibody production and response diminishes, and immune memory is also affected. The incidence of autoimmune and malignant diseases also increases (Gurka, 1989).

Malnutrition

Malnutrition affects the ability to fight disease. Especially in protein and caloric deficiencies, there is a decrease in immunocompetent white blood cells. Cell-mediated immunity and complement activity are particularly diminished. The thymus gland and lymph nodes atrophy, particularly in the presence of iron deficiency (Gurka, 1989). The malnourished patient is more susceptible to infection, especially by fungi, viruses, and intracellular bacteria (Fidler and Keen, 1988). In critical care, malnutrition is common. Inadequate intake caused by endotracheal tubes, nasogastric suction, or surgical status as well as anorexia, nausea, and vomiting caused by drugs, treatment, or illness contribute to malnutrition in the critically ill.

Malignancy

Malignancies, or neoplastic diseases, that cause secondary immunodeficiency include Burkitt's lymphoma, chronic lymphocytic leukemia, acute leukemia, multiple myeloma, and Hodgkin's disease. In these and other malignancies, therapeutic treatment such as chemotherapy and radiation also severely compromise immunity (Golightly and Dolan, 1991). Radiation destroys both B and T lymphocytes and causes shrinkage of lymphoid tissue. The resulting decreased resistance to infection may last for a year or longer (Dattwyler, 1991; Fidler and Keen, 1988). Chemotherapy also causes a decrease in lymphocytes. Most chemotherapeutic drugs alter the proliferation and differentiation of stem cells, which results in decreased white blood cells (Gurka, 1989).

Chronic Disease

Most patients with chronic disease are in a debilitated state, which places them at risk for infection. In renal disease or renal failure, a decrease in circulating lymphocytes is seen. This in conjunction with the presence of uremic toxins, acidosis, and malnutrition often seen depresses the immune response (Golightly, 1991; Gurka, 1989). Diabetes also results in an increased susceptibility to infection. High blood sugars, neuropathy, and vascular insufficiency contribute to this increased risk (Bullock, 1988b).

Pharmacological Agents

Drugs other than chemotherapeutics can cause immune system depression. The chronic abuse of alcohol results in a decrease in granulocytes and diminished cell-mediated immunity. Antibiotics can alter the normal bacterial flora of the gastrointestinal and respiratory tracts, which allows pathogenic organisms to attach and invade more easily. Steroids cause an increase in neutrophils while decreasing monocytes and eosinophils. They also may diminish production of IgG. When used on a long-term basis, cell-mediated immunity is impaired. Interleukin-2 is decreased, and the migration of T lymphocytes and macrophages is affected (Dattwyler, 1991).

Therapeutic Immunosuppression

In transplantation, immunosuppression is the ultimate goal, preventing the body from recognizing the transplanted tissue as nonself, or foreign. Advances in immunosuppressive drug therapy have improved the survival and quality of life for transplant recipients. Though the drugs may vary somewhat depending on the tissue or organ transplanted, kidney, bone marrow, heart, lung, liver, and pancreas transplants all require some degree of immunosuppression. Drugs used for immunosuppression include corticosteroids, antimetabolites, monoclonal and polyclonal antibodies, and others such as cyclosporine. Corticosteroids affect lymphocytes, especially T cells. Thus, their chronic use impairs cell-mediated immunity. An antimetabolite used in transplants is azathioprine (Imuran), which seems to primarily affect T cells. Antibodies used are those that have been synthesized in animals injected with human blood cells. Antilymphocyte serum (ALS) suppresses humoral and cell-mediated immunity; antithymocyte globulin (ALG) depresses primarily T cells. OKT3, a monoclonal antibody, is also used to depress T-cell function. Cyclosporine (CSA) is another immunosuppressant; it inhibits T-lymphocyte function but leaves humoral immunity and phagocytosis intact (Dattwyler, 1991).

Besides placing the patient at greater risk for infection, immunosuppressants have other deleterious side effects, and require close nursing supervision during administration. Monitoring for patient response and side effects is very important.

Infectious Diseases

There are a number of infectious diseases that result in immunocompromise. Measles, tuberculosis, acute viral infections, and cytomegalovirus (CMV) are examples. Acquired immunodeficiency syndrome, or AIDS, is currently one of the nation's greatest health problems.

AIDS. Presently an incurable, fatal disease, AIDS has become an epidemic in this country. Nurses see AIDS in all settings of health care, including critical care. AIDS also exists as a "hidden" disease, since many individuals may have been exposed or carry the disease unknowingly (for example, patients who received blood transfusions prior to 1985). Though the incidence of AIDS continues to climb, these patients are living longer with a better quality of life because of advances in treatment.

AIDS was first recognized as a syndrome in 1981, when the Centers for Disease Control (CDC) reported an increased incidence of a rare pneumonia and cancer in homosexual males. By 1982, the syndrome was noted to affect those other than homosexuals; patients with hemophilia A were infected. In 1984, the causative virus was isolated by a physician in California, and named human T-cell leukemia/lymphoma virus (HTLV-3). At the same time, the virus was discovered in France, and named lymphadenopathy-associated virus (LAV). The virus was renamed human immunodeficiency virus (HIV) in 1987 (Coletti et al., 1989).

Pathophysiology. AIDS affects the body's immune response; it is manifested by recurrent opportunistic infections and/or rare malignancies that are seldom seen in immunocompetent individuals. AIDS is primarily a dysfunction of cell-mediated immunity, as the HIV virus causes a deficiency in T_4 (T-helper) lymphocytes. T_4 Lymphocytes are infected by the HIV virus, which then reproduces within and kills the lymphocyte (Fidler and Keen, 1988). HIV also infects cells in the brain, spinal cord, and peripheral nerves (Holloway, 1988; Scherer, 1990).

HIV, a retrovirus, replicates in the T-helper cells. A retrovirus is a virus that transcribes its genetic material, RNA, into DNA by using an enzyme called reverse transcriptase. HIV does not survive long outside the body. The virus is transmitted through intimate contact with body fluids, blood, or blood products. This transmission can occur through rectal or vaginal intercourse with an infected person, intravenous drug use with contaminated equipment, transfusion with contaminated blood or blood products, accidental exposure through needle sticks or breaks in the skin, or from mother to fetus during gestation or childbirth (Table 12–13). Transmission via breast-feeding has occurred but is rare (Barrick, 1990). Transmission is dose related, and is not known to be spread by casual contact (Ceccio, 1988). The virus must enter the blood stream to cause infection (Barrick, 1990). Those infected with the virus may remain asymptomatic for 3 to 5 years or longer (Barrick, 1988); AIDS is actually the final stage in HIV infection (Holloway, 1988).

AIDS is more common in males, in those living in urban areas, and is disproportionately higher in blacks and Hispanics. Whereas homosexuals comprise the majority of those infected, the incidence in that population is declining. Transmission is primarily through sexual intercourse in males, and through intravenous drug use in females. Children are infected primarily through being born to infected mothers (Barrick, 1990). The incidence of HIV is rising in rural areas. Those considered at high risk for contracting HIV are homosexual males with a history of multiple partners, heterosexuals with frequent, multiple partners, intravenous drug abusers, and patients requiring multiple blood transfusions (Fidler and Keen, 1988). The risk to those requiring transfusions has been greatly decreased through the development of screening and heat treatment of blood products, which inactivates HIV (Barrick, 1990; Beaufoy et al., 1988; Ceccio, 1988).

The Centers for Disease Control has developed a classification system for HIV infection. Group I is the first stage of infection; acute flu-like symptoms develop and antibodies can be detected in serum. In group II, patients are asymptomatic though the virus continues to multiply and T-helper cells are killed. This stage can last for years. In group III, patients become symptomatic with generalized lymphadenopathy. Group IV is manifested through other diseases, including malignancies, opportunistic infections, and neurological involvement (Centers for Disease Control, 1986). Universal precautions as recommended by the Centers for Disease Control are displayed in Table 12–14.

Clinical Manifestations. In AIDS, severe immunodeficiency results in various opportunistic infections and malignancies. The signs and symptoms of AIDS vary greatly depending on the particular opportunistic infections or malignancies present and the degree of patient immunosuppression (Table 12–15). AIDS is diagnosed by clinical signs of opportunistic infections (Table 12–16), malignancies, wasting syndrome, or de-

Table 12–13. RISK FACTORS/TRANSMISSION OF HIV

Rectal or vaginal intercourse with frequent, multiple partners
IV drug abuse/sharing needles
Transfusion with contaminated blood or blood products
Transmission from mother to fetus during gestation or childbirth; or to newborn during breast-feeding
Occupational exposure to infected blood or body fluids through needle sticks or sharp instruments

Table 12–14. UNIVERSAL PRECAUTIONS TO PREVENT TRANSMISSION OF HIV IN HEALTH CARE SETTINGS

1. Gloves should be worn whenever touching blood or body fluids, mucous membranes, or nonintact skin; whenever handling any items or surfaces soiled with blood or body fluids; whenever performing venipuncture or other vascular access procedures. Gloves should be changed after contact with each patient.
2. Masks, protective eyewear, or face shields should be worn for any procedure in which droplets of blood or body fluids might be generated, or when splattering might occur.
3. Gowns or aprons should be worn for any patient care or procedure in which splattering of blood or body fluids might occur.
4. Hands and skin surfaces should be washed immediately and thoroughly after any contact with blood or body fluids. Hands should be washed immediately after removing gloves.
5. Needles, scalpels, and other sharp instruments should be handled with extreme care during procedures, cleaning, and disposal to prevent accidental injuries. Needles should not be recapped, broken, removed, or otherwise manipulated; they should be placed in a puncture-resistant container for disposal. Puncture-resistant containers should be placed near to patient care areas for ready access and changed before becoming overfull.
6. Mouthpieces, resuscitation bags, or ventilation devices should be readily accessible for emergency use.

Note: Universal blood and body fluid precautions should be used consistently for *all* patients.

Blood and body fluids that universal precautions apply to include: blood and other body fluids containing visible blood; semen and vaginal secretions; cerebrospinal, synovial, pleural, peritoneal, pericardial, and amniotic fluids.

Adapted from Centers for Disease Control. Recommendations for prevention of HIV transmission in health-care settings. MMWR, 36(2S):3–18, 1987.

mentia in combination with laboratory studies showing immunodeficiency not attributable to other causes (Barrick, 1988; Holloway, 1988). The diagnosis is confirmed by the presence of HIV antibodies detected by enzyme linked immunosorbent assay (ELISA) and confirmed by the Western blot test.

Laboratory findings in AIDS include a positive HIV antibody test, decreased WBC and lymphocyte counts, depressed T_4 lymphocyte count, an abnormal T_4/T_8 ratio (<1.0), and thrombocytopenia (Holloway, 1988).

Acute illness can be gradual or sudden and will include complaints of fatigue, malaise, fever, night sweats, lymphadenopathy, anorexia, persistent diarrhea, weight loss, cough, and shortness of breath (Barrick, 1988; Holloway, 1988). The

Table 12–15. SYMPTOMS OF HIV INFECTION AND/OR AIDS

Fever
Night sweats
Fatigue, weakness
Generalized lymphadenopathy
Malaise
Anorexia
Weight loss
Diarrhea
Dementia
Peripheral neuropathy
Malignancies: Kaposi's sarcoma (KS), lymphoma
Opportunistic infections (see Table 12–16)

most common manifestations of AIDS are pneumonia caused by the protozoan *Pneumocystis carinii* and a rare malignancy known as Kaposi's sarcoma (Coletti et al., 1989).

Pneumocystis carinii pneumonia (PCP) is the predominant pulmonary infection in AIDS. Patients present with hypoxemia and diffuse infiltrates on chest x-ray. Diagnosis is made by sputum induction, bronchoscopy with bronchoalveolar lavage, transbronchial biopsy, or open lung biopsy of tissue to identify the organism (Singer et al., 1990). Treatment of PCP includes the administration of sulfamethoxazole-trimethoprim (Bactrim, Septra) and/or pentamidine (Coletti et al., 1989). These drugs have improved the prognosis and survival in PCP, but have deleterious side effects such as neutropenia (Bullock, 1988b).

Another pulmonary pathogen is cytomegalovirus (CMV). Patients present similarly to those with PCP; diffuse infiltrates on chest x-ray and hypoxemia. Mortality with CMV infection is high, especially if the patient also has PCP. Gancyclovir is used to treat CMV infections (Singer et al., 1990).

Kaposi's sarcoma (KS) is a malignant tumor of the endothelium. On the skin, it appears as a purplish brown lesion, usually on the extremities. Kaposi's sarcoma may also affect tissue in the lymph nodes, lung, gastrointestinal tract, liver, or bone. Diagnosis is made by tissue biopsy, and it is treated with chemotherapeutics such as vinblastine, vincristine, adriamycin, or bleomycin. Other malignancies frequently seen in AIDS are non-Hodgkin's lymphomas, leukemias, and squamous cell carcinoma of the mouth and rectum (Coletti et al., 1989).

Neurological manifestations of AIDS can be caused by opportunistic infections of the brain

Table 12-16. OPPORTUNISTIC INFECTIONS IN AIDS

Pathogen	Target Site/Effect	Treatment
Protozoan		
Pneumocystis carinii	Lung/pneumonia	Trimethoprim-sulfamethoxazole (Bactrim, Septra) Pentamidine isethionate
Toxoplasma gondii	CNS/infection	Pyrimethamine, sulfadiazine
Cryptosporidium	GI tract/profuse diarrhea	Antimotility drugs, fluid/electrolyte replacement
Viral		
Cytomegalovirus (CMV)	Eye/retinitis, lung/pneumonitis, GI tract/colitis	Gancyclovir
Herpes simplex 1 and 2	Oral, genital, perirectal mucosa/painful lesions	Acyclovir (Zovirax)
Herpes zoster	Cutaneous/painful lesions	Acyclovir (Zovirax)
Epstein-Barr	Oral mucosa/hairy leukoplakia	
Fungal		
Candida	Oral, esophageal mucosa/thrush, painful swallowing	Nystatin, clotrimazole, ketoconazole
Cryptococcus neoformans	Meninges/meningitis, disseminated illness	Amphotericin B (Fungizone) flucytosine (Ancobon)
Bacterial		
Mycobacterium avium	Liver, lung/disseminated illness	Ansamycin, clofazimine (Lamprene)
Mycobacterium tuberculosis	Lung/TB, disseminated illness	Isoniazid (INH), rifampin

and spinal cord, malignancies, pharmacological therapies, or direct infection of the central nervous system with HIV. AIDS dementia complex, probably caused by direct infection with HIV, is the most frequent cause of neurological symptoms in AIDS patients (Scherer, 1990). Symptoms include problems with memory and cognition, personality changes, apathy, and social withdrawal. AIDS dementia progresses over months. In direct HIV infection, Zidovudine (Retrovir, formerly called azidothymidine [AZT]) is the drug used in treatment; it is an antiviral agent that inhibits replication of the virus and is known to cross the blood-brain barrier (Scherer, 1990).

Other common disorders in AIDS include cryptococcal meningitis, treated with amphotericin B; toxoplasmosis, treated with pyrimethamine and sulfadiazine; candidiasis, treated with nystatin; and herpes simplex or herpes zoster, treated with acyclovir. *Cryptosporidium* is a frequent cause of diarrhea; treatment primarily consists of antidiarrheal medications.

Medical/Nursing Management. Medical treatment of AIDS is aimed at the early detection and treatment of opportunistic infections (see Table 12-16) and malignancies, the management of symptoms, and prevention of complications (Coletti et al., 1989). In addition to specific medications, orders may include chest physiotherapy, respiratory support, oxygen, nutritional support, intravenous fluids for hydration, analgesics, and physical therapy.

Research concerning HIV and the treatment of AIDS continues to be vastly important, with many areas open to investigation. These areas include the use of antiviral agents, immune modulators, and the possible development of a vaccine. Zidovudine is an antiviral agent—it is approved for the treatment of HIV infection and is in wide use. Immune modulators being investigated include alpha and gamma interferon and interleukin-2. Use of these drugs is aimed at boosting the depressed immune system by increasing the number of T cells or enhancing their function. Vaccination is an important and controversial area of HIV research. Development of a vaccine for HIV is difficult because HIV exists in many antigenic forms, and is able to alter its antigenic coating.

Nursing care of the patient with AIDS is complex, especially in critical care. The list of nursing diagnoses, actual and potential, is long, and depends on the particular manifestations seen (Table 12-17). Basic goals are prevention of infection, optimal gas exchange, maintenance of adequate hydration and optimal nutritional status, maintenance of skin and mucous mem-

Table 12–17. NURSING DIAGNOSES IN AIDS

Potential for infection
Impaired gas exchange
Impaired tissue integrity
Altered nutritional status: less than body requirements
Alteration in bowel elimination: diarrhea
Alteration in comfort: pain
Anxiety
Alteration in thought processes
Knowledge deficit
Altered self-concept
Potential for fluid volume deficit
Potential for injury
Social isolation
Fluid volume deficit

brane integrity, relief of pain and promotion of comfort and rest, reduced anxiety, and alert and oriented mental status.

Potential for infection related to immunosuppression, disease process, malnutrition, chemotherapy, opportunistic pathogens. Thorough handwashing should be carried out before, during, and after any patient contact. Monitor vital signs and hemodynamic parameters at least every 4 hours and PRN; any temperature elevation should be immediately investigated. Auscultate breath sounds for adventitious sounds. Provide pulmonary toilet at least every 2 hours while awake, including spirometry, chest physiotherapy, and postural drainage. Use strict aseptic technique for any invasive procedures, suctioning, or dressing changes. Promote good body and oral hygiene, keeping skin clean and dry. Assess skin, axillae, groin areas, and mucous membranes for signs of infection or breakdown; any signs of opportunistic infections such as thrush, herpes, diarrhea, or mental changes should be reported. Frequently assess IV sites, incisions, and wounds for redness, swelling, heat, or tenderness, although these signs may be masked. Obtain wound, urine, sputum, and throat cultures as indicated and as ordered. Follow laboratory studies (CBC, urinalysis, cultures) for increases or decreases in WBC and differential counts or the presence of bacteria. Maintain adequate fluid balance and optimal nutritional status. Other signs to assess for are chills, dyspnea, and diaphoresis. Note that usual signs of infection may be absent in any immunocompromised patient and that fever often is the only indicator; thorough baseline documentation and frequent assessment are necessary to detect subtle changes that may indicate dangerous infection.

Impaired gas exchange related to pulmonary infection. Assess pulmonary status every 4 hours and PRN; auscultate for adventitious sounds, note rate, depth, and rhythm of respirations. Observe for dyspnea, cough, sputum production, or use of accessory muscles for respiration. Monitor arterial blood gases for signs of hypoxemia, acidosis, signs of hyperventilation (respiratory alkalosis), or changes from baseline. Assess patient for cyanosis and tachycardia. Administer oxygen therapy and/or respiratory support as ordered and monitor response. Pulmonary toilet should be performed at least every 2 hours while awake, including spirometry, chest physiotherapy, and postural drainage. Obtain sputum cultures if infection is suspected. Administer antibiotics, other antimicrobials as ordered, with close observation for side effects.

Impaired tissue integrity related to invasive lines and/or procedures, diarrhea, malnutrition, malignant lesions (KS), chemotherapy, or immobility. Assess skin and mucous membranes for signs of infection or breakdown, noting color, temperature, presence of lesions, and moisture. Provide meticulous hygiene to prevent breakdown and infection, keeping skin clean, dry, though moisturized. Perform frequent oral care with nonirritating, nondrying solutions and soft bristled brushes. Avoid trauma to skin; turn at least every 2 hours, and provide padding for bony prominences. If possible, use air-fluidized or alternating pressure mattress to prevent pressure. Encourage mobility as appropriate.

Altered nutritional status: less than body requirements related to diarrhea, malabsorption, anorexia, painful oral lesions, NPO status. Assess patient for baseline height and desired weight. Record caloric and protein intake, I&O, and daily weights. Provide dietary consultation if needed, and encourage preferred foods to be brought by significant others. Monitor laboratory studies, especially total protein, serum albumin, hematocrit, and hemoglobin. Administer vitamin, mineral, and caloric supplements as ordered. Encourage small, frequent, high-protein and high-calorie meals and snacks. Administer antiemetics 30 minutes before meals as needed. Provide meticulous oral hygiene and relief measures for painful oral lesions. Determine need for supplements or diet changes. Administer enteral feedings, hyperalimentation as ordered, with close observation for response.

Alteration in bowel elimination: diarrhea related to gastrointestinal infection, antibiotics, cytotoxic drugs, enteral feedings. Assess patient for diarrhea, noting frequency, amount, consistency, and the presence of blood, fat, mucus, or undigested particles. Monitor bowel sounds at least every shift. Administer anti-infectives and antidiarrheals as ordered, noting response. Monitor strict I&O, and maintain adequate hydration status through fluid replacement as necessary. Assess for electrolyte disturbances (such as monitor labs, and patient for dysrhythmias, weakness, cramps). Obtain stool cultures as ordered, and monitor for microbial growth. Encourage optimal nutrition. Adjust rate/strength of enteral feedings if necessary. Keep perineum clean and dry; assess and treat for excoriation and breakdown.

Alteration in thought processes related to CNS infection, malignancy, pharmacological interventions. Assess baseline mental, emotional, and neurological status. Monitor for neurological changes such as headache, confusion, dizziness, visual disturbances. Note mood alterations, problems with memory or cognition. Reorient the patient as necessary, and protect from injury. Promote calm environment; provide information in simple, easy to understand terms; reinforce as needed. Provide emotional support and reassurance to patient and significant others.

Alteration in comfort: pain related to infections, neuropathy, lesions, chemotherapy, procedures, immobility, and/or treatments. Assess pain for location, duration, intensity, precipitating factors, and character. Administer analgesics, anti-inflammatory drugs as needed and ordered; anticipate need and monitor for response. Position patient for comfort, providing support with pillows/padding. Change position every 2 hours and as needed. Provide meticulous skin care and oral hygiene. Promote calm, restful environment; reduce stressors as able. Administer massage and heat/cold applications as effective. Encourage diversional activities, relaxation, and imagery techniques.

Anxiety related to diagnosis, uncertain outcome of disease, fear of death or procedures, reaction of significant others to diagnosis. Assess patient's/family's/significant other's level of anxiety; determine positive coping mechanisms. Establish rapport and atmosphere of mutual acceptance. Encourage open, honest communication and expression of feelings. Be available to patient and significant others; provide reassurance without false hope. Provide information regarding disease process, treatments, medications, and procedures. Orient patient and significant others to critical care environment. Encourage patient and significant other to participate in planning and implementation of care. Remain with patient during procedures or periods of anxiety; encourage relaxation and imagery techniques.

Nursing concerns regarding AIDS are many, and include the nurse as well as the patient. The prevention of transmission of HIV in the clinical setting is of vast importance. Universal precautions should be practiced at all times with all patients, by all members of the health care team (see Table 12–14). Handwashing continues to be the single most important action taken. As discussed above, protection of the immunosuppressed AIDS patient from infection is of primary importance. Assessments must be ongoing and thorough. Staff must have access to ongoing support, as caring for AIDS patients is demanding as well as challenging, and poses quite an emotional strain. The risk of exposure also places a constant emotional strain on nurses. Continuing education must be available that addresses prevention of transmission, current research, and treatments. Support of staff, education, and research will continue to improve AIDS patient outcome.

Treatment of the Immunocompromised Patient

Whatever the cause of the immunodeficiency, the patient has the potential to develop infection, which is the leading cause of death in these patients. It is important to remember that immunosuppressed patients will not respond to infection typically; the signs and symptoms of infection will vary greatly and may be absent or masked. Close monitoring through thorough assessment, early detection and treatment, and prevention of complications are goals in treating the immunocompromised patient.

Medical and surgical treatments are aimed at the cause of symptoms and the prevention of complications. In primary immunodeficiencies, B- and T-cell defects are treated with specific replacement therapy or bone marrow transplants (Fidler and Keen, 1988). In secondary immunodeficiencies, the underlying condition is treated. Malnutrition is corrected, immunosuppressants are stopped if possible, and medications are given to treat infections or other disease states.

A detailed, documented database containing the patient's history, physical examination, and laboratory studies is paramount. Other nursing goals, as in AIDS, are aimed at prevention of infection, nutritional support, maintenance of skin and mucous membrane integrity, fluid and electrolyte balance, and renal function, emotional support, alleviation of discomfort, and promotion of rest (Dattwyler, 1991). See Nursing Care Plan for the Immunocompromised Patient.

Summary

All patients in critical care have the potential for alterations in function of the hematological and immunological systems. A thorough understanding of normal anatomy and physiology provides the critical care nurse with a basis on which to build. Nurses play a key role in the assessment and management of patients with serious alterations in the hematological and immunological systems, such as DIC and AIDS.

References

Anderson, G., and Bullock, B. L. (1988): Normal and altered erythrocyte function. In: B. L. Bullock and P. P. Rosendahl (eds.). *Pathophysiology: Adaptations and Alterations in Function.* 2nd ed. Boston: Scott, Foresman, pp. 211–227.

Barrick, B. (1988): Caring for AIDS patients: A challenge you can meet. *Nursing '88* 18(11):50–59.

Barrick, B. (1990): AIDS: Light at the end of a decade. *American Journal of Nursing* 90(11):36–40.

Belcher, A. E. (1989): Hematolymphatic system. In: J. M. Thompson, G. K. Mcfarland, J. E. Hirsch, S. M. Tucker, and A. C. Bowers (eds.). *Mosby's Manual of Clinical Nursing.* 2nd ed. St. Louis: C. V. Mosby, pp. 1400–1445.

Beaufoy, A., Goldstone, I., and Riddell, R. (1988): AIDS: What nurses need to know. *The Canadian Nurse* 84(7):16–27.

Bullock, B. L. (1988a): Normal immunologic response. In: B. L. Bullock, and P. P. Rosendahl (eds.). *Pathophysiology: Adaptations and Alterations in Function.* 2nd ed. Boston: Scott, Foresman, pp. 149–159.

Bullock, B. L. (1988b): Immunodeficiency. In: B. L. Bullock and P. P. Rosendahl (eds.). *Pathophysiology: Adaptations and Alterations in Function.* 2nd ed. Boston: Scott, Foresman, pp. 160–166.

Bullock, B. L. (1988c): Normal and altered leukocyte function. In: B. L. Bullock and P. P. Rosendahl (eds.). *Pathophysiology: Adaptations and Alterations in Function.* 2nd ed. Boston: Scott, Foresman, pp. 228–240.

Bullock, B. L. (1988d): Normal and altered coagulation. In: B. L. Bullock and P. P. Rosendahl (eds.). *Pathophysiology: Adaptations and Alterations in Function.* 2nd ed. Boston: Scott, Foresman, pp. 241–253.

Ceccio, C. M. (1988): AIDS: Scientific update, treatment, and nursing care. *Orthopaedic Nursing* 7(5):13–24.

Centers for Disease Control (1986): Classification system for human T-lymphocyte virus. MMWR 35:334–339.

Coletti, M., German, M., Zeller, J. M., and Balkstra, R. (1989): Immunologic system. In: J. M. Thompson, G. K. Mcfarland, J. E. Hirsch, S. M. Tucker, and A. C. Bowers (eds.). *Mosby's Manual of Clinical Nursing.* 2nd ed. St. Louis: C. V. Mosby, pp. 1302–1399.

Cotran, R. S., Kumar, V., and Robbins, S. L. (1989): *Robbins Pathological Basis of Disease.* 4th ed. Philadelphia: W. B. Saunders.

Dattwyler, R. J. (1991): Immunomodulation: Therapeutic manipulation of the immune system. In: J. T. Dolan (ed.). *Critical Care Nursing: Clinical Management Through the Nursing Process.* Philadelphia: F. A. Davis, pp. 1181–1203.

Dolan, J. T. (1991): *Critical Care Nursing: Clinical Management Through the Nursing Process.* Philadelphia: F. A. Davis.

Fidler, M. R. (1988): Immunologic anatomy and physiology. In: M. R. Kinney, D. R. Packa, and S. B. Dunbar (eds.). *AACN's Clinical Reference for Critical-Care Nursing.* 2nd ed. New York: McGraw-Hill, pp. 1171–1201.

Fidler, M. R., and Keen, M. F. (1988): The immunocompromised patient. In: M. R. Kinney, D. R. Packa, and S. B. Dunbar (eds.). *AACN's Clinical Reference for Critical-Care Nursing.* 2nd ed. New York: McGraw-Hill, pp. 1249–1269.

Golightly, M. G. (1991): Clinical application: Immunodeficiency disorders. In: J. T. Dolan (ed.). *Critical Care Nursing: Clinical Management Through the Nursing Process.* Philadelphia: F. A. Davis, pp. 1213–1226.

Golightly, M. G., and Dolan, J. T. (1991): Assessment of immunologic function. In: J. T. Dolan (ed.). *Critical Care Nursing: Clinical Management Through the Nursing Process.* Philadelphia: F. A. Davis, pp. 1176–1180.

Gurka, A. M. (1989): The immune system: Implications for critical care nursing. *Critical Care Nurse* 9(7):24–35.

Guyton, A. C. (1986): *Textbook of Medical Physiology.* 7th ed. Philadelphia: W. B. Saunders.

Harvey, M. A. (1986): *Study Guide to Core Curriculum for Critical Care Nursing.* Philadelphia: W. B. Saunders.

Holloway, N. M. (1988): *Nursing the Critically Ill Adult.* 3rd ed. Menlo Park, CA: Addison-Wesley.

Jackson, B. S. (1988a): Hematopoietic data acquisition. In: M. R. Kinney, D. R. Packa, and S. B. Dunbar (eds.). *AACN's Clinical Reference for Critical-Care Nursing.* 2nd ed. New York: McGraw-Hill, 1136–1142.

Jackson, B. S. (1988b): Hyperviscosity and anemias. In: M. R. Kinney, D. R. Packa, and S. B. Dunbar (eds.). *AACN's Clinical Reference for Critical-Care Nursing.* 2nd ed. New York: McGraw-Hill, pp. 1143–1155.

Jackson, B. S., and Jones, M. B. (1988a): Coagulopathies. In: M. R. Kinney, D. R. Packa, and S. B. Dunbar (eds.). *AACN's Clinical Reference for Critical-Care Nursing.* 2nd ed. New York: McGraw-Hill, pp. 1156–1167.

Jackson, B. S., and Jones, M. B. (1988b). Hematologic anatomy and physiology. In: M. R. Kinney, D. R. Packa, and S. B. Dunbar (eds.). *AACN's Clinical Reference for Critical-Care Nursing.* 2nd ed. New York: McGraw-Hill, pp. 1113–1135.

Jennings, B. M. (1985): The hematologic system. In: J. G. Alspach, and S. M. Williams (eds.). *Core Curriculum for Critical Care Nursing.* Philadelphia: W. B. Saunders, pp. 495–561.

Kuhar, P. A., and Hill, K. M. (1991): White clot syndrome: When heparin goes haywire. *American Journal of Nursing* 91(3):59–60.

Miller, F., and Habicht, G. (1991): Immune system: Underlying principles. In: J. T. Dolan (ed.). *Critical Care Nursing: Clinical Management Through the Nursing Process.* Philadelphia: F. A. Davis, pp. 1155–1175.

Parrillo, J. E. (1991): *Current Theory in Critical Care Medicine.* Philadelphia: B. C. Decker.

Rick, M. E. (1991): Hemorrhagic and thrombotic disorders. In: J. E. Parrillo (ed.). *Current Therapy in Critical Care Medicine.* Philadelphia: B. C. Decker, pp. 288–292.

Scherer, P. (1990): How AIDS attacks the brain. *American Journal of Nursing* 90(1):44–52.

Singer, P., Askanazi, J., Akiva, L., Bursztein, S., and Kvetan, V. (1990): Reassessing intensive care for patients with the acquired immunodeficiency syndrome. *Heart and Lung* 19(4):387–394.

Thelan, L. A., Davie, J. K., and Urden, L. D. (1990): *Textbook of Critical Care Nursing: Diagnosis and Management.* St. Louis: C. V. Mosby.

Young, L. M. (1990): DIC: The insidious killer. *Critical Care Nurse* 10(10):26–33.

Recommended Reading

Alspach, J. G., and Williams, S. M. (1985): *Core Curriculum for Critical Care Nursing.* Philadelphia: W. B. Saunders.

Centers for Disease Control (1990): HIV prevalence, projected AIDS case estimates: Workshop, October 31–November 1, 1989. JAMA 263(11):1477, 1480.

Crow, S. (1983): Nursing care of the immunosuppressed patient. *Infection Control* 4(6):465–467.

Damrosch, S., Abbey, S., Warner, A., and Guy, S. (1990): Critical care nurses' attitudes toward, concerns about, and knowledge of the acquired immunodeficiency syndrome. *Heart and Lung* 19(4):395–400.

Davey, R. J. (1991): Blood product therapy. In: J. E. Parrillo (ed.). *Current Therapy in Critical Care Medicine.* Philadelphia: B. C. Decker, pp. 292–296.

Deloor, R. M., and Schreiber, M. J. (1985): The hematologic system. In: S. Millar, L. K. Sampson, and M. Soukop (eds.). *AACN Procedure Manual for Critical Care.* 2nd ed. Philadelphia: W. B. Saunders, pp. 410–430.

Dossey, B. M., Guzzetta, C. E., and Kenner, C. V. (1990): *Essentials of Critical Care Nursing: Body-Mind-Spirit.* Philadelphia: J. B. Lippincott.

Esparaz, B., and Green, D. (1990): Disseminated intravascular coagulation. *Critical Care Nursing Quarterly* 13(2):7–13.

Fidler, M. R., and Keen, M. F. (1988): Hypersensitivity and anaphylaxis. In: M. R. Kinney, D. R. Packa, and S. B. Dunbar (eds.). *AACN's Clinical Reference for Critical-Care Nursing.* 2nd ed. New York: McGraw-Hill, pp. 1235–1248.

Fidler, M. R., and Morgan, M. S. (1988): Immunologic data acquisition. In: M. R. Kinney, D. R. Packa, and S. B. Dunbar (eds.). *AACN's Clinical Reference for Critical-Care Nursing.* 2nd ed. New York: McGraw-Hill, 1202–1234.

Fischbach, F. T. (1988): *A Manual of Laboratory Diagnostic Tests.* New York: J. B. Lippincott.

Gurevich, I. (1985): The competent internal immune system. *Nursing Clinics of North America* 20(1):151–161.

Harrington, L., and Hufnagel, J. M. (1990): Heparin-induced thrombocytopenia and thrombosis syndrome: A case study. *Heart and Lung* 19(1):93–98.

Johanson, B. C., Wells, S. J., Hoffmeister, D., and Dungca, C. U. (1988): *Standards for Critical Care.* 3rd ed. St. Louis: C. V. Mosby.

Kenner, C. V., Guzzetta, C. E., and Dossey, B. M. (1985): *Critical Care Nursing: Body-Mind-Spirit.* 2nd ed. Boston: Little, Brown.

Kinney, M. R., Packa, D. R., and Dunbar, S. B. (1988): *AACN's Clinical Reference for Critical-Care Nursing.* 2nd ed. New York: McGraw-Hill.

Lewis, A. (1988): *Nursing Care of the person with AIDS/ARC.* Rockville, MD: Aspen.

McLeod, M., and Silverthorn, K. (1988): AIDS and the ICU nurse. *The Canadian Nurse* 84(7):28–30.

Millar, S., Sampson, L. K., and Soukop, M. (1985): *AACN Procedure Manual for Critical Care.* Philadelphia: W. B. Saunders.

Moran, T. A. (1989): AIDS: Current implications and impact on nursing. *Journal of Intravenous Nursing* 12(4):220–226.

Suchak, B. A., and Barbon, C. B. (1989): Disseminated intravascular coagulation: A nursing challenge. *Orthopaedic Nursing* 8(6):61–69.

Swearingen, P. L. (1988): Acquired immunodeficiency syndrome. In: *Manual of Critical Care: Applying Nursing Diagnoses to Adult Critical Care Illness.* St. Louis: C. V. Mosby, pp. 477–488.

Swearingen, P. L. (1988): Disseminated intravascular coagulation. In: *Manual of Critical Care: Applying Nursing Diagnoses to Adult Critical Care Illness.* St. Louis: C. V. Mosby, pp. 418–422.

Taber, J. (1989): Nutrition and HIV infection. *American Journal of Nursing* 89(11):1446–1451.

Thompson, J. M., Mcfarland, G. K., Hirsch, J. E., Tucker, S. M., and Bowers, A. C. (1989): *Mosby's Manual of Clinical Nursing.* 2nd ed. St. Louis: C. V. Mosby.

Waltzer, W. C. (1991): Clinical application: Clinical organ transplant. In: J. T. Dolan (ed.). *Critical Care Nursing: Clinical Management Through the Nursing Process.* Philadelphia: F. A. Davis, pp. 1204–1212.

Chapter 13

Joanne M. Krumberger, R.N., M.S.N., CCRN

Gastrointestinal Alterations

Objectives

- Review anatomy and physiology of the gastrointestinal system.
- Describe general assessment of the gastrointestinal system.
- Discuss nutritional assessment and therapies to provide optimal nutrition.
- Compare pathophysiology, assessment, nursing diagnoses, outcomes, and interventions for acute upper gastrointestinal bleeding, acute pancreatitis, and hepatic failure.
- Formulate a plan of care for the patient with acute upper gastrointestinal bleeding, acute pancreatitis, and hepatic failure.

Body cells require water, electrolytes, and nutrients (carbohydrates, fats and proteins) to obtain the energy necessary to fuel body functions. The primary function of the alimentary tract (oropharyngeal cavity, esophagus, stomach, small and large intestines) and accessory organs (pancreas, liver, and gallbladder) is to provide the body with a continual supply of nutrients. Additionally, food must move through the system at a slow enough rate for digestive and absorptive functions to take place, but also fast enough to meet body needs. This requires appropriate and timely movement of nutrients through the gastrointestinal (GI) tract (motility), the presence of specific enzymes to break down nutrients (digestion), and transport mechanisms to move the nutrients into the blood stream (absorption). Each part is adapted for specific functions, including passage of food, food storage, digestion, and absorption. In this chapter, a brief physiological review of each section of the GI system and a general assessment of the GI system serve as an introduction and provide the foundation for the discussion of the most frequent gastrointestinal disorders encountered in the critical care setting: acute upper gastrointestinal bleeding, acute pancreatitis, and liver failure. The remainder of the chapter reviews the pathophysiology of the disorder, nursing and medical assessments, select nursing diagnoses, nursing and medical interventions, and patient outcomes. Complete nursing plans of care for select nursing diagnoses are provided. These serve as good summaries of the most common patient care problems and collaborative interventions. Nutritional assessment and nutritional support therapies will also be presented, as altered nutrition is a common nursing diagnosis in patients with GI disorders.

Anatomy and Physiology of the GI System

GI TRACT

The anatomic structure of the gastrointestinal system is shown in Fig. 13-1. It comprises the alimentary canal (beginning at the oropharynx and ending at the anus), and accessory organs (liver, pancreas, and gallbladder) that empty their products into the canal at certain points. A review of the anatomy of the gut wall is provided as an introduction to this section because it provides the foundation for the understanding of absorption of nutrients and GI protective mechanisms.

Gut Wall

Beginning in the esophagus and extending to the rectum, the GI tract is composed of multiple tissue layers.

Mucosa. The innermost layer, the mucosa, is the most important physiologically. It is this layer that is exposed to food substances, and therefore plays a role in nutrient metabolism. The mucosa is also protective. The cells in this layer are connected by tight junctions that produce an effective barrier against large molecules and bacteria and serve to protect the GI tract from bacterial colonization. The goblet cells in the mucosa secrete mucus, which provides lubrication for food substances and protects the mucosa from excoriation.

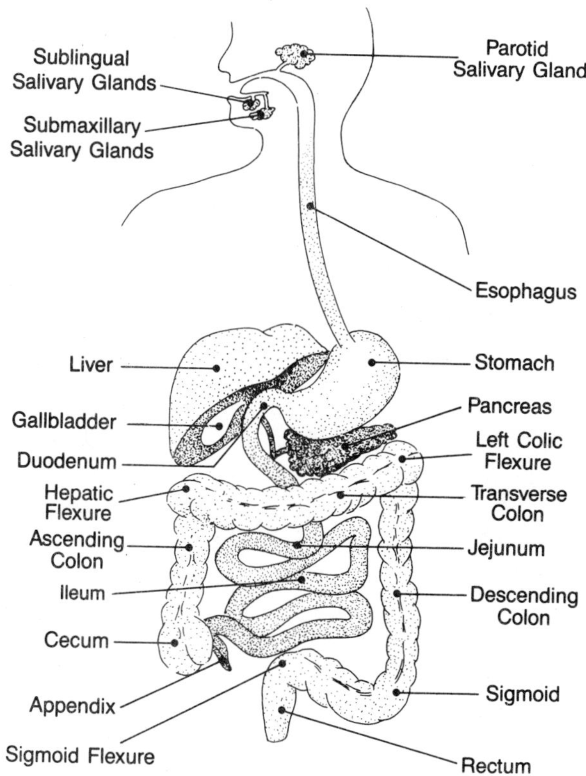

Figure 13-1. The gastrointestinal system.

Gastric Mucosal Barrier. In the stomach, the special architecture of cells of the mucosa and the mucus that is secreted is known as the gastric mucosal barrier. This physiological barrier is impermeable to hydrochloric acid, which is normally secreted in the stomach, but can be permeable to other substances such as salycilates, alcohol, steroids, and bile salts. It is the disruption of this barrier by these types of substances that is thought to play a role in ulcer development. Additionally, these cells have a special feature in that they do regenerate rapidly, which explains how disruptions in the mucosa can be quickly healed.

Submucosa. The second layer of the gut wall, the submucosa, comprises connective tissue, blood vessels, and nerve fibers. The muscularis externa is the major muscular layer of the wall. The serosa is the outermost layer.

Beneath the mucosa, submucosa, and muscularis externa are various nerve plexuses that are innervated by the autonomic nervous system. Disturbances in these neurons in a given segment of the GI tract cause a lack of motility.

Oropharyngeal Cavity

Mouth. Food substances are ingested into the oral cavity primarily according to the intrinsic desire for food called hunger. Food in the mouth is initially subject to mechanical breakdown by the act of chewing (mastication). Chewing of food is important for digestion of all foods, but particularly for fruits and raw vegetables because they require the cellulose membranes around their nutrients to be broken down. The muscles of chewing are innervated by the motor branch of the fifth cranial nerve.

Saliva is the major secretion of the oropharynx and is produced by three pairs of salivary glands: submaxillary, sublingual, and parotid. Saliva is rich in mucus, which provides lubrication of food. Salivary amylase, a starch-digesting enzyme, is also secreted. Stimuli such as sight, smell, thoughts, and taste of food stimulate salivary gland secretion. Parasympathetic stimulation will promote a copious secretion of watery saliva. Conversely, sympathetic stimulation will produce a scanty output of thick saliva. The normal daily secretion of saliva is 1200 ml.

Pharynx. Swallowing is a complex mechanism involving oral, or voluntary, pharyngeal, and esophageal stages. It is made more complex because the pharynx serves several other functions, the most important of which is respiration. The pharynx participates in the function of swallowing for only a few seconds at a time to aid in the propulsion of food, which is triggered by the presence of fluid or food in the pharynx. Table 13-1 outlines the three broad stages of swallowing.

Esophagus

Once fluid or food enters the esophagus, it is propelled through the lumen by the process of peristalsis, which involves the relaxation and contraction of esophageal muscles stimulated by the bolus of food. This occurs repeatedly until the food reaches the lower esophageal sphincter, which is the last centimeter of the esophagus. This area is normally contracted and thus prevents the reflux of gastric contents into the esophagus that would damage the lining by gastric acid and enzymes. Waves of peristalsis cause this sphincter to relax and allow food to enter the stomach. Mucosal layers in the esophagus secrete mucus, which protects the lining from damage by gastric secretions or food, and serves as a lubricant.

Stomach

Anatomically, the stomach is located at the distal end of the esophagus. It is divided into four regions: the cardia, fundus, body, and antrum (Fig. 13-2). The muscular walls form multiple folds that allow for greater expansion of the stomach. The opening at the distal end of the stomach opens into the small intestine and is surrounded by the pyloric sphincter. The motor functions of the stomach include storage of food until it can be accommodated by the lower GI tract; mixing of food with gastric secretions until it forms a semifluid mixture called chyme; and slow emptying of the chyme into the small intestine at a rate that allows for proper digestion and absorption. Motility is accomplished through peristalsis. The pyloric sphincter at the distal end of the stomach functions to prevent duodenal reflux.

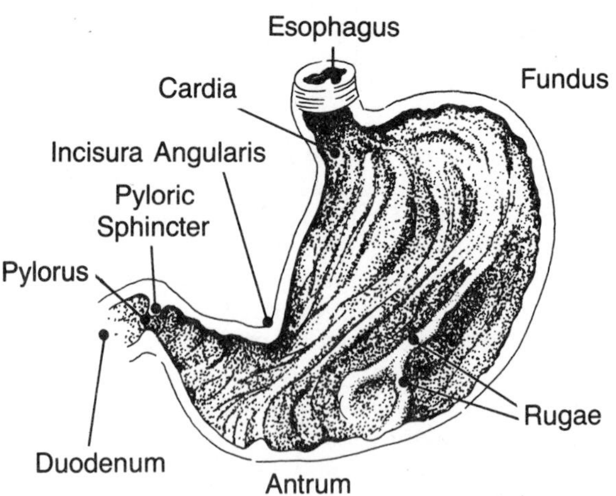

Figure 13-2. The stomach.

Gastric secretions are produced by mucus-secreting cells that line the inner surface of the stomach and by two types of tubular glands: the oxyntic, or gastric, glands and the pyloric glands. Table 13-2 summarizes the major gastric secretions.

An oxyntic gland is composed of three types of cells: mucous neck cells, which secrete mostly mucus; the peptic, or chief, cells, which secrete pepsinogen; and oxyntic, or parietal cells, which secrete hydrochloric acid. Mucous cells secrete a

Table 13-1. SWALLOWING STAGES

Voluntary/(Oral) Stage
Initiates swallowing process; usually stimulated by bolus of food in the mouth near the pharynx
Pharyngeal: Involuntary
Passage of food through pharynx to esophagus
Esophageal: Involuntary
Promotes passage of food from pharynx to stomach

Table 13-2. GASTRIC SECRETIONS

Gland/Cells	Secretion
Cardiac Gland	Mucus
Pyloric Gland	Mucus
Fundic (Gastric) Gland	
Mucus Neck Cells	Mucus
Parietal Cells	Water Hydrochloric Acid Intrinsic Factor
Chief Cells	Pepsinogen Mucus

very viscid and alkaline mucus that coats the stomach mucosa, providing protection and lubrication for food transport. The parietal cells secrete hydrochloric acid solution, which functions to begin digestion of food in the stomach. Hydrochloric acid is very acidic (pH 0.8), and the rate of secretion is normally 2–3 mEq/hr. There are known stimulants of hydrochloric acid secretion that increase its secretion rate 10-fold, including vagal stimulation, gastrin, and the chemical properties of chyme. Histamine, which stimulates the release of gastrin, also stimulates hydrochloric acid secretion. Current drug therapies for ulcer disease utilize histamine (H_2) receptor blockers that block the effects of histamine and therefore hydrochloric acid stimulation. The acidic environment of the stomach promotes the conversion of pepsinogen, a proteolytic enzyme secreted by gastric chief cells, to pepsin. Pepsin begins the initial breakdown of proteins. Pepsin is only active in a highly acidic environment, pH <5, and therefore hydrochloric acid secretion is essential for protein digestion.

An essential protein secreted only by the stomach's parietal cells is intrinsic factor. Intrinsic factor is necessary for the absorption of vitamin B_{12} in the ileum. Vitamin B_{12} is critical to the formation of red blood cells and a deficiency causes anemia.

In addition to hydrochloric acid and pepsinogen secretion, the stomach secretes fluid rich in sodium and potassium and other electrolytes. Therefore, losses of these fluids via vomiting or gastric suction will place the patient at risk for fluid and electrolyte imbalances, as well as acid-base disturbances (Table 13–3).

Table 13–3. ELECTROLYTE/ACID-BASE DISTURBANCES ASSOCIATED WITH THE GI TRACT

Fluid Loss	Imbalances
Gastric Juice	Metabolic Alkalosis Potassium Deficit Sodium Deficit Fluid Volume Deficit
Small Intestine Juice	Metabolic Acidosis Potassium Deficit Sodium Deficit Fluid Volume Deficit
Large Intestine Juice (recent ileostomy)	Metabolic Acidosis Potassium Deficit Sodium Deficit Fluid Volume Deficit
Biliary or Pancreatic Fistula	Metabolic Acidosis Sodium Deficit Fluid Volume Deficit

Small Intestine

The first 10 to 12 inches of the small intestine is called the duodenum. This anatomical area is physiologically important in that pancreatic juices and bile from the liver empty into this structure. The duodenum also contains an extensive network of mucus-secreting glands called Brunner's glands. The function of this mucus is to protect the duodenal wall from digestion by gastric juice. Secretion of mucus by Brunner's glands is inhibited by sympathetic stimulation, which leaves the duodenum unprotected from gastric juice. This is thought to be one of the reasons why this area of the GI tract is the site for over 50% of peptic ulcers.

The next 7 to 8 feet of the small intestine is called the jejunum, and the remaining 10 to 12 feet consists of the ileum. The opening into the first part of the large intestine is protected by the ileocecal valve, which prevents reflux of colonic contents back into the ileum.

The movements of the small intestine include mixing contractions and propulsive contractions. The net movement of chyme in the small intestine is 3 to 5 hours from the pylorus to the ileocecal valve, although this activity is greatly increased after meals. Digestion and absorption of foodstuffs occur primarily in the small intestine. The anatomical arrangement of villi and microvilli in the small intestine greatly increases the surface area of the this area, accounting for its highly digestive and absorptive capabilities. Located on the entire surface of the small intestine are small pits called crypts of Lieberkühn, which produce intestinal secretions at a rate of 2000 ml/day. These secretions are neutral in pH and supply the watery vehicle necessary for absorption to occur.

In the small intestine, digestion of carbohydrates, fats, and proteins begins with degradation by pancreatic enzymes that are secreted into the duodenum. Pancreatic juice contains enzymes for digesting all three major types of food: proteins, carbohydrates, and fats (Table 13–4). It also contains large quantities of bicarbonate ions (HCO_3), which play an important role in neutralizing acidic chyme that is emptied from the stomach into the duodenum. Pancreatic juice is primarily secreted in response to the presence of chyme in the duodenum.

Table 13–4. PANCREATIC ENZYMES AND THEIR ACTIONS

Enzyme	Action
Trypsin*	Digests Proteins
Chymotrypsin*	Digests Proteins
Carboxypolypeptidase*	Digests Proteins
Ribonuclease	Digests Proteins
Deoxyribonuclease	Digests Proteins
Pancreatic Amylase	Digests Carbohydrates
Pancreatic Lipase	Digests Fats
Cholesterol Esterase	Digests Fats

* Becomes activated only after secreted into the intestinal tract.

The small intestine also handles water, electrolyte, and vitamin absorption. Up to 10 L of fluid enters the GI tract daily and fluid composition of stool is only around 200 ml. Sodium is actively reabsorbed in the small intestine. Chloride is absorbed in the ileum and HCO_3 is secreted. Potassium is absorbed as well as secreted in the GI tract. Vitamins, with the exception of B_{12}, and iron are absorbed in the upper part of the small bowel. As mentioned earlier, Vitamin B_{12} is absorbed in the terminal ileum in the presence of intrinsic factor.

Large Intestine

The large intestine, or colon, is anatomically divided into the ascending colon, transverse colon, descending colon, and rectum (Fig. 13–3). The functions of the colon are absorption of the water and electrolytes from the chyme and storage of fecal material until it can be expelled. The proximal one-half of the colon functions primarily in absorptive activities, whereas the distal one-half is concerned with storage. The characteristic contractile activity in the colon is called haustrations, which serves to propel fecal material through the tract. A mass movement will move a mass of feces into the rectal vault and then the urge to defecate will be elicited. The mucosa of the large intestine is lined with crypts of Lieberkühn, but the cells contain very few enzymes. Rather, mucus is secreted, which protects the colon wall against excoriation and serves as a medium for holding fecal matter together.

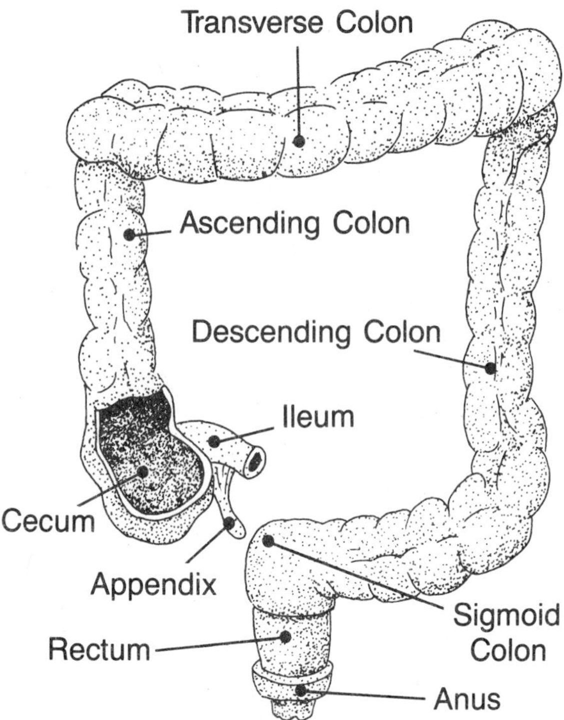

Figure 13–3. The intestinal system.

ACCESSORY ORGANS

Pancreas

The pancreas is located in both upper quadrants of the abdomen, with the head in the upper right quadrant and the tail in the upper left quadrant. The head and tail are separated by a midsection called the body of the pancreas (Fig. 13–4). Because the pancreas lies retroperitoneally, it cannot be palpated, and this explains why diseases of the pancreas can cause pain that radiates to the back. Additionally, there is not a well-developed pancreatic capsule, and this may explain why inflammatory processes of the pancreas can freely spread and affect the surrounding organs (stomach and duodenum).

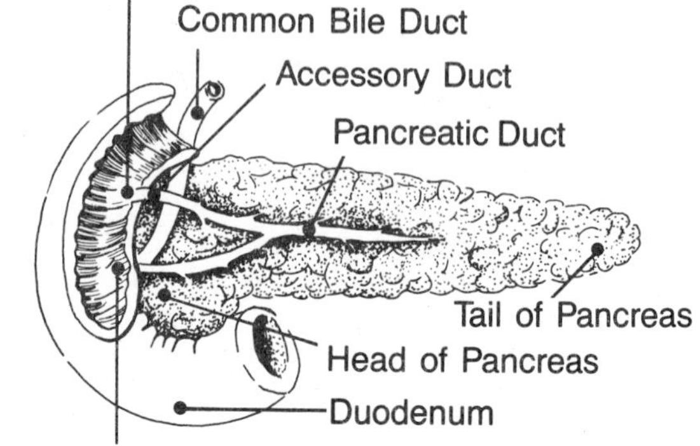

Figure 13–4. The pancreas.

The pancreas has both exocrine (production of digestive enzymes) functions and endocrine (production of insulin and glucagon) functions. The cells of the pancreas, called acini, secrete the major pancreatic enzymes essential for normal digestion (Table 13–4). Trypsinogen and chymotrypsinogen are secreted in inactive form to prevent autodigestion of the gland. Bicarbonate is also secreted by the pancreas and plays an important role in enabling the pancreatic enzymes to work to break down foodstuffs. After breakdown by pancreatic enzymes, food is further digested by enzymes in the small intestine and absorbed into the blood stream. The presence of acid in the stomach stimulates the duodenum to produce the hormone secretin, which stimulates pancreatic secretions. Protein substances in the duodenum stimulate the production of cholecystokinin (CCK).

The endocrine functions of the pancreas are accomplished by groups of alpha and beta cells that compose the islets of Langerhans. Beta cells secrete insulin and alpha cells secrete glucagon. Both are essential to carbohydrate metabolism. When beta cells are affected by disease, blood glucose levels become elevated.

The exocrine and endocrine functions of the pancreas are essential to digestion and carbohydrate metabolism, respectively. Therefore, pancreatic dysfunction can predispose the patient to malnutrition, and accounts for many problems in the clinical setting.

The pancreatic response to low flow states (decreased cardiac output) or hypotension is often ischemia of the pancreatic cells. This ischemia is thought to play a role in the release of cardiotoxic factors (myocardial depressant factor), which are known to decrease cardiac output. Pancreatic ischemia can also result in acute pancreatitis, which will be discussed later in the chapter.

Liver

The liver is the largest internal organ of the body, and is located in the right upper abdominal quadrant. The basic functional unit of the liver is the liver lobule (Fig. 13–5). Hepatic cells are arranged in cords that radiate from the central vein into the periphery. Blood from portal arterioles and venules empties into channels called sinusoids. Lining the walls of the sinusoids are specialized phagocytic cells called Kupffer cells. These cells remove bacteria and other foreign material from the blood.

The liver has a rich blood supply, receiving blood from both the hepatic artery and portal vein, which drains structures of the GI tract. The blood supplied to the liver by these two vessels accounts for approximately 25% of the cardiac output.

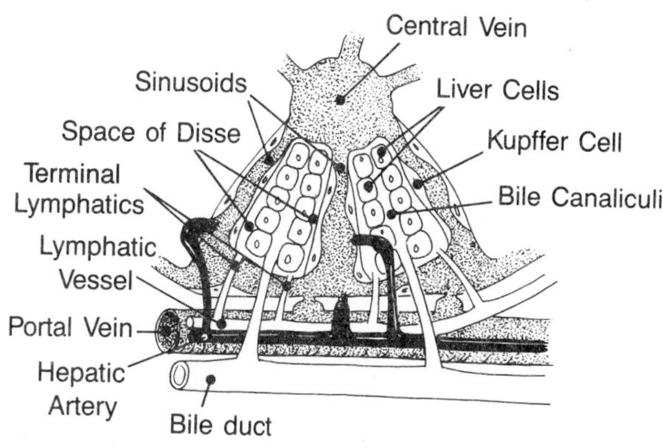

Figure 13–5. The normal liver lobule.

The liver performs over 400 functions. The following discussion of hepatic functions is based on the classification by Guyton (1986) and includes vascular, secretory, and metabolic functions. These actions are summarized in Table 13–5.

Vascular Functions

Blood Storage. Resistance to blood flow (hepatic vascular resistance) in the liver is normally low. Any increase in pressure in the veins drain-

Table 13–5. FUNCTIONS OF THE LIVER

Vascular Functions
Blood Storage
Blood Filtration
Secretory Functions
Production of Bile Salts
Secretion of Bilirubin
Conjugation of Bilirubin
Metabolic Functions
Carbohydrate Metabolism
Fat Metabolism
Protein Metabolism
Synthesis of Blood Clotting Components (Factors II, VI, VII, VIII, IX, X)
Removal of Activated Clotting Factors
Detoxification of Drugs, Hormones, and Other Substances
Storage Functions
Blood
Glucose
Vitamins (A, B_{12}, D, E, K)
Fat

ing the liver causes blood to accumulate in the sinusoids and causes the sinusoids to distend to handle the increased blood volume. The liver sinusoids can store up to 400 ml of blood. This can serve as a compensatory mechanism in cases of hypovolemic shock in which blood from the liver can be shunted into the circulation to increase blood volume.

Filtration. As mentioned earlier, Kupffer cells that line the sinusoids cleanse the blood of bacteria and foreign material that has been absorbed through the GI tract. These cells are extremely phagocytic, and thus normally prevent almost all bacteria from reaching the systemic circulation.

Secretory Functions

Bile Production. The secretion of bile is a major function of the liver. Bile is composed of water, electrolytes, bile salts, phospholipids, cholesterol, and bilirubin. Approximately 500 to 1000 ml of bile is produced daily. Bile salts emulsify fats and foster their absorption. The bile salts are reabsorbed in the terminal portion of the ileum and then transported back to the liver where they can be used again. Bile travels to the gallbladder via the common bile duct where it is stored and concentrated.

Bilirubin Metabolism. Bilirubin, a physiologically inactive pigment, is a metabolic end product of the degradation of hemoglobin. Bilirubin enters the circulation bound to albumin in the plasma and is "free," or unconjugated, in this state. It is this portion of the bilirubin that is reflected in the "indirect" serum bilirubin level. Accumulation of unconjugated bilirubin is toxic to cells. Conjugation of bilirubin by the liver and the binding of bilirubin to albumin prevent this from occurring. Approximately 80% of bilirubin transported to the liver is conjugated in hepatic cells and the rest is conjugated with other substances. Almost all bilirubin is secreted into bile. Some conjugated bilirubin does return to the blood and is reflected in the "direct" serum bilirubin level. Excess bilirubin accumulation in the blood results in jaundice. There are several causes of jaundice, including hepatocellular, hemolytic, and obstructive. Hemolytic jaundice results from increased red blood cell destruction; i.e., blood incompatibilities and sickle cell disease. Viral hepatitis is the most common cause of hepatocellular jaundice (jaundice caused by hepatic cell damage). Cirrhosis and liver cancer can also decrease the liver's ability to handle bilirubin. Obstructive jaundice is usually caused by gallbladder disease; e.g., gallstones.

Metabolic Functions

Carbohydrate Metabolism. The liver plays an important role in the maintenance of normal blood glucose concentration. When the concentration of glucose increases above normal levels, it is stored as glycogen (glycogenesis). When blood glucose levels fall, glycogen stored in the liver is split to form glucose (glycogenolysis). If blood glucose levels drop below normal and glycogen stores are depleted, the liver can make glucose from proteins and fats (gluconeogenesis).

Protein Metabolism. All nonessential amino acids are produced in the liver. All amino acids must be deaminated (removal of NH_4) to be used for energy by cells or converted into carbohydrates or fats. Ammonia is released and then removed from the blood by conversion to urea in the liver. The urea that is secreted by the liver into the blood stream is excreted by the kidneys.

With the exception of gamma globulins, the liver also produces all plasma proteins in the blood. The major types of plasma proteins are albumins, globulins, and fibrinogen. Albumin functions to maintain blood osmotic pressure and prevents plasma loss from the capillaries. Globulins are essential for cellular enzymatic reactions. Fibrinogen helps form blood clots.

Fat Metabolism. Almost all cells in the body are capable of lipid metabolism; however, the liver metabolizes fats so rapidly that it is the primary site for these functions. The liver is also the primary site for the conversion of excess carbohydrates and proteins to triglycerides.

Production and Removal of Blood Clotting Factors. In addition to fibrinogen, the liver is the site of synthesis of prothrombin (factor II), accelerator globulin (factor V), and factors VII, VIII, IX, and X. Factors II, VII, IX, and X are vitamin K dependent. The liver also removes active clotting factors from the circulation, and therefore prevents clotting in the macro- and microvasculature.

Detoxification. Drugs, hormones, and other toxic substances are metabolized by the liver to inactive forms for excretion. This is usually accomplished by converting the fat-soluble compounds to water-soluble compounds. They can then be excreted via the bile or the urine.

Vitamin and Mineral Storage. Excess stores of vitamins A, B_{12}, D, E, and K are stored in the liver. The liver also contains up to 30% of the total body iron supply. Magnesium is also stored in the liver.

Gallbladder

The gallbladder is a saclike structure that lies beneath the right lobe of the liver. Its primary function is to store and concentrate bile. The gallbladder can hold approximately 70 ml of bile. Bile salts are secreted into the duodenum when nutrients are ingested. The gallbladder is connected to the duodenum via the common bile duct. Bile flow is controlled by contraction of the gallbladder and relaxation of the sphincter of Oddi, which is located at the junction of the common bile duct and the duodenum. Contraction of the gallbladder is controlled by hormonal (cholecystokinin) and central nervous system signals and is initiated by the presence of food in the duodenum. Bile salts function to emulsify fats and also assist in the absorption of fatty acids.

NEURAL INNERVATION OF THE GI SYSTEM

Functions of the GI system are influenced by neural and hormonal factors. The autonomic nervous system exerts multiple effects. In general, parasympathetic cholinergic fibers or drugs that mimic parasympathetic effects are stimulatory to GI secretion and motility, whereas sympathetic stimulation or adrenergic drugs tend to be inhibitory. Parasympathetic and sympathetic fibers also innervate the gallbladder and pancreas. Another neural regulator of gastric secretions is stimulated by sight, smell, and thoughts of food, as well as food in the mouth. In this phase (cephalic), the brain centers reflexively cause parasympathetic stimulation of gastric secretions by chief and parietal cells.

HORMONAL CONTROL OF THE GI SYSTEM

The GI tract is considered the largest endocrine organ in the body. Hormones that influence GI function include those produced by specialized cells in the GI tract as well as by other endocrine organs (pancreas and gallbladder). Gastrointestinal hormones modulate such activities as motility, secretion, absorption, and maturation of GI tissues. Table 13–6 summarizes the more common GI hormones and their actions.

BLOOD SUPPLY OF THE GI SYSTEM

Blood supply to organs within the abdomen is referred to as splanchnic circulation. The GI system receives proportionally the largest percentage of the cardiac output. Approximately one-third of the cardiac output supplies these tissues. The superior and inferior mesenteric and celiac arteries supply the stomach, small and large intestines, pancreas, and gallbladder. The liver has a dual blood supply and receives part of its blood supply from the hepatic artery. Circulation to the GI system is unique in that venous blood draining the system empties into the portal vein, which then perfuses the liver. The portal vein supplies approximately 70 to 75% of liver blood flow.

Owing to the large percentage of cardiac output that perfuses the GI tract, it is a major source of blood flow during times of increased need; i.e., during exercise or as a compensatory mechanism in hemorrhage. Conversely, prolonged occlusion or hypoperfusion of a major artery supplying the

Table 13–6. ACTIONS OF GASTROINTESTINAL HORMONES

Action	Gastrin	CCK	Secretin	Gastric Inhibitory Peptide
Acid Secretion	Stimulates	Stimulates	Inhibits	Inhibits
Gastric Motility	Stimulates	Stimulates	Inhibits	—
Gastric Emptying	Inhibits	Inhibits	Inhibits	Inhibits
Intestinal Motility	Stimulates	Stimulates	Inhibits	—
Mucosal Growth	Stimulates	Stimulates	Inhibits	—
Pancreatic HCO_3 Secretion	Stimulates	Stimulates	Stimulates	0
Pancreatic Enzyme Secretion	Stimulates	Stimulates	Stimulates	0
Pancreatic Growth	Stimulates	Stimulates	Stimulates	—
Bile HCO_3 Secretion	Stimulates	Stimulates	Stimulates	0
Gallbladder Contraction	Stimulates	Stimulates	Stimulates	—

0 = no effect; dash = not yet tested

GI tract can lead to mucosal ischemia and eventually necrosis. Necrosis of intestinal villi can destroy the GI tract's barrier to harmful toxins and bacteria. These bacteria can then enter the blood supply and cause septic shock.

General Assessment of the GI System

A comprehensive assessment of the abdomen includes a history, inspection, auscultation, percussion, and palpation. Of most import is the timing of auscultation, which should be done prior to any manipulation of the abdomen to avoid altering the frequency of bowel sounds. Optimal positioning of the patient to relax the abdomen should be done prior to beginning auscultation. Make the patient comfortable in a supine position with the arms at sides or folded at the chest. Placing a pillow under the knees also helps relax the abdominal wall.

Mapping of the abdomen for descriptive purposes is usually done using the four-quadrant method by drawing imaginary lines crossing at the umbilicus: right upper, right lower, left upper, and left lower. Symptoms such as pain may also be described using these landmarks.

HISTORY

An assessment of the GI system begins with a nursing history unless an emergency situation exists requiring immediate physiological assessment and intervention. The patient should be questioned about any past problems with indigestion, difficulty swallowing (dysphagia), pain on swallowing, nausea and vomiting, heartburn, belching, abdominal distention or bloating, diarrhea, constipation, or bleeding. All symptoms should be explored in terms of when symptoms became apparent, any precipitating factors, what treatment was sought, factors that relieved or made the symptoms worse, and finally whether the symptom is current.

A careful pain assessment should also be done, and is a challenging aspect of the history. Pain receptors in the abdomen are less likely to be localized and are mediated by common sensory structures projected to the skin. Therefore, it is often difficult to distinguish pain of a peptic ulcer or cholecystitis from that of a myocardial infarction. Abdominal pain is most often caused by engorged mucosa, pressure in the mucosa, distention, or spasm. Visceral pain is more likely to cause pallor, perspiration, bradycardia, nausea and vomiting, weakness, and hypotension, and should also be assessed. Increasing intensity of pain, especially after a therapeutic regimen, is always significant and usually signifies complicating factors such as increasing inflammation, gastric distention, hemorrhage into tissue or the peritoneal space, or peritonitis from perforation or anastomosis leakage. It is always best to get the description of the location and type of pain in the patient's own words.

A history of any GI surgeries, including the names and dates, should also be discussed. A current list of medications is also important, especially since many drugs have gastrointestinal side effects.

INSPECTION

General inspection of the abdomen should focus on the following characteristics:

Skin Color and Texture

Look for pigmentation of skin (jaundice), lesions, discolorations, old or new scars, and hair pattern. General nutrition and hydration status may also be discerned.

Symmetry and Contour of Abdomen

Note the size and shape of the abdomen and visible protrusions and adipose distribution. Abdominal distention, particularly in the presence of pain, should always be investigated as it usually indicates trapped air or fluid within the abdominal cavity. Abdominal distention is always abnormal.

Masses/Pulsations

Look for any obvious abdominal masses. These are best seen on deep inspiration. Pulsations, if they are seen, usually originate from the aorta.

Peristalsis/Movement

Motility of the stomach may be reflected in movement of the abdomen in lean individuals, and therefore would be a normal sign. However, strong contractions are abnormal and indicate disease.

AUSCULTATION

Bowel sounds are high-pitched gurgling sounds caused by air and fluid as they move through the GI tract. They are best heard using the diaphragm of the stethoscope and should be systematically assessed in all four quadrants of the epigastrium. Note the frequency and character of the sounds. The frequency of bowel sounds has been estimated at from 4 to 34 per minute, and they are usually irregular. Therefore, the abdomen must be auscultated at least 5 minutes before a conclusion of complete absence of bowel sounds can be made. Table 13–7 reviews common etiologies of increased and decreased bowel sounds as they relate to critical illness.

Vascular sounds such as bruits may also be heard and indicate dilated, tortuous, or constricted vessels. Venous hums may also normally be heard from the inferior vena cava. A hum in the periumbilical region in a patient with cirrhosis indicates an obstructed portal circulation. Peritoneal friction rubs may also be heard and may indicate infection, abscess, or tumor in the abdomen.

PERCUSSION

Percussion is aimed at detecting fluid, gaseous distention, or masses in the abdomen. Tympany will predominate because of the presence of gas within the GI tract. Solid masses will percuss as dull. Organ borders of the liver, spleen, and stomach may also be ascertained. Abnormal findings are usually confirmed by radiological tests in the critical care setting.

PALPATION

Palpation is used to evaluate the major organs with respect to shape, size, position, mobility, consistency, and tension. Palpation is performed last because it often elicits pain and/or muscle spasm. It is important to monitor this aspect of the physical examination by watching the patient's face. Deep abdominal tenderness and/or rebound tenderness need to be differentiated. Rigidity or guarding of the abdomen should also be noted. Masses in the liver, spleen, kidneys, gallbladder, and descending colon can also be felt through palpation.

Table 13-7. ETIOLOGIES OF INCREASED AND DECREASED BOWEL SOUNDS

Decreased Bowel Sounds	Increased Bowel Sounds
Peritonitis	Early Pyloric or Intestinal Obstruction
Gangrene	Bleeding Ulcers or Electrolyte Disturbances
Reflux Ileus	Varices
Surgical Manipulation of Bowel	Diarrhea
Late Bowel Obstruction	Subsiding Ileus

■ Nutritional Assessment and Therapies

ASSESSMENT

Adequate nutritional support of the critically ill patient is an aspect of nursing care and needs to be considered early in the patient's illness. Increased morbidity and mortality rates, delayed wound healing, and altered normal immune responses have all been associated with malnutrition.

Body homeostasis requires that there is balance between energy supply and expenditure. The basal metabolic rate (BMR) is the energy a person requires to perform physiological processes at rest. Logically, stressors such as fever, trauma, and sepsis impact negatively on energy balance (increase BMR) and need to be considered in the care of the critically ill patient. Nitrogen balance is also important and reflects whether or not the body is building protein. Anabolism reflects a positive nitrogen balance, or that the body is building protein. Catabolism, or a negative nitrogen balance, represents body breakdown of protein. Most critically ill patients by virtue of their injury or disease process are in a catabolic state, and this needs to be considered in the assessment and when instituting nutritional therapies.

Complete nutritional assessment consists of history taking and anthropometric and biochemical measurements and allows for quantification of nutritional health. The parameters the nurse most commonly uses to assess nutritional balance in a critically ill patient are albumin and nitrogen balance. Normal serum albumin is 4.0 to 5.2. Nitrogen balance is calculated using the following calculation:

$$\text{Nitrogen Balance} = \frac{\text{Protein Intake}}{6.25} - \text{Urinary Urea Nitrogen} + 4$$

If the number calculated is zero, nitrogen balance is present. If the number is positive, protein synthesis is occurring. If the number is negative, protein catabolism exists and the patient is malnourished. A diet history may also help to determine nutritional state before illness.

The final step in performing a nutritional

assessment is to determine the individual caloric needs of the patient. This is normally calculated using a basal energy requirements calculation (Harris-Benedict) Table 13–8.

NUTRITIONAL THERAPIES

Total Parenteral Nutrition

Total parenteral nutrition (TPN) is a very successful way to provide nutrients to patients who are unable to maintain adequate nutritional status by oral intake. Formulas for TPN contain all known essential nutrients, including water, protein, carbohydrate, fat, electrolytes, vitamins, and trace elements. The proportion of these elements as well as the total calories are individualized to the patient. The mixture usually comprises 20 to 30% glucose and 3.5 to 5.0% amino acids. The ratio of glucose, which supplies calories, to nitrogen or amino acids is about 200:1, which will maintain nitrogen balance and promote weight gain, wound healing, and anabolism. Electrolytes are also added to the solution, including sodium, potassium, and chloride. Fats are supplied either by IV supplement or are mixed in the TPN bag. Adjustments in the formula are made as the patient's energy expenditure changes during the course of the illness.

Nurses are responsible for the administration of TPN therapy. Major complications of TPN include sepsis, and fluid and electrolyte imbalance. Maintaining sterility of the TPN set-up is essential. All tubing should be changed at least every 24 to 48 hours. No IV push or piggyback medications should be given in the same line. Intravenous site care should be meticulous. Because TPN solution is hyperosmolar, it is usually administered through a central line, which can become infected without meticulous care by nursing and medicine. Monitoring fluid and electrolyte balance, and for early signs of infection, is an important nursing aspect of care related to this therapeutic modality. Glucose overfeeding and other electrolyte imbalances can also be complications of TPN therapy. Therefore, serum glucose and other electrolytes need to be monitored. Patients on TPN should have blood sugars measured by finger stick every 6 hours until glucose tolerance is assessed. When the blood sugar stabilizes, blood sugars can be monitored less frequently. Occasionally, insulin needs to be administered with TPN therapy, especially in patients in whom insulin secretion and regulation may be impaired. It is also important to remember that TPN needs to be weaned slowly to prevent hypoglycemic reactions.

Table 13–8. BASAL ENERGY REQUIREMENTS CALCULATION (BEE)* (Harris-Benedict Equation)

Women

$$BEE = 655 + (9.6 \times Wt) + (1.8 \times Ht) - (4.7 \times Age)$$

Men

$$BEE = 66 + (13.7 \times Wt) + (5 \times Ht) - (6.8 \times Age)$$

* Used to determine caloric requirements; weight in kilograms; height in centimeters; age in years

Enteral Nutrition

Enteral nutrition refers to the delivery of nutrients into the GI tract. It is most commonly selected for patients with neuromuscular impairment, patients who cannot meet their nutritional needs by oral intake alone, patients who are hypercatabolic, or patients who are unable to eat as a result of their underlying illness; i.e., intensive care unit patients on ventilators or with hypoperfusion states. Enteral nutrition depends on an intact bowel that is able to absorb nutrients.

To accommodate diverse patient needs, many types of enteral formulas have been developed. All contain protein, carbohydrates, and fat, but the proportion of each differs. The osmolality or ionic concentration is important in selecting a formula for enteral feedings. Isotonic solutions have approximately the same osmolality as normal plasma. These formulas are usually initially administered at full strength and the rate of administration increased as tolerated. Hypertonic formulas have osmolalities greater than normal plasma. These solutions are initially administered at full strength and a slow rate (25 ml/hr) or at half strength at 50 ml/hr. Rate and strength of formulas can be advanced, but never at the same time. Patients receiving hypertonic solutions must be assessed for severe diarrhea, electrolyte depletion, and dehydration.

The mouth is the ideal method of enteral nutrition, but for patients who are unable to consume food orally, a variety of routes are available for administration of enteral nutrition. The most common is the nasogastric tube. Tube length is dependent on placement in the GI tract. A 36-inch tube is standard and reaches the stomach if inserted via the nose.

Feeding schedules may be either intermittent or continuous. The stomach is normally a reservoir for intermittently receiving food. Therefore, an intermittent schedule is recommended by most authorities. Feedings delivered in this manner are delivered by gravity and regulated with a roller clamp to infuse over 40 to 60 minutes. Delivery of tube feeding using a syringe is not recommended because of the risk of pulmonary aspiration. Feedings delivered into the small intestine should be delivered by constant infusion since normally the intestinal mucosa receives nutrients from the stomach in peristaltic waves. Enteral feeding pumps are recommended for delivery.

Complications associated with enteral feedings include:

- Feeding tube obstruction
- Pulmonary complications caused by improper tube placement or aspiration
- Gastrointestinal symptoms: diarrhea, abdominal distention, delayed gastric emptying, cramping, and constipation
- Metabolic complications: hyperglycemia, hypercapnia, and electrolyte imbalance

Table 13–9 reviews common enteral feeding complications and select nursing interventions. The most common complication of tube feedings is diarrhea. It can be caused by multiple factors, including concomitant drug therapy; the formula's lactose, lipid, or fiber content; the osmolality of the feeding; and bacterial contamination. Pulmonary complications are potentially the most serious and can result from improper tube placement or aspiration.

In summary, enteral feedings are a safe form of nutritional therapy. The most common complications are gastrointestinal in nature. The nurse is responsible for prevention of these complications and this can be accomplished through

Table 13–9. TUBE FEEDING COMPLICATIONS AND SELECT NURSING INTERVENTIONS

Mechanical Complications

1. Tube obstruction
   a. Flush feeding tube with at least 30 ml of water every 4 hr during continuous feedings, after medications, after intermittent feedings, before and after checking residuals.
   b. Use polyurethane tube.
   c. Used medications in elixir form whenever possible.
   d. If tube becomes obstructed, irrigate with either water or cola.

Pulmonary Complications

1. Improper tube placement
   a. Verify the position of all small-bore feeding tubes by x-ray.
   b. Identify patients at risk for malposition; i.e., impaired gag/cough reflex, patients who are obtunded, heavily sedated, or those receiving neuromuscular blocking agents.

Note: Air insertion into tube with auscultation can be misleading. Attempting to aspirate gastric contents is also insufficient because small-bore tubes collapse easily

2. Aspiration
   a. Monitor residuals every 4 hours and temporarily discontinue feedings if volume is greater than 100–150 ml/hr for 2 consecutive hours.
   b. Monitor for abdominal distention with abdominal girth measurements.
   c. Assess bowel sounds
   d. Monitor for tube position every 4 hours. Mark feeding tube at exit site.
   e. To prevent reflux, keep head of bed elevated 30–40 degrees during feedings. Discontinue feedings for 10–15 min prior to rolling patient's head flat for therapies.
   f. Color tube feedings with dye. Monitor pulmonary secretions. Secretions can also be tested with glucose oxidase reagent strips.

Gastrointestinal Complications

1. Diarrhea
   a. Review medications the patient is receiving.
   b. Dilute hypertonic oral suspensions before administering.
   c. Administer fiber-enriched formulas or bulking agents to normalize stool consistency (i.e., Metamucil).
   d. Prevent bacterial contamination:
      i. When possible, use full-strength, ready-to-use formula.
      ii. Use meticulous handwashing techniques in handling all formulas and supplies.
      iii. Avoid touching inside of delivery sets.
      iv. Wash delivery sets with soapy water and rinse after intermittent feedings. Change delivery sets every 24 hr.
      v. Limit hang time of formulas at room temperature to 8–12 hr (Exception: prefilled sets; read manufacturer recommendations).

Metabolic Complications

1. Hyperglycemia
   a. Monitor urine sugar and acetone every 4–6 hr until stable.
   b. Monitor blood glucose every 24 hr.
   c. Observe for signs and symptoms of hyperglycemia. Administer insulin as ordered, usually per sliding scale.
   d. Use delivery methods which ensure administration of feeding at a constant rate.
2. Hypercapnia.
   a. Use formulas with lower carbohydrate and higher fat content for respiratory-compromised and ventilator-dependent patients.
   b. Monitor respiratory status.
3. Electrolyte imbalance
   a. Monitor fluid status closely.
   b. Monitor serum sodium, potassium, and phosphate.

careful monitoring. Based on the current research base, the following recommendations are made:

1. All patients placed on tube feedings should have standing orders or protocols that provide guidelines for confirming correct tube placement, handling of formulas, administration of formulas, and managing complications.

2. Fine-bore tubes need to be carefully assessed as they are easily dislodged. Food coloring should be added to all feedings to help detect aspiration or tube displacement. Check for gastric residual every 4 hours.

3. Use good handwashing technique in the preparation of delivery sets or in reconstituting formulas (such as half-strength). Rinse delivery set with water before adding new formula. Limit hang time of formulas at room temperature to 8 to 12 hours. Change delivery sets every 24 hours.

4. Monitor blood sugars by finger stick every 6 hours until blood sugars are stable. Institute daily weights, daily electrolyte panels, BUN, and glucose until stabilized. Monitor trace elements every week.

5. Use a controller pump to administer feedings at a constant rate. Flush feeding tubes every 4 hours during continuous feedings, after giving intermittent feedings, and after medications.

6. Provide ongoing nutritional assessments.

Acute Upper Gastrointestinal Bleed

PATHOPHYSIOLOGY

There are many causes of acute upper GI bleeding that would necessitate admission of a patient to the critical care unit. Table 13–10 reviews the most common causes of this GI emergency.

Peptic Ulcer Disease

Duodenal and gastric ulcers are the most common cause of upper GI bleeding. Duodenal and gastric ulcers are characterized by a break in the mucosa extending through the muscularis mucosae. The ulcer crater is usually surrounded by either acute or chronic inflamed cells. Over time, the inflamed tissue is replaced by necrotic tissue, then granulation tissue, and finally scar tissue.

The role of gastrin, which stimulates excess secretion of acid, is important in the pathogenesis of duodenal ulcer disease. Research indicates that parietal cell mass in this patient population is 1.5 to 2.0 times greater than in persons with no ulcer disease. In patients with normal acid secretion, impaired mucosal resistance to acids is being studied as an etiology. Duodenal ulcer disease is also associated with several chronic diseases, including chronic pulmonary disease, cirrhosis, renal failure and transplantation, renal stones, and coronary artery disease. Duodenal ulcer disease is estimated to be 1.5 to 3.0 times more common in males than females.

Table 13–10. CAUSES OF UPPER GI BLEEDS

Duodenal Ulcer
Gastric Ulcer
Cushing's Ulcer
Curling's Ulcer
Stress Ulcer
Mallory-Weiss Tear
Gastritis
Esophagitis
Esophageal or Gastric Varices

Risk factors for development of this disease have also been widely studied. Although certain foods, beverages, and spices may cause dyspepsia (Table 13–11), there are no supportive data that indicate that diet causes or reactivates duodenal ulcers. Furthermore, a cause and effect relationship between a bland diet or milk consumption on duodenal ulcer disease has not been substantiated.

Known risk factors for duodenal ulcer disease are listed in Table 13–12. Alcoholic beverages are acid secretion stimulants and in high concentrations cause damage to the gastric mucosal barrier. The use of alcoholic beverages is associated with duodenal lesions and upper gastrointestinal bleeding.

Aspirin and other nonsteroidal anti-inflammatory drugs (NSAIDs) may cause acute gastric mucosal damage, chronic ulcers, and precipitate upper gastrointestinal bleeding.

Table 13–11. DIETARY STIMULANTS OF ACID SECRETION

Unrefined Wheat
Coffee
Coca Cola
Tab
Acid-Neutralized Coffee
7-Up
Beer
Tea

Table 13-12. KNOWN RISK FACTORS FOR DUODENAL ULCER DISEASE

Alcohol
Drugs
  Aspirin
  NSAID
  ?Corticosteroids (>30 days; >1g)
Smoking
Genetic Predisposition
  Acid hypersecretion
  Altered mucosa
Defense Mechanism
?Stress

Cigarette smoking is causally linked to duodenal ulcer disease. Studies indicate that smoking impairs ulcer healing, is associated with recurrences, and increases patient risk for complications. Mortality rates for patients who smoke are also higher.

There is also strong evidence that supports a genetic link for duodenal ulcer disease. Twenty to 50% of duodenal ulcer patients report a positive family history (Sleisenger and Fordtran, 1989).

Emotional factors also influence gastric function; however, the specific role of personality types and responses to stressful events as mediated by the central nervous system has not been clearly linked to duodenal ulcer disease and needs further study.

The cause of gastric ulcers is poorly understood. It is not known whether acid and pepsin damage the mucosa or whether acid and pepsin cause the ulceration once mucosal damage occurs. Gastric mucosal ischemia is also believed to be an important pathogenesis of acute mucosal injury (see stress ulceration below). Abnormalities in mucus production and/or bicarbonate secretion have also been widely studied. Theoretically, gastric ulcer patients might secrete lower than normal amounts of mucus or bicarbonate, or they may produce an inferior quality of mucus. Gastric ulcers tend to recur frequently, usually at the same site.

Stress Ulcers

A stress ulcer is an acute gastric mucosal erosion that commonly occurs in patients placed in intensive care units. The lesions are associated with patients who have sustained severe trauma, who have long-term sepsis, in patients who have been severely burned (Curling's ulcer), in patients with cranial or central nervous system disease (Cushing's ulcer), and finally in patients who chronically ingest drugs that have known adverse effects on the gastric mucosa. Abnormalities range from small surface hemorrhages to deep ulcerations with massive gastrointestinal hemorrhage and occasionally perforation. Massive upper gastrointestinal bleeding usually occurs 3 to 7 days after the initial insult and significantly increases the mortality rate for the critically ill patient.

Factors associated with stress ulcers are reviewed in Table 13-13. Acid hypersecretion is not associated with all etiologies of stress ulcers, but some amount of acid is necessary for the formation of an ulcer. Cardiogenic shock directly impairs oxygen supply to the stomach, and therefore may impair vascular perfusion of the stomach, causing mucosal anoxia. Stress may reduce both the quality and the quantity of mucus in the stomach. Mucus, a natural defense mechanism in the stomach, delays the diffusion of H^+ ions into the mucosa. Lowered mucosal pH (<3.5) and decreased regeneration of mucosal cells also have been implicated in the development of stress ulcers.

Mallory-Weiss Tear

A Mallory-Weiss tear is an arterial bleed from an acute longitudinal tear in the gastroesophageal mucosa and accounts for 10 to 15% of upper GI bleeding episodes. It is associated with long-term NSAID ingestion and with excessive alcohol intake. The upper GI bleed usually occurs after episodes of forceful retching. Bleeding usually spontaneously resolves; however, lacerations of the esophagogastric junction may cause a massive GI bleed.

Esophageal Varices

In chronic cirrhotic liver failure, as liver cells die, there is a resultant increase in the portal venous pressure, which is called portal hypertension. As a result, part of the venous blood in the splanchnic system may be diverted from the liver to the

Table 13-13. PATHOGENESIS OF STRESS ULCERS

Acid Hypersecretion
Gastric Anoxia (Hypotension)
Altered Mucosal Defense Mechanisms
Decreased Mucosal pH

systemic circulation by the development of connections to neighboring low-pressure veins. This is termed collateral circulation. The most common sites for the development of these collateral channels are in the submucosa of the esophagus and rectum, in the anterior abdominal wall, and in the parietal peritoneum. Figure 13–6 shows the liver with collateral circulation. The normal portal venous pressure is 2 to 6 mm Hg. As pressure rises in these veins, they become distended with blood, the vessels enlarge, and varices develop. Formation of varices requires that this pressure increase to over 10 mm Hg. The most common sites for the development of these varices are in the esophagus and the upper portion of the stomach. In summary, esophageal and gastric varices represent massively dilated submucosal veins that divert splanchnic venous blood from the high-pressure portal system. These varices tend to have a low tolerance for pressure and thus tend to bleed. It is estimated that between 13 and 70% of patients with varices will bleed (Galambos, 1985).

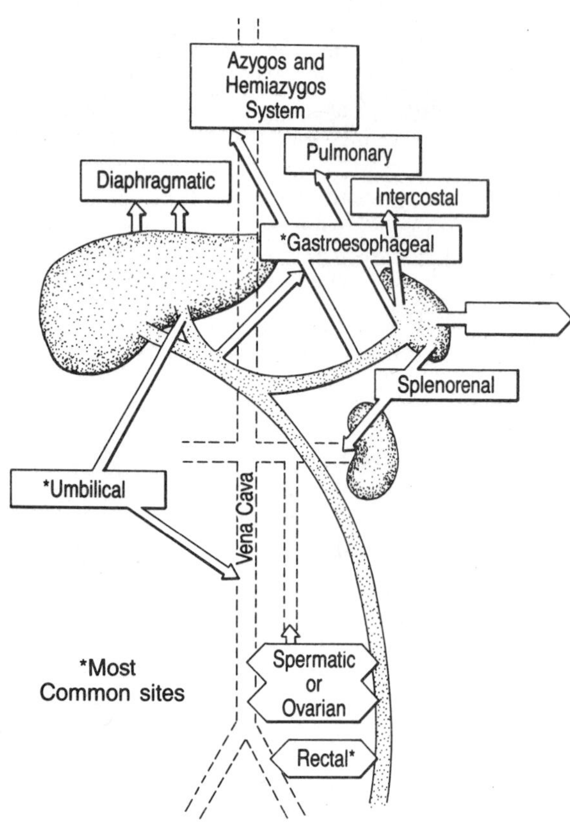

Figure 13–6. The liver and collateral circulation.

ASSESSMENT

Clinical Presentation

Patients manifest blood loss from the gastrointestinal tract in several ways. Hematemesis is bloody vomitus that is either bright red, which indicates a fresh bleed, or "coffee-ground," which is an older bleed (blood that has been in the stomach long enough for the gastric juices to act on it). Blood may also be passed via the colon. Melena is shiny, black, foul-smelling vomitus or stool and results from the degradation of blood by stomach acids or intestinal bacteria. Bright red or maroon blood, hematochezia, can also be passed from the rectum. Gastrointestinal blood loss can also be occult; detected only by testing the stool with a chemical reagent (guaiac). However, stool and nasogastric drainage can test guaiac positive for up to 10 days after a bleed and are associated with chronic bleeds. Hematemesis, melena, or hematochezia indicates an episode of acute upper GI bleeding. Hematemesis results from large amounts of blood collecting in the stomach accompanied by nausea. Hematochezia is usually a sign of lower GI bleeding. When hematochezia is from an upper GI source, it is associated with a massive bleed (greater than 1000 ml). Upper GI bleeding may also be accompanied by mild epigastric pain or abdominal distress, although it is not very common. Pain is thought to arise from the acid bathing the ulcer crater.

Finally, patients may present with clinical signs and symptoms of blood loss, such as hypotension, tachycardia, dizziness, dyspnea, restlessness and anxiety, decreased level of consciousness, decreased urine output, and shock. Table 13–14 summarizes the common presenting manifestations of an acute upper GI bleed. Rapid assessment of the patient is undertaken to determine the seriousness of the bleed; i.e., is it acute or chronic; and to determine whether the patient is hemodynamically stable or unstable. Patients with acute upper GI bleed will commonly have signs or symptoms of hypovolemic shock (Chapter 7).

Nursing Assessment

Assessment of the severity of blood loss is a first priority, and includes frequent monitoring of vital signs and head-to-toe assessments of body systems for signs of shock. Blood pressure and heart rate depend upon the amount of blood loss, the suddenness of the blood loss, and the degree of cardiac and vascular compensation (Sleisenger

Table 13-14. CLINICAL SIGNS AND SYMPTOMS OF UPPER GI BLEED

Hematemesis
Melena
Hematochezia
Abdominal Discomfort
Signs and Symptoms of Hypovolemic Shock
  Hypotension
  Tachycardia
  Cool, clammy skin
  Changes in level of consciousness
  Decreased urine output
  Decreased gastric motility

and Fordtran, 1989). Vital signs should be monitored at least every 15 minutes. As blood loss exceeds 1000 ml, the shock syndrome progresses, causing decreased blood flow to the skin, lungs, liver, and kidneys. As a result of decreased blood flow to the skin, the patient will be cool and clammy. Decreased blood flow to the lungs will cause hyperventilation to maintain adequate oxygenation. As blood flow decreases to the liver, waste products will accumulate in the blood, as reflected in an increasing BUN. Urine output is a very sensitive measure of tissue perfusion and blood flow, and therefore output must be measured at least every hour. Abdominal assessment may reveal a soft or distended abdomen. Bowel sounds most often are hyperactive owing to the sensitivity of the bowel to blood. Hypotension is an advanced sign of shock. As a rule, a systolic pressure under 100 mm Hg or a postural drop in blood pressure greater than 10 mm Hg reflects a blood loss of at least 1000 ml—25% of the total blood volume. As blood pressure falls, it can be assumed that more blood has been lost. Rarely, a central venous pressure (CVP) or pulmonary artery catheter will be inserted to evaluate the patient's hemodynamic response to the blood loss. The CVP and/or pulmonary capillary wedge pressure (PCWP) will be lowered in the patient with hemorrhagic shock. The ECG may also show ST segment depression or flattening of the T waves, which indicates decreased coronary blood flow.

In addition to the physical examination, it is important to take a history to ascertain if there have been previous episodes of bleeding or surgery for bleeding, a family history of bleeding, or a current illness that may lead to bleeding such as coagulopathies, cancer, or liver disease. Concurrent diseases also impact on the patient's response to the hemorrhage and treatment modalities. Patterns of drug or alcohol ingestion and other risk factors need to be assessed and may also help ascertain the etiology.

Medical Assessments

Laboratory Studies

The common laboratory studies ordered for a patient with an acute GI bleed are listed in Table 13-15. A complete blood count is always ordered. It is important to remember, however, that the hematocrit (Hct) does not change substantially during the first few hours after an acute GI bleed. During this time, it is important not to underestimate the severity of the bleed, which is best done with the vital signs as mentioned above. Only when extravascular fluid enters the vascular space to restore volume does the hematocrit drop. This is further complicated by fluids and blood that will be administered during the resuscitation period. Platelet and white blood cell counts may also be increased, reflecting the body's attempt to restore homeostasis. An electrolyte profile will also be ordered. Decreases in potassium and sodium are common owing to the accompanying vomiting. Later, serum sodium levels may increase as a result of the loss of vascular volume. Glucose is often elevated on ac-

Table 13-15. LABORATORY TESTS FOR UPPER GI BLEED

Complete Blood Count
  Hemoglobin—normal, then decreases
  Hematocrit—normal, then decreases
  WBC count—elevated
  Platelet Count—initially elevated, then decreased
Electrolyte Panel
  Serum K—decreases, then increases
  Serum Na—elevated
  Serum Ca—normal or decreased
  Serum BUN, Creatinine—elevated
  Serum ammonia—possible elevation
  Serum glucose—hyperglycemia common
  Serum lactate—elevated
Hematology Profile
  PT, PTT—usually decreased
Serum Enzymes
  Elevated
Arterial Gases
  Respiratory alkalosis/Metabolic acidosis
Gastric Aspirate for pH and Guaiac
  Possibly acidotic pH; Guaiac+

count of the stress response. Increases in the BUN and creatinine reflect decreased perfusion to the liver and kidneys, respectively. Liver functions tests, a clotting profile, and serum ammonia will be ordered to rule out preexisting liver disease. An arterial blood gas (ABG) analysis will be ordered to evaluate the patient's acid-base and oxygenation status. Respiratory alkalosis is common with GI bleed owing to the effects of the sympathetic nervous system on the lungs and patient anxiety. As shock progresses, the patient may present with metabolic acidosis as a result of anaerobic metabolism. Hypoxemia may also be present as a result of decreased circulating hemoglobin levels.

Barium X-rays and Endoscopy

The history and physical examination are not definitive diagnostic examinations since they do not define the bleeding lesion that is necessary before definitive treatment can be initiated. The two most frequently used tests are the barium x-ray and endoscopy. In a patient who is admitted to the critical care unit, endoscopy is the procedure of choice. Endoscopy allows for direct mucosal inspection with the use of a fiberoptic scope. Flexible scopes allow this test to be performed at the bedside, which is preferable in an unstable critically ill patient. Endoscopic evaluation of the source of the bleed will not be undertaken until the patient has been hemodynamically stabilized with conventional medical therapies (see section on intervention). Barium x-rays can be performed to help define the presence of peptic ulcers, sites of bleeding, tumors, and inflammatory processes.

NURSING DIAGNOSES

The actual and potential nursing diagnoses most commonly seen in patients with an acute GI bleed include:

1. Fluid volume deficit related to decreased circulating blood volume
2. Anxiety related to hemorrhage, pain or discomfort, hospitalization, fear of the unknown
3. Altered tissue perfusion related to decreased circulating blood volume
4. Knowledge deficit related to disease process, therapeutic interventions
5. Impaired gas exchange related to loss of oxygen-carrying capacity
6. Potential for fluid volume excess related to fluid overload from treatment regimen

Additionally, patient problems that can result from the disease process or treatment regimen include:

1. Altered electrolyte balance related to loss of blood and gastric contents, administration of fluids and blood products
2. Hepatic encephalopathy related to altered cerebral metabolism from increased circulating ammonia

See the Nursing Care Plan for the Patient with an Acute Upper GI Bleed.

COLLABORATIVE MANAGEMENT; NURSING AND MEDICAL CONSIDERATIONS

The management of acute GI bleeds is initially focused on hemodynamically stabilizing the patient and then moves to diagnosing the cause of bleeding and initiation of specific and supportive therapies (Table 13–16). The nurse's specific role during the initial management of acute GI bleeds includes patient assessments, carrying out ordered medical therapeutics, monitoring the patient's physiological and psychosocial responses to the interventions, monitoring for complications of the disease process or treatment regimen, and supportive care. Patient and family support during the acute phase is a nursing priority. Explanations of diagnostic tests, medical therapies, and the intensive care environment are extremely important to patients who are often anxious about their diagnosis and the outcome.

Hemodynamic Stabilization

Patients who are hemodynamically unstable need to have immediate venous access using large-bore

Table 13–16. MANAGEMENT OF UPPER GI BLEED

- Hemodynamic Stabilization
  - Colloids
  - Crystalloids
  - Blood/Blood Products
- Definitive and Supportive Therapies
  - Gastric Lavage
  - Pharmacological Therapies
    - Antacids
    - H_2 blockers
  - Endoscopic Therapies
    - Sclerotherapy
    - Heater probe
    - Laser
  - Surgical Therapies

NURSING CARE PLAN FOR THE PATIENT WITH AN ACUTE GI BLEED

Nursing Diagnosis	Outcome	Intervention
Fluid volume deficit related to decreased circulating blood volume	Normal circulating body fluid volume Control or resolution of hemorrhage Preload indicators WNL Stable Hct and Hgb Stable weight Balanced I/O	Monitor vital signs for hemodynamic instability; orthostatic changes Measure preload indicators; CVP, PCWP Monitor ECG, skin, urine output, daily weights, frequency, amount and characteristics of GI secretions Monitor response to fluid replacement Monitor labs; serial Hct, Hgb, BUN, K, Na Monitor nature of bowel sounds Monitor for clinical manifestations of perforation; severe persistent abdominal pain; board-like abdomen Lavage prn as ordered until clear Administer medications, parenteral fluids Prepare for endoscopy, assist as necessary, monitor for complications
Altered tissue perfusion related to decreased circulating blood volume	Absence of signs and symptoms of decreased perfusion Absence of decreased sensorium, chest pain, renal failure Stable hemodynamics Urine output >30 ml/hr Skin warm/dry Bowel sounds WNL	Monitor for hypoperfusion and hemodynamic instability Monitor VS every 15 min until stable Measure CVP, PCWP, CO every 1 hr until stable Monitor for presence of tachycardia, chest pain, ST segment elevation, diaphoresis, cool/clammy extremities Measure urine output every 4 hr Monitor for alterations in level of consciousness Assess for nature of bowel sounds, decreased Monitor for increased bilirubin Notify physician of changes, abnormalities
Anxiety related to hospitalization, hospital regimen	Patient/family demonstrates decreased anxiety with nursing intervention; i.e., explanations of environment Patient/family verbalizes understanding of disease, medical and nursing interventions used	Assess level of anxiety Explain ICU environment and all procedures Provide reassurance to patient and family Approach patient and family in a calm concerned manner Structure ICU environment to provide rest; limit stimuli as possible Describe disease process and all therapeutics instituted Anticipate treatments and procedures and provide explanations and reassurance Provide for patient comfort Liberalize or restrict family visitation as necessary Involve patient/family in planning care Encourage patient/family verbalization of fears or concerns
Potential for fluid volume excess related to fluid overload from treatment regimen	Normal respiratory pattern Absence of lung congestion or pulmonary edema	Carefully monitor hemodynamic response to all fluids given Monitor breath sounds at least every hr during fluid administration Monitor for: sudden restlessness or anxiety, dyspnea, tachycardia, coughing, coarse crackles throughout all lung fields, productive white or pink-tinged frothy sputum, dysrhythmias, abnormal ABGs, acute changes in blood pressure, increased CVP, jugular vein distention Record accurate I/O Daily weights Document and report any abnormalities
Potential for infection related to contaminated surgical wound or translocation to blood (post-op surgical)	Free of infection Afebrile Wound clean, dry, without redness, swelling, erythema, pain, purulent drainage	Use aseptic technique for all dressing changes Monitor appearance of incision and surrounding tissue; note any redness, warmth, swelling, or complaints of pain or tenderness Document and report all wound drainage, color, amount, odor Culture any suspicious drainage Monitor WBC count, temperature trends Monitor nutritional status, nitrogen balance, albumin levels

continued

NURSING CARE PLAN FOR THE PATIENT WITH AN ACUTE GI BLEED *Continued*		
Nursing Diagnosis	Outcome	Intervention
		Teach patient/family S&S of wound infection for discharge planning
Potential for ineffective breathing pattern related to obstruction of the airway by the Sengstaken-Blakemore tube	Prevention of or early detection of airway obstruction	Maintain prescribed pressures in all balloon ports Deflate balloon ports as ordered (*always* deflate the esophageal balloon before the gastric balloon) Maintain traction on ports as ordered Keep patient on bed rest with HOB elevated Sedate patient as necessary; provide for safety Irrigate nasogastric tube every 2 hr and prn to maintain patency; note gastric contents Suction nasopharynx frequently Keep scissors at bedside and cut entire tube and remove if there is an episode of sudden respiratory distress, or the gastric balloon deflates prior to esophageal balloon Cleanse and lubricate all skin in contact with tube or traction device

intravenous tubes and fluid started. To restore vascular volume, fluids need to be infused as rapidly as the patient's cardiovascular status will allow and until the vital signs return to baseline. The physician may order colloids, crystalloids, or albumin initially to achieve this purpose. The nurse's role is to gain venous access and initiate prompt fluid resuscitation. Because the blood pressure is the most sensitive measure of adequacy of vascular volume, frequent monitoring of vital signs, at least every 5 to 15 minutes, needs to be a priority. Often intra-arterial lines are inserted for continuous blood pressure monitoring. A parameter the nurse can use to assess the adequacy of fluid administration is reversal of the signs of hemorrhagic shock. These would include normal skin color and temperature, absence of tachycardia, and adequate urine output. The goal of fluid therapy is to improve the circulation of red blood cells. Oxygen may also be started, which will assist in tissue oxygenation.

Patients who continue to bleed or who have an excessively low Hct (<25%) and clinical symptoms may be resuscitated with blood and blood products. The physician's decision to use blood products will be based on laboratory data and clinical examination. Blood is transfused to improve oxygenation (with red blood cells) and/or to improve coagulation (platelets/plasma). It is important to remember that a Hct may not initially be reflective of actual blood volume during the first 24 to 72 hours after a bleed and until vascular volume is restored. A reasonable goal for the management of blood transfusions is a Hct of 30%, but this goal will be individualized for the patient based on clinical assessments. One unit of packed red blood cells (PRBCs) can be expected to increase the hemoglobin (Hgb) by 1 g and the Hct by 2 to 3%, but this is influenced by the patient's intra-vascular volume status, and by whether the patient is currently actively bleeding.

Maintenance of bed rest with the head of the bed elevated is important supportive care to prevent further bleeding and to decrease the risk of aspiration. Exertion increases intra-abdominal pressure, which predisposes the patient to further bleeding. Keeping the head of the bed elevated also serves to prevent reflux of gastric contents into the esophagus. Clearing the nasopharynx of secretions is also a nursing priority to prevent aspiration, particularly in patients who have an altered level of consciousness and impaired swallowing reflexes. Suction and intubation equipment needs to be readily accessible.

In addition to monitoring the effects of fluid resuscitation and blood product administration, the nurse also monitors for complications of the therapy. In patients with preexisting cardiovascular, pulmonary, or renal disease, central venous or pulmonary artery pressure monitoring may be instituted to prevent fluid administration overload. Frequent assessments of breath sounds by the nurse during fluid administration will help prevent this complication. Careful monitoring for complications of blood transfusion therapy is also important. These include hypercalcemia, hyperkalemia, infection, increased ammonia levels, hypothermia, and anaphylactic reactions.

Recognition of Potential Complications

Perforation of the gastric mucosa is the major GI complication of peptic ulcer disease. The nurse needs to be familiar with the signs and symptoms of acute perforation, which are reviewed in Table 13–17. The most common signs of this complication are an abrupt onset of abdominal pain followed rapidly by signs of peritonitis. The goal for the management of this patient is preparation for emergent surgery. Fluid and electrolyte resuscitation, and treatment of any immediate complications, will be priorities. These patients will almost always have nasogastric tubes placed for gastric decompression. Broad-spectrum antibiotics are also usually ordered prior to surgery. Antacids and histamine blockers may or may not be indicated depending on the etiology of the upper GI bleed. Mortality rates for patients with perforations range from 10 to 40% depending on the age and condition of the patient at the time of surgery.

Gastric Lavage

Gastric lavage may be ordered, but this is a controversial therapy in the treatment of an upper GI bleed. Physicians in favor of gastric lavage claim it helps indicate the rapidity of the bleed, whether there is active bleeding in the GI tract, and serves to cleanse the stomach in preparation for endoscopy. If lavage is ordered, 1000 to 2000 ml of normal saline is usually instilled via nasogastric tube and then gently removed by manual or intermittent suction until the secretions are clear. Research indicates that room-temperature lavage is the most effective, since ice lavage may cause hydrochloric acid to diffuse back into the submucosa and cause increased bleeding (Stern, 1985). Room-temperature solutions also prevent hypothermia and are better tolerated by patients. After lavage, the nasogastric tube may be left in or removed. Some research indicates that nasogastric tubes left in place may increase hydrochloric acid secretion in the stomach and cause increased bleeding. Eighty to 90% of upper gastrointestinal bleeds are self-limiting and will stop with lavage therapy alone or on their own. In addition, it is important for the nurse to carefully document the nature of the nasogastric secretions or vomitus; i.e., color, amount, and pH.

Table 13–17. SIGNS OF ACUTE GASTRIC PERFORATION

Abrupt Onset of Severe Abdominal Pain
Abdominal Tenderness
Boardlike Abdomen
Usually Absent Bowel Sounds
Leukocytosis
Presence of Free Air on X-Ray

Pharmacological Therapies

Pharmacological agents are utilized to decrease gastric acid secretion or to reduce acid effects on gastric mucosa. The most common agents utilized include antacids, histamine antagonists (H_2 blockers), and mucosal barrier enhancers. Table 13–18 summarizes these major drugs, including actions, dose and route, side effects, and nursing implications.

Antacids. These act as a direct alkaline buffer to control the pH of the gastric mucosa. Antacids are usually ordered every 1 to 2 hours

Table 13–18. PHARMACOLOGICAL INTERVENTIONS FOR UPPER GI BLEED

Antacids
Mechanism of action: Acid neutralizer
Dosage: 30–60 ml every 1–2 hr or adjust to pH
Side effects: Depend on antacid used. See medication formulary for specific drug side effects. Most common include diarrhea, constipation
Nursing Considerations: Monitor patients in renal failure closely

H-2 Blockers

Tagamet, Cimetadine
Mechanism of action: Competitively inhibits the action of histamine at the histamine H_2 receptors of the parietal cells
Dose: Parenteral: 300 mg every 6 hr. Excreted in urine.
Side Effects: Confusional states, decreased WBC count, nephritis, pancreatitis, somnolence, rash, diarrhea, thrombocytopenia, arthralgias, drug interactions
Nursing considerations: Monitor closely in patients with renal failure, monitor for complications with other drugs, monitor platelet counts

Ranitidine (Zantac)
Mechanisms of action: histamine H_2 receptor antagonist
Dose: 50 mg every 6–8 hr
Side effects: Leukopenia, thrombocytopenia, malaise, dizziness, depression, tachycardia, diarrhea, constipation, hepatitis, arthralgias
Nursing considerations: Monitor closely in patients with hepatic and renal failure, monitor platelet count

initially. If a nasogastric tube is left in place, antacids may be ordered to maintain the gastric pH above 5. The nurse is responsible for obtaining the gastric pH, antacid administration, and monitoring for side effects of the therapy. The major side effects of antacids include diarrhea, electrolyte disturbances (increased Mg^+ and Na^+), and metabolic alkalosis.

Histamine Blockers. These act to block all factors that stimulate the parietal cells in the stomach to secrete hydrochloric acid. The two most common H_2 blockers on the market are cimetadine and ranitidine. A more recent complication associated with all drugs that increase gastric pH is microbial colonization of the stomach, which may predispose patients to tracheal colonization in intubated patients. This may possibly increase the risk for nosocomial pneumonia.

Mucosal Barrier Enhancers. These serve to act on the gastric mucosa to reduce the effects of acid secretion. Prostaglandins are known to improve the mucosal barrier. Sucralfate is a drug used in the treatment of duodenal ulcers and acts to form a protective barrier over the ulcer site. Colloidal bismuth binds to the ulcer base and also stimulates mucus secretion, which acts to prevent further mucosal damage.

Penicillins. A bacterium, *Helicobacter pylori,* has recently been associated with the development of ulcers in peptic ulcer disease. Penicillins, which are effective against this bacterium, may be ordered in the prophylactive treatment of bleeding gastric ulcers, particularly in patients who have recurrent bleeds.

Endoscopic Therapies

Several endoscopic therapies have been developed to control peptic ulcer bleeding. The advantage of these therapies is that they can be applied at the time of diagnosis. Sclerotherapy involves injecting the bleeding ulcer with a necrotizing agent. The most common agents used are morrhuate sodium and tetradecylsulfate. These agents work by traumatizing the endothelium, causing necrosis and eventual sclerosis of the bleeding vessel. Thermal methods of endoscopic therapy include the heater probe, laser photocoagulation, and electrocoagulation. All of these therapies act to tamponade the vessel to stop active bleeding. Because they are performed at the bedside, the nurse assists with the procedures and monitors for untoward effects. Maintenance of airway and breathing during endoscopic procedures is of major concern. Placement of the patient in a left lateral reverse Trendelenburg position can help prevent respiratory complications. Other common complications of sclerotherapy include fever and oozing from the bleeding site. A more serious complication when morrhuate sodium is used is the development of adult respiratory disease syndrome (ARDS), which is thought to occur from the exposure of lung tissue to fatty substances liberated from the necrotizing agent used to sclerose the bleeding vessel.

Surgical Therapies

Surgery may be considered for patients who have a massive GI bleed that is immediately life threatening, in patients who continue to bleed despite medical therapies, and in the case of perforation or unremitting pyloric obstruction.

The purpose of emergency surgery in patients with a massive upper GI bleed is to prevent death from exsanguination. The patient usually will be admitted to an ICU for initial management; i.e., fluid and cardiorespiratory resuscitation to stabilize the patient as much as possible in preparation for the emergent surgery. The most common reason for emergency surgery is massive rebleeding that occurs within 8 hours of admission to the hospital.

Patients may also become surgical candidates if they continue to bleed despite aggressive medical intervention. Criteria for delayed surgery varies from institution to institution, but is usually considered in patients who require greater than 8 U of blood within a 24-hour period.

Impaired emptying of solids or liquids from the stomach into the small intestine (gastric outlet obstruction) may also necessitate surgical intervention. The major symptoms of obstruction include vomiting and continued ulcer pain that is localized in the epigastrium.

Surgical therapies for peptic ulcer disease include gastric resections (antrectomy, gastrectomy, gastroenterostomy, vagotomy), or combined surgeries to restore GI continuity (Billroth I, Billroth II) or to prevent GI complications of the surgery (vagotomy and pyloroplasty). An antrectomy may be performed for duodenal ulcers to decrease the acidity of the duodenum by removing the antrum, which secretes gastric acid. A vagotomy decreases acid secretion in the stomach by dividing the vagus nerve along the esophagus. A pyloroplasty may be performed in conjunction with a vagotomy to prevent stomach atony, a common complication of the vagotomy procedure. A Billroth I procedure involves a vagotomy, antrectomy, and anastomosis of the stomach to the duodenum. A Billroth II involves a vagotomy, a resection of the antrum, and anastomosis of the stomach to the jejunum (Fig. 13–7). A perforation can be treated by simple closure by use of patch to cover the gastric mucosal hole (omental patch), or by excising the ulcer and suturing the surrounding tissue.

Postoperative nursing care is focused on prevention and monitoring of potential complications. Fluid and electrolyte imbalances are commonly related to the fluids lost during the surgical procedure and the drains that are left in place to either decompress the stomach (nasogastric tube) or to drain the surgical site. Additionally, the GI system may not function normally for a period of time postoperatively, resulting in nausea, vomiting, and diarrhea. The provision of adequate nutrition, which is essential for proper wound healing, is necessary. In cases of prolonged ileus postoperatively, total parenteral nutrition may be considered. Monitoring for proper wound healing is also a nursing concern. Signs and symptoms of wound infection (erythema, swelling, tenderness, drainage, fever, increased white blood cell count) need to be documented and reported accordingly. A systemic infection may result from peritonitis in the case of perforation where stomach or intestinal contents spill into the peritoneum. Rupture of the anastomosis postoperatively may also lead to this complication. Pain is also an important postoperative nursing concern. Abdominal incisions are associated with more postoperative discomfort because of their anatomical location. In addition, postoperative lung infections are more common in patients with abdominal incisions because the patient tends to splint respirations because of incisional pain. Deep breathing and coughing exercises are also more painful in this patient population.

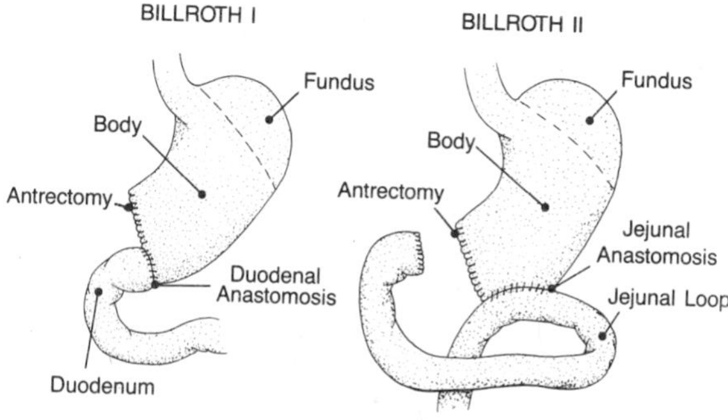

Figure 13–7. Billroth I and II.

Specific nursing diagnoses associated with the postoperative care of the upper GI bleed patient include:

1. Potential for infection; wound
2. Potential for infection related to inflammation of the peritoneum
3. Potential for altered nutrition related to dysfunctional bowel
4. Altered comfort related to incision
5. Impaired gas exchange/ineffective airway clearance related to anesthesia, surgery, decreased activity, pain, splinting, nasogastric tube

TREATMENT OF VARICEAL BLEEDS

Hemorrhaging esophageal and/or gastric varices are usually a medical emergency as they usually cause massive upper GI bleeding. The patient typically presents with hemodynamic instability and signs and symptoms of shock. Often, the cause of the bleed is unknown unless the patient has a known history of cirrhosis or has previously bled from varices. Initial treatment of this population will therefore be the same. Top priorities will include hemodynamic stabilization and establishment of a patent airway. Gastric lavage may be used to clear the stomach and to document the amount of blood loss. Diagnosis of the etiology of the bleed per endoscopy will be the next priority before definitive treatment for the varices can be undertaken.

Vasopressin

Vasopressin (Pitressin) (Table 13–19) is a synthetic antidiuretic hormone and introduction of this hormone into the blood stream can reduce bleeding in 35 to 60% of patients bleeding from varices. It acts directly on gastrointestinal smooth muscle as a vasoconstrictor. Vasopressin lowers portal venous pressure by vasoconstriction, and decreases venous blood flow. Ultimately, it decreases pressure and flow in liver collateral circulation channels to decrease bleeding. Vasopressin is administered in a dose of 0.2 to 0.4 U/min via an infusion pump. Because it is a vasoconstrictor, vasopressin should be infused via a central line. Vasopressin may be administered up to 36 hours, and then is usually slowly weaned if no signs of rebleeding exist.

The critical care nurse's assessments are important during vasopressin administration because while its major action is to constrict splanchnic blood flow, it has many harmful systemic effects. Continuous ECG and blood pres-

Table 13–19. VASOPRESSIN (PITRESSIN) THERAPY

Mechanism of Action
Vasoconstrictor: constricts splanchnic vascular bed, contracts intestinal smooth muscle, and lowers portal vein pressure.
Dose
Most commonly used IV, although may be given intra-arterially. IV infusion is started at 0.2 units/min initially. May be increased to 0.4 units/min. Maximum recommended dose is 0.9 unit/min. Vasopressin should be continued for at least 24 hr after bleeding is controlled.
Side Effects
GI: nausea and vomiting; cramping.
Cardiovascular: hypertension; cardiac dysrhythmias; exacerbation of heart failure.
Neurological: tremors; headache; vertigo.
Integumentary: pallor, localized gangrene.
Nursing Considerations
Monitor for angina.
Infuse through a central line.

sure monitoring is essential because of the constriction effects vasopressin has on the coronary arteries. Chest pain, dysrhythmias, and other symptoms of coronary ischemia are common side effects of this drug. Renal vasoconstriction is another side effect that may induce renal failure and associated complications. Strict intake and output, daily weights, and serum laboratory values need to be closely monitored. Concurrent liver failure and its associated fluid imbalances further complicate the picture. Because vasopressin is an antidiuretic hormone, its mechanism of action will also induce water retention. Consequently, ascites and edema associated with liver failure often will worsen.

Balloon Tamponade

If bleeding continues despite vasopressin therapy, balloon tamponade with a Sengstaken-Blakemore tube (SBT) may be considered (Fig. 13–8). The adult SBT has three lumens. One for gastric aspiration similar to a nasogastric tube, one for inflating the esophageal balloon, and one for inflating the gastric balloon. A variation of this tube is the Minnesota tube, which has an additional fourth lumen that allows for esophageal aspiration. Inflation of the balloon ports applies pressure to the vessels supplying the varices to decrease blood flow, thereby stopping the bleed.

The tip of the balloon is inserted into the stomach and the gastric balloon is inflated and clamped. The tube is then withdrawn until resistance is felt so that pressure is exerted at the gas-

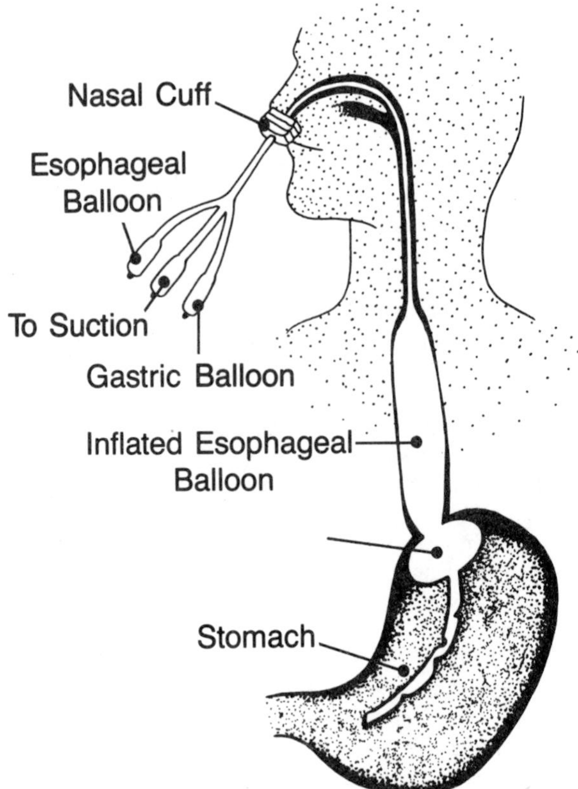

Figure 13–8. Sengstaken-Blakemore tube.

troesophageal (GE) junction. Correct positioning and traction are maintained by use of an external traction source or nasal cuff around the tube at the mouth or nose. External traction can be attached to a helmet or to the foot of the bed. Proper amounts of traction are essential as too little traction will let the balloon fall away from the gastric wall and thereby not put enough pressure on the bleeding vessels. Too much traction can cause discomfort, gastric ulceration, or vomiting. If bleeding does not stop with inflation of the gastric balloon, the esophageal balloon will be inflated and clamped. Normal inflation pressure is 20 to 45 mm Hg. The esophageal balloon can remain inflated up to 48 hours without tissue damage occurring.

The critical care nurse is responsible for maintaining balloon lumen pressures and patency of the system. X-ray confirmation of the gastric balloon port below the GE junction is necessary. Ideally, the balloons should be deflated every 8 to 12 hours to decompress the esophagus and gastric mucosa. The status of the bleeding varices can also be assessed at this time, and the nurse must be prepared for hematemesis during this procedure. Of most importance is that the esophageal balloon must be deflated before the gastric balloon or else the entire tube will displace upward and occlude the airway.

Spontaneous rupture of the gastric balloon and upward migration of the tube and occlusion of the airway are other possible complications that need to be assessed. Esophageal rupture may also occur, and is characterized by the abrupt onset of severe pain. In the event of either of these two life-threatening emergencies, all three lumens should be cut and the entire tube removed. For this reason, scissors are generally kept at the patient's bedside at all times.

Other complications of the SBT include ulcerations of the esophageal or gastric mucosa. Additionally, sores can develop around the mouth and nose related to the traction devices. Frequent cleansing and lubrication of these areas can help prevent skin breakdown. The nasopharynx also will require frequent suctioning because of increased secretions from the irritating tube and a decreased swallowing reflex. The nasogastric tube should also be irrigated at least every 2 hours to ensure patency and to keep the stomach empty. This will help to prevent aspiration. Additionally, blood that is allowed to accumulate in the stomach of a patient with liver failure is problematic as it will stimulate increased ammonia production that cannot be handled by the patient. Ammonia intoxication may ensue.

Sclerotherapy

Sclerotherapy is another option in the treatment of bleeding varices. (See discussion above.) After identifying the varices, the sclerosing agent is injected into the varix and surrounding tissue. Usually, several applications of the sclerosing agent are needed several days apart to decompress the bleeding varix.

Surgical Interventions

Permanent decompression of portal hypertension can only be achieved through surgical procedures that divert blood around the blocked portal system. These are called portal-caval shunts. In these types of surgery, a connection is made between the portal vein and the inferior vena cava, which diverts blood flow into the vena cava to decrease portal pressure. There are several variations of this procedure, including the end-to-side shunt and the side-to-side shunt (Fig. 13–9). While the end-to-side shunt is technically the easiest, it does divert all blood from the gut directly into the general circulation before detoxification can

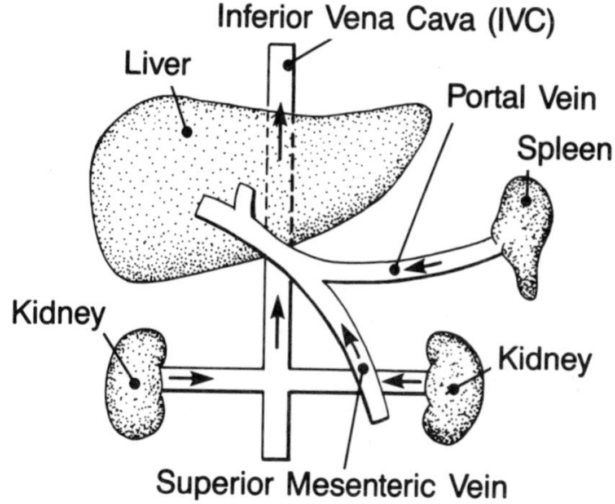

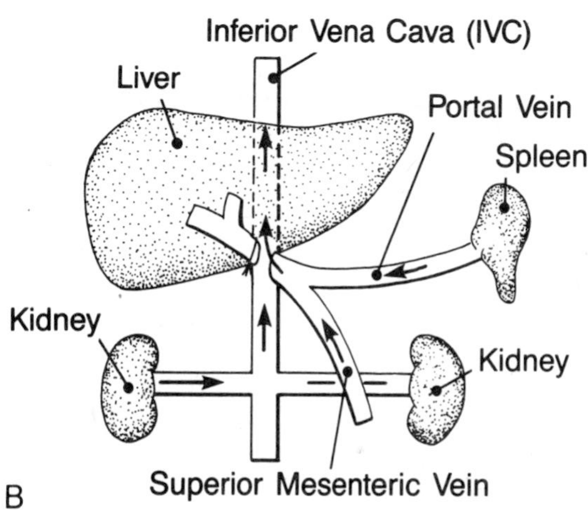

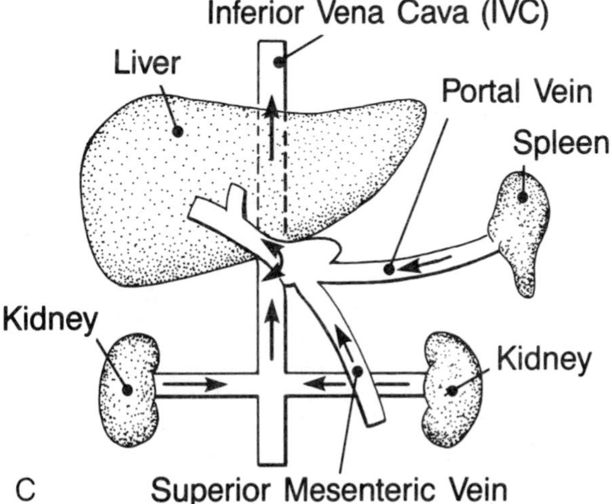

Figure 13–9. Types of portal-caval shunts. *A* Shows normal portal circulation; *B* shows an end-to-side shunt; and *C* shows a side-to-side shunt.

occur, increasing the risk of portal encephalopathy. The side-to-side shunt attempts to prevent this complication by allowing some of the portal blood to flow back into the liver for detoxification.

Other surgical techniques for reduction of portal pressure include splenorenal and mesocaval shunts. The major complication of these procedures is a high thrombosis rate. Portal systemic shunting reduces portal hypertension and therefore decreases bleeding from esophageal varices. The nurse needs to be aware that a temporary increase in ascites occurs following all of these procedures, and careful assessments and interventions are needed in the care of this patient population (see liver failure section).

PATIENT OUTCOMES

Expected patient care outcomes for each nursing diagnosis for the patient experiencing an acute GI bleed include the following:

Fluid Volume Deficit

* Normal circulating body fluid volume
* Control or resolution of hemorrhage
* Preload indicators within normal limits (CVP and PCWP)
* Stable Hct and Hgb
* Stable weight/balanced I/O

Anxiety

* Patient demonstrates decreased level of anxiety with nursing intervention; i.e., teaching, explanations
* Patient demonstrates understanding of disease, medical and nursing interventions

Decreased Tissue Perfusion

* Absence of signs of decreased perfusion of body organs
* Absence of decreased sensorium
* Urine output greater than 30 ml/hr
* Absence of renal failure
* Stable hemodynamics
* Bowel sounds within normal limits
* Skin warm, dry

Knowledge Deficit

* Patient/family understands patient's condition; treatment regimen
* Patient/family asks appropriate questions; voice concerns

Potential for Fluid Volume Excess

* Normal respiratory pattern
* Absence of congestion; pulmonary edema

Altered Electrolyte Balance

* Electrolyte values within normal limits

Encephalopathy

* Absence or resolution of altered thought processes
* Ammonia levels controlled

Potential for Infection (Surgical Patient)

* Free of infection
* Afebrile
* Wound clean, dry, and intact

Altered Comfort (Surgical Patient)

* Patient is comfortable

Potential for Ineffective Breathing Pattern (Patient with Sengstaken-Blakemore Tube)

* Normal respiratory pattern
* SBT patent

■ Acute Pancreatitis

Acute pancreatitis is defined as an acute inflammatory disease of the pancreas. The intensity of the disease ranges from mild cases in which the patient will generally present with abdominal pain and elevated blood amylase to extremely severe types that result in multiple organ failure. In 85 to 90% of patients, the disease is self-limiting (mild acute pancreatitis) and they generally recover rapidly. However, the disease can run a fulminant course and is associated with a mortality rate of over 50% (Sabesin, 1987). Management of this more severe form of the disease requires intensive nursing and medical care.

PATHOPHYSIOLOGY

Acute pancreatitis appears to be an autodigestive disease, which means that the organ is damaged by the enzymes that it produces. Many pancreatic juices are secreted into the duodenum and are essential to normal carbohydrate, fat, and protein metabolism. The way in which the enzymes become activated to initiate the autodigestion process has been widely studied, but the exact mechanism remains unknown. Some theories propose that a toxic agent may alter the way in which the pancreas secretes enzymes. Another theory proposes that duodenal contents containing activated enzymes enter the pancreatic duct, causing inflammation. Another theory implicates biliary stones that cause obstruction of the biliary ducts and therefore hypertension of the pancreas as the mechanism. Regardless of how the enzymes are activated, enzymatic damage to pancreatic cells (acinar cells) is the outcome of the disease process. Trypsinogen, phospholipase A, and elastase have been proposed as the primary enzymes responsible for the autodigestive process.

Acute pancreatitis has been classified by the gradation of the lesions found in the pancreas. In the mild form, there are areas of fat necrosis in and around pancreatic cells along with interstitial edema. Frank pancreatic necrosis is absent. This mild form may progress to a more severe form with extensive fat necrosis in and around the pancreas, pancreatic cellular necrosis, and hemorrhage in the pancreas itself. It is the hemorrhagic form of this acute inflammatory disease that is associated with a high mortality rate.

Both endocrine and exocrine functions of the pancreas are impaired in mild and severe manifestations of the disease. Endocrine functions include the secretion of insulin and glucagon. The secretion of carbohydrate, fat, and protein enzymes necessary for digestion of foodstuffs are the exocrine functions of the pancreas. Hyperglycemia, hypoglycemia, and nutritional depletion, therefore, are common effects of all forms of acute pancreatitis.

In a great majority of patients, acute pancreatitis resolves spontaneously within 5 to 7 days, with return of normal pancreatic endocrine and exocrine functions. Conversely, severe pancreatitis can affect every organ system in the body. Table 13–20 reviews the major systemic complications of acute fulminating pancreatitis.

It appears that as pancreatic cells are damaged, more digestive enzymes are released, which in turn causes more pancreatic damage. Local effects of pancreatitis include inflammation of the pancreas, inflammation of the peritoneum around the pancreas, and fluid accumulation in the peritoneal cavity. A major systemic effect of enzyme release into the circulatory system is vasodilation, which in turn can cause hypotension and shock. The release of trypsin is known to cause abnormalities in blood coagulation and clot lysis. Disseminated intravascular coagulation and GI bleeding/infarction can be the result. The release of other enzymes (phospholipases) is thought to cause the many pulmonary complications associated with acute pancreatitis. Acute respiratory failure and ARDS are the two most common. Acute renal failure is thought to be a consequence of alterations in the renin-angiotensin mechanism. Death during the first 2 weeks of acute pancreatitis usually results from pulmonary or renal complications.

Other serious metabolic complications of acute pancreatitis include hypocalcemia and hyperlipidemia, which are thought to be related to the areas of fat necrosis found in the pancreas with acute inflammation. Hypocalcemia is a serious complication and almost always indicates the

Table 13–20. SYSTEMIC COMPLICATIONS OF ACUTE PANCREATITIS

- Pulmonary
  - Arterial hypoxemia
  - Atelectasis, pneumonia, pleural effusion
  - ARDS
- Cardiovascular
  - Hypovolemic shock
  - Myocardial depression
  - Cardiac dysrhythmias
- Hematological
  - Coagulation abnormalities
  - DIC
- Gastrointestinal
  - GI bleeding
  - Pancreatic pseudocyst
  - Pancreatic abscess
- Renal
  - Azotemia, oliguria
  - Acute renal failure
- Metabolic
  - Hypocalcemia
  - Hyperlipidemia
  - Hyperglycemia
  - Metabolic acidosis
- CNS
  - Pancreatic encephalopathy
  - Retinopathy
- Peripheral
  - Arthritis

Adapted from Pitchumoni, C.S., Agarwal, N., and Jain, J.K.: Systemic complications of acute pancreatitis. *American Journal of Gastroenterology* 83(6):597–603, 1988.

more serious manifestation of acute pancreatitis. Various hormone imbalances, particularly parathyroid hormone imbalance, are also commonly found.

Pancreatic pseudocysts occur in up to 20% of cases of acute pancreatitis and are a part of the necrotizing process. A pseudocyst is a collection of inflammatory debris and pancreatic secretions. The pseudocyst can rupture and hemorrhage or become infected, causing bacterial translocation and sepsis. Less commonly found systemic complications of the disease such as arthritis, visual disturbances, disorientation, agitation, and delusions have also been reported in the literature (Pitchumoni et al., 1988).

Acute pancreatitis has a number of causes, but the most common are alcohol abuse and gallstone disease. Alcohol is known to change the composition of pancreatic juice, particularly by increasing the amounts of trypsinogen. Table 13-21 lists a number of other causes of this disease. A large number of drugs may initiate acute pancreatitis either when taken in toxic doses or as a result of a drug reaction. A high triglyceride level is another important cause of pancreatitis, which can be prevented in susceptible individuals. Pancreatitis due to blunt or penetrating abdominal trauma or following endoscopic exploration of the biliary tree has also been reported.

Table 13-21. CAUSES OF ACUTE PANCREATITIS

- Alchohol
- Biliary Disease
  - Gallstones
  - Common Bile Duct Obstruction
- Drugs
  - Thiazide diuretics
  - Furosemide
  - Estrogen
  - Procainamide
  - Tetracycline
  - Sulfonamides
- Hypertriglyceridemia
- Perforation of esophagus, intestine, stomach
- Opiate Administration
- Penetrating Duodenal Ulcer
- Surgery
- Trauma
- Infectious Agents
- Carcinoma
- Tumors
  - Pancreas
  - Lung
- Radiation Injury
- Ectopic Pregnancy
- Ovarian cyst
- Hypercalcemia
- Heredity
- Idiopathic

ASSESSMENT

History/Physical Examination

A diagnosis of acute pancreatitis can only be made based on careful clinical examination and laboratory and radiological tests. Common presenting signs and symptoms and laboratory and radiological findings in acute pancreatitis are listed in Table 13-22. Nurses are responsible for initial and ongoing clinical assessments, monitoring, recording, and reporting of physical and laboratory data.

In 95% of cases, patients with acute pancreatitis present with complaints of severe abdominal pain (Given, 1984). It is most often mid-epigastric, but may be generalized or localized in the left upper quadrant, often radiating to the back. It usually begins abruptly, and commonly after a large meal or alcohol binge. The pain associated with acute pancreatitis is often steady and severe, but may increase gradually for several hours. The patient may curl up with both arms over the abdomen to relieve the pain. On physical examination, abdominal tenderness and/or guarding

Table 13-22. SIGNS AND SYMPTOMS OF ACUTE PANCREATITIS

Clinical Symptoms
- Pain
- Nausea and vomiting
- Fever
- Dehydration
- Abdominal guarding, distention
- Grey Turner's sign
- Cullen's sign

Laboratory Diagnostics
- Serum and urine amylase—elevated
- Serum lipase—elevated
- WBC count—elevated
- Hct—elevated with dehydration; decreased with hemorrhagic pancreatitis
- Calcium—decreased
- Potassium—decreased
- Albumin—decreased
- Glucose—elevated with islet cell damage
- Bilirubin, SGOT/LDH—elevated with liver disease
- Alkaline phosphatase—elevated with biliary disease

may be present. Distention of the upper abdomen and tympany may also be present.

Nausea and vomiting are also common presenting symptoms. A hallmark sign of acute pancreatitis is severe abdominal pain that is unrelieved by retching or vomiting. The vomitus will characteristically consist of gastric and duodenal contents. Fever is also a common symptom, but is usually less than 39°C. The presence of a temperature greater than 39°C may indicate cholecystitis, peritonitis, or intra-abdominal abscess and is associated with more severe forms of the disease.

In severe acute hemorrhagic pancreatitis, the patient will exhibit overt signs of dehydration and hypovolemic shock. Patients with more severe pancreatic disease may also have ascites, jaundice, or palpable abdominal masses. A bluish discoloration of the flanks (Grey Turner's sign) or around the umbilical area (Cullen's sign) indicates the presence of hemorrhagic pancreatitis and accumulation of blood in these areas. These signs usually do not appear for 1 to 2 weeks as more of the pancreatic gland is destroyed. Measurement of abdominal girth at least every 4 hours needs to be instituted in patients in whom hemorrhagic pancreatitis is suspected to detect internal bleeding.

Diagnostic Tests

The clinical diagnosis of acute pancreatitis requires laboratory and radiological testing because the clinical history, presenting signs and symptoms, and physical examination mimic many other gastrointestinal and cardiovascular disorders. As an example, the pain associated with acute pancreatitis is like that associated with peptic ulcer disease, gallbladder disease, intestinal obstruction, and an acute myocardial infarction. This is due to the fact that pain receptors in the abdomen are poorly differentiated as they exit the skin surface.

Serum lipase and amylase tests are the most specific for acute pancreatitis because as the pancreatic cells and ducts are destroyed, these enzymes are released. However, there are problems in using these values as pure indicators of the disease. Serum amylase and lipase levels are usually elevated during the first 24 to 48 hours from the onset of symptoms. In mild pancreatitis, these levels may be close to normal, and if a few days have elapsed since the beginning of symptoms, enzymes may be completely normal in the presence of acute pancreatitis. To complicate the diagnosis, elevated serum amylase is not specific to acute pancreatitis. Other conditions associated with an elevated amylase level are listed in Table 13–23. Serum amylase measurement is much more specific if isoenzymes are elevated (isoamylase) or urinary amylase is measured. Serum amylase may be falsely lowered in patients with elevated blood serum triglycerides. Other pancreatic enzymes such as lipase, trypsin, elastase, and phospholipase A are being studied for use in laboratory diagnosis, but as of yet they are not more accurate than amylase, which is currently the most widely used. If a patient has symptoms associated with acute pancreatitis and the serum amylase is at least 3 times normal, it is very likely that the patient has acute pancreatitis (Sabesin, 1987).

Advances in the diagnosis of acute pancreatitis have been in the development of improved computed tomography (CT) imaging modalities and magnetic resonance imaging (MRI), which are used to confirm the diagnosis. These imaging techniques have proven superior to the previously used sonography and CT scans as mild edematous pancreatic changes were not usually identifiable on these scans. Gastrointestinal complications of acute pancreatitis such as pancreatic pseudocyst, abscess or perforation, and obstruction of the biliary tree are also distinguishable using any of the above techniques. Additionally, radiographs of the chest and abdomen are also initially done when the patient presents with acute abdominal pain to rule out intestinal ileus, perforation, pericardial effusion, and pulmonary disease. Abdominal films may also reveal intes-

Table 13–23. OTHER CONDITIONS ASSOCIATED WITH INCREASED SERUM AMYLASE

Salivary Gland Disease
Renal Insufficiency
Diabetic Ketoacidosis
Intra-abdominal Disease (perforations, obstructions, aortic disease, peritonitis, appendicitis)
Biliary Tract Disease
Pregnancy
Cerebral Trauma
Pneumonia
Tumors
Chronic Alcoholism
Burns
Shock
Gynecological Disorders
Prostatic Disease

tinal gas-filled loops, which are signs of paralytic ileus.

Other common laboratory abnormalities associated with acute pancreatitis include an elevated white blood cell count due to the inflammatory process and an elevated serum glucose due to beta cell damage and pancreatic necrosis. Hypokalemia may be present because of associated vomiting. In the presence of acute renal failure as a systemic complication, hyperkalemia may predominate. Hypocalcemia is common with severe disease, and usually indicates pancreatic fat necrosis. Serum albumin and protein levels may be decreased owing to the movement of fluid into the extracellular space. Elevations in serum bilirubin, LDH, SGOT, and prothrombin time are common in the presence of concurrent liver disease. Triglycerides may be extremely elevated and may be a causative factor in the development of the acute autodigestive process. Arterial blood gas analysis may show hypoxemia and retained CO_2 levels, which would indicate associated respiratory failure that is a common complication of the acute process.

Predicting the Severity of Acute Pancreatitis

As mentioned earlier, patients with acute pancreatitis can present with mild or fulminant disease. As a consequence, a lot of research has addressed identifying criteria for predicting the prognosis of patients with acute pancreatitis. The most widely used in this country are those of Ranson (1985) (Table 13–24). The number of signs present during the first 48 hours of admission directly relate to the patient's chance of significant morbidity and mortality. The overall mortality rate is 10%, but exceeds 50% in hemorrhagic pancreatitis. In Ranson's (1985) research, patients with less than three signs have a 1% mortality rate, 15% for three to four signs, 40% if five to six signs are present, and 100% if seven or more signs are positive. The scale has a 96% accuracy rate and does aid in comparing results of research on this disease from different hospital centers.

Table 13–24. RANSON CRITERIA FOR PREDICTING SEVERITY OF ACUTE PANCREATITIS

At admission or on Diagnosis
- Age >55 years (over 70)
- Leukocyte count >16,000/μl (>18,000)
- Serum glucose >200 mg/dl (>220)
- Serum lactic dehydrogenase >350 IU/ml (>400)
- Serum aspartate aminotransferase >250 IU/dl

During initial 48 hr
- Fall in hematocrit >10%
- Blood urea nitrogen level rise >5 mg/dl (>2)
- Serum calcium <8 mg/dl
- Base deficit >4 mEq/liter (>5)
- Estimated fluid sequestration >6 L (>4)
- Arterial PaO_2 <60 mm Hg

When criteria values for non-alcoholic acute pancreatitis differ from those in alcohol-related disease, they are given in parentheses.

From Ranson, J.C.: Risk factors in acute pancreatitis. *Hospital Practice* 20(4):69–73, 1985.

NURSING DIAGNOSES

Actual or potential nursing diagnoses associated with acute pancreatitis or due to systemic complications of the disease process include:

1. Altered comfort related to the inflammatory process in the pancreas, obstruction of the pancreatic duct, and decreased blood supply
2. Fluid volume deficit related to fluid shift into the peritoneum and retroperitoneal space; serum, blood, plasma, albumin loss into the peritoneum; dehydration from nausea, vomiting, and fever
3. Altered nutrition: less than body requirements related to loss of exocrine functions of the pancreas, low intake; alcoholism
4. Impaired gas exchange: potential related to respiratory insufficiency, atelectasis, ARDS from elevated concentrations of active pancreatic enzymes
5. Potential for infection related to peritonitis from leakage of pancreatic enzymes into the peritoneal cavity, formation of pancreatic pseudocyst or abscess

MEDICAL AND NURSING MANAGEMENT

Nursing and medical priorities for the management of acute pancreatitis include (1) fluid resuscitation and electrolyte replacement to maintain or replenish vascular volume and electrolyte balance; (2) supportive therapies that are aimed at decreasing gastrin release from the stomach and preventing the gastric contents from entering the duodenum (resting the pancreas while maintaining the nutritional status of the patient); (3) analgesics for pain control; and (4) treatment of systemic complications, the most common being respiratory. The manifestation of the disease process, i.e., mild versus severe disease, will affect each of these priority areas and will be addressed in each section.

Fluid Replacement

In patients with mild or severe acute pancreatitis, some amount of fluid collects in the retroperitoneal space and peritoneal cavity. Initially, most patients present with some degree of dehydration, and in severe cases overt hypovolemic shock. Some patients may have sequestered up to 12 L of fluid upon presentation. Hypovolemia and shock are major causes of death early in the disease process. Fluid replacement then becomes a high priority in the treatment of acute pancreatitis. In some cases, aggressive fluid resuscitation fails to reverse the shock process.

The solutions ordered by the physician for fluid resuscitation are usually colloids or Ringer's lactate; however, fresh frozen plasma and albumin may also be used. Some research has been done to study the advantage of using one solution over the other, but none proved to be more effective. Regardless of which solution is used, fluid replacement serves to perfuse the pancreas, which is thought to decrease the severity of the progression of the disease. Also, the kidneys remain perfused and may prevent the development of acute renal failure as a complication.

Critical assessments to evaluate fluid replacement include accurate monitoring of intake and output and daily weights. Often a Foley catheter will be placed to measure hourly urine outputs as a fall in urine output to less than 30 ml/hr is an early and sensitive measure of hypovolemia and hypoperfusion. Vital signs, including blood pressure and heart rate, are also sensitive measures of volume status. Expected patient outcomes need to be individualized, but reasonable goals would be to maintain BP >100 systolic without orthostatic drop, and a HR <100. Warm extremities would be an indicator of adequate peripheral circulation.

Patients with more severe manifestations of the disease may have pulmonary artery pressure monitoring to assist in evaluating fluid status and response to treatment. The pulmonary capillary wedge pressure would be the most sensitive measure of adequacy of volume status and left ventricular filling pressure. A PCWP between 11 and 14 is a realistic goal for most patients.

Patients with severe disease who fail to respond to fluid therapy alone (hypotension continues) may need medications to support blood pressure. The drug of choice is dopamine, which may be started at a low dose (2–5 μg/kg/min). An advantage of this drug is that at low doses, it maintains renal perfusion while supporting blood pressure. Patients with acute hemorrhagic pancreatitis may also need packed red blood cells in addition to fluid therapy to restore intravascular volume.

Electrolyte Replacement

Hypocalcemia (<8 mg/dl) is a common electrolyte imbalance occurring in about one-third of patients with acute pancreatitis (Sleisenger and Fordtran, 1989). It is associated with a high mortality rate (see Ranson's prognostic signs in Table 13–24). The exact mechanism for this metabolic complication is not completely understood, but it is thought to be related to decreased binding with proteins in the plasma. Calcium is essential for catalyzing impulses for nerves and muscles, for maintaining the integrity of cell membranes and vessels, for normal blood clotting, and for bones and teeth. Calcium is also essential for increasing contractility in the heart. An ECG sign of hypocalcemia is lengthening of the QT interval. Severe hypocalcemia (<6 mg/dl) may cause tetany, seizures, and respiratory distress. Patients with severe hypocalcemia should be placed on seizure precautions with respiratory support equipment on hand (e.g., oral airway, suction). The nurse is responsible for monitoring calcium levels, for administering replacement, and for monitoring the patient's response to any calcium given. Calcium replacements should be infused via a central line because peripheral infiltration may cause tissue necrosis. The patient also needs to be monitored for calcium toxicity. Symptoms include lethargy, nausea, shortening of the QT interval, and decreased excitability of nerves and muscles. Hypomagnesemia may also be present with hypocalcemia and magnesium may need to be replaced as well. Correction of serum magnesium levels is often required before calcium levels will return to normal.

Potassium is another electrolyte that may need to be replaced early in the treatment regimen owing to the vomiting associated with acute pancreatitis. Potassium is also abundant in pancreatic juices. Hypokalemia is associated with cardiac dysrhythmias, muscle weakness, hypotension, and irritability. Potassium should be diluted and administered slowly over 1 hour via an infusion pump.

Hyperglycemia is surprisingly a less common complication of acute pancreatitis and is related to impaired secretion of insulin by islet cells in the pancreas or release of glucagon by alpha cells. In some cases, hyperglycemia may be associated with dehydration or other electrolyte imbalances.

Sliding scale regular insulin may be ordered, and needs to be administered very cautiously because glucagon levels are only transiently elevated in acute pancreatitis.

Resting the Pancreas

Nasogastric suction is used in most patients with acute pancreatitis to suppress pancreatic exocrine secretion by preventing the release of secretin from the duodenum. Normally, secretin, which stimulates pancreatic secretion production, is stimulated when there is acid in the duodenum. Nausea, vomiting, and abdominal pain may also be decreased when an nasogastric tube is placed to suction early in treatment (Sabesin, 1987). A nasogastric tube is also necessary in patients with ileus, severe gastric distention, and a decreased level of consciousness to prevent complications due to pulmonary aspiration. Oral intake should not be allowed until the abdominal pain subsides and serum amylase levels have returned to normal. Starting oral intake prior to this may cause the abdominal pain to return and may induce further inflammation of the pancreas by stimulating the autodigestive disease process. This will increase the risk of pancreatic abscess formation. In patients with mild pancreatitis, oral fluids can usually be restarted within 3 days to a week, with slow advancement of solids as tolerated.

Prolonged NPO (nothing per mouth) status is difficult for patients. Frequent mouth care and maintenance of skin integrity around the nasogastric tube through lubrication are important nursing concerns to prevent injury and maximize patient comfort. Bed rest is also used to decrease pancreatic secretion stimulation by decreasing the patient's basal metabolic rate.

Nutritional Support

Patients with severe manifestations of the disease may be on prolonged NPO status with nasogastric suction because of paralytic ileus, persistent abdominal pain, pancreatic pseudocyst or abscesses, or other systemic complications. These patients are candidates for total parenteral nutrition (TPN). Because patients with acute pancreatitis often have hyperlipidemia as a part of their disease process, lipid supplementation may not be ordered.

Comfort Management

Pain control is a nursing priority in patients with acute pancreatitis not only because it produces extreme patient discomfort, but because pain will increase the patient's metabolism and increase pancreatic secretions. The pain of pancreatitis is due to the edema and distention of the pancreatic capsule, obstruction of the biliary system, and peritoneal inflammation from pancreatic enzymes. Pain may be severe, constant, and last for many days and is related to the degree of pancreatic inflammation.

Careful pain assessment for a baseline needs to be done early after the patient's admission, including information about the onset, intensity, duration, and location (local or diffuse). Analgesics will need to be ordered by the physician to control abdominal pain. It is important to remember in this case that some analgesics cause spasm of the sphincter of Oddi, which holds the duodenum in place, and will exacerbate the pain associated with acute pancreatitis. Morphine is one such drug, and therefore hydromorphone (Dilaudid) and meperidine (Demerol) are considered the drugs of choice. Pain medications should be routinely administered at least every 3 to 4 hours to prevent uncontrollable abdominal pain. Use of a pain-rating scale, i.e., on a scale of 1 to 10, may also help in determining the amount of analgesia to administer and in evaluating the patient's response to medication. As mentioned before, insertion of a nasogastric tube to low intermittent suction may help ease pain considerably. Patient positioning may also be useful in relieving some of the discomfort and should be facilitated by the nurse as the patient's hemodynamic status allows.

Pharmacological Interventions

Various pharmacological therapies have been researched in the treatment of acute pancreatitis. A variety of drugs to rest the pancreas have been studied, specifically anticholinergics, glucagon, somatostatin, cimetidine, and calcitonin, but have not been shown to be effective. Histamine blockers and antacids are useful in preventing stress ulcers in critically ill patients, which would be appropriate for this patient population.

Antibiotics have also been studied to treat the inflammation of the pancreas with the idea of preventing pancreatic pseudocysts or abscesses. Antibiotics were not proven to be effective and now are generally utilized only with a confirmed infection.

5-Fluoruracil and propylthiouracil decrease the metabolism of pancreatic cells and the production of enzymes and may be utilized during the acute phase. Bile salts may also be ordered to facilitate digestion and absorption of nutrients.

Treatment of Systemic Complications

Multisystem complications of acute pancreatitis are related to the pancreas's ability to produce many vasoactive substances that affect organs throughout the body. These complications are summarized in Table 13–20.

Peritoneal lavage has been used since the 1960s for the treatment of systemic complications associated with severe acute pancreatitis. The theory behind using this therapy is that it removes toxic substances that are released by the damaged pancreas into the peritoneal fluid. Examples include trypsinogen, kinins, histamines, and prostaglandins. These substances are thought to mediate many of these systemic effects. Peritoneal lavage removes these substances before they can be absorbed and exert their effect. Clinical trials studying the effects of lavage on patient outcome have not demonstrated a decreased mortality rate. Presently, it is usually used when standard therapies mentioned above have not been working during the first few days of hospitalization.

The procedure for peritoneal lavage involves placement of a peritoneal dialysis catheter. Isotonic solution with dextrose, heparin, and potassium are added. An antibiotic may also be used in the solution. Two liters of solution are infused at a time over 15 to 20 minutes and then are drained by gravity. This cycle is repeated every 1 to 2 hours for 48 to 72 hours. If peritoneal lavage is effective, the hemodynamic response by the patient is usually immediate.

Close monitoring of respiratory status during peritoneal lavage is essential as accumulation of fluid in the peritoneum will cause restricted movement of the diaphragm, a muscle used for inspiration. Hyperglycemia may be another effect of this therapy as dextrose may be absorbed from the fluid into the blood stream.

Pulmonary complications are very common in patients with both mild and severe manifestations of the disease. Arterial hypoxemia, atelectasis, pleural effusions, and pneumonia have been identified in many patients with acute pancreatitis. Ranson (1985) found evidence of arterial hypoxemia in patients with mild disease without clinical or x-ray findings to support the pulmonary dysfunction. Arterial blood gases should be drawn every 8 hours for the first few days to monitor for this complication. Treatment for hypoxemia includes vigorous pulmonary care such as deep breathing and coughing and frequent position changes. Oxygen therapy may also be used to improve overall oxygenation status. Pulmonary emboli have also been documented as a complication of acute pancreatitis. Careful fluid administration to prevent fluid overload and pulmonary congestion is also necessary.

Patients with severe disease may develop overt respiratory failure. Radiologically and clinically, it is indistinguishable from adult respiratory distress syndrome (ARDS).

Close monitoring and management of other complications of acute pancreatitis such as coagulation abnormalities and hemorrhage, cardiovascular failure and dysrhythmias, and acute renal failure are also important. Coagulation defects in acute pancreatitis are similar to disseminated intravascular coagulation (DIC), and are treated in the same way. Disseminated intravascular coagulation in acute pancreatitis is associated with a high mortality rate. The cardiac depression associated with acute pancreatitis may vary, but as mentioned, hypovolemic shock is a grave presentation. Astute cardiovascular monitoring and volume replacement is needed to reverse this serious complication. Impaired renal function has been documented in many patients. Diuretics and vasodilators may be used to treat this complication.

Gastrointestinal complications of acute pancreatitis include pancreatic pseudocyst and abdominal abscess. A pseudocyst should be suspected in any patient who has persistent abdominal pain and nausea and vomiting, a prolonged fever, and elevated serum amylase. A CT scan can be helpful in diagnosing the location and size of the pseudocyst. Signs and symptoms of an abdominal abscess include increased WBC count, fever, abdominal pain, and vomiting. A CT scan will provide a definitive diagnosis.

Surgical Management

A pancreatic resection for acute necrotizing pancreatitis may be performed to prevent systemic complications of the disease process. In this procedure, dead or infected pancreatic tissue is surgically removed. In some cases, the entire pancreas will be removed. Usually the indication for surgical intervention is clinical deterioration of the patient despite conventional treatments or the presence of peritonitis (Teerenhovi et al., 1988).

Surgery may also be indicated for pseudocysts; however, surgery is usually delayed as some pseudocysts have been known to resolve spontaneously. Surgical treatment of a pseudocyst can be done through internal or external drainage or needle aspiration. Acute surgical intervention may be required if the pseudocyst becomes infected or perforates.

Surgical treatment of the abdominal abscess is always necessary because without it the patient mortality rate is near 100% (Wilson et al., 1988).

Surgery may also be performed in the case in which gallstones are thought to be the cause of the acute pancreatitis. A cholecystectomy would most likely be performed.

PATIENT OUTCOMES

Expected outcomes for the patient with acute pancreatitis include:

1. Restoration of normal fluid balance as evidenced by a balanced I/O, stable weight, normal PCWP, urine output >30 ml/hr
2. Restoration and maintenance of hemodynamic stability as evidenced by a return of BP to baseline, absence of tachycardia
3. Pain is maintained at tolerable levels for the patient as evidenced by subjective and objective cues that pain is diminished
4. Nutritional balance is maintained/restored as evidenced by a serum albumin >4 mg/dl; positive nitrogen balance; stable weight
5. Pulmonary gas exchange is maintained as evidenced by a $PaO_2 > 60$ mm Hg; clear lung fields; absence of atelectasis, pneumonia, pulmonary edema, or pleural effusion
6. Early detection and reporting of systemic complications of acute pancreatitis, including hypovolemic shock; acute respiratory failure; cardiac failure; renal failure; and pancreatic complications

See the Nursing Care Plan for the Patient with Acute Pancreatitis.

Hepatic Failure

PATHOPHYSIOLOGY

Hepatic, or liver, failure results when the liver is unable to perform its many functions. These functions are reviewed in Table 13–5. Liver failure can result from necrosis or a decrease in the blood supply to liver cells. This most often is caused by hepatitis or inflammation of the liver. Liver failure can also result from chronic liver disease in which healthy liver tissue is replaced by fibrotic tissue. This form of liver failure is called cirrhosis. Finally, liver cells can be replaced by fatty cells or tissue and is known as fatty liver disease.

Hepatitis

Hepatitis is an acute inflammation of liver cells, or hepatocytes. Other white blood cells in the liver may also be inflamed. This inflammation is accompanied by edema, and early in the course of the disease, there is no real disturbance in the architecture of the liver. The normal liver architecture is pictured in Figure 13–10 and is char-

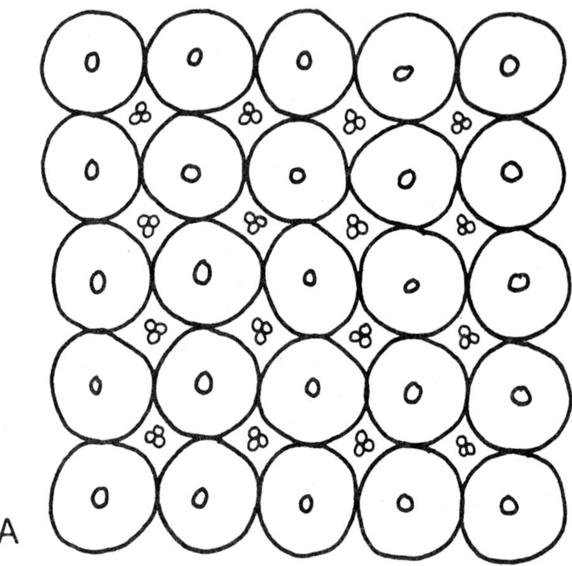

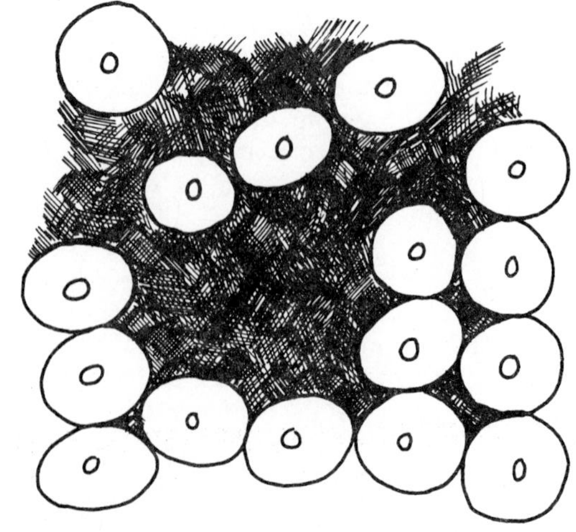

Figure 13–10. Liver architecture in cirrhosis. *A*, Normal liver. *B*, Changes occurring in cirrhosis.

NURSING CARE PLAN FOR THE PATIENT WITH ACUTE PANCREATITIS

Nursing Diagnosis	Outcome	Intervention
Fluid volume deficit related to loss of fluid into peritoneal cavity, dehydration from nausea and vomiting, fever, NG suction, defects in coagulation	BP >100 systolic, >60 MAP, or returned to baseline HR <100 PCWP WNL Urine Output >30 ml/hr Extremities warm, dry Stable hematocrit and hemoglobin Absence of bleeding Afebrile	Monitor hemodynamic status closely, vital signs, PA pressures, urine output, I/O, daily weight, peripheral circulation Administer fluid replacements, blood or blood products, and monitor patient response to treatment Monitor for signs and symptoms of hemorrhage; hematocrit and hemoglobin; Cullen's sign or Turner's sign; measure abdominal girth every 4 hours Monitor temperature and administer antipyretics or apply cooling blanket as needed
Altered comfort related to interruption of blood supply to the pancreas, edema and distention of the pancreas, peritoneal irritation	Pain is within tolerable levels	Perform a pain assessment noting onset, duration, intensity, and location Control pain with drug of choice (meperidine). Avoid morphine, which causes spasm of the sphincter of Oddi, and the ampulla of Vater, which increases pain. Schedule pain medication to prevent severe pain episodes Differentiate pain from cardiac origin Keep activities at a minimum. Maintain bed rest restriction. Position patient to optimize comfort Administer sedation as needed
Altered nutrition; less than body requirements related to nausea and vomiting; depressed appetite; alcoholism; impaired nutrient metabolism due to pancreatic injury and altered production of digestive enzymes	Positive nitrogen balance Normal serum albumin Stable weight	Assess nutritional status through clinical exam and laboratory analysis Calculate caloric needs and compare to actual intake Provide adequate nutritional intake as needed. Offer nutritional supplements as needed Administer TPN as ordered. Prevent complications by attention to aseptic technique in the handling and administration of TPN and catheter care. Monitor for signs and symptoms of infection. Monitor glucose and other electrolytes to detect electrolyte complications of therapy
Impaired gas exchange related to atelectasis; pleural effusions, ARDS, fluid overload during fluid administration, pulmonary emboli, splinting from pain	PaO_2 >60 $PaCO_2$ within normal limits or at baseline Absence or resolution of pulmonary complications	Monitor pulmonary status closely. Auscultate breath sounds every 4 hr and PRN. Monitor respiratory rate Administer vigorous pulmonary hygiene; coughing and deep breathing; humidification therapy Note secretions for amount, color, consistency, and odor Administer oxygen as prescribed. Monitor ABGs according to clinical status Administer analgesia to prevent pain due to splinting Reposition patient frequently to maximize ventilation and perfusion and to prevent pooling of secretions
Electrolyte imbalance related to prolonged nausea and vomiting, gastric suction, autodigestive process, therapeutic regimen	Calcium, magnesium, potassium, and glucose WNL	Monitor electrolyte balance carefully and administer replacements according to unit protocol Assess fluid balance evaluating electrolyte values

acterized by a basic functional unit of the liver called a lobule. The liver lobule is uniquely made in that it has its own blood supply, allowing the liver cells to be exposed continuously to blood. As the inflammation progresses, the normal pattern of the liver is disturbed by the inflammatory process. This interrupts the normal blood supply to liver cells, causing necrosis and breakdown of healthy cells. Blood backs up in the portal system, causing increased pressure. This is known as portal hypertension. Liver cells do have the capacity to regenerate. Over time, liver cells that become damaged can be removed from the body's immune system and are replaced with healthy liver cells. Therefore, most patients with hepatitis recover with normal liver function.

Hepatitis most often is caused by a viral disease. Two viruses have been identified: the hepatitis A virus (HAV) and the hepatitis B virus (HBV). There is a third classification of hepatitis known as non-A, non-B, or hepatitis C, in which the exact viral pathogen has yet to be identified. Hepatitis D virus is a small virus and must occur in combination with HBV.

Types

Hepatitis A. Hepatitis A (HA) is the most common type of viral hepatitis. The virus infects the liver and is eliminated by the feces. This virus is primarily spread through oral ingestion of food, water, and shellfish that have been infected by fecal contaminates. Hepatitis A was previously known as infectious hepatitis. This disease is usually mild in presentation, and therefore many individuals may have had the disease without being aware of it.

Hepatitis B. Hepatitis B (HB) is usually a more serious form of hepatitis. Persons are considered infectious as long as antigens for the virus are found in the blood stream. It is spread primarily by blood, blood products, and body fluids or secretions such as semen and saliva. Hepatitis B was formally called serum hepatitis. The virus can spread percutaneously, through mucous membranes, or through contact with infected fluids. Modes of transmission of HB are summarized in Table 13–25. Health care providers are at risk for contracting this form of hepatitis. Of most importance, HB can result in the development of a carrier state, chronic hepatitis, cirrhosis, and cancer of the liver.

Hepatitis Non-A, Non-B (Hepatitis C). Hepatitis non-A, non-B (HNANB) is transmitted through blood or blood products. It also can be spread through sexual contact and is frequently seen in the male homosexual population. Hepatitis NANB is also commonly the form transmitted through blood transfusions. The virus can be mild, and often the patient is asymptomatic. It rarely progresses to fulminant hepatic failure.

Hepatitis D. Hepatitis D (HDV) always occurs in the presence of HB and relies on the virus to spread. The HDV is transmitted in the same way as the HBV.

Table 13–25. MODES OF TRANSMISSION FOR HEPATITIS B

Blood
Blood Products
Semen
Saliva
Percutaneously Through Mucous Membranes
Direct Contact with Infected Fluids/Objects

Assessment

Hepatitis A. HA is diagnosed by the presence of hepatitis A antibodies in the blood. These antibodies occur within 2 to 6 weeks and remain in the blood serum indefinitely. These initial antibodies are of the immunoglobulin M (IgM) class and indicate a current infection. Later, they are replaced by the IgG class and indicate immunity to HA.

Common signs and symptoms of HA include

* Brown urine
* Depression
* Loss of appetite
* Nausea and vomiting
* Fever
* Weakness, chills
* Headache
* Right upper quadrant discomfort or pain
* Irritability
* Clay-colored feces

In addition to clinical signs and symptoms, liver function tests will be elevated and coagulation tests disturbed. Common liver function tests are listed in Table 13–26.

Early in HA, there is an incubation period in which the patient is asymptomatic but is contagious. Hepatitis A is most contagious before signs and symptoms occur. Once symptoms are apparent, because many symptoms are typical of a flulike illness, the virus may be misdiagnosed. Some patients may become jaundiced, which will bring them to the hospital. Generally, signs and symptoms of HA develop 2 to 7 days before the onset of jaundice. Acute symptoms can progress or disappear once jaundice is present. Usually, the patient recovers within 4 to 6 months from the onset of symptoms. Recovery is determined by a return to normal of liver function tests and the absence of clinical symptoms. Occasionally, a relapse can occur, but the symptoms are less severe. Chronic liver disease or a carrier state usually does not follow in this type of hepatitis.

Hepatitis B. Diagnosis of HB is made through the presence of antigen-antibody systems

Table 13-26. COMMON LIVER FUNCTION TESTS

Serum or Plasma	Alteration
Albumin	Decreased
Ammonia	Increased
Bile Pigments	
Total bilirubin	Increased
Direct or conjugated bilirubin	Increased
Cholesterol	Increased
Coagulation tests	
Prothrombin time (PT)	Prolonged
Partial thromboplastin time (PTT)	Prolonged
Enzymes	
Alkaline phosphatase	Increased
Glutamic oxaloacetic transaminase (SGOT)	Increased
Glutamic pyruvic transaminase (SGPT)	Increased
Urine	
Bilirubin	Increased
Urobilinogen	Increased

in the blood. Hepatitis B surface antigens (HBsAGs) can be found from 1 to 10 weeks following exposure to the virus. Patients are considered infectious as long as HBsAGs are present. Several other antigen-antibody systems can be used to diagnose HB. These include HBeAG and HBcAG. These antibody complexes are detectable throughout the acute stages of the illness.

The incubation period for HB can last from 6 weeks to 6 months. Clinical signs and symptoms of the acute phase are the same as for HA. Patients with HB, however, have more of a chance of developing fulminant hepatic failure, which is characterized by sudden degeneration of the liver and loss of all normal liver functions. The functional sequelae of fulminant hepatic failure will be presented later in this section. The most important clinical sign is a decrease in liver size. Other signs of impending fulminant hepatic failure are listed in Table 13–27. The mortality rate for this complication is up to 5%. Patients who do survive usually do not have any residual liver failure.

Table 13-27. SIGNS AND SYMPTOMS OF FULMINANT HEPATIC FAILURE

Hyperexcitability
Insomnia
Irritability
Vomiting
Decreased Level of Consciousness

Hepatitis Non-A, Non-B. Diagnosis of HNANB is made when laboratory testing for HA and HB are negative, yet clinical signs and symptoms of hepatitis are present and liver function tests are abnormal. This virus has an incubation period of 2 weeks to 6 months. Clinical signs and symptoms are similar to those listed for HA.

Nursing Diagnoses

Nursing diagnoses associated with viral hepatitis include:

1. Activity intolerance related to fatigue, fever, flulike symptoms
2. Altered nutrition; less than body requirements, related to loss of appetite, nausea, vomiting, loss of liver metabolic functions
3. Potential for infection related to loss of liver cell function to phagocytize bacteria

Collaborative Management

There is no definitive treatment for acute inflammation of the liver. Goals for medical and nursing care include provision of rest and assisting the patient in obtaining optimal nutrition.

Rest is important, particularly in the early stages of hepatitis. The patient's severe fatigue will usually require bed rest. Most patients can be cared for at home unless the disease becomes prolonged or fulminant failure develops. If the patient is hospitalized, the nurse can assist the individual in spacing activities to ensure adequate rest. Medications to help the patient rest or to decrease agitation are usually not ordered by the physician as most drugs require clearance by the liver, which is impaired during the acute phase.

Maintenance of the nutritional status of the patient is a nursing priority. Loss of appetite, nausea, and vomiting may persist for weeks. A high-carbohydrate, low-protein diet is usually recommended. Patients will usually avoid fatty, greasy foods. Nursing measures such as administering antiemetics may be helpful, although all hepatotoxic drugs should be avoided. Small frequent meals and supplements should be offered. Evaluation of nutritional status needs to be ongoing, including assessments of intake, output, daily weights, serum albumin, and nitrogen balance. Patients need to be instructed not to take any over-the-counter drugs that can cause liver damage. Table 13–28 lists common hepatotoxic drugs. Alcohol should also be avoided.

Table 13–28. COMMON HEPATOTOXIC DRUGS

Analgesics
- Acetaminophen (Tylenol)
- Salicylates (Aspirin)

Anesthetics
- Ethrane
- Fluothane
- Penthrane

Anticonvulsants
- Phenytoin (Dilantin)
- Phenobarbital (Luminal)

Antidepressants
- Monoamine Oxidase (MAO) Inhibitors
- Amitriptyline (Elavil)
- Doxepin (Sinequan)

Antimicrobial Agents
- Isoniazid (INH)
- Nitrofurantoin (Macrodantin)
- Rifampin
- Sulfonamides (Gantrisin, Silvadene)
- Tetracycline

Antipsychotic Drugs
- Haloperidol (Haldol)
- Chlorpromazine (Thorazine)
- Fluphenazine (Prolixin)
- Prochlorperazine (Compazine)
- Promethazine (Phenergan)
- Thioridazine (Mellaril)

Cardiovascular Drugs
- Methyldopa (Aldomet)
- Quinidine sulfate

Hormonal Agents
- Antithyroid Drugs
- Oral contraceptives
- Oral hypoglycemics
  - Tolbutamide (Orinase)
  - Chlorpropamide (Diabinese)

Sedatives
- Chlordiazepoxide (Librium)
- Diazepam (Valium)

Others
- Cimetidine (Tagamet)

Special precautions must be taken while caring for the patient with hepatitis to prevent spread of the virus. These include:

* The use of gloves while handling all items that are contaminated with patient's body secretions
* Disposable patient care items should be used; i.e., thermometers, dishes, eating utensils
* A private room and bathroom are required for patients who are fecally incontinent
* Gowns should be used when providing direct patient care
* Linen or any hospital equipment that is contaminated with feces or blood needs to be double bagged and labeled

Teaching the patient and family handwashing and personal hygiene techniques is important. Counseling may be needed for individuals in whom transmission via a sexual route is suspected.

Prophylaxis for hepatitis A and hepatitis B virus are available. Immune globulin (IG) can be administered to individuals both before and after exposure to the virus. Preexposure prophylaxis is recommended to persons traveling to countries where hepatitis A is prevalent. A hepatitis B vaccine was developed in the early 1980s. A series of three injections to produce antibodies against HBsAG is now used. It is highly recommended for all health care personnel.

Patient Outcomes

Resolution of hepatitis can be evaluated based on the following criteria:

1. Patient is able to tolerate increasing levels of activity
2. Absence of abdominal discomfort/pain
3. Liver function tests return to baseline
4. Serological tests indicate absence of active virus
5. Nutritional status maintained
6. Absence of infection

Cirrhosis

Cirrhosis causes severe alterations in the structure and function of liver cells. It is characterized by inflammation and liver cell necrosis that may be focal or diffuse. Fat deposits may also be present. The enlarged liver cells cause compression of the liver lobule, leading to increased resistance to blood flow and portal hypertension. Necrosis is followed by regeneration of liver tissue, but not in a normal fashion. Fibrous tissue is layed down over time, which distorts the normal architecture of the liver lobule. These fibrotic changes are usually irreversible, resulting in chronic liver dysfunction.

There are four types of cirrhosis: (1) alcoholic cirrhosis (Laënnec's), (2) biliary cirrhosis, (3) cardiac cirrhosis, and (4) postnecrotic cirrhosis. Laënnec's cirrhosis, which results from chronic alcohol abuse, is the most common type in the United States. Alcohol is known to be toxic to the liver; however, not all alcoholics go on to develop cirrhosis. Other alcohol-induced injuries of the liver include fatty liver and alcoholic hepatitis. These may occur independently or along with the cirrhosis. Acetaldehyde, a toxic metabolite of alcohol ingestion, causes liver cell damage and death. Fibrotic tissue replaces liver cells and ultimately causes the liver to shrink. In end-stage disease, almost all liver cells are replaced by this tissue, which is unable to carry out the normal functions of the liver.

Biliary cirrhosis is caused by a decrease in bile flow, most commonly due to long-term obstruction of bile ducts. It eventually leads to degeneration and fibrosis of the ducts.

Cardiac cirrhosis is most commonly caused by severe long-term right-sided congestive heart failure. Decreased oxygenation of liver cells and cellular death characterizes this disease.

Postnecrotic cirrhosis can be a result of exposure to hepatotoxins, chemicals, an infection, or be due to a metabolic disorder. It results in massive death of liver cells, and is also associated with the development of liver cancer.

Fatty Liver

Fatty liver is defined as an accumulation of excessive fats in the liver and it is morphologically distinguishable from cirrhosis. Alcohol abuse is the most common cause of this disorder. Other etiologies include obesity, diabetes, hepatic resection, starvation, and TPN. Damage caused by the fat deposits may result in liver dysfunction, failure, and death.

ASSESSMENT OF HEPATIC FAILURE

Presenting Clinical Signs

Initial clinical signs of hepatic failure are vague, including weakness, fatigue, loss of appetite, weight loss, abdominal discomfort, nausea and vomiting, and a change in bowel habits. As destruction in the liver progresses, the systemic effects of the disease become apparent as liver function becomes impaired. This results in loss of the normal vascular, secretory, and metabolic functions of the liver (see Table 13–5). The functional sequelae of liver disease can be divided into three categories: (1) portal hypertension, (2) reduced liver metabolic processes, and (3) impaired bile formation and flow. These derangements and their clinical manifestations are summarized in Table 13–29.

Table 13–29. CLINICAL SIGNS AND SYMPTOMS OF LIVER DISEASE

- Cardiac
  - Hyperdynamic circulation
  - Portal hypertension
  - Dysrhythmias
  - Activity intolerance
  - Edema
- Dermatological
  - Jaundice
  - Spider angiomas
  - Pruritus
- Electrolyte Disturbances
  - Hypokalemia
  - Hyponatremia (dilutional)
  - Hypernatremia
- Endocrine
  - Increased aldosterone
  - Increased antidiuretic hormome
- Fluid Disturbances
  - Ascites
  - Water retention
  - Decreased volume in vascular space
- Gastrointestinal
  - Abdominal discomfort
  - Decreased appetite
  - Diarrhea
  - GI bleeding
  - Varices
  - Malnutrition
  - Nausea and vomiting
- Hematological
  - Anemia
  - Impaired coagulation
  - DIC
- Immune System
  - Increased Susceptibility to Infection
- Neurological
  - Hepatic Encephalopathy
- Pulmonary Findings
  - Dyspnea
  - Hyperventilation
  - Hypoxemia
  - Ineffective breathing patterns
- Renal
  - Hepatorenal Syndrome

Portal Hypertension

Portal hypertension causes two main clinical problems for the patient: a hyperdynamic circulation and the development of esophageal and/or gastric varices. Liver cell destruction causes shunting of blood and increased cardiac output. Vasodilation is also present, which in effect causes decreased perfusion to all body organs even though the cardiac output is very high. This is known as high-output failure, or hyperdynamic circulation. Clinical signs and symptoms of this disorder are identical to heart failure and include jugular vein distention, rales, and decreased perfusion to all organs. Initially, the patient may have hypertension, flushed skin, and bounding pulses. Blood pressure will eventually fall. Dysrhythmias are also common. Increased portal venous pressure causes the formation of channels to shunt blood to decrease pressure. These channels or varices are problematic because they can bleed, causing a massive upper gastrointestinal bleed (see section on upper GI bleed).

Impaired Metabolic Processes

The liver is the most complex organ in terms of all of its metabolic processes. Liver failure causes altered carbohydrate, fat, and protein metabolism; decreased synthesis of blood clotting factors; decreased removal of activated clotting components; decreased metabolism of vitamins and iron; decreased storage functions; and decreased detoxification functions.

Altered carbohydrate metabolism may result clinically in unstable blood sugar. The serum glucose is usually elevated above 200. This is termed cirrhotic diabetes. Altered carbohydrate metabolism may also result in malnutrition and a decreased stress response.

Altered fat metabolism may result in a fatty liver. Fat is used by all cells for energy, and altered metabolism may cause fatigue and decreased activity tolerance for many patients. Alterations in skin integrity, which are common with chronic liver disease, are also thought to be related to this metabolic dysfunction. Bile salts are also not adequately produced, which leads to an inability of fats to be metabolized by the small intestine. Malnutrition can result.

Protein metabolism is also decreased. Albumin synthesis is decreased and serum albumin will fall. Albumin is necessary for colloid osmotic pressure to hold fluid in the intravascular space and for nutrition. Low albumin is also thought to be associated with the development of ascites, one complication of hepatic failure. Globulin is another protein that is essential for transporting substances in the blood. Fibrinogen is an essential protein necessary for normal clotting. This coupled with a decreased synthesis of many blood clotting factors predisposes the patient to bleeding. Clinical signs and symptoms can range from bruising and nose and gingival bleeding to frank hemorrhage. The patient may also develop disseminated intravascular coagulation. These patients can also have a decreased platelet count.

Kupffer cells in the liver play an important role in fighting infections throughout the body. Loss of this function predisposes the patient to severe infections, particularly gram-negative sepsis.

The liver also removes activated clotting factors from the general circulation to prevent widespread clotting in the system. Loss of this function predisposes the patient to emboli, particularly to the lungs.

Decreased metabolism and storage of vitamins A, B_{12}, and D and iron, glucose, and fat predispose the patient to many nutritional deficiencies. A well-known function of the liver to detoxify drugs, ammonia, and hormones is also lost. Loss of ammonia conversion to urea in the liver is responsible for many of the neurological alterations seen in liver failure as ammonia is allowed to directly enter the central nervous system. These range from minor sensory-perceptual changes such as tremors, slurred speech, and impaired decision-making to dramatic confusion or profound coma.

Hormonal imbalances are common in liver disease. Most important physiologically is the activation of aldosterone and antidiuretic hormone. These are thought to contribute to some of the fluid and electrolyte disturbances commonly found. Sodium and water retention and portal hypertension lead to a third-spacing of fluid from the intravascular space into the peritoneal cavity (ascites). The resultant decrease in plasma volume will cause activation of compensatory mechanisms in the body to release antidiuretic hormone and aldosterone. This causes further water and sodium retention. The renin-angiotensin system is also activated, which causes systemic vasoconstriction. The kidneys are most affected and urine output will decrease because of impaired perfusion. Sexual dysfunction is also common in patients with liver disease, which can lead to self-concept alterations in patients. Dermatological lesions that occur in some patients with liver failure, called spider angioma, are thought to be related to an endocrine imbalance. These vascular lesions (Fig. 13–11) may be venous or arterial and represent the progression of liver disease.

The inability of the liver in failure to metabolize drugs is well known. All drugs metabolized by the liver need to be restricted. The administration of such drugs could cause acute liver failure in a patient with chronic disease. A fecal

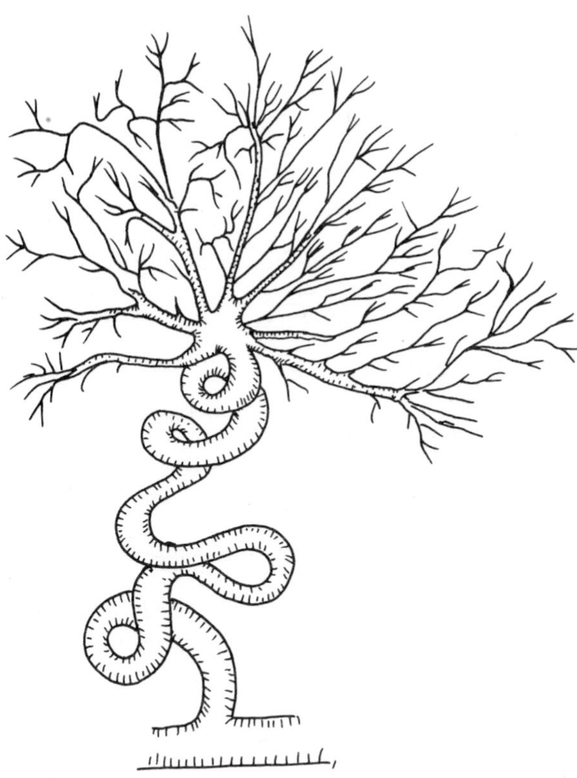

Figure 13–11. Spider angioma.

odor to the breath (fetor hepaticus) is thought to be due to an accumulation of methylmercaptan in the body.

Impaired Bile Formation and Flow

The liver's inability to metabolize bile is reflected clinically in an elevated serum bilirubin and staining of tissue by bilirubin or jaundice. Jaundice will generally be present with any bilirubin over 3 mg/dl.

NURSING DIAGNOSES

The following nursing diagnoses, actual and potential, can be derived from assessment data in a patient with liver failure:

1. Decreased activity tolerance related to impaired liver metabolism; decreased nutritional intake
2. Fluid volume deficit related to bleeding from esophageal or gastric varices; decreased production of clotting factors; and decreased effective vascular volume from ascites
3. Altered nutrition, less than body requirements related to impaired carbohydrate, protein, and fat metabolism; decreased protein intake; impaired absorption of fat-soluble vitamins and vitamin B_{12}
4. Ineffective breathing pattern related to elevation of the diaphragm from ascites; impaired thought processes from altered ammonia detoxification
5. Altered thought processes related to impaired handling of ammonia and drugs, protein intake, diuretic therapy to treat ascites; GI bleeding with increased protein load; dehydration and shock
6. Impaired renal tissue perfusion, related to decreased effective vascular volume from ascites; accumulation of nephrotoxic drugs from impaired liver metabolism

MEDICAL AND NURSING MANAGEMENT

Nursing and medical management of the patient in liver failure are aimed at liver and system supportive therapies and early recognition and treatment of complications associated with the disease process

Diagnostic Tests

Laboratory findings in patients with liver disease (see Table 13–26) are a direct result of destruction of hepatic cells (liver enzymes) or from the effects of reduced metabolic processes.

In addition, parenchymal tests such as a liver biopsy can be performed to study directly the liver cell architecture. The liver will characteristically be small with a marked decrease in functioning hepatic cell structures. This allows for a definitive diagnosis of the cause of the hepatic failure. An ultrasound may be helpful in detecting impaired bile flow.

Hepatic drug clearance tests of known substances are also used to study liver function. The most common are dyes that are injected into the blood and then the clearance is measured at specific time intervals.

Supportive Therapies

Hemodynamic instability and decreased perfusion to core organs may be the end result of portal hypertension and hyperdynamic circulation. Invasive monitoring may be used in the very critically ill patient, but must be considered in terms of the potential for infection in a patient with an impaired immune response. Vasoactive drugs plus fluids may be ordered to support blood pressure and kidney perfusion, which require close monitoring by the nurse. Portal hypertension also predisposes the patient to esophageal and gastric varices, which have the potential to bleed. This was discussed in the previous section on upper gastrointestinal bleed.

The patient with liver failure is also at risk for bleeding complications because of decreased synthesis of clotting factors. Patients with a prolonged PT and PTT and decreased platelet count should be protected from injury through the use of padded side rails and assistance with all activity. Needle sticks should be kept to a minimum. Therapeutic touch in providing all nursing cares will also reduce the risk for bleeding. Blood products may be ordered in severe cases. Disseminated intravascular coagulation is a more severe complication that may also develop in these patients. Gastrointestinal bleeding needs to be prevented in these patients because of the associated increase in protein load, which is not tolerated well. Antacids and histamine (H_2) blockers may be ordered to prevent gastritis and bleeding from stress ulcers.

Treatment of Complications

Ascites

Impaired handling of salt and water by the kidneys, as well as other abnormalities in fluid homeostasis, predisposes the patient to an accumulation of fluid in the peritoneum, or ascites. Ascites is problematic because as more fluid is retained, it pushes up on the diaphragm, impairing the patient's breathing pattern. Nursing assessment of respiratory status through respiratory rate, breath sounds, and ABG monitoring is critical. Frequent monitoring of abdominal girths and daily weights will alert the nurse to fluid accumulation. Abdominal girths should be measured at the level of the umbilicus. Positioning the patient in a semi-Fowler's position also allows for free diaphragm movement. Frequent deep-breathing and coughing exercises and changes in position are important to prevent this complication. Some patients may require elective intubation until medical management of the ascites is accomplished.

Ascites is medically managed through bed rest, a low-sodium diet, fluid restriction, and diuretic therapy. Diuretics must be administered cautiously, however, because if the intravascular volume is depleted too quickly, acute renal failure may be induced. Close monitoring of serum creatinine, BUN, and urine output are important for the early detection of this potential complication. Careful monitoring of electrolyte balance, particularly serum potassium and sodium, is also important in diuretic administration. Head-out-of-water body immersion has also been used to expand the circulatory blood volume prior to the administration of diuretic therapy to enhance the effect of the diuretic.

Paracentesis is another medical therapy to treat ascites in which ascitic fluid is withdrawn through percutaneous needle aspiration. Close monitoring of vital signs during this procedure is necessary, especially as fluid is withdrawn. Major complications include sudden loss of intravascular pressure and tachycardia. One to two liters of fluid are generally withdrawn at one time to prevent these complications. The amount, color, and character of fluid obtained should be documented. Often a specimen of the fluid is sent for analysis. Abdominal girth should be remeasured after the procedure. Salt-poor albumin may also be administered to increase colloid osmotic pressure and decrease loss of fluid into the peritoneal cavity.

Peritoneovenous shunt is a surgical procedure used to relieve ascites that is resistant to other therapies. The Leveen shunt is inserted by placing the distal end of a tube under the peritoneum and tunneling the other end under the skin into the jugular vein or superior vena cava. (Fig. 13–12). A valve that opens and closes according to pressure gradients allows ascitic fluid to flow into the superior vena cava. The patient's breathing normally triggers the valve. During inspiration, pressure will increase in the peritoneum and decrease vena cava pressure, allowing fluid to flow from the peritoneum into the general circulation. Major complications of this therapy include hemodilution, clotting of the shunt, wound infection, leakage of ascitic fluid from the incision, and bleeding problems.

A variation of this procedure is the Denver shunt, which involves placement of a pump in addition to the peritoneal catheter. Fluid is allowed to flow through the pump from the peritoneum into the general circulation at a uniform rate. The pump also allows the physician or nurse to squeeze the pump percutaneously to increase flow or to clear the catheter of any solid matter.

Portal Systemic Encephalopathy

Portal systemic encephalopathy (PSE) is a functional derangement of the central nervous system that causes altered levels of consciousness and

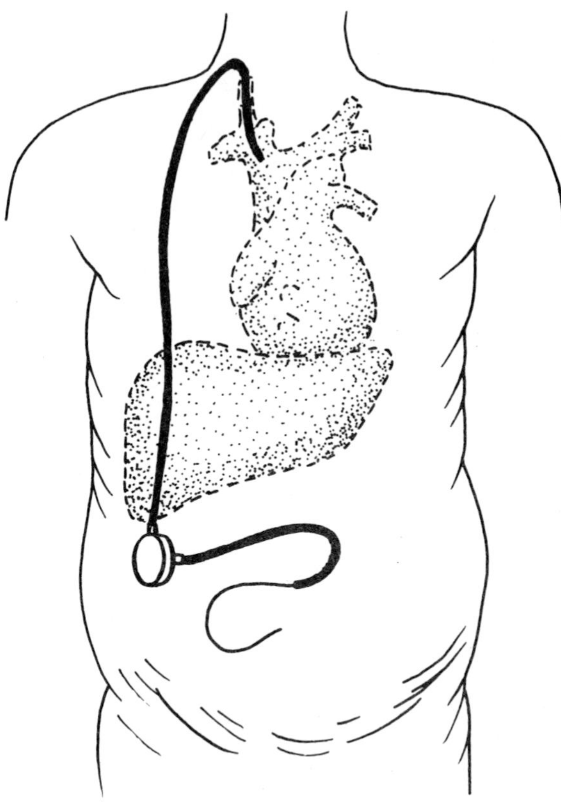

Figure 13–12. LeVeen shunt.

cerebral manifestations from confusion to coma. Impaired motor ability is also often present. Asterixis is a flapping tremor of the hand that is an early sign of PSE that can be assessed by the nurse.

The exact cause of portal systemic encephalopathy is unknown, but it is thought to be abnormal ammonia metabolism. Elevated serum ammonia levels are thought to interfere with normal cerebral metabolism. In acute liver failure, signs and symptoms of this disorder may appear rapidly, whereas in chronic failure, they often occur over time. There are many conditions that may precipitate the development of PSE, including fluid and electrolyte and acid-base disturbances, increased protein intake, portal-systemic shunts, blood transfusions, GI bleeding, and many drugs such as diuretics, analgesics, narcotics, and sedatives. Progression of PSE can be divided into stages (Table 13–30).

Measures to decrease ammonia production are necessary in the treatment of PSE. Protein intake needs to be limited to 20 to 40 g/day. Neomycin and lactulose are two drugs that can be administered to reduce bacterial breakdown of protein in the bowel.

Table 13–30. STAGES OF PORTAL SYTEMIC ENCEPHALOPATHY

Stage 1
- Tremors
- Slurred speech
- Impaired decision-making

Stage 2
- Drowsiness
- Loss of sphincter control
- Asterixis

Stage 3
- Dramatic confusion
- Somnolent

Stage 4
- Profound coma
- Unresponsive to pain

Neomycin is a broad-spectrum antibiotic that destroys normal bacteria found in the bowel. This decreases protein breakdown and ammonia production. Neomycin is given orally every 4 to 6 hours. This drug is toxic to the kidneys, and therefore cannot be given to patients in renal failure. Daily renal function studies need to be monitored when administering neomycin.

Lactulose creates an acidic environment in the bowel that causes the ammonia to leave the blood stream and enter the colon. Ammonia is trapped in the bowel. Lactulose also has a laxative effect that allows for elimination of the ammonia. Lactulose is given orally or via a rectal enema.

Restriction of medications that are toxic to the liver is another important treatment.

Nursing measures to protect the patient with an altered mental status from harm is a priority. Many patients with PSE may need to be sedated to prevent harm to themselves or to others. Orazepam (Serax), diazepam (Valium), or lorazepam (Ativan) may be used judiciously, as they are less dependent on liver function for excretion.

Hepatorenal Syndrome

Acute renal failure that occurs with liver failure is called hepatorenal syndrome (HRS). The pathophysiology of this disorder is not well understood, but it is associated with end-stage cirrhosis and ascites, decreased albumin, and portal hypertension. Decreased urine output and elevated serum creatinine usually occur acutely. The prognosis

NURSING CARE PLAN FOR THE PATIENT WITH HEPATIC FAILURE		
Nursing Diagnosis	**Outcome**	**Intervention**
Fluid volume deficit related to variceal hemorrhage, third spacing of peritoneal fluid (ascites), coagulation abnormalities	Absence/resolution of bleeding Hematocrit/hemoglobin, coagulation factors, protein, albumin WNL Vital signs returned to baseline	See the Nursing Care Plan for the Patient with Upper GI Bleed related to varices for specific nursing interventions Monitor blood counts and coagulation function tests Protect patient from injury. Pad side rails and assist with activities of daily living. Monitor for bleeding from IV sites, mucous membranes, petechiae Limit punctures for blood draws, IVs Guaiac all specimens for occult blood Administer fluid and blood products as ordered and monitor patient response Administer vitamin K and other coagulation products
Altered nutrition; less than body requirements related to altered liver metabolism of food nutrients, insufficient intake, impaired absorption of fat-soluble vitamins, vitamin B_{12} deficiency, and anemia	Sufficient protein intake for liver regeneration No blood accumulation of nitrogen waste products (BUN WNL) Liver function tests WNL Serum albumin WNL Positive nitrogen balance	Limit protein intake Monitor serum BUN Administer vitamins synthesized by the liver: A, B, D, and K Monitor nutritional status through serum albumin, nitrogen balance, daily weights Consider enteral feeding or TPN if PO intake is insufficient
Ineffective breathing pattern and impaired gas exchange related to dyspnea form ascites, increased risk of pulmonary infections from decreased activity of Kupffer cells	Effective lung expansion Absence of dyspnea ABGs WNL or returned to baseline	Monitor patient's ongoing respiratory status, including respiratory rate, breath sounds, depth of respirations Monitor ABGs for increasing CO_2 and decreasing PaO_2 Encourage patient to cough and deep breathe. Perform chest physiotherapy; i.e., percussion, vibration, suctioning as needed Administer O_2 as ordered according to clinical assessment Administer sedatives and analgesics cautiously so as not to impair respiratory effort Monitor fluid status and treat ascites; accurate I/O; measure abdominal girths every 4 hr; monitor daily weights; restrict fluids and sodium; administer diuretics as ordered Assist with paracentesis as needed
Altered thought processes related to impaired handling of ammonia, aggressive diuretic therapy, diet, medications that require liver metabolism, decreased perfusion states	Absence of or resolution of hepatic encephalopathy Stable BUN	Prevent increased ammonia production via protein restriction; prevent and treat infection, dehydration, electrolyte, or acid-base disturbances; judicious use of sedative narcotic tranquilizers; cautious administration of diuretic therapy Administer lactulose and neomycin and monitor Reduce risk of GI bleeding through antacid and H_2 blocker administration Monitor patient response to therapy (ammonia levels) and through careful neurological assessments Reorient patient and provide for safety during periods of impaired mentation; prevent hazards related to immobility

for the patient with HRS is generally poor because therapies to improve renal function usually are ineffective. General medical therapies to improve liver function while supporting renal function are the goals. Fluid administration and diuretic therapy are used to improve urine output. Drugs toxic to the kidney are discontinued. Occasionally, hemodialysis may be used to support renal function if there is a chance for an improvement in liver function.

PATIENT OUTCOMES

Patient outcomes for the patient with liver failure include

1. Absence/resolution of bleeding
2. Hct/Hgb returned to baseline
3. Coagulation functions tests within normal limits
4. Sufficient intake of protein for liver re-

generation, but not so much that it causes increased/accumulation of nitrogen waste products

5. Serum albumin/protein within normal limits
6. Absence of ascites
7. Weight stable
8. Adequate oxygenation and ventilation
9. Resolution of encephalopathy
10. Creatinine/BUN stable

See the Nursing Care Plan for the Patient with Hepatic Failure.

Summary

Acute upper GI bleed, acute pancreatitis, and liver failure account for the major potentially life-threatening emergencies that require careful and astute assessments and care by the critical care nurse and medical team. Priorities for care include initial assessments and resuscitation, diagnostic testing to make a definitive diagnosis, and prompt interventions to stabilize or reverse the pathophysiological process and prevent complications. Nursing's scope of care specifically includes ongoing assessments and monitoring, documenting and reporting patient responses to diagnostics and treatment regimens, early detection of complications, and supportive care. Patient/family teaching of the ICU routine and all therapies instituted is also a priority. As appropriate, discharge teaching of the underlying pathological process and dietary, medication, and activity regimens may also be initiated in the ICU. Successful management of all of these patient populations requires a collaborative effort of all disciplines.

References

Given, B. A. (1984): *Gastroenterology in Clinical Nursing.* St. Louis: C. V. Mosby.

Galambos, J. T. (1985): Portal hypertension. *Seminars in Liver Disease* 5(3):277–285.

Pitchumoni, C. S., Agarwal, N., and Jain, J. K. (1988): Systemic complications of acute pancreatitis. *American Journal of Gastroenterology* 83(6):597–603.

Ranson, J. C. (1985): Risk factors in acute pancreatitis. *Hospital Practice* 20(4):69–73.

Sabesin, S. (1987): Countering the dangers of acute pancreatitis. *Emergency Medicine* 10:71–96.

Sleisenger, M., and Fordtran, J. (1989): *Gastrointestinal Disease.* 4th ed. Philadelphia: W. B. Saunders.

Stern, A. I. (1985): The gastric mucosal barrier. *Medical Journal of Australia* 142:9–10.

Teerenhovi, H. et al. (1988): Influence of pancreatic resection on systemic complications in acute necrotizing pancreatitis. *British Journal of Surgery* 75(8):793–795.

Wilson, C., McArdle, C. S., Carter, C. C. et al. (1988): Surgical treatment of acute necrotizing pancreatitis. *British Journal of Surgery* 75(11):1119–1123.

Recommended Reading

Brown, A. (1991): Acute pancreatitis: Pathophysiology, nursing diagnoses, and collaborative problems. *Focus on Critical Care* 18, 121–130.

Curtas, S. et al. (1989): Evaluation of nutritional status. *Nursing Clinics of North America* 24(3):301–313.

Decker, S. I. (1985): Life-threatening consequences of a GI bleed. *RN* 10:18–27.

Fain, J. A., and Amato-Vealey, E. (1988): Acute pancreatitis: A GI emergency. *Critical Care Nurse* 8(5):47–63.

Gitnick, G. (1987): *Handbook of Gastrointestinal Emergencies.* New York: Elsevier.

Jeffres, S. (1989): Complications of acute pancreatitis. *Critical Care Nurse* 9(4):38–50.

Keith, J. S. (1985): Hepatic failure: Etiologies, manifestations and management. *Critical Care Nurse* 5:60–80.

Ricci, J. A. (1987): Alcohol induced upper gastrointestinal hemorrhage: Case studies and management. *Critical Care Nurse* 7(1):56–67.

Chapter 14

Joanne Krumberger; R.N., M.S.N., CCRN
Linda Waite; R.N., M.N.

Endocrine Crises

Objectives

- Identify pancreas, adrenal, and thyroid disorders that are seen in critical care units.
- Describe the feedback mechanisms for regulation of cortisol, thyroid hormone, and insulin.
- Compare pathophysiology, assessment, nursing diagnoses, outcomes, and interventions for hyperglycemic crisis, hypoglycemic crisis, adrenal crisis, thyroid storm, and myxedema coma.
- Compare and contrast diabetic ketoacidosis and hyperosmolar hyperglycemic nonketotic coma.
- Formulate a plan of care for the patient with hyperglycemic crisis, hypoglycemic crisis, adrenal crisis, thyroid storm, and myxedema coma.

The endocrine glands form a communication network that links all body systems. Hormones from these glands control and regulate metabolic processes governing such activities as energy production, fluid and electrolyte balance, and stress reactions. This system is closely linked and integrated by the nervous system. In particular, the hypothalamus and pituitary glands play a major role in hormonal regulation. The hypothalamus manufactures and secretes several releasing or inhibiting hormones that are conveyed to the pituitary and stimulate or inhibit release of specific hormones. This system is governed by feedback control mechanisms that regulate the level of hormones within the body. Positive feedback systems stimulate release of a controlling hormone when serum hormone levels are low. Negative feedback systems inhibit the release of controlling hormones when hormone levels are high. Figures 14–1 and 14–2 provide examples of how these feedback systems work to control circulating levels of cortisol and thyroid hormones. These same feedback systems also control secretion/inhibition of hormones outside hypothalmic-pituitary control, such as insulin (Fig. 14–3).

Diseases involving the hypothalamus, pituitary gland, or the primary endocrine organs, i.e., pancreas, adrenal gland, or thyroid gland, can interfere with normal feedback mechanisms and the secretion of hormones and result in disease states. Crisis states can occur when these diseases are untreated or undertreated, the patient is stressed, or as the result of a multitude of other factors. This chapter deals with such crises that occur as a result of dysfunction of the pancreas, adrenal gland, and thyroid gland.

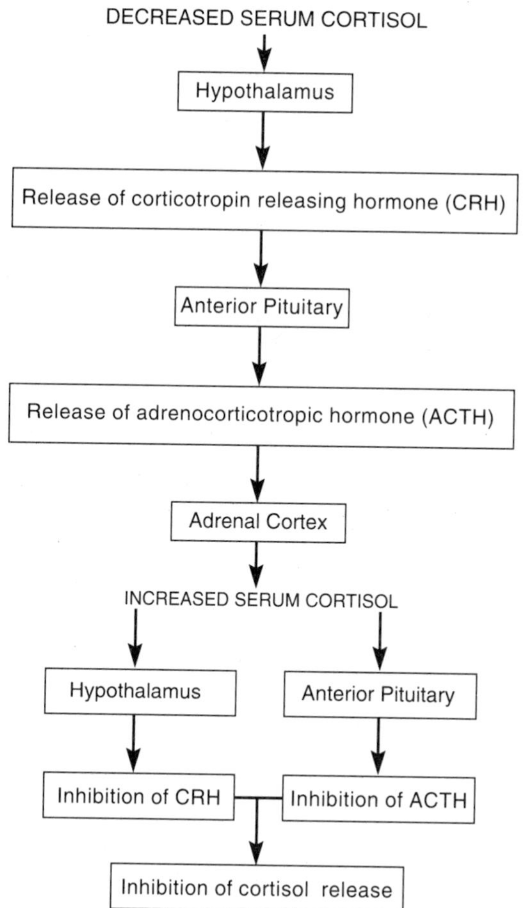

Figure 14–1. Feedback systems for cortisol regulation.

Pancreatic Endocrine Emergencies

The three major endocrine disorders associated with the pancreas are diabetic ketoacidosis (DKA), hyperosmolar hyperglycemic nonketotic coma (HHNC), and hypoglycemia, which are acute complications of diabetes mellitus. An understanding of the normal physiology of insulin as well as the pathophysiology, critical assessments, and collaborative treatment regimens of the above-mentioned disorders is essential to the management and nursing care of these patients.

Insulin is normally released from the pancreas by beta cells of the islets of Langerhans in response to increases in blood glucose. Other stimulants of insulin secretion include gastrin, secretin, cholecystokinin, and arginine. Insulin is essential to normal carbohydrate, protein and fat metabolism. Table 14–1 summarizes the physiological activity of insulin. Insulin is necessary for cellular uptake of glucose by most cells in the body, including muscle, fibroblasts, mammary glands, the anterior pituitary, lens of the eye, and the aorta. These cells constitute the largest percentage of body mass and expend the most energy. Insulin is not required for glucose to enter liver cells, kidney tubules, nerve tissue, erythrocytes, and intestinal mucosa.

Without insulin, glucose fails to enter cells, accumulates in the blood (hyperglycemia), and triggers a variety of physiological processes as the cells without glucose begin to starve. Insulin is also anabolic in that it works with other hormones (thyroid, sex, and growth hormones) to promote growth. An excess in circulating insulin

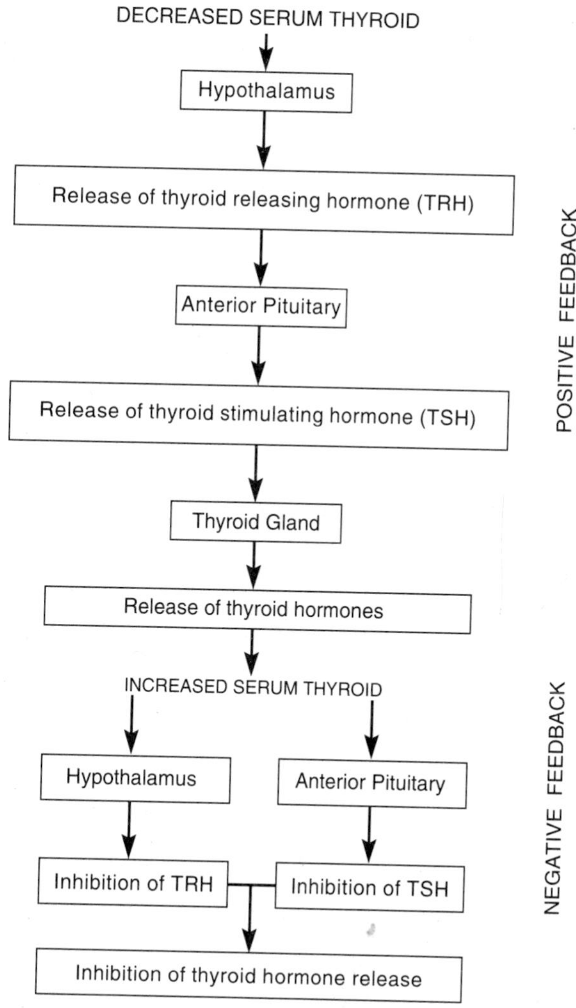

Figure 14–2. Feedback systems for thyroid hormone regulation.

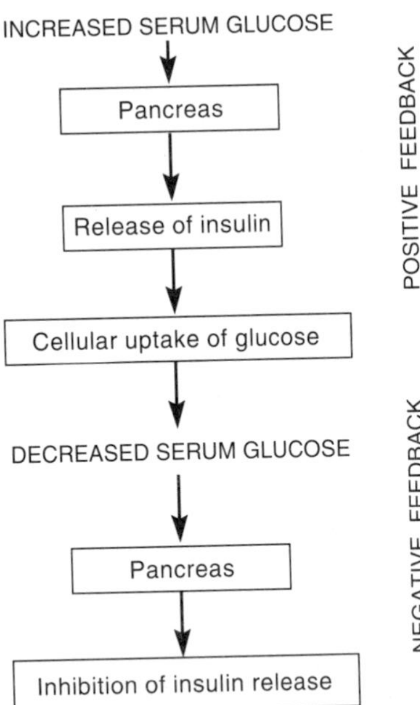

Figure 14–3. Feedback systems for insulin regulation.

greater than the body's requirement results in decreased serum glucose and primarily changes in level of consciousness as glucose is the preferred fuel of the central nervous system.

DIABETES MELLITUS

Diabetes Mellitus (DM) is a metabolic disease that is caused by ineffective uptake of glucose by cells. There are several types of diabetes, the two most common being insulin-dependent DM (Type I, IDDM) and non–insulin-dependent DM (Type II, NIDDM). Type I DM usually has a juvenile or early adult onset, and is characterized by little or no endogenous insulin production. Type II DM usually occurs in older adults, and is associated with below normal, normal, or above normal insulin production.

The acute complications of diabetes mellitus include diabetic ketoacidosis, hyperosmolar hyperglycemic nonketotic coma, and hypoglycemia.

Table 14–1. PHYSIOLOGICAL ACTIVITY OF INSULIN

Carbohydrate Metabolism
- Increases glucose transport across cell membrane in muscle, fat, and hepatic tissue
- Within liver and muscle, promotes formation of glycogen, the storage form of glucose
- Inhibits gluconeogenesis in liver, thus sparing amino acids and glycerol for protein and fatty acid synthesis

Fat Metabolism
- Increases triglyceride synthesis
- Increases fatty acid transport into adipose tissue
- Inhibits lipolysis of triglycerides stored in adipose tissue
- Stimulates fatty acid synthesis from glucose and other substrates

Protein Metabolism
- Increases amino acid transport across cell membrane of muscle and liver
- Augments protein synthesis
- Inhibits proteolysis

Hyperglycemic Crises

Pathogenesis

Etiology DKA. A number of factors can trigger diabetic ketoacidosis (DKA) (Table 14–2), the most common being infections and severe stress states. Many patients present with DKA as the initial indication of previously undiagnosed diabetes mellitus (Type I, IDDM). The condition may also occur in patients with known DM who fail to administer enough insulin or have increased insulin requirements. Patients using an insulin pump may also develop DKA because of a malfunctioning pump system or infection of the catheter. Lack of knowledge regarding the disease process, insulin administration, or lack of compliance with the therapeutic regimen must also be assessed as a possible etiology. Diabetic ketoacidosis characteristically develops over a short period of time and patients seek medical help early because of the pathophysiological effects.

Pathophysiology of DKA. Diabetic ketoacidosis is an endocrine emergency resulting from a sustained relative or absolute insulin deficiency. It is also usually associated with increased levels of insulin-antagonistic hormones (glucagon, cortisol, catecholamines, and growth hormone). The physiological consequences of insulin deficiency include increased fatty acid release, decreased glucose uptake by cells, and increased amino acid release from cells. Hyperglycemia also causes an osmotic diuresis due to fluid shifts from areas of higher-concentration intracellular and extracellular spaces, and results in fluid volume deficits and electrolyte losses (sodium, chloride, potassium, magnesium, phosphate). Glycosuria is common as serum glucose exceeds renal threshold. With decreased insulin levels, metabolism of ketones formed by the liver as a result of fatty acid oxidation is impaired. These ketoacids accumulate in the blood and body fluids—a condition called ketosis. Metabolic acidosis due to an

Table 14–2. PRECIPITATING FACTORS FOR DIABETIC KETOACIDOSIS

- Infections
  - Pneumonia
  - Urinary Tract
  - Upper Respiratory
  - Meningitis
  - Pancreatitis
  - Cholecystitis
- Vascular Disorders
  - Myocardial Infarction
  - Cerebral Vascular Accident
- Drugs
  - Thiazide Diuretics
  - Dilantin
  - Steroids
  - Epinephrine
  - Psychotropics
  - Analgesics
  - β-Blockers
- Insulin
  - Omission (new-onset DM, noncompliance in a known diabetic, inadequate dosage of insulin)
  - Increased demand (i.e., increased growth in children)
  - Malfunction of insulin pump
  - Infection at catheter site (infusion pump)
- Stress (unmet increased requirements for insulin due to physical or emotional stress. Also associated with increased secretion of insulin-antagonistic hormones)
  - Infection
  - Trauma
  - Surgery
  - Growth spurts
  - Acute illness
- Development of Insulin Resistance
  - During menstruation
  - During pregnancy
- Endocrine Disorders
  - Hyperthyroidism
  - Cushing's Disease
  - Pheochromocytoma

accumulation of ketoacids and lactic acids from decreased perfusion is present.

Protein stores are broken down by the liver into amino acids and then into glucose and nitrogen to provide energy. Without insulin, the glucose liberated cannot be used, and this further increases serum blood glucose, increases urine glucose (glycosuria) and worsens the osmotic diuresis. As nitrogen accumulates in the periphery, blood urea nitrogen (BUN) will rise. Breakdown of protein stores also stimulates the loss of intracellular potassium, increasing potassium in the serum. Potassium may accumulate in the serum (hyperkalemia) owing to potassium shifts from the cell to the serum with acidosis or be lost owing to osmotic diuresis (hypokalemia). It is important to note that no matter what the serum level of potassium, total body potassium deficits are common and must be considered in the overall management of DKA.

As the concentration of glucose in the plasma increases, the kidney begins to excrete glucose as a response (glycosuria). This will cause an osmotic diuresis with urinary losses of water, sodium, potassium, magnesium, calcium, and phosphorus. This causes an increase in serum osmolality, which in turn causes more fluid to shift from the intracellular to extracellular space and worsens the dehydration. This hyperosmolarity is also thought further to impair insulin secretion as well as promote insulin resistance. The glomerular filtration rate in the kidney also decreases in response to these severe fluid volume deficits. Decreased glucose excretion (which increases serum glucose) and hyperosmolality result. The altered neurological status frequently seen in these patients is partly due to cellular dehydration and the hyperosmolar state.

The absence or lack of insulin causes an enhanced decomposition of fat (lipolysis), increased free fatty acid mobilization from peripheral adipose tissue stores, and the development of ketosis from impaired metabolism of ketones. As ketone and H^+ ions accumulate and acidosis worsens, the body will attempt to buffer this. Normally this would be done by bicarbonate, but the patient with DKA often has diminished bicarbonate levels because of osmotic diuresis. Carbonic acid will then accumulate. Acidosis in DKA characteristically develops very quickly. The respiratory system will attempt to compensate for excess carbonic acid by blowing off carbon dioxide, which is also an acid. This explains the rapid, deep breathing seen in these patients, which are called Kussmaul respirations. In addition to carbonic acid, patients with DKA may have an accumulation of lactic acids (lactic acidosis) from the loss of volume from the osmotic diuresis. Dehydration may cause decreased perfusion to core organs, causing hypoxemia and worsening of the lactic acidosis.

Excess lactic acid results in what is called an increased anion gap (increased body acids). Sodium, potassium, chloride, and bicarbonate are responsible for maintaining a normal anion gap, which is normally less than 12 mEq/L. Ketone accumulation will cause an increase in anion gap above 12 (Table 14–3).

Table 14–3. EQUATION FOR ANION GAP

$$Na - (Cl^- + HCO_3^-)$$

Normal value 12–14; elevated value indicates accumulation of acids associated with DKA.

Many enzymatic reactions within the body function only within a limited range of pH. As the patient becomes more acidotic and enzymes become more ineffective, body metabolism will be slowed. This causes a further decrease in ketone metabolism and acidosis will be worsened. The stress response also contributes to the metabolic alterations as the liver is stimulated by hormones (glucagon, catecholamines, cortisol, and growth hormones) to break down protein stores, increasing serum glucose and nitrogen. Some of these hormones also decrease the ability of glucose to be used by cells for energy, compounding the problem. The central nervous system alterations seen in DKA are thought to be influenced by the acidosis.

In summary, cells without glucose will starve and begin to use existing stores of fat and protein to provide energy for body processes (gluconeogenesis). Fats are broken down faster than they can be metabolized, which will result in an accumulation of ketone acids, a by-product of fat metabolism in the liver. Ketone acids will accumulate in the blood stream where hydrogen (H^+) ions will dissociate from the ketones, causing a metabolic acidosis. The more acidic the patient becomes, the less able he/she is to metabolize these ketones. Acetone is also formed during this process and is responsible for the "fruity breath" found in these patients. These pathophysiological processes are reviewed in Table 14–4.

Etiology of HHNC. Hyperosmolar hyperglycemic nonketotic coma is usually precipitated by inadequate insulin secretion or action, and is more commonly seen in a newly diagnosed Type II non–insulin-dependent diabetic. Some patients may have no history of diabetes mellitus. The majority of patients are elderly with decreased compensatory mechanisms to maintain homeostasis in hyperosmolar states. A major illness mediated through glucose overproduction due to the stress response may contribute to the development of HHNC. High-caloric parenteral and enteral feedings that exceed the patient's ability to metabolize the glucose have been known to induce HHNC. Several drugs have also been associated with the development of the disorder. The major etiologies of HHNC are reviewed in Table 14–5.

Table 14–4. PHYSIOLOGICAL CONSEQUENCES OF DIABETIC KETOACIDOSIS

	Insulin Deficiency	
Carbohydrate	***Fat***	***Protein***
Decreased glucose use in cells requiring insulin for glucose entry	Increased lipolysis due to lack of inhibition of lipases	Increased catabolism
Overproduction of glucose by liver (gluconeoformation genesis)	Increased fatty acids to liver (unable to metabolize)	Ketone
Hyperglycemia (hyperosmolality)	Ketone formation	
Glycosuria		
Osmotic Diuresis		
Fluid Volume Deficit	Ketonuria	
Electrolyte Imbalance	Acidosis	

Pathophysiology of HHNC. Hyperosmolar hyperglycemic nonketotic coma, also known as hyperglycemic nonacidotic diabetic coma, is a pancreatic endocrine emergency characterized by

Table 14–5. ETIOLOGIES OF HYPEROSMOLAR HYPERGLYCEMIC NONKETOTIC COMA

- Newly diagnosed non–insulin-dependent diabetes
- Elderly
- Major Illnesses
  - Sepsis
  - Pancreatitis
  - Uremia
  - Stroke
  - Burns
  - Acute myocardial infarction
  - Gastrointestinal hemorrhage
- Stress
- High-calorie parenteral or enteral feedings
- Medications
  - Thiazide Diuretics
  - Glucocorticoids
  - Sympathomimetics
  - Phenytoin
  - Chlorpromazine
  - Cimetidine
  - Calcium Channel Blockers
  - Immunosuppressive Agents
  - β-Blockers
  - Diazoxide

profound hyperglycemia, hyperosmolality, and severe dehydration, which is associated with minimal ketosis resulting from insulin deficiency.

Hyperglycemia results from decreased utilization and increased production of glucose. The hyperglycemic state causes an osmotic movement of water from higher concentration of solutes (intracellular space) to lesser concentration of solutes (extracellular space). This results in expansion of the extracellular fluid volume and intracellular dehydration. The osmotic diuresis and resultant intracellular and extracellular dehydration in HHNC is generally more severe than that found in DKA because HHNC generally develops very insidiously over a period of weeks to months. By the time these patients seek medical attention, they are profoundly dehydrated and hyperosmolar. Alterations in neurological states as a consequence are common and are due to cellular dehydration. As a result, the mortality rate associated with HHNC is higher than with DKA. Additionally, these patients are older and commonly have other medical problems that affect morbidity and mortality.

Ketoacidosis is usually not seen in patients with HHNC. It is believed that insulin levels in these patients may remain high enough to prevent lipolysis and ketone formation. Glucose counterregulatory hormones that promote lipolysis are lower in HHNC than those found in patients with DKA (Graves, 1990). Table 14–6 reviews the major pathophysiological events associated with HHNC.

Table 14–6. PATHOPHYSIOLOGY OF HYPEROSMOLAR HYPERGLYCEMIC NONKETOTIC COMA

Insulin Deficiency (inadequate supply, inadequate insulin action, or increased glucose load)

↓

Decreased Glucose Utilization
Increased Gluconeogenesis

↓

Hyperglycemia

↓

Osmotic Diuresis

↓

Intracellular Dehydration
Glycosuria
Loss of Water and Electrolytes
Increased Serum Osmolality
Decreased Renal Function (increased BUN)

↓

Shock

Assessment of DKA and HHNC

Clinical Presentation. The presenting symptoms seen in DKA and HHNC are similar, and it is most helpful to discuss the similarities and highlight the differences in these two disorders (Table 14–7). Signs of DKA and HHNC are related to the degree of dehydration present and the electrolyte imbalances. The osmotic diuresis that occurs from hyperglycemia results in signs of increased thirst (polydipsia) and increased urine output (polyuria). Increased hunger (polyphagia) may also be an early sign. It is important to point out that the elderly have a decreased sense of thirst, so this may not be seen in patients who typically develop HHNC. Signs of intravascular dehydration are also common as these disease processes continue and may include

* Hypotension (orthostatic)
* Tachycardia
* Warm, dry skin
* Dry mucous membranes
* Loss of skin turgor
* Soft eyeballs

As intracellular and intravascular volumes are depleted, vomiting can become a problem, which further worsens total body dehydration. As a result, urine output will fall. Patients will also report symptoms of weakness and anorexia. The lungs will be clear to auscultation, even in the presence of pneumonia. Abdominal pain and tenderness are also common presenting symptoms, particularly in DKA, and are associated with dehydration and underlying pathophysiology such as pyelonephritis, duodenal ulcer, appendicitis, and metabolic acidosis. Pain associated with DKA will most commonly disappear with treatment of dehydration. Weight loss may also occur because of fluid losses and an inability to metabolize glucose.

Typically, dehydration is more profound in patients with HHNC because of the length of illness and patient age. The hypotonic osmotic diuresis also tends to be more severe, causing profound losses of water and electrolytes, and resulting in intracellular and extracellular fluid volume deficits.

Altered states of consciousness range from restlessness, confusion, and agitation to somnolence and coma. Generally, altered states of consciousness are more pronounced in patients with HHNC. The level of consciousness is related to the severity of hyperglycemia and serum hyperosmolarity. Deep tendon reflexes may also be de-

Table 14–7. MANIFESTATIONS OF DIABETIC KETOACIDOSIS AND HYPEROSMOLAR HYPERGLYCEMIC NONKETOTIC COMA

	DKA	HHNC
Pathophysiology	Insulin deficiency resulting in cellular dehydration and volume depletion, acidosis, and protein catabolism	Insulin deficiency resulting in dehydration, hyperosmolality, and impaired renal function
Health History	History of Type I DM (use of insulin)	History of Type II DM (non-insulin-dependent)
	Signs and symptoms of hyperglycemia prior to admission	Signs and symptoms of hyperglycemia prior to admission
	Can also occur in Type II DM in severe stress	Occurs most frequently in elderly, with preexisting renal and cardiovascular disease
Onset	Develops quickly	Develops insidiously
Clinical Presentation	Flushed, dry skin	Flushed, dry skin
	Dry mucous membranes	Dry mucous membranes
	Decreased skin turgor	Decreased skin turgor (may not be present in elderly)
	Tachycardia	Tachycardia
	Hypotension	Hypotension
	Kussmaul respirations	Shallow respirations
	Acetone breath	
	Altered level of consciousness	Altered level of consciousness (generally more profound and may include absent deep tendon reflexes, paresis, and positive Babinski sign)
	Polydipsia	
	Polyuria	
	Nausea and vomiting	
	Anorexia	
Diagnostics	Elevated plasma (average: 675 mg/dl) and urine glucose levels	Elevated plasma glucose (usually >1000 mg/dl)
	Arterial pH <7.30	Arterial pH >7.30
	Decreased bicarbonate	Bicarbonate >15 mEq/L
	Positive serum and urine ketoacids	Absence of significant ketosis
	Azotemia	Azotemia
	Electrolytes vary with state of hydration; often hyperkalemic on presentation despite marked body deficit	Electrolytes vary with state of hydration; often hypernatremic which contributes to hyperosmolality
	Plasma hyperosmolality increased due to hemoconcentration	Plasma hyperosmolality (>330 mOsm/kg)

creased. Seizures and focal neurological signs may also be present and often cause misdiagnosis in patients with HHNC. Aphasia, paresis, and a positive Babinski reflex may also be present with HHNC.

As mentioned above, in DKA, the absence of sufficient insulin, glucose utilization is profoundly impaired and inhibits the peripheral of uptake of glucose as well as protein synthesis and lipogenesis (Graves, 1990). Glucose can still be used in non-insulin-dependent tissues and free fatty acids are mobilized and transported to the liver for metabolism. The liver becomes overwhelmed and is unable to oxidize the excessive amount of ketones. The excessive production and decreased metabolism of ketone bodies result in ketonuria and loss of bicarbonate, resulting in metabolic acidosis. Nausea is an early sign of DKA, and is thought to be a result of retained ketones. Increases in the rate and depth of breathing (Kussmaul respirations) are common as the patient attempts to compensate for the metabolic acidosis. Later in the disease process, the respiratory status of the patient may be influenced by the neurological status precipitating impaired breathing patterns of gas exchange. Acetone breath from fat metabolism may also be noted. A decreased level of consciousness is also associated with the severe acidotic state (pH < 7.15). The flushed face associated with DKA is common in carbonic acid accumulation and is due to superficial vasodilation.

Laboratory Evaluation. A number of diagnostic studies will be ordered by the physician to evaluate for DKA and HHNC, to rule out other potential diseases, and to detect complications.

In DKA, the serum glucose is generally greater than 300 mg/dl, averaging 675 mg/dl. A well-hydrated patient in ketoacidosis may present with a serum glucose less than 300 mg/dl. Glycosuria will be present with a serum glucose >170 to 200 mg/dl. Serum osmolality will be increased from the high concentration of glucose. Increased serum and urine ketones are also present from fat metabolism. Dehydration from osmotic diuresis will be reflected by hemoconcentration (increased blood values due to decreased plasma volume). Therefore, the hematocrit, hemoglobin, and creatinine levels will often be elevated. The BUN will also be increased owing to hemoconcentration and from the breakdown of protein stores. The WBC count may be elevated from an infection or from the stress response.

Potassium (K^+) may be normal, elevated, or subnormal depending on the hydration status of the patient. Most often the patient presents with hyperkalemia, although total body stores of K^+ will be quite depleted. Additionally, in an acidotic state, which is a hallmark sign of DKA, K^+ will be forced out of the cell into the serum. It may accumulate there, causing hyperkalemia, or be lost via osmotic diuresis or from vomiting. Hyperkalemia can be life threatening (>6.5 mEq/dl) with the development of heart blocks, bradydysrhythmias, sinus arrest, ventricular fibrillation, or asystole. During treatment of acidosis, or with the administration of insulin, K^+ may be forced back into the cell and may cause a decrease in serum K^+ or hypokalemia. This is associated with ventricular dysrhythmias. Regardless of serum potassium levels, total body stores of potassium are generally low owing to osmotic diuresis. Phosphate levels may also fall with treatment. Sodium (Na^+) may be elevated from hormonal effects during stress, low from the hyperglycemic state, or normal.

Arterial blood gas analysis will commonly reflect a metabolic acidosis (low pH and low bicarbonate). The $PaCO_2$ may also be low, reflecting the attempt by the respiratory system to compensate for the acidosis. As the patient's level of consciousness deteriorates, the patient may develop severe breathing disturbances that will cause a precipitous increase in the $PaCO_2$ and a concurrent fall in pH. Severe acidosis is associated with cardiovascular collapse, which can result in death.

In HHNC, the laboratory results are similar to those in DKA but with three major differences. The serum glucose in HHNC is generally more elevated with a reported mean of 1166 mg/dl (Graves, 1990). Plasma osmolality is also higher than found in DKA and is associated with the degree of dehydration found. Ketosis is usually absent or very mild in comparison to DKA. Serum electrolyte concentrations, as described above, may be low, normal, or elevated, and generally are not reliable indicators of total body stores. Generally, profound total body electrolyte losses are expected. Table 14–8 summarizes the laboratory findings in DKA and HHNC.

Table 14–8. DIAGNOSTIC FINDINGS IN DKA AND HHNC

Serum	
Glucose	Elevated (generally higher in HHNC)
Potassium	Initially may be normal, elevated, or decreased depending on hydration status Most commonly elevated in DKA, although body stores are depleted Decreased with initiation of therapy
Hydrogen ions	Elevated only in DKA causing metabolic acidosis
Sodium	Normal, elevated, or decreased depending on hydration status Most commonly elevated in HHNC
Chloride	Elevated with acidosis (DKA only)
Phosphorous	Total body levels depleted Initial serum value may be normal, elevated, or decreased Serum level falls with treatment
Magnesium	Total body levels depleted Initial serum value may be normal, elevated, or decreased Serum level falls with treatment
Osmolality	Elevated due to dehydration (generally higher in HHNC)
Creatinine	Elevated due to hemoconcentration
BUN	Elevated due to protein breakdown and hemoconcentration
Chloride	Decreased with initiation of therapy
Amylase	Elevated due to hemoconcentration
Bicarbonate	Decreased (DKA only)
pH	Decreased due to accumulation of acids and dehydration (DKA only)
WBC count	Elevated due to infection or stress response
Anion Gap	Elevated (DKA only)
Urine	
Glucose	Elevated
Ketones	Elevated (DKA only)

Nursing Diagnoses of DKA and HHNC

The nursing diagnoses that may apply to a patient with DKA and HHNC based on assessment data include:

1. Fluid volume deficit related to hyperglycemia and osmotic diuresis, effects of vomiting
2. Ineffective breathing patterns; impaired gas exchange related to Kussmaul respirations to compensate for acidosis (DKA only); effects of level of consciousness on respiratory status
3. Sensory/perceptual alterations related to metabolic and electrolyte abnormalities
4. Electrolyte imbalance related to hyperglycemia, osmotic diuresis, vomiting, acidosis, treatment regimen
5. Acid-base imbalance: acidosis (DKA only) related to ketone and hydrogen ion accumulation, hypoperfusion from dehydration, decreased bicarbonate reserve
6. Knowledge deficit related to disease process, monitoring, and treatment regimen

Collaborative Management of DKA and HHNC

The primary objectives in the treatment of DKA and HHNC include respiratory support, fluid and electrolyte replacement, administration of insulin to correct hyperglycemia, correction of acidosis in DKA, monitoring, prevention of complications, and patient teaching and support.

Respiratory Support. Assessment of the airway, breathing, and circulation are the first priorities in managing these life-threatening disorders. Airway and breathing may be supported through the use of oral airways and oxygen therapy. In more severe cases, the patient may be intubated. Prevention of aspiration by head of bed elevation and perhaps nasogastric tube suction may be considered in a patient with impaired mentation who is actively vomiting.

Fluid Replacement. Dehydration may have progressed to shock by the time of admission. Immediate intravenous access and rehydration needs to be accomplished. In DKA, the total water deficit approximates 6 L, but may be as high as 10 L. In HHNC, fluid requirements are usually greater, ranging from 8 to 12 L.

Monitoring for signs and symptoms of hypovolemic shock are a priority. Vital signs will need to be recorded at least every hour initially along with the urine output. Unstable patients will require constant monitoring and recording of hemodynamic parameters at least every 15 minutes. Central venous pressure or pulmonary artery pressure monitoring may also be instituted to evaluate fluid requirements and monitor patient response to treatment. This is particularly true of patients with HHNC, who tend to be elderly and have concurrent cardiovascular and renal disease. Accurate intake, hourly recording of urine output, and daily weights are also essential. Changes in mentation may also indicate a change in fluid status. Ongoing assessment of the level of consciousness, including response to pain, motor response, reflexes, and neurological signs, will alert the nurse to a change in mentation.

Normal saline (0.9% NS) is usually the fluid of choice for initial fluid replacement as long as the patient is hypotensive and in shock because it best replaces extracellular fluid volume deficits. A rate of 1 L/hr is usually begun until the patients has stabilized. Once the patient has a normal blood pressure, hypotonic saline (0.45% NS) is used to replace intracellular fluid deficits. The goal is generally to replace one-half of the estimated fluid deficit over the first 8 hours. Lactated Ringer's may be used to avoid excess administration of chloride. The second half of the fluid deficit should be replaced during the next 16 hours of therapy. As the plasma glucose approaches 250 to 300 mg/dl, 5% glucose should be added to the replacement fluid. This prevents hypoglycemia, and allows for the continued use of insulin. Glucose also prevents the development of cerebral edema, a complication of therapy.

Fluid overload from overaggressive fluid replacement can be prevented by monitoring of breath sounds and cardiovascular assessments. Signs and symptoms of fluid overload are reviewed in Table 14–9. Rapid fluid administration may also contribute to cerebral edema, which is a complication associated with DKA. The rapid fall in plasma glucose with rapid fluid administration and concurrent insulin therapy (see next section) may result in movement of water into brain cells, causing brain swelling.

Insulin Therapy. Replacement of insulin is

Table 14–9. SIGNS AND SYMPTOMS OF FLUID OVERLOAD

Tachypnea
Rales
Neck Vein Distention
Tachycardia
Increased PCWP, CVP

definitive therapy for DKA and HHNC to restore normal glucose uptake by cells, while preventing complications of excess insulin administration: hypoglycemia, hypokalemia, and hypophosphatemia (Graves, 1990). Regular insulin IV is preferred. Most patients are initially bolused with 0.3 to 0.4 Us of regular insulin per kilogram of body weight (Butts, 1987). This is usually followed by an insulin drip via an infusion pump at between 5 and 10 Us/hr. The advantages of an insulin drip include smooth administration of insulin with a predictable pattern for the fall of blood glucose and ease of administration. Some physicians prefer intramuscular injections of insulin for maintenance after the initial IV bolus. However, if no appreciable change in serum glucose level occurs within 2 hours, intravenous therapy is usually insituted.

Serum glucose levels need to be monitored every 1 to 2 hours while on continuous insulin drip therapy. Serum blood glucose, reagent pads, or glucometers can be used as long as one consistent method is used. As soon as the serum glucose reaches 300 mg/dl, the insulin drip will usually be decreased and the primary IV solution changed to 5% glucose with hypotonic saline (D5/0.45 NS) to prevent hypoglycemia and cerebral edema, and to replace intracellular fluid volume deficits. Once serum glucose levels stabilize, the patient is generally managed with IV insulin drips or with subcutaneous insulin based on a sliding scale. Serum glucose levels may then be monitored every 6 to 8 hours. There are a variety of machines used in some settings that continuously monitor blood glucose and administer glucose or insulin based on the result.

As discussed above, it is important that serum glucose is not lowered too rapidly as cerebral edema may occur as a complication. This may result in seizures and coma. Any patient who exhibits an abrupt change in the level of consciousness after initiation of insulin therapy needs to have his or her blood glucose drawn and protective measures instituted to prevent harm. Seizure precautions should also be started. Treatment of acute cerebral edema usually involves administration of an osmotic diuretic such as 20% mannitol solution and high-dose glucocorticoids.

Electrolyte Replacement. Potassium, phosphate, chloride, and magnesium replacements may be required, especially during insulin administration. Osmotic diuresis in DKA and HHNC results in total body potassium depletion ranging from 400 to 600 mEq (Shafrir et al., 1987). Potassium deficit may be greater in HHNC. In the absence of renal disease, potassium monitoring and replacement should begin with fluid therapy. Twenty to 40 mEq of potassium is usually added to each liter of fluid administered. This may be augmented by additional doses of potassium per minibag. Potassium therapy needs to be individualized for each patient.

Total body phosphorus levels are also depleted owing to osmotic diuresis. This may result in impaired respiratory and cardiac functions. For this reason, potassium phosphate is often used in treating part of the potassium deficit. Phosphate replacements should not be used in patients with renal failure.

Urinary losses of magnesium are also common. Replacements are usually given as 1 to 2 g magnesium sulfate 10% solution IV over 15 to 30 minutes. Intramuscular magnesium therapy may also be instituted.

Treatment of Acidosis. Acidosis is generally only a feature of DKA and is not treated with bicarbonate until the serum pH is 7.10 or less. By correcting fluid and electrolyte imbalances and administering insulin, the kidneys will begin again to conserve bicarbonate to restore acid-base homeostasis, and ketone formation will cease. When required, intravenous bicarbonate will be used to bring the pH up to 7.10, but not to correct pH. Usually, the bicarbonate is added to the hypotonic normal saline. Too rapid correction of acidosis may cause central nervous system acidosis and severe hypoxemia at the cellular level. Serum arterial blood gas (ABG) analysis should be frequently done to assess for changes in pH, bicarbonate, $PaCO_2$, and oxygenation status.

Patient/Family Teaching. Education of patients is a key area in the prevention of DKA in particular. Discharge goals for patients and family members include being able to

Describe the pathophysiology, diagnosis, and therapeutic regimen for diabetes

Describe the early signs and symptoms of hyperglycemia and ketoacidosis

Discuss signs and symptoms of infections that require medical attention

Demonstrate or describe prescribed therapies used to control diabetes (e.g., glucose monitoring, diet, exercise, insulin administration)

Properly demonstrate how to document serum glucose, insulin dosage/time, site of injection, diet, and exercise

List situations that may require an increase or decrease in insulin requirements

The teaching plan should be formulated with input from the patient and family. The importance of regular diet, exercise, rest/sleep, and relaxation needs to be emphasized. Teaching sessions may also be used to allow for verbalization of feelings and coping strategies related to the impact of diabetes on the lifestyle. The patient should also be encouraged to wear or carry a Medic-Alert bracelet or wallet card at all times.

Outcome Criteria for DKA/HHNC

Outcomes for the patient with DKA or HHNC include:

1. Fluid balance
2. Electrolyte balance
3. Hemodynamic stability
4. Serum glucose <200 mg/dl
5. Serum osmolality within normal limits
6. Patient alert and oriented
7. Normal respiratory parameters
8. Nutritional balance
9. Information to comply with discharge regimen
10. ABGs within normal limits or returned to baseline (DKA)

See the Nursing Plan for the Patient with Hyperglycemic Complications of a Pancreatic Endocrine Disorder.

Hypoglycemia

Pathogenesis

Etiologies. Hypoglycemia, or decreased serum blood glucose level, needs to be closely monitored in patients on insulin therapy, especially in situations in which the insulin dose is greater than the body's requirements or rotation of sites from a hypertrophied area to one with unimpaired absorption. Other causes of hypoglycemia include: insufficient caloric consumption from a missed or delayed meal or snack, insufficient nutrition, decreased intake due to nausea and vomiting, anorexia, or interrupted tube feedings or total parenteral nutrition (TPN). Weight loss and recovery from stress (infections, illness) decrease requirements for exogenous insulin. Strenuous exercise that is not compensated by an increase in intake of food, or a decrease in insulin dose, also precipitates hypoglycemia.

Careful assessment of the patient with renal and liver dysfunctions and concurrent hypoglycemic medication administration is necessary. Decreased degradation or excretion of hypoglycemic medications prolongs or potentiates the effects of these medications. It is also important to keep in mind those drugs that potentiate the action of antidiabetic medications such as propranolol and oxytetracycline. In summary, hypoglycemia ensues when glucose uptake and utilization are too rapid (i.e., exercise), when glucose release and availability are inadequate (i.e. decreased intake), and when there is excessive insulin release (i.e., taking too much insulin). The major etiologies of hypoglycemia are reviewed in Table 14–10.

Pathophysiology. A hypoglycemic episode is defined as a decrease in plasma glucose level to 50 mg/dl or below. Glucose production falls behind glucose utilization and results in a change of the level of consciousness. Additionally, there is a rise in insulin-antagonistic hormones, including glucagon, epinephrine, cortisol, and growth hormone.

Cognitive/perceptual changes are common as glucose is the preferred energy source for the brain. Headache, impaired mentation, irritability, inability to concentrate, and dizziness are predominate findings. Prolonged hypoglycemia may lead to irreversible brain damage.

Other systemic clinical manifestations of hypoglycemia are caused by activation of the sympathetic nervous system and the resultant release of epinephrine that is triggered by a progressive decrease in the glucose supply to the brain. Sys-

Table 14–10. ETIOLOGIES OF HYPOGLYCEMIA

Excess Insulin/Oral Hypoglycemics
- Insulin
- Oral Hypoglycemics
- Islet cell tumors (insulinomas)
- Liver disease (impaired metabolism of insulin)
- Renal disease (impaired inactivation of insulin)
- Autoimmune phenomenon
- Drugs which potentiate action of antidiabetic medications (Propranolol, Oxytetracycline)
- Elderly patients on sulfonylureas

Underproduction of Glucose
- Heavy alcohol
- Poor nutrition
- Drugs: aspirin, disopyramidine (Norpace), haloperidol (Haldol)
- Underproduction by liver
- Hormonal causes

Too Rapid Utilization of Glucose
- GI surgery
- Extrapancreatic tumor
- Strenuous exercise

NURSING CARE PLAN FOR THE PATIENT WITH HYPERGLYCEMIC COMPLICATIONS OF AN ENDOCRINE DISORDER

Nursing Diagnosis	Outcome	Intervention
Fluid volume deficit related to osmotic diuresis and total body water loss, ketosis and increased lipolysis, vomiting	Normal serum glucose Hemodynamic stability: BP, HR, CVP, PCWP WNL Normal sinus rhythm Urine output >30ml/hr Balanced I/O Stable weight Warm, dry extremities Presence of normal skin turgor Moist mucous membranes	Assess fluid status: Vital signs every 1 hr until stable Intake/output measurements every 1-2 hr Skin turgor; signs of dehydration Consider insensible fluid losses via skin and lungs Daily weights Initiate therapy for dehydration: IV fluid administration as ordered: monitor for signs and symptoms of fluid overload during administration; monitor effects Monitor neurological status closely during fluid administration
Electrolyte imbalance related to lack of insulin, fluid shifts, acid/base imbalance, vomiting/NG suction	Glucose 70-100 mg/dl Serum electrolytes WNL: Sodium Potassium Calcium Phosphorus Osmolality WNL	Monitor blood glucose every 1 hr via serum blood glucose or finger sticks, titrate insulin therapy; monitor for signs and symptoms of hypoglycemia Serum electrolytes every 1-2 hr until stable Assess etiologies of electrolyte loss (i.e., diuresis, vomiting, NG suction) Replace electrolytes as needed, individualize according to serum values Monitor for signs and symptoms of hypokalemia (peaked *T* wave on ECG; ST segment changes Add glucose to maintenance IVs once blood sugar is at 300 mg/dl Seizure precautions as necessary
Ineffective breathing pattern/impaired gas exchange related to acidosis (DKA), decreased level of consciousness	Normal respiratory rate and pattern RR 10-25/min Tidal volume >5 ml/kg Normal $Paco_2$ on ABG analysis (DKA) Resolution of hyperglycemia	Assess airway and breathing upon admission Provide support as appropriate: e.g., airway, intubation equipment Assess respiratory status every 4 hr; every 1-2 hr in patients with impaired level of consciousness Correlate ABG results with clinical exam Prevent aspiration in patients with impaired level of consciousness; HOB elevated; NG decompression
Sensory/perceptual alteration related to hyperglycemia, acidosis, electrolyte imbalance	Patient is alert Oriented to person, place, and time Appropriate behavior	Monitor neurological status every 1 hr until stable, then every 2 hr Monitor for weakness, increasing confusion, lethargy, drowsiness, obtundation Provide orientation cues Seizure precautions as appropriate Provide for safety and hazard related to immobility with alterations in consciousness: Provide mouth and skin care Turn every 1-2 hr Perform passive ROM Provide for elimination
Knowledge deficit related to disease process, treatment regimen, complications of DKA	Patient/family is able to: Describe pathophysiology and causes of DKA Discuss and is compliant with diet, exercise regimen prescribed List signs and symptoms of hypoglycemia, hyperglycemia	Assess patient/family ability to learn information; psychomotor and sensory skills if reagent strip monitoring or insulin self-administration is prescribed; demonstrate use of insulin pump as appropriate Design a teaching program that includes information on pathophysiology of DKA; causes of DKA; diet and exercise restrictions; signs and symptoms of hyperglycemia and hypoglycemia, including interventions; signs and symptoms of infection Demonstrate methods for blood glucose monitoring; i.e., finger

continued

NURSING CARE PLAN FOR THE PATIENT WITH HYPERGLYCEMIC COMPLICATIONS OF AN ENDOCRINE DISORDER *Continued*

Nursing Diagnosis	Outcome	Intervention
	List signs and symptoms of infections that require medical follow-up Demonstrate glucose monitoring mechanism prescribed Demonstrate self-administration of insulin as appropriate	sticks with glucometer or reagent strip, sugar and acetone of urine; have patient return demonstration until proficient Demonstrate method of insulin administration; discuss dosage, frequency, action, duration, sites, side effects Discuss situations that would require adjustment of insulin dose Consult with dietician if weight reduction program is appropriate Encourage use of diabetic identification bracelet Provide written materials for all content taught; provide means for the patient to get questions answered after discharge Schedule follow-up teaching session after discharge

temic signs of epinephrine release include cool, clammy skin, pallor, tremors, palpitations, and tachydysrhythmias.

Assessment

Clinical Presentation. The most common signs and symptoms of hypoglycemia are summarized in Table 14–11. Symptoms of hypoglycemia can be categorized by symptoms from autonomic nervous system stimulation characteristic of a rapid decrease in serum glucose, and those symptoms reflective of an inadequate supply of glucose to neural tissues associated with a slower, more prolonged decline in glucose. Subjective symptoms of impaired mentation predominate because of the brain's requirement for constant glucose for energy.

With a rapid decrease in serum glucose levels, there is activation of the sympathetic nervous system mediated by epinephrine release from the adrenal medulla. This compensatory "fight or flight" mechanism may result in symptoms such as tachycardia, diaphoresis, pallor, and dilated pupils. The patient may also report feelings of apprehension, nervousness, headache, tremulousness, and general weakness.

Slower and more prolonged declines in serum glucose result in symptomatology related to an inadequate glucose supply to neural tissues (neuroglucopenia). These may include restlessness and difficulty in thinking and speaking. Visual disturbances and paresthesias may also be present. The patient may also have profound changes in the level of consciousness and/or convulsions. Personality changes and psychiatric manifestations can also be reported.

Laboratory Evaluation. The confirming laboratory sign of hypoglycemia is a serum or capillary blood glucose level less than 50 mg/dl. The glucose level should be checked on all high-risk individuals with the above-mentioned clinical signs. In patients with a known history of DM, a thorough history of past experiences of hypoglycemia, including associated signs and symptoms, should be elicited during the admission of the patient.

Table 14–11. SIGNS AND SYMPTOMS OF HYPOGLYCEMIA

Decrease in Blood Sugar	
Rapid	***Prolonged***
Activation of Sympathetic Nervous System	Inadequate Glucose Supply to Neural Tissues (CNS)
Epinephrine Release from Adrenal Medulla	Neuroglycopenia
Nervousness	Headache
Apprehension	Restlessness
Tachycardia	Difficulty Speaking
Palpitations	Difficulty Thinking
Pallor	Visual Disturbances
Diaphoresis	Altered Consciousness
Dilated Pupils	Coma
Tremulousness	Convulsions
Fatigue	Change in Personality
General Weakness	Psychiatric Reactions
Headache	Maniacal Behavior
Hunger	Catatonia
	Acute paranoia

Nursing Diagnoses

The nursing diagnoses applicable to the patient with a hypoglycemic episode include:

1. Altered electrolyte balance: hypoglycemia, related to excess circulating insulin as compared to glucose
2. Altered mental status related to decreased fuel (glucose) to brain cells
3. Potential for injury: seizures, related to altered neuronal function associated with hypoglycemia
4. Knowledge deficit related to prevention, recognition, and treatment of hypoglycemia

Collaborative Management

After confirming plasma or capillary glucose levels, 10 to 20 g of carbohydrate needs to be administered. Common food substances that contain at least 15 g of carbohydrate are listed in Table 14–12. Intravenous glucose is more commonly administered in the ICU (50% dextrose injections). If venous access is not available and the patient cannot take glucose by mouth, glucagon can be administered intramuscularly. Infusions of 10% dextrose may also be started to maintain serum glucose levels between 100 and 200 mg/100 dl. Glucose levels should be reassessed 15 to 30 minutes after treatment and repeated as necessary. Ongoing assessment of vital signs and ECG during the acute phase is also a priority.

Neurological assessments should be done to detect any changes in cerebral function related to hypoglycemia. It is important to document baseline neurological status, including mental status, cranial nerve function, sensory/motor function, and deep tendon reflexes. There is a potential for seizure activity related to altered neuronal cellular metabolism during the hypoglycemic phase. Patients should be assessed for seizure activity. Description of the seizure event and associated symptoms would be important to note. Seizure precautions should be instituted, including padded side rails, oral airway, oxygen and suction available at bedside, and removal of potentially harmful objects from the environment. Hypoglycemia is also associated with dysrhythmias in susceptible patients.

Patient and family teaching about hypoglycemic episodes may also be appropriate in the critical care setting. The patient and family need to be instructed on the causes, symptoms, treatment, and prevention of hypoglycemia. Principles regarding diet, insulin or oral hypoglycemics, and exercise may need to be incorporated into the teaching plan as appropriate. Instruction on use of home blood glucose monitoring may also be needed.

Table 14–12. FOOD SOURCES OF CARBOHYDRATES (15g)
4 oz sweetened carbonated beverage
4 oz unsweetened fruit juice
1 cup skim milk
1 tablespoon honey
Glucose gels or tablets (follow manufacturer's instructions)

Outcome Criteria

Outcomes for the patient with a hypoglycemic episode include:

1. Plasma/capillary glucose within normal limits
2. Absence of signs and symptoms of hypoglycemia
3. Alert/oriented; reversal of mental status changes
4. Absence of seizure activity
5. Patient/family is able to identify causes of hypoglycemia, state symptoms of hypoglycemia, state type and amount of foods that may be used to treat hypoglycemia, perform home blood glucose monitoring

Acute Adrenal Crisis

Acute adrenal crisis represents a life-threatening endocrine emergency. Individuals who have suppression of or an absolute lack of secretion of corticosteroids are potential candidates for this disorder. The manifestations of acute adrenal crisis result from insufficient secretion by the adrenal cortex of glucocorticoids (primarily cortisol) and/or mineralcorticoids (primarily aldosterone). The deficiency of glucocorticoids is especially significant as their influence on the defense mechanisms of the body and its response to stress make them essential for life. An insufficiency of adrenal androgens may also exist, but the manifestations are not clinically significant.

Cortisol is normally released in response to stimulation by adrenocorticotropic hormone (ACTH) from the anterior pituitary gland. In turn, ACTH is stimulated by corticotropin-releasing hormone from the hypothalamus, which is influenced by circulating cortisol levels, circadian rhythms, and stress. Circadian rhythms affect ACTH, and thus cortisol levels, diurnally, creating peak levels of cortisol in the morning and the lowest levels around midnight. This normal rhythm can be overridden by stress. During stress, plasma cortisol may increase as much as 10 times its normal level. Increased release of cortisol increases blood glucose concentration by promoting glycogen breakdown and gluconeogenesis in the liver, increases lipolysis and free fatty acid production, increases protein degradation, and inhibits the inflammatory and immune responses. These and additional effects are summarized in Table 14–13.

Aldosterone secretion is stimulated by angiotensin, which is converted by renin to angiotensin I and then to angiotensins II and III. The renin-angiotensin system is primarily activated by decreased sodium, increased potassium, decreased extracellular fluid (ECF) volume, and decreased blood pressure. When stimulated, aldosterone acts in the kidneys on the ascending loop of Henle, the distal convoluted tubule, and the collecting ducts to increase sodium ion reabsorption and increase potassium and hydrogen ion excretion. Because reabsorption of sodium creates an osmotic gradient across the renal tubular membrane, antidiuretic hormone (ADH) is activated, causing water to be reabsorbed with sodium. The physiology of aldosterone is summarized in Table 14–14.

Table 14–13. PHYSIOLOGY OF GLUCOCORTICOIDS (CORTISOL)

Controlled by adrenocorticotrophic hormone (ACTH) from anterior pituitary and corticotropin releasing hormone (CRH) from hypothalamus
ACTH stimulated by:
- Corticotropin-releasing hormone
- Circulating levels of cortisol
- Circadian rhythm
- Stress

Effects of glucocorticoids:
- Protein metabolism: promotes gluconeogenesis; stimulates protein breakdown and inhibits protein synthesis
- Fat metabolism: increases lipolysis and free fatty acid production; promotes fat deposits in face and cervical area
- Opposes action of insulin (decreases glucose transport and utilization in cells)
- Inhibits inflammatory response
  - Suppresses mediator release (kinins, histamine, prostaglandins, leukotrienes, serotonin)
  - Stabilizes cell membrane and inhibits capillary dilatation
  - Decreases formation of edema
  - Inhibits leukocyte migration and phyagocytic activity
- Immunosuppression
  - Decreases proliferation T lymphocytes and killer cell activity
  - Decreases complement production and immunoglobulins
- Increases circulating erythrocytes
- GI effects: increases appetite; increases rate of acid and pepsin secretion in stomach
- Increases uric acid excretion
- Decreases serum calcium
- Sensitizes arterioles to effects of catecholamines—maintains blood pressure
- Increases renal glomerular filtration rate and secretion of water

Table 14–14. PHYSIOLOGY OF MINERALCORTICOIDS (ALDOSTERONE)

Controlled by renin-angiotensin system
Renin-angiotensin system triggered by
- Decreased renal perfusion pressure
- Low plasma volume
- Increased potassium
- Decreased sodium
- Decreased blood pressure

Effects
- Reabsorption of sodium
- Excretion of potassium and hydrogen

PATHOGENESIS

Etiology

Hypofunction of the adrenal gland results from either primary or secondary mechanisms that suppress corticosteroid secretion. Primary mechanisms, resulting in Addison's disease, are those that cause destruction of the adrenal gland itself. At least 90% of the adrenal cortex must be destroyed before clinical signs and symptoms appear. Primary disorders result in deficiencies of both glucocorticoids and mineralcorticoids. Some of the mechanisms that can cause primary adrenal deficiency include autoimmune destruction of the gland (idiopathic), infections, hemorrhagic destruction, and granulomatous infiltrations.

Secondary mechanisms that can produce adrenal insufficiency are those that interfere with ACTH secretion or simply suppress normal secretion of corticosteroids. These generally result in deficiencies of only glucocorticoids, since stimulation of the mineralcorticoids is not dependent on ACTH secretion. Mechanisms that can produce secondary adrenal insufficiency include long-term steroid use, and pituitary and hypothalmic disorders. A more detailed listing of possible causes of primary and secondary adrenal insufficiency are listed in Table 14–15.

The most common group of patients seen in acute adrenal crisis are those who are currently on or have been recently withdrawn from corticosteroid therapy. Corticosteroids are utilized in the treatment of various inflammatory, allergic, and immunoreactive disorders such as rheumatoid arthritis, asthma, lupus erythematosus, ulcerative colitis, and thrombocytopenic purpura. Other disorders in which corticosteroids are used are listed in Table 14–16. Chronic use of these steroids suppresses the normal CRH–ACTH–adrenal feedback systems (see Fig. 14–1). This can result in adrenal suppression depending on the individual response, specific drug, dose, frequency, and duration of therapy. Adrenal suppression has been found to exist in patients who have received glucocorticoid therapy in doses that exceed three times the usual replacement dose for more than 10 days (Bagdade, 1986). Longer-acting agents such as dexamethasone are more likely to produce suppression than shorter-acting steroids such as hydrocortisone. It may take several months before normal secretion of corticosteroids returns in patients who have been tapered off corticosteroids in the previous 9 months. These individuals may be unable to respond adequately to stress. Thus, it is important to be familiar with disorders that may be treated with corticosteroids, as the resulting adrenal suppression may prevent a normal stress response in these individuals, and this puts them at risk for the development of acute adrenal crisis.

Table 14–15. CAUSES OF ADRENAL INSUFFICIENCY

Primary
- Autoimmune disease (idiopathic and polyglandular)
- Granulomatous disease (tuberculosis, sarcoidosis, histoplasmosis, blastomycosis)
- Metastatic cancer
- Hemorrhagic destruction (anticoagulation, trauma, sepsis)
- Sepsis (meningococcal or staphylococcal)
- Autoimmune deficiency syndrome
- Drugs: ketoconazole, aminoglutethimide, trimethoprim (suppress adrenals); phenytoin, barbiturates, rifampin (increased steroid degradation)
- Developmental/genetic abnormality

Secondary
- Long-term steroid use
- Pituitary tumors, hemorrhage, radiation, metastatic cancer
- Infiltrative disorders (sarcoidosis)
- Postpartum hemorrhage (Sheehan's syndrome)
- Trauma or surgery
- Hypothalmic disorders

Table 14–16. THERAPEUTIC USES OF CORTICOSTEROIDS

- Replacement therapy in patients with primary or secondary adrenal cortical insufficiency
- Symptomatic treatment of inflammatory, allergic, or immunologic disorders including:
  - Rheumatic: rheumatoid arthritis, osteoarthritis, acute gouty arthritis, ankylosing spondylitis, systemic lupus erythematosus
  - Allergic: allergic rhinitis, bronchial asthma, dermatitis, serum sickness, drug hypersensitivity, anaphylactic shock
  - Ophthalmic: conjunctivitis, keratitis, iritis, uveitis, acute optic neuritis, chorioretinitis, allergic corneal marginal ulcers
  - Gastrointestinal: ulcerative colitis, regional enteritis, chronic active hepatitis
  - Hematological/Neoplastic: thrombocytopenic purpura, hemolytic anemia, leukemia, Hodgkin's disease, multiple myeloma
  - Other: nephrotic syndrome, gout, hypercalcemia, multiple sclerosis, tuberculosis, meningitis
- Supportive use in actue disorders
  - Septic shock
  - Neurological emergencies (to treat cerebral edema): head trauma, cerebral hypoxia, tumors, hemorrhage, infection
  - Pulmonary disorders: asthma, chronic bronchitis, ARDS

Patients with acquired immune deficiency syndrome (AIDS) are a relatively new category of patients at risk for developing adrenal insufficiency. The adrenal glands may be the site of cytomegalovirus infection in as many as 50% of patients with AIDS (Knowlton, 1989). Although adrenal involvement is common, it is rare that AIDS patients have over 90% destruction of the adrenal gland. However, some of the drugs utilized to treat AIDS patients, specifically trimethoprim and ketoconazole, are also known to suppress adrenal function, placing them at risk (Knowlton, 1989; Reasner, 1990).

Addison's disease, or primary adrenal insufficiency, is a less common cause for adrenal insufficiency or adrenal crisis than either of the above. Damage of the adrenal gland in 50 to 70% of individuals with Addison's disease is the result of idiopathic autoimmune destruction (McCance and Huether, 1990). Tuberculosis is now a rare cause of adrenal insufficiency in the United States. The autoimmune form of the disease is frequently associated with other autoimmune diseases such as Hashimoto's thyroiditis, pernicious anemia, idiopathic hypoparathyroidism, and diabetes mellitus Type I.

Hemorrhagic destruction of the adrenal glands has been reported in the course of anticoagulation, after surgical procedures, or during infection. Anticoagulation therapy with heparin can cause selective hypoaldosteronism and, more rarely, cases of hemorrhage resulting in both mineral and glucocorticoid deficiencies. A common complication of meningococcal meningitis is massive adrenal hemorrhage, which can result in lethal adrenal insufficiency.

Acute adrenal crisis can be precipitated in any patient with chronic adrenal insufficiency by providing inadequate hormone replacement during times of acute stress such as infection, trauma, or surgery or after sudden withdrawal of steroids in a patient after long-term therapy. During periods of stress the adrenal cortex is able to increase the production of cortisol up to 10 times the normal rate if necessary. Individuals with inadequate adrenal cortex function are unable to increase production, and thus go into an acute life-threatening crisis.

Pathophysiology

Acute adrenal crisis is produced by an absolute or relative lack of cortisol (glucocorticoid) and aldosterone (mineralcorticoid). A deficiency of cortisol results in decreased production of glucose, decreased metabolism of protein and fat, decreased appetite, decreased intestinal motility and digestion, and decreased vascular tone and the effects of catecholamines. If the patient with deficient cortisol is stressed, this deficiency can produce profound shock because of significant decreases in vascular tone and the diminished effects of catecholamines.

Deficiency of aldosterone results in decreased sodium and water retention, decreased circulating volume, and increased potassium and hydrogen ion reabsorption. These effects are seen in patients with underlying primary adrenal insufficiency but not secondary adrenal insufficiency (decreased ACTH) because aldosterone secretion is not dependent on ACTH.

ASSESSMENT

When collecting the patient database, look for patients who are at risk, have predisposing factors, or have physical findings associated with chronic adrenal insufficiency. Some of the historical data to look for includes:

1. Drug history: steroids in past year, phenytoin, barbiturates, rifampin
2. Illness history: infection, cancer, autoimmune disease, diseases treated with steroids, radiation to head or abdomen
3. Family history: autoimmune disease, Addison's disease
4. Nutrition: weight loss, appetite
5. Miscellaneous: fatigue, dizziness, weakness, darkening of skin, low blood glucose that does not respond to therapy, salt craving (dramatic craving such as drinking pickle juice or eating salt from shaker)

Clinical Presentation

Neurological System. Neurological signs and symptoms in acute adrenal crisis are related to decreased glucose levels, decreased protein metabolism, decreased volume/perfusion, and decreased sodium. Patients may complain of headaches, fatigue that worsens as the day progresses, and severe weakness. They may also suffer from mental confusion, listlessness, lethargy, apathy, psychoses, and emotional lability.

Cardiovascular System. Cardiovascular signs and symptoms in acute adrenal crisis are related to hypovolemia (decreased water reabsorption), decreased vascular tone (decreased effectiveness of catecholamines), and hyperkalemia. Assess the patient for hypotension (orthostatic or lying down), tachycardia, decreased cardiac output, weak, rapid pulse, dysrhythmias, and cold, pale skin. The chest x-ray may show decreased heart size. Changes in the ECG may result if hyperkalemia is significant, and can include peaked T waves, widened QRS, long PR interval, and/or decreased P wave amplitude. Hypovolemia and vascular dilatation may be severe enough in crisis to produce hemodynamic collapse and shock.

Gastrointestinal (GI) System. The GI signs and symptoms in acute adrenal crisis are related to decreased digestive enzymes and decreased intestinal motility and digestion. Anorexia is always present and nausea and vomiting and abdominal pain are present in the majority of patients (Reasner, 1990).

Genitourinary System. Decreased circulation to the kidneys from decreased circulating volume and hypotension causes a decrease in the glomerular filtration rate and decreased renal perfusion. Decreased urine output may occur as a result.

Integumentary System. Patients with chronic primary adrenal insufficiency may have hyperpigmentation, especially in areas such as the mucous membranes, scars, and over joints. This is related to the increased secretion of melanocyte-stimulating hormone (MSH) that occurs with increases in ACTH secretion. Women with chronic primary adrenal insufficiency may also suffer from loss of pubic and axillary hair related to decreased levels of adrenal androgens.

Laboratory Evaluation

Typical laboratory findings in the patient with acute adrenal crisis may include hypoglycemia, hyponatremia, hyperkalemia, increased BUN, and metabolic acidosis. Hypercalcemia or hyperuricemia are possible owing to volume depletion. A summary of laboratory and physical findings can be found in Table 14–17.

Table 14–17. CLINICAL MANIFESTATIONS IN ADRENAL CRISIS

Manifestation	Mechanism
Decreased Cortisol (primary and secondary)	
Signs and Symptoms	
Headache, lethargy, severe weakness, mental fatigue	Decreased glucose to brain Decreased metabolism protein
Anorexia, nausea and vomiting, abdominal pain, decreased appetite	Decreased digestive enzymes Decreased intestinal motility and digestion
Tachycardia, sweating, tremors	Decreased glucose
Orthostatic hypotension/hypotension	Decreased vascular tone r/t, decreased effect catecholamines
Increased pigmentation (primary), loss of pubic and axillary hair (women)	Increased secretion MSH Decreased androgens
Lab Findings	
Hypoglycemia	Decreased cortisol
Eosinophilia, lymphocytosis	Decreased cortisol
Elevated BUN	Decreased excretion
Decreased Aldosterone (primary)	
Signs and Symptoms	
Hypotension	Decreased circulating volume
Decreased heart size	Decreased circulating volume
Headache, lethargy	Decreased sodium
Dysrhythmias	Increased potassium
ECG changes; peaked T waves, long PR, widened QRS, decreased P amplitude	Increased potassium,
Cold, pale skin	Decreased tissue perfusion
Weak, rapid pulse	Decreased circulating volume
Decreased cardiac output	Decreased circulating volume
Decreased urine output	Decreased circulating volume
Lab Findings:	
Hypovolemia	Decreased sodium and water retention
Hyponatremia	
Hyperkalemia	Increased potassium reabsorption
Metabolic acidosis	Increased potassium and hydrogen ion reabsorption

Table 14–18. COSYNTROPIN STIMULATION TEST

Obtain baseline blood sample for cortisol level
Administer 0.25 mg cosyntropin (synthetic ACTH) IV
Obtain serum cortisol level 1 hr later
To cover adrenal insufficiency may give dexamethasone (Decadron), 8 mg IV (does not affect serum cortisol)
Normal response: Two- to three fold increase in cortisol over baseline or cortisol level >20 μg/dl

Data from Hamburger, S., et al.: *Endocrine & Metabolic Emergencies.* Bowie, Maryland, Robert J. Brady, 1984; Knowlton, A.I.: Adrenal insufficiency in the intensive care setting. *J. Intensive Care Med.* 4(1):35–45, 1989; and Reasner, C.A.: Adrenal disorders. *Crit. Care Nurs.* 2. 13(3):67–73, 1990.

Diagnosis of adrenal insufficiency is made by evaluating plasma cortisol levels. A decreased plasma cortisol is indicative of adrenal insufficiency, but does not differentiate between primary or secondary adrenal insufficiency. A plasma cortisol of less than 15 μg/dl in a severely ill patient is consistent with the diagnosis of adrenal insufficiency (Bagdade, 1986). A "normal" plasma cortisol level in a stressed patient is considered abnormally low; i.e., it should be high during stress, and may indicate adrenal insufficiency. The ACTH levels will vary depending on whether the adrenal insufficiency is primary (increased) or secondary (decreased), and can assist in diagnosis. In acute adrenal crisis, there is no time to wait for the laboratory results to confirm the diagnosis before beginning treatment. If possible, a cosyntropin (a synthetic ACTH; Cortrosyn) stimulation test is done to determine adrenal insufficiency. The technique for performing this test is outlined in Table 14–18. Notice that a corticosteroid, such as dexamethasone, is given to the patient during the test to provide the patient with the necessary glucocorticoid support while the test is being run.

Adrenal crisis features are nonspecific and may inadvertently be attributed to other medical disorders. Signs and symptoms will also vary depending on whether the patient is deficient in both glucocorticoids and mineralcorticoids (primary) or only glucocorticoids (secondary). Because of the emergent nature of this condition, the diagnosis should be considered in any patient acutely ill with fever, vomiting, hypotension, shock, decreased sodium, increased potassium, or hypoglycemia.

NURSING DIAGNOSES

The nursing diagnoses which may apply to a patient with acute adrenal crisis based on the assessment data include:

1. Fluid volume deficit related to deficiency of aldosterone hormone (mineralcorticoid) and decreased sodium and water retention
2. Altered tissue perfusion, decreased related to cortisol deficiency resulting in decreased vascular tone, decreased effectiveness of catecholamines
3. Sensory/perceptual alterations related to decreased glucose levels, decreased protein metabolism, decreased perfusion, and decreased sodium
4. Altered nutrition: less than body requirements, related to deficiency of cortisol and resultant decreased metabolism of protein and fats, decreased appetite, and decreased intestinal motility and digestion
5. Knowledge deficit related to long-term corticosteroid management
6. Activity intolerance related to use of endogenous protein for energy needs and loss of skeletal muscle mass as evidenced by early fatigue, weakness, and exertional dyspnea

COLLABORATIVE MANAGEMENT

As stated earlier, adrenal crisis requires immediate recognition and intervention if the patient is to survive. Primary objectives in the treatment of adrenal crisis include identifying and treating the precipitating cause, replacement of fluid and electrolytes, hormonal replacement, and patient/family education.

Replace Fluid and Electrolytes

Fluid losses should be replaced with 5% dextrose and normal saline until signs and symptoms of hypovolemia stabilize. This not only will reverse the volume deficit, but will provide glucose to minimize the hypoglycemia. The patient may need as much as 5 L of fluid in the first 12 to 24 hours to maintain an adequate blood pressure, urine output, and replace the fluid deficit.

Hyperkalemia frequently responds to volume expansion and glucocorticoid replacement and may require no further treatment. In fact, the patient may become hypokalemic during therapy and require potassium replacement. The acidosis will also usually correct itself with volume expansion and glucocorticoid replacement. However, if the pH is <7.1 or $HCO_3 < 10$ mEq/L, the patient may require supplementary sodium bicarbonate.

Hormonal Replacement

If adrenal insufficiency has not been previously diagnosed and the patient is unstable, dexamethasone phosphate (Decadron), 4 mg IV bolus, then 4 mg every 8 hours can be given until the cosyntropin test has been done. Dexamethasone will not interfere with serum cortisol levels.

Initially, glucocorticoid replacement is the most important hormonal replacement. Hydrocortisone sodium succinate (Solu-Cortef) is the drug of choice because it has both glucocorticoid and mineralcorticoid activities in high doses. An initial IV bolus of 100 to 300 mg is given followed by a continuous intravenous infusion to provide an additional 100 mg every 8 hours. Providing a continuous infusion is important because the short half-life of the drug would leave the patient deficient if only given in bolus form. The infusion is usually continued for at least 24 hours or until the patient has stabilized. Cortisone acetate, 50 mg IM, may also be given every 12 hours until stable to provide coverage in case the intravenous route is faulty.

Once the patient improves, the dose of hydrocortisone is decreased 20 to 40% daily until a maintenance dose is achieved. The patient can be switched to oral replacement once oral intake is resumed. At these lower doses (<300 mg hydrocortisone/day), the patient with primary adrenal insufficiency may require mineralcorticoid replacement. Fludrocortisone, 0.1 to 0.2 mg daily, is then added. Table 14–19 describes in more detail the drugs utilized in treatment of acute adrenal crisis.

Patient/Family Education

In a patient with known adrenal insufficiency and/or on corticosteroid therapy, adrenal crisis is preventable. Education of patients and family/significant others is the key to prevention. In addition, patients should wear medical identification bracelets to facilitate treatment. Discharge goals include the patient/significant other will be able to

Table 14–19. DRUGS USED TO TREAT ADRENAL CRISIS

Hydrocortisone Sodium Succinate (Solu-Cortef)
Class
Corticosteroid, glucocorticoid, mineralcorticoid
Action
Same effects as cortisol (see Table 14-13)
Anti-inflammatory and immunosuppressive effects
Salt-retaining (mineralcorticoid) effects in high doses
Dose
Individualized; adrenal crisis: 100-300 mg IV bolus; 100 mg every 8 hr in continuous IV infusion
Side Effects
Vertigo, headache, paresthesia, insomnia
Menstrual abnormalities
Fluid and electrolyte disturbances
Hypertension, congestive heart failure
Peptic ulcers, nausea, and vomiting
Immunosuppression, impaired wound healing
Increased serum glucose
Cushingoid state
Nursing considerations
Institute prophylactic measures against GI bleeding
Be aware of multiple drug-drug interactions, especially with IV route: oral contraceptives, phenytoin, digoxin, phenobarbital, theophylline, insulin, anticoagulants, salicylates
Avoid abrupt discontinuation of corticosteroid therapy
Monitor serum glucose and electrolytes closely
Watch for signs and symptoms of fluid overload (may worsen hypertension or congestive heart failure)
Watch closely for signs of infection (drug may mask)
Maintain adequate nutrition to avoid catabolic effects of corticosteroids
Provide meticulous skin care and institute protective measures

Cortisone Acetate (Cortone)
Class
Corticosteroid, glucocorticoid, mineralcorticoid
Action
Same as hydrocortisone
Dose
Individualized; adrenal crisis: 50 mg IM every 12 hr
Side Effects
Same as hydrocortisone
Nursing Considerations
Same as hydrocortisone; not used to treat acute adrenal crisis

Dexamethasone (Decadron)
Class
Corticosteroid, glucocorticoid
Action
Has only glucocorticoid effects
Dose
Give only during cosyntropin test 4 mg IV bolus; 4 mg IV every 8 hr until test done
Side Effects
Same as hydrocortisone
Nursing Considerations
Same as hydrocortisone

Fludrocortisone Acetate (Florinef)
Class
Corticosteroid, mineralcorticoid
Action
Increases sodium reabsorption in renal tubules and increases potassium and hydrogen excretion
Dose
0.1-0.2 mg/day PO
Side Effects
Increased blood volume, edema, hypertension, CHF, headaches, weakness or extremities
Nursing Considerations
Assess for signs of fluid overload, CHF
Monitor serum sodium and potassium levels closely
Use only in conjunction with glucocorticoid therapy
Restrict sodium intake if edema or fluid overload
Not used to treat acute crisis, but added as glucocorticoid is decreased toward maintenance level

---

Describe the pathophysiology and therapeutic regimen for chronic adrenal insufficiency. Describe the rationale for and long-term effects of corticosteroid therapy

Identify the signs and symptoms associated with acute adrenal insufficiency

List minor stress situations which may require doubling of steroid administration

List major stress situations which require notification of the physician

Verbalize an understanding of the rationale for tapering doses of steroids rather than abruptly terminating administration

Demonstrate administration of intramuscular doses of cortisol and describe situations in which this would be appropriate

Table 14-20 contains a summary of treatment of adrenal crisis.

OUTCOME CRITERIA

Patient care outcomes for the patient with adrenal crisis include:

1. Fluid and electrolyte balance
2. Adequate central and peripheral perfusion
3. Hemodynamic stability
4. Mentation return to baseline
5. Normal protein and fat metabolism
6. Adequate nutritional balance and stable weight

Table 14-20. TREATMENT OF ADRENAL CRISIS

Identify and treat precipitating event
Replace fluid and electrolytes
- D5/NS until hypotension improves
- Acidemia usually corrects with volume expansion (if pH < 7.1, $HCO_3 < 10$ mEq/L, give $NaHCO_3$)
- Hyperkalemia responds to volume expansion and glucocorticoids
- *Note:* May become hypokalemic with volume expansion and may need replacement

Hormonal replacement
- Hydrocortisone (Solu-Cortef): 100–300 mg IV immediately; add 100 mg to IV and give continuous infusion every 6–8 hr
- Cortisone acetate; 50 mg IM every 12 hr (in case IV route faulty)
- Continue IV replacement at least 24 hr after recovery from acute phase
- After stabilized, decrease hydrocortisone dose 20–40%/day until maintenance dose reached (25.0–37.5 mg/day)
- When dose < 100–150 mg/day, may need to add fludorcortisone acetate (oral mineralcorticoid)

Patient education
- ID bracelet
- Awareness of signs and symptoms of insufficiency
- Doubling dose with minor stress

7. Patient/family able to state activities necessary to prevent adrenal crisis
8. Demonstrates increased physical activity

See the Nursing Care Plan for the Patient in Acute Adrenal Crisis.

Thyroid Crises

Thyroid disorders, like adrenal insufficiency, are disorders that if previously diagnosed and adequately treated, do not generally result in crisis states. However, if patients with thyroid disorders, especially undiagnosed thyroid disorders, are stressed either physiologically or psychologically, the results can be life threatening.

Thyroid hormones if deficient or excessive can produce dysfunction in all body systems. The thyroid hormones, thyroxine (T_4) and triiodothyronine (T_3), are secreted by the thyroid gland under the influence of the anterior pituitary gland via secretion of thyroid-stimulating hormone (TSH) from the hypothalamus. Regulation of these hormones occurs via the positive and negative feedback mechanisms discussed earlier (see Fig. 14–2). Thyroxine accounts for 90% of circulating thyroid hormone, but half of all thyroid activity comes from T_3. Triiodothyronine is five times more potent, acts quicker, and enters cells more easily than T_4. Triiodothyronine is derived from conversion of T_4 to T_3 in nonthyroid tissue. Certain conditions and drugs can block the conversion of T_4 to T_3, creating potential thyroid imbalance. Possible causes for blocked conversion are listed in Table 14–21.

Table 14-21. CAUSES OF BLOCKAGE OF T_4 TO T_3 CONVERSION

- Severe illness: chronic renal failure, cancer, chronic liver disease
- Trauma
- Malnutrition, fasting
- Drugs: glucocorticoids, propranolol (Inderal), propylthiouracil, amiodarone
- Radiopaque dyes

To understand the pathogenesis, clinical manifestations, and management of thyroid disease, and particularly thyroid crises, it is necessary to understand the effects thyroid hormone has on the body. Table 14–22 lists some of the physiological effects of thyroid hormone.

THYROID STORM

Pathogenesis

Etiology

Hyperthyroidism is a common and usually benign illness. The three most common types of

Table 14-22. PHYSIOLOGICAL EFFECTS OF THYROID HORMONE

Major Effects
- Increases metabolic activities of all tissues
- Increases rate of nutrient use for energy production
- Increases rate of growth
- Increases activities of other endocrine glands

Other Effects
- Regulates protein synthesis and catabolism
- Regulates body heat production and dissipation
- Increases gluconeogenesis and utilization of glucose
- Maintains appetite and secretion of GI substances
- Maintains calcium metabolism
- Stimulates cholesterol synthesis
- Maintains cardiac rate, force, and output
- Affects respiratory rate, oxygen utilization, and carbon dioxide formation
- Affects red blood cell production
- Affects CNS development and cerebration
- Necessary for muscle tone and vigor and normal skin constituents

NURSING CARE PLAN FOR THE PATIENT IN ACUTE ADRENAL CRISIS		
Nursing Diagnosis	**Outcome**	**Intervention**
Fluid volume deficit related to deficiency of aldosterone hormone (mineralcorticoid), decreased sodium and water retention	Fluid balance restored Electrolyte balance restored: Na 135–145 mEq/L; K 3.5–5.0 mEq/L Urine output >30 ml/m BP WNL/returned to baseline Warm, pink skin HR 60–100	Administer IV fluids and electrolytes as ordered (glucose in normal saline) until signs and symptoms of hypovolemia stabilized; initial fluids will be administered rapidly; monitor for signs of overload. Monitor vital signs, orthostatic changes, hemodynamics (preload indicators with hemodynamic catheter in place; CVP/PCWP), central and peripheral perfusion (mean arterial pressure/cardiac output) Monitor fluid balance (intake and output)/daily weight Monitor heart rate and rhythm at least every 1 hr (every 15 min in unstable patients) Monitor glucose, potassium, and sodium every 2–4 hr until stable Monitor renal function: BUN, creatinine, urine output, specific gravity, urine sodium, and potassium Administer scheduled doses of IV glucocorticoids and assess response Avoid abrupt changes in position (to upright) until fluid balance is restored Explain diagnostic tests to patient/family Prevent adrenal crisis by ensuring patients at risk to receive exogenous cortisol in stress states Assess for reversal of defining characteristics: hydration restored to oral mucous membranes, absence of orthostasis, normal skin turgor, denies thirst, normal urine output
Altered tissue perfusion; decreased related to cortisol deficiency resulting in decreased vascular tone, decreased effectiveness of catecholamines	Adequate central and peripheral perfusion and hemodynamic stability as evidenced by: Palpable peripheral pulses (2+) Warm/dry skin Adequate urine output (30 ml/hr) Usual mentation BP >90 systolic; mean arterial pressure >60 mm Hg CI >2.5 L/min/m² CVP 6–12 cm H_2O SVR 800–1200 dynes/sec Absence of respiratory distress	Monitor changes in mental status (anxiety, confusion, lethargy, coma), personality changes Inspect skin for pallor, mottling, cyanosis; note color and temperature (especially in cannulated extremities) Provide skin care, change position every 1.5–2.0 hr/keep skin clean dry Monitor respiratory rate Monitor for changes in blood pressure Assess gastrointestinal function; decreased bowel sounds, nausea and vomiting, abdominal distention, anorexia; insert NG as needed Monitor lab data: serum and urine electrolytes, BUN, creatinine Note hourly changes in urine output; record specific gravity
Sensory/perceptual alterations related to decreased glucose levels, decreased protein metabolism, decreased perfusion, decreased sodium	Mentation returned to baseline Alert/oriented	Assess level of consciousness, ability to speak, response to stimuli/commands Observe behavioral responses: disorientation, confusion, irritability Provide a quiet environment; speak in calm, quiet voice Provide for consistent caregivers whenever possible Encourage family/significant others to stay with patient Provide frequent reality orientation Provide for environmental safety, quiet environment, soft restrains, minimize stressful situations, promote rest Monitor electrolytes; BUN, liver function tests Administer and assess effects of drugs

continued

NURSING CARE PLAN FOR THE PATIENT IN ACUTE ADRENAL CRISIS *Continued*		
Nursing Diagnosis	**Outcome**	**Intervention**
Altered nutrition; less than body requirements related to deficiency of cortisol and resultant decreased metabolism of protein and fat, decreased appetite, decreased intestinal motility and digestion	Normal protein and fat metabolism is restored Adequate nutrition is reestablished as evidenced by positive nitrogen balance; weight WNL	Note admission weight/height, daily weight Document oral intake, food history, calorie counts Promote optimal environment during attempts at oral intake; provide assistance with eating as necessary Assess presence/character of bowel sounds; assess GI losses; i.e., vomiting, diarrhea Assure parenteral/enteral nutrition solutions are delivered as prescribed; assess function and tolerance Provide small frequent meals Refer to nutritional team/registered dietitian Provide antacids/histamine antagonists as ordered Assess metabolic response to nutritional support; monitor lab studies
Knowledge deficit related to long-term corticosteroid management	Patient/family able to state activities necessary to prevent adrenal crisis: Describe pathophysiology and therapeutic regimen for chronic adrenal insufficiency Describe rationale for and long-term effects of corticosteroid therapy Identify signs and symptoms associated with acute adrenal insufficiency Identify minor stress situations that may require doubling of corticosteroid administration List major stress situations which require physician notification Verbalize understanding and rationale for tapering of corticosteroids rather than withdrawing abruptly	Provide medication instructions: action, name, dose, schedule, importance of adherence, life-long need for drug Instruct patient/family on administration of corticosteroids in stress states: Define stress: identification and reduction of; minor vs severe Instruct patient to call physician for temporary increase in glucocorticoid dose; double dose for minor stress If vomiting, instruct patient to call physician (for parenteral administration); instruct in parenteral hydrocortisone at home Instruct patient to inform all health care providers of corticosteroid use; carry ID card Instruct patient/family of importance of gradual corticosteroid tapering. To seek medical attention in event of stress state (*Note:* Patients who have been on long-term corticosteroid therapy should receive glucocorticoids during periods of stress for at least 1 year after the drugs are discontinued)
Activity intolerance related to use of endogenous protein for energy needs and loss of skeletal muscle mass as evidenced by early fatigue and weakness, exertional dyspnea	Demonstrates increased physical activity as evidence by: BP, HR, RR, WNL Verbalizes decreased fatigue	Provide passive/active ROM exercises to patient if bedridden Assist with ambulation, ADLs Monitor patient response to increased activity: monitor BP, heart rhythm, respirations; note tachycardia, dysrhythmias, dyspnea, diaphoresis, pallor Check vital signs before and immediately after each activity Assess for other causes of fatigue; i.e., treatments, medications Restrict activity; space with rest periods Provide for nutrition (see above) Encourage verbalization of feelings regarding limitations

hyperthyroidism are toxic diffuse goiter, toxic multinodular goiter, and toxic uninodular goiter. The vast majority of patients with hyperthyroid crises (thyroid storm) have either toxic diffuse goiter or an unusually large toxic multinodular goiter.

The most common form of hyperthyroidism is toxic diffuse goiter, also known as Graves' disease. It occurs most frequently in young (third or fourth decade), previously healthy women. A family history of hyperthyroidism is often present. Its cause is unknown, but it is believed to be an autoimmune disease, since all of the affected patients have abnormal immunoglobulins. These immunoglobulins attack thyroid tissue, producing thyroid inflammation, diffuse enlargement, and hyperplasia of the gland.

Toxic multinodular goiter is the second most common cause of hyperthyroidism. It also occurs more commonly in women, but they are generally older than those with toxic diffuse goiter (fourth to seventh decade). Crises in patients with toxic multinodular goiter are more commonly associated with heart failure or severe muscle weakness.

These and other possible causes of hyperthyroidism are listed in Table 14–23.

Thyroid storm usually occurs in untreated or inadequately treated patients with hyperthyroidism. Few cases arise in patients who have had previously normal thyroids. Most of these individuals have had Graves' disease for at least several months. The crisis is often precipitated by stress related to an underlying illness, general anesthesia, or surgery. Nonsurgical causes are the most frequent precipitating events; i.e., diabetic ketoacidosis, trauma, burns, infection, or severe emotional stress. Mortality is more often the result of the underlying illness rather than the thyrotoxic state.

Pathophysiology

The mechanisms that produce thyroid storm are not clearly understood, particularly since thyroid hormone levels in these patients are no higher than in those with uncomplicated hyperthyroidism. One theory regarding pathogenesis of thyroid storm is that thyroid hormones sensitize the body to catecholamines and/or act as pseudocatecholamines when the patient with hyperthyroidism is stressed (Gavin, 1991; Johnson, 1983). It may also be that peripheral tissues simply can no longer respond to the increased circulating thyroid hormones present in hyperthyroidism, precipitating a crisis. Another theory is that there is a sudden increase in thyroid hormone, but it is transient (Gavin 1991; Johnson, 1983). This transient rise may be the result of vigorous palpation of the thyroid gland, reduction or withdrawal of antithyroid drugs, or ingestion of excessive thyroid hormone. Recent studies indicate that part of the enhanced sympathetic activity that occurs is also due to an increased number of β-adrenergic receptors (Gavin, 1991).

Certain enzymes may be the key to the dramatic increase in metabolic rate that occurs in thyroid storm. Thyroid hormones normally increase the synthesis of enzymes that stimulate cellular mitochondria and energy production. When excess thyroid hormone is present, as in thyroid storm, the increased activity of these enzymes produces excessive thermal energy and fever (Gavin, 1991).

Thyroid hormone plays a major role in regulating body metabolism, and as a result has effects on most of the body systems. Thus, hyperthyroidism can produce a hyperdynamic, hypermetabolic state that results in disruption of many major body functions. To understand the pathophysiology of thyroid storm requires an understanding of the disruptions that occur in hyperthyroidism. Thyroid crisis is really just a magnification of these disruptions. Common findings in patients with hyperthyroidism are listed in Table 14–24 and discussed below.

Table 14–23. CAUSES OF HYPERTHYROIDISM

Most Common
- Toxic diffuse goiter (Graves' disease)
- Toxic multinodular goiter
- Toxic uninodular goiter

Other Causes
- Factitious hyperthyroidism
- T_3 toxicosis
- Exogenous iodine in patient with preexisting thyroid disease: exposure to iodine load from radiographic contrast dyes, medications (amiodarone, organidine)
- Thyroiditis (transient)

Rare Causes
- Metastatic thyroid cancer
- Malignancies with circulating thyroid stimulators
- TSH-producing pituitary tumors
- Acromegaly

Associated with other disorders*
- Pernicious anemia, idiopathic Addison's disease, myasthenia gravis, sarcoidosis, Albright's syndrome

* Presence of these disorders in patient in crisis should increase likelihood that patient has hyperthyroidism.

ASSESSMENT

Clinical Presentation

The extent of signs and symptoms in thyroid storm is variable and nonspecific. Diagnosis may be delayed because it may be difficult to see the relationship between the diverse signs and symptoms and attribute them to the hyperthyroid state. Thyroid storm has an abrupt onset and is best characterized as a state of unregulated hy-

Table 14–24. CLINICAL MANIFESTATIONS OF THYROID STORM AND MYXEDEMA COMA

Thyroid Storm	Myxedema Coma
Increased metabolic rate	Decreased metabolic rate
Nervousness, delirium, emotional lability	Difficulty concentrating, lethargy, somnolence
Fine tremor	Perceptive hearing loss, vertigo
Exaggerated reflexes	Slow speech, coarse voice
Increased temperature, heat intolerance	Decreased temperature, cold intolerance
Increased perspiration	Decreased perspiration
Palpitations	Distant heart sounds
Tachycardia	Bradycardia
Widened pulse pressure	Pericardial effusion
Dysrhythmias	Mucinous edema
Dyspnea	Dyspnea on exertion
Increased respiratory rate	Decreased respiratory rate
Weight loss	Weight gain
Increased appetite	Decreased appetite
Increased bowel movements	Decreased bowel movements
Smooth, moist skin	Coarse, dry skin
Fine hair	Dry, brittle hair

permetabolism. The most prominent clinical features are severe fever, marked tachycardia, tremors, delirium, stupor, and coma. If allowed to go untreated, patients will succumb in 1 to 2 days to extreme hyperpyrexia and cardiovascular collapse.

Neurological Disturbances. Thyroid hormone normally maintains central nervous system cerebration. The hypermetabolism and resulting increased cerebration produced by excess thyroid hormone causes hyperactivity of the nervous system both psychologically and physiologically. Patients may be seen with signs and symptoms such as increased irritability, decreased attention span, agitation, nervousness, wide mood swings, and fear or paranoia. Thyroid storm may be heralded by the onset of delirium, overt psychosis, convulsions, stupor, or coma. However, in the elderly patient, these signs and symptoms may be masked, and depression or apathy may be seen instead.

Muscle weakness is produced by increased protein catabolism. It can result in fine rhythmic tremors of the tongue, eyelids, or even eyeballs; peripheral tremors, especially with activity; thoracic muscle weakness causing dyspnea; and proximal muscle weakness.

Temperature regulation is lost, resulting in increased cold tolerance, heat intolerance, fever, and excessive sweating. Cold tolerance is more common in young patients. Older patients may naturally lose their ability to shiver and be less uncomfortable in the cold. The patient's body temperature may be elevated as high as 106°F.

Cardiovascular Disturbances. Thyroid hormone plays a role in maintaining cardiac rate, force of contraction, and cardiac output. The increase in metabolism and the stimulation of catecholamines produced by thyroid hormone causes a hyperdynamic heart. Contractility, heart rate, and cardiac output increase. These effects are magnified by the body's increased demand for oxygen and nutrients. In thyroid storm, the increased demands on the heart may be so severe as to produce heart failure and cardiovascular collapse if the crisis is not recognized and treated.

The increase in heat production and metabolic end products also causes the blood vessels of the skin to dilate. This enhances oxygen and nutrient delivery to the peripheral tissues and accounts for the patient's warm, moist, pink skin.

Patients experience palpitations, tachycardia (out of proportion to the fever), and a widened pulse pressure. A prominent third heart sound may be heard as well as a systolic murmur over the pulmonic and/or aortic areas. Occasionally a rub may be heard. The most common dysrhythmias seen are frequent premature atrial contractions, atrial fibrillation, or atrial flutter. In an elderly patient with underlying heart disease, thyroid storm may be heralded by worsening of angina or severe congestive heart failure. Hyperthyroidism should be suspected in the patient who while asleep has sinus tachycardia, or in the patient with atrial fibrillation that does not slow in response to digoxin.

Pulmonary Disturbances. Thyroid hormone affects respiratory rate and depth, oxygen utilization, and carbon dioxide formation. Tissue oxygen needs increase as a result of hypermetabolism. This increased need for oxygen stimulates the respiratory drive, increasing respirations. However, increased protein catabolism reduces protein in respiratory muscles (diaphragm and intercostals), producing weakness and decreased lung vital capacity. As a result, even with increased respirations, muscle weakness may prevent the patient from meeting the oxygen demand and cause hypoventilation, CO_2 retention, and respiratory failure.

Gastrointestinal Disturbances. Increased metabolism and accelerated protein and fat degradation increase appetite and cause weight loss. Thyroid hormone also increases gastrointestinal motility, resulting in decreased absorption, especially of vitamins, and an increase in frequency of stools. Diarrhea is not common but may occur. Elderly patients, on the other hand, may be constipated. Abdominal pain, nausea, jaundice, vomiting, and diarrhea may be prominent manifestations of the patient in thyroid storm.

Skeletal Muscle Disturbances. Muscle protein degradation in skeletal muscles exceeds protein synthesis, causing generalized muscle wasting, weight loss, fatigue, and weakness. The extreme energy expenditure of hypermetabolism also contributes to this process. The weakness tends to be most prominent in the proximal muscles of the limbs, making it difficult for patients to climb stairs or rise from chairs.

Integumentary Disturbances. Inadequate protein synthesis also affects the skin, hair, and nails. Patients with hyperthyroidism typically have thin, fine, silky fragile hair; soft, friable nails; and thin skin. They can also develop petechiae caused by rupture of fragile blood vessels. Some of these skin changes may vary with the age or sex of the patient. Young women generally have the more classic findings identified above. Young men may not notice texture changes in their skin, but rather an increase in acne and sweating. An elderly patient with dry atrophic skin may not have significant skin changes with hyperthyroidism.

Hematopoietic Disturbances. Thyroid hormone has affects on red cell production. Splenomegaly is present in up to half the patients with toxic diffuse goiter. Poor vitamin B_{12} absorption can produce pernicious anemia, resulting in weakness, fatigue, dyspnea, and pallor. The red blood cells being produced are abnormally large and may rupture as they pass through small capillaries and liberate free bilirubin and causes the skin to turn pale yellow (jaundice). White blood cell and neutrophil counts vary. About 10% of the patients will have a decrease in neutrophils. Others will have an increased white blood cell count indicating underlying infection.

Ophthalmic Disturbances. Ophthalmic changes in hyperthyroidism are most likely to indicate evidence of thyroid disease, but may be nonspecific. Exophthalmos is found almost exclusively in toxic diffuse goiter (Fig. 14–4), but severity of eye findings is highly variable. Changes may be as mild as upper lid retraction and lid lag or as severe as extraocular muscle palsies and sight loss.

The ability of the patient to survive thyroid storm is determined by the severity of the hyperthyroid state and the patient's general health. The severity of the hyperthyroid state is not necessarily indicated by the serum levels of thyroid hormone, but more by tissues/organ responsiveness to the hormone; i.e., the degree of the impairment of key organ functions. General health factors that should be considered include age, nutritional status, chronic illness, underlying illness, or stressful event, and concomitant drug therapy. In the elderly, some signs may be masked. A history of weight loss and the presence of such cardiac abnormalities as atrial fibrillation and congestive heart failure may be the only clues.

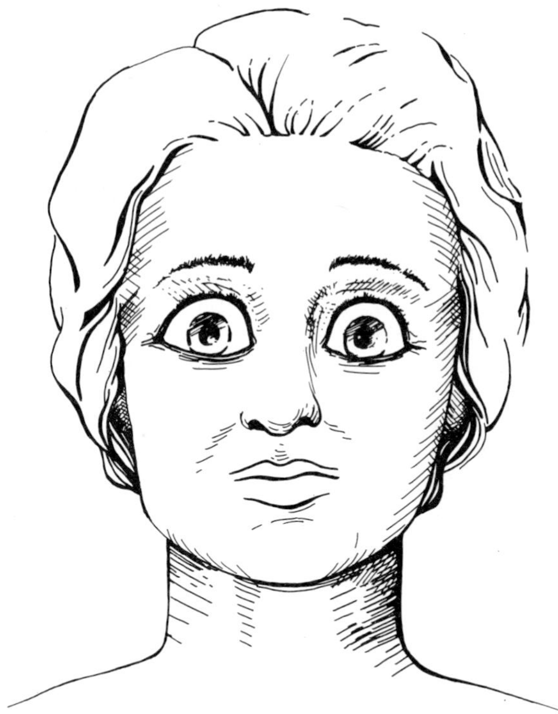

Figure 14–4. Exophthalmos.

Laboratory Evaluation

There are no laboratory tests that separate thyroid storm from uncomplicated hyperthyroidism. Both T_3 and T_4 levels should be drawn as well as resin T_3 uptake. Resin T_3 uptake is an indirect measure of free T_4 levels (free T_4 is the portion that is biologically active) and will be elevated in hyperthyroid states. Although an elevation of thyroid hormones is to be expected, these levels will generally be no higher than those normally found in uncomplicated hyperthyroidism. In any event, the patient must be treated before these results will be available.

Possible laboratory abnormalities that may result from thyroid storm are listed in Table 14–25.

Table 14–25. LABORATORY MANIFESTATIONS OF THYROID STORM AND MYXEDEMA COMA

Thyroid Storm	Myxedema Coma
Increased T_3, T_4	Decreased T_3, T_4
Increased resin T_3 uptake	Decreased resin T_3 uptake
Anemia	Anemia
Hyperglycemia	Hypoglycemia
Leukocytosis	Leukocytosis absent
Increased/decreased sodium	Decreased sodium
Decreased potassium	Respiratory acidosis
Increased calcium	Decreased platelet count
Increased BUN	Increased cholesterol
Abnormal liver function tests	Increased triglycerides

NURSING DIAGNOSES

The nursing diagnoses that may apply to a patient with thyroid storm are based on assessment data and include:

1. Decreased cardiac output related to increased metabolic demands on the heart, hyperthermia, extreme tachycardia, dysrhythmias, congestive heart failure
2. Hyperthermia related to loss of temperature regulation, increased metabolism, increased heat production
3. Ineffective breathing pattern related to muscle weakness, decreased vital capacity resulting in hypoventilation and CO_2 retention, increased oxygen need
4. Altered nutrition; less than body requirements related to increased peristalsis, decreased absorption
5. Potential impaired skin integrity related to thin skin, fragile blood vessels
6. Activity intolerance related to muscle weakness, muscle wasting, tremors, fatigue, extreme energy expenditure
7. Sensory/perceptual alterations related to hypermetabolism and increased cerebration, agitation, delirium, psychosis
8. Knowledge deficit related to disease process, therapeutic regimen, prevention of complications

COLLABORATIVE MANAGEMENT

As stated earlier, thyroid storm requires immediate intervention if the patient is to survive. The primary objectives in treatment of thyroid storm include identifying and treating the precipitating cause, inhibiting thyroid hormone biosynthesis, blocking thyroid hormone release, antagonizing peripheral effects of thyroid hormone, providing supportive care, and patient/family education.

Inhibition of Thyroid Hormone Biosynthesis

Two drugs may be used to inhibit thyroid hormone biosynthesis—propylthiouracil (PTU) and methimazole (Tapazole). Propylthiouracil is the drug of choice because in large doses it will inhibit conversion of T_4 to T_3 in peripheral tissues, resulting in a more rapid reduction of circulating thyroid hormone levels. Neither of these drugs is available in intravenous form and must be given orally. The patient in thyroid crisis should receive propylthiouracil, 800–1200 mg PO as a loading dose, and 400 to 600 mg PO daily until thyroid storm is controlled. Methimazole is administered in a 80- to 120-mg PO loading dose and 40 mg PO daily. Both drugs can produce agranulocytosis and bleeding tendencies and have additional potential side effects of paresthesias, vertigo, drowsiness, nausea, and headaches.

The big drawback to both PTU and methimazole is that they lack immediate effect. They do not block the release of thyroid hormone already stored in the thyroid gland and may take weeks or even months to lower thyroid hormone levels to normal.

Blockage of Thyroid Hormone Release

Iodide agents have the ability to inhibit the release of thyroid hormone from the thyroid gland and at high doses may also inhibit thyroid production. Lugol's solution or saturated solution of potassium iodide (SSKI) up to 30 drops PO daily may be given. Sodium iodide, 1 g IV every 8 to 12 hours, or 1 to 2 g in an IV drip over 8 to 12 hours, may also be used. These drugs must be given 1 to 2 hours after antithyroid drugs (PTU or methimazole) are given to prevent the iodide from being used to synthesize more thyroxine. Possible side effects of iodide agents include metallic taste, inflammation of the salivary glands, rhinitis, headaches, diarrhea, and gastritis.

Lithium carbonate also has the ability to inhibit release of thyroid hormone but is more toxic, so it is only used in patients with an iodide allergy. Serum thyroxine levels will fall approximately 30 to 50% with any of these drugs, with stabilization in 3 to 6 days.

Antagonism of Peripheral Effects of Thyroid Hormone

Because it may take days or longer for the above treatments to have full effect, immediate action is necessary to minimize the dramatic effects thyroid storm produces in the major organ systems. The mortality rate of thyroid storm has been significantly reduced with the introduction of β-blockers to block the peripheral effects of thyroid hormone. The drug of choice to accomplish this is propranolol (Inderal). Propranolol will markedly reduce the effects of thyroid hormone on the cardiovascular system, decreasing cardiac output, decreasing heart rate, and diminishing supraventricular dysrhythmias. It also has the added ability to partially inhibit peripheral conversion of T_4 to T_3. Propranolol may be given intravenously in 1- to 2-mg boluses every 10 to 15 minutes up to 15 to 20 mg. The intravenous route is indicated if the patient is comatose, unable to take oral medications, and/or the heart rate is greater than 140/min. Oral doses range from 160 to 320 mg daily in divided doses. The dose is individualized to the patient's response. Results should be seen within minutes using the intravenous route and within 1 hour using the oral route. Intravenous effects should last 3 to 4 hours. However, propranolol is contraindicated in patients with chronic lung disease (asthma, emphysema), hypotension, pulmonary edema, or heart block. Caution must also be used in patients who are on insulin or oral hypoglycemic agents, patients on monoamine inhibitors, and pregnant women.

If unable to use propranolol, guanethidine and reserpine may be used instead. Reserpine will decrease hyperthermia, tachycardia, and the psychological aberrations within 4 to 6 hours. Problems with reserpine include its slow onset, nervous system depression, flushing, and diarrhea. Guanethidine takes several days to take effect and can produce orthostatic hypotension and deplete myocardial catecholamines.

Drugs used to treat thyroid storm are summarized in Table 14–26.

Supportive Care

1. Fluid and electrolyte deficits should be corrected with adequate hydration with glucose and multivitamins.

2. Fever should be treated with external cooling measures and acetaminophen. Aspirin should be avoided as it increases the level of free thyroxine.

3. Stress doses of glucocorticoids are given to cover possible adrenal insufficiency and minimize the effects of increased glucocorticoid turnover and degradation that occur in thyroid crisis. Hydrocortisone, 200 to 300 mg IV initially, followed by 300 mg daily via IV drip, is given. Dexamethasone, 8 to 10 mg daily in three doses, can also be used.

4. Digoxin is given to patients in congestive heart failure or with tachydysrhythmias. Recent research indicates calcium blockers such as verapamil and diltiazem may also be effective in controlling heart rate and rhythm (Isley, 1990).

5. If able to eat, patients should be given high-calorie, high-protein diets to support them during this state of hypermetabolism and protein catabolism. If patients are unable to eat, hyperalimentation or enteral feeding should be instituted.

6. Dialysis and plasmapharesis have also been utilized with some success to remove large amounts of protein-bound thyroid hormone.

Patient/Family Education

Education of patients and family/significant others is crucial in identifying and preventing episodes of thyroid storm. Teaching will vary depending on the long-term therapy chosen for each patient; e.g., drugs versus radioactive iodine or surgery. For the patient receiving drug therapy, discharge goals include the patient/significant other will be able to

Describe the pathophysiology and therapeutic regimen for hyperthyroidism

Identify the signs and symptoms associated with development of hyperthyroid crisis

Describe situations that require notification of the physician

Describe the rationales for and appropriate administration of drugs used in treatment

Identify signs and symptoms of side effects associated with the therapeutic regimen (agranulocytosis, hypothyroidism)

Table 14–27 contains a summary of treatment for thyroid storm.

Table 14–26. DRUGS USED TO TREAT THYROID STORM

Propylthiouracil (PTU)

Class

Antithyroid drug

Action

Inhibits synthesis of thyroid hormones; inhibits peripheral conversion of T_4 to T_3

Dose

800–1200 mg PO loading dose; 400–600 mg every day until thyroid storm controlled

Side Effects

Granulocytopenia, thrombocytopenia, bleeding
Paresthesias, vertigo, drowsiness, depression, headaches
Nausea and vomiting, epigastric distress
Skin pigmentation, urticaria, rash
Loss of hair, edema

Nursing Considerations

Monitor for bleeding tendencies, decreased platelet count
Provide small, frequent meals if GI problems
Monitor for neurological changes and provide safety measures
Provide frequent skin care

Methimazole (Tapazole)

Class

Antithyroid drug

Action

Inhibits thyroid hormone synthesis

Dose

90–120 mg PO loading dose; 40 mg daily

Side Effects

Same as propylthiouracil

Nursing Considerations

Same as propylthiouracil

Lugol's Solution/Saturated Solution of Potassium Iodide (SSKI)

Class

Thyroid suppressant

Action

Inhibits synthesis of thyroid hormones and their release into the circulation

Dose

30 drops PO daily

Side Effects

Rash, metallic taste, burning mouth, sore teeth/gums
Inflammation of salivary glands
Headaches
Gastritis, diarrhea
Allergic reactions

Nursing Considerations

Monitor for allergic reactions; acute toxicity (vomiting, abdominal pain, diarrhea, circulatory collapse)
Provide frequent mouth care; dilute with fruit juice or water to improve taste
Provide small, frequent meals if GI problems
Give 1–2 hr after antithyroid drugs

Sodium Iodide

Class

Thyroid suppressant

Action

Same as Lugol's solution

Dose

1 g every 8–12 hr IV

Side Effects

Same as above
Iodide toxicity: edema of larynx, multiple hemorrhages of skin/mucous membranes, serum sickness, pulmonary edema

Nursing Considerations

Monitor for allergic/toxic reactions
Provide good mouth care
Provide small, frequent meals if GI problems
Give 1–2 hr after antithyroid drugs

Propranolol (Inderal)

Class

β Adrenergic blocker

Action

Blocks β-adrenergic receptors in heart and juxtaglomerular apparatus: decreases sympathetic influence, causing decreased cardiac contractility, decreased heart rate, decreased renin release, and decreased blood pressure; also partially inhibits peripheral conversion T_4 to T_3

Dose

IV: 1–2 mg bolus every 10–15 min up to 15–20 mg/PO: 160–320 mg daily in divided doses
Dose individualized to patient response

Side Effects

Bradycardia, CHF, cardiac dysrhythmias, hypotension
Dizziness, vertigo, tinnitis, fatigue
Bronchospasm, dyspnea, rhinitis
GI upset: pain, nausea, vomiting, anorexia

Nursing Considerations

Contraindicated in patients with chronic lung disease, hypotension, pulmonary edema, or heart block
Caution in patients on insulin or oral hypoglycemic agents, monoamine inhibitors, and pregnant women
Continuous cardiac montioring and frequent blood pressure monitoring necessary when giving intravenously
Give with food if administering orally
Assess for side effects and consult with physician if they occur

Reserpine

Class

Sympathetic adrenergic neuroblocking drug

Action

Depletes catecholamine stores, reducing heart rate and blood pressure; also has sedative and tranquilizing effects

Dose

1–5 mg IM loading dose; then 1.0–2.5 mg every 4–6 hr

Side Effects

Cutaneous flushing
Diarrhea
Central nervous system depression
Orthostatic hypotension

Nursing Considerations

Monitor for central nervous system effects
Monitor blood pressure closely

Guanethidine (Ismelin)

Class

Sympathetic adrenergic neuroblocking agent

Action

Depletes catecholamine stores and blocks catecholamine release, reducing blood pressure

Dose

1–2 mg/kg PO daily

Side Effects

Dizziness
Weakness
Syncope
Hypotension
Diarrhea
Fluid retention and edema

Nursing Considerations

Same as reserpine

Table 14-27. TREATMENT OF THYROID STORM

Identify and treat precipitating cause
Inhibit hormone biosynthesis
Propylthiouracil (PTU): 800–1200 mg PO loading; 400–600 mg PO daily until thyrotoxicosis controlled OR Methimazole (Tapazole): 90–120 mg PO loading dose; 40 mg PO daily
Block thyroid hormone release
Lugol's solution: 30 drops daily PO
Sodium iodide: 1 g IV over 30 min every 8–12 hr
Give 1–2 hr after PTU or methimazole loading dose
Antagonize peripheral effects of thyroid hormone
Propranolol (Inderal): 1–2 mg IV boluses every 10–15 min up to 15–20 mg IV; 160–320 mg daily PO; individualized to response
If propranolol contraindicated, give reserpine or guanethidine
Supportive therapy
Correct fluid and electrolyte imbalance
Treat hyperthermia (no aspirin)
Hydrocortisone: 200–300 mg IV loading; then 300 mg IV drip over 24 hr
Digoxin for CHF or tachydysrhythmia. Calcium blockers may be better at controlling heart rate and rhythm
High-calorie, high-protein diet
Patient/family education

Outcome Criteria

Outcomes for the patient with thyroid storm include:

1. Stable hemodynamic parameters and metabolic rate
2. Temperature within normal range
3. Effective breathing pattern
4. Nutritional needs met and weight maintained
5. Skin intact without petechiae
6. Return to baseline activity level
7. Return to baseline mentation and personality
8. Patient/significant others will verbalize an understanding of the patient's illness, anticipated treatment, and potential complications

See the Nursing Care Plan for the Patient with Thyroid Storm.

MYXEDEMA COMA

Pathogenesis

Etiology

Underlying causes for myxedema coma consist of those that produce hypothyroidism. Most cases occur in patients with either long-standing autoimmune disease of the thyroid (Hashimoto's thyroiditis) or patients who have received surgical or radioactive iodine treatment for Graves' disease and have received inadequate hormone replacement. It is rarely associated with hypothyroidism produced by pituitary or hypothalmic disorders. These and other less common causes of hypothyroidism are listed in Table 14–28.

Myxedema coma is the end stage of improperly treated, neglected, or undiagnosed hypothyroidism. It is a life-threatening emergency with a mortality rate as high as 50% despite appropriate therapy. Much of this mortality rate can be attributed to underlying illnesses. Patients who develop myxedema coma in most cases are elderly females. It is rarely seen in young individuals. It occurs more frequently in winter as a result of the increased stress of exposure to cold in an individual unable to maintain body heat. It is also associated with other types of physiological or psychological stress or underlying illness. Known precipitating factors include exposure to cold, infection, trauma, critical illness, and administration of central nervous system depressants such as narcotics, barbiturates, or anesthesia. Common underlying illnesses include infection, anemia, heart failure, ascites, pleural and pericardial effusions, seizures, and aspiration.

Pathophysiology

Myxedema coma in the absence of an associated stress or illness is uncommon, with infection being the most frequent stressor. The addition of

Table 14-28. CAUSES OF HYPOTHYROIDISM

Primary Thyroid Disease
Autoimmune (Hashimoto's thyroiditis)
Radioactive iodine treatment of Graves' disease
Thyroidectomy
Congenital enzymatic defect in thyroid hormone biosynthesis
Inhibition of thyroid hormone synthesis or release
- Antithyroid drugs
- Iodides
- Lithium carbonate
- Oral hypoglycemic agents

Idiopathic thyroid atrophy
Secondary (Pituitary)/Tertiary (Hypothalamus) Disease
Tumors
Infiltrative disease (sarcoidosis)
Hypophysectomy
Pituitary irradiation
Head injury
Pituitary infarction

NURSING CARE PLAN FOR THE PATIENT WITH THYROID STORM

Nursing Diagnosis	Outcome	Intervention
Decreased cardiac output related to increased metabolic demands on heart, extreme tachycardia, dysrhythmias, congestive heart failure	Stable hemodynamic parameters and metabolic rate as evidenced by: Cardiac output 4-8 L/min; cardiac index 2.5-4 L/min/m^2 Pulmonary artery pressures, wedge pressure, and CVP within normal range Return to baseline BP for patient Heart rate 60-100 beats/minute Control of dysrhythmias Urine output >30 ml/hr	Control temperature (see nursing diagnosis of hyperthermia below) Assess/monitor for signs and symptoms of cardiac compromise Blood pressure, pulse pressure Apical pulse, sleeping heart rate Pulmonary artery and wedge pressures, CVP Cardiac output, cardiac index, SVR Respiratory rate, breath sounds, secretions Dysrhythmias Heart sounds: S_1, S_2, gallop, murmur Complaints of chest pain, palpitations, SOB; signs of ischemia Hourly urine output Provide adequate hydration, monitor hemodyamic response to fluid therapy Monitor electrolyte status Monitor potassium and calcium levels Watch for signs/symptoms of hypokalemia or hypercalcemia Administer digoxin as ordered and monitor response Minimize demand on heart by controlling activity Assess for previous history of chronic lung disease, heart block, pulmonary edema (propranolol contraindicated) Administer and monitor effects of drugs utilized to combat thyroid hormone effects Assess response to propranolol: BP, HR, CO, PAP, PAWP, CVP Assess response to antithyroid drugs and monitor for toxic effects (see Table 14-26).
Hyperthermia related to loss of temperature regulation, increased metabolism, increased heat production	Temperature return to normal range: —37°C; 98.6°F	Monitor patient's temperature every 1 hr; continuously with probe if possible Assess fluid status: hourly I/O, daily weight, diaphoresis, skin turgor, mucous membranes Utilize cooling measures to decrease temperature: Administer acetaminophen (no aspirin) Ice packs (axillae and groins) Cooling mattress Minimal covers Control room temperature Administer and monitor effects of drugs utilized to combat thyroid hormone effects Administer antibiotics if infection a precipitator
Ineffective breathing pattern related to muscle weakness and decreased vital capacity resulting in hypoventilation and CO_2 retention, increased oxygen need from hypermetabolism	Effective breathing pattern as evidenced by: Normal respiratory rate, depth, and pattern Normal $PaCO_2$ (35-45 mm Hg) and pH (7.35-7.45) on ABG analysis or return to patient baseline $PaO_2 > 60$ mm Hg on ABG analysis Normal vital capacity, tidal volume Resolution of muscle weakness Patient reports breathing easier	Assess respiratory status every 4 hr; every 1-2 hr in patient with altered level of consciousness Assess airway and breathing effort, use of accessory muscles Assess rate and depth of respiration Auscultate breath sounds Obtain ABGs as ordered and PRN Obtain pulmonary function parameters: tidal volume, vital capacity Assess subjective complaints of shortness of breath, dyspnea on exertion Provide supportive measures to facilitate respiratory effort Support airway as appropriate: airway, supplementary oxygen, suctioning, intubation equipment/ventilator Position patient for ease of respiratory effort; i.e., head of bed elevated Provide quiet, restful environment Allow frequent rest periods

NURSING CARE PLAN FOR THE PATIENT WITH THYROID STORM *Continued*

Nursing Diagnosis	Outcome	Intervention
		– Minimize activity to decrease oxygen need – Send sputum for culture and sensitivity – Administer antibiotics if ordered Administer and monitor effects of drugs utilized to combat thyroid hormone effects
Altered nutrition; less than body requirements related to increased peristalsis, decreased absorption, increased requirements	Body weight will stabilize at patient's normal level Nutritional needs met as evidenced by: Serum albumin 3.5–5.5 g/dl Serum glucose 70–110 mg/dl	Assess effects of thyroid hormone on GI system – Bowel sounds; abdominal pain – Nausea and vomiting – Increased number/frequency of bowel movements, diarrhea – Normal vs current weight (i.e., recent weight loss) – Serum albumin level – Fatigue, weakness – Liver function tests, BUN Provide adequate nutrition and calories – Provide high-calorie, high-protein diet – Avoid foods that increase peristalsis such as tea, coffee, fibrous and highly seasoned foods – Monitor adequacy of patients' intake; take measures to supplement if necessary, i.e., tube feedings, hyperalimentation – Weigh patient daily on same scale at same time of day – Provide multivitamin and mineral supplements as needed – Provide frequent, small feedings – Monitor BUN, creatinine to assess positive nitrogen balance – Minimize activity to decrease energy requirement Provide adequate glucose to support energy needs – Provide adequate dextrose in intravenous fluids – Administer hydrocortisone as ordered – Monitor for signs and symptoms of hyperglycemia (polyuria, polydipsia, weakness, fatigue, lethargy) – Monitor serum glucose levels Administer and monitor effects of drugs utilized to combat thyroid hormone effects
Potential impaired skin integrity related to thin skin, fragile blood vessels	Skin intact without breakdown or petechiae	Provide pressure relief measures; i.e., eggcrate, air mattress, heel pads Turn and reposition every 2 hr Cleanse skin frequently to maintain minimal moisture Check skin for signs of bleeding and pressure areas Provide frequent mouth care
Activity intolerance related to muscle weakness, muscle wasting, tremors, fatigue, anemia, and extreme energy expenditure	Patient will return to baseline activity level	During acute crisis, minimize physical activity – Provide all daily cares for patient – Maintain on bed rest Allow for adequate rest/sleep periods – Minimize group interruptions – Assess patient's normal sleep patterns/habits and try to accommodate them – Maintain quiet, calm environment – Administer sedatives if ordered and assess effectiveness – Assess for and provide patient with calming diversional activities Provide adequate nutrition Increase activity gradually after acute crisis abates; monitor physical response to activity Administer oxygen during activity Administer and monitor effects of drugs utilized to combat thyroid hormone effects

continued

NURSING CARE PLAN FOR THE PATIENT WITH THYROID STORM *Continued*

Nursing Diagnosis	Outcome	Intervention
Sensory/perceptual alterations related to hypermetabolism and increased cerebration, agitation, delirium, psychosis	Return to baseline mentation and behavior Return to normal personality (per family/significant others)	Assess for degree of physiological/psychological dysfunction Orientation Irritability, nervousness, agitation Memory, attention span Mood swings, fear, paranoia Convulsions, stupor, coma Tremors: tongue, eyelids, peripheral Muscle weakness Minimize effects of environment on mental status Reorient patient frequently Maintain quiet environment, minimizing extraneous stimuli Provide simple, brief explanations of activities, procedures, or equipment Provide meaningful, relaxing stimuli to patient Minimize physiological effects of hypermetabolism Initiate protective measures for patient with convulsions/agitation/delusions: padded siderails, soft restraints, close supervision Provide all care if level of consciousness decreased Minimize physical exertion required by patient Assist patient with daily cares as needed Administer and monitor effects of drugs utilized to combat thyroid hormone effects
Knowledge deficit related to disease process, therapeutic regimen, prevention of complications	Patient/family member/significant other will verbalize an understanding of the patient's illness, anticipated treatment, and potential complications	Assess patient/family current level of knowledge and readiness to learn Design teaching program which includes the following information as appropriate Pathophysiology of hyperthryoidism Signs and symptoms associated with hyperthyroid crisis Situations that require notification of physician Rationale for and appropriate administration of drugs Signs and symptoms of side effects associated with therapeutic regimen (agranulocytosis, hypothyroidism) Provide written materials for all content taught. Provide means for the patient to get questions answered after discharge Schedule follow-up teaching session after discharge

stress to an already hypothyroid patient further accelerates the metabolism and clearance of whatever thyroid hormone is present in the body. Thus, he or she is in a situation of increased hormone utilization but decreased hormone production, which precipitates a crisis state.

As in hyperthyroidism, low levels of thyroid hormone also disrupt the normal physiology of most body systems. Hypothyroidism produces a hypodynamic, hypometabolic state. Myxedema coma is a magnification of these disruptions initiated by some type of stressor, as indicated above. Myxedema coma takes many months to develop and should be suspected in patients with known thyroid history, with a surgical scar on the lower neck, or in those who are unusually sensitive to medications or narcotics. Common findings in patients with hypothyroidism and myxedema coma are listed in Table 14–24 and discussed below.

Assessment

Clinical Presentation

Many patients may have had vague signs and symptoms of hypothyroidism for several years. The earliest signs may be fatigue, weakness, muscle cramps, and intolerance to cold. Again, the clinical picture of myxedema coma varies with the rate of onset and severity. Diagnosis is based on the clinical signs and symptoms, a high index of suspicion, and a careful history and physical examination. Many of the manifestations are attributable to the development of mucinous edema. This interstitial edema is the result of water retention and decreased protein.

Neurological Disturbances. The decreased metabolic rate and resulting decreased cerebration produces both psychological and physiological changes. Difficulty concentrating, slowed mentation, depression, lethargy, somnolence, and coma can all be seen. Grand mal seizures can be seen in 25 to 30% of patients in myxedema coma (Hamburger et al., 1984). Speech may be slow and deliberate and the patient may have a coarse, raspy, hoarse voice as a result of mucinous edema of the vocal cords. Mucinous edema can also produce hearing loss and vertigo. Personality changes such as paranoia and delusions may develop.

Patients with hypothyroidism are unable to maintain body heat owing to the decreased metabolic rate and production of thermal energy. Because of this, patients may present in crisis after being stressed by exposure to cold. Hypothermia is present in 80% of the patients in myxedema coma, with temperatures as low as 24°C (Meek, 1980). Patients with temperatures less than 32°C have a grave prognosis. If the patient with myxedema coma has a temperature greater than 36°C, underlying infection should be suspected.

Cardiovascular Disturbances. Cardiac function is depressed and results in decreased contractility, decreased stroke volume, decreased heart rate, and decreased cardiac output. About one-third of the patients will develop pericardial effusions, which may make heart tones distant (Hamburger et al., 1984). The ECG will have decreased voltage as a result of the pericardial effusion. Because of the diminished adrenergic stimulation produced by low thyroid levels, about half of patients with myxedema coma will be hypotensive with a systolic blood pressure below 100 mm Hg (Hamburger et al., 1984). However, these patients may also be hypertensive because of atherosclerotic disease.

Pulmonary Disturbances. Respirations are depressed, producing hypoventilation and carbon dioxide retention. Patients may experience dyspnea on exertion because they are unable to increase respiratory efforts with activity. As part of the picture of generalized mucinous edema and fluid retention, these patients may also develop pleural effusions or upper airway edema, further restricting their breathing.

Gastrointestinal Disturbances. Decreased thyroid levels decrease appetite, decrease peristalsis, and interfere with carbohydrate metabolism. Patients frequently experience anorexia, decreased bowel sounds, constipation, and paralytic ileus. Fluid retention and the decreased metabolic rate, however, result in weight gain and ascites.

Skeletal Muscle Disturbances. Slowed motor conduction produces decreased tendon reflexes and sluggish awkward movements. Thyroid hormone also maintains calcium metabolism, so hypothyroidism results in increased bone density because of decreased calcium mobilization.

Integumentary Disturbances. Patients typically have dry, flaky, cool, coarse skin; dry, coarse hair; and brittle nails. They may also have a yellow tint to their skin that results from depressed hepatic conversion of carotene to vitamin A. Generalized mucinous edema develops, especially in the eyelids, periorbital tissue, and dorsa of the hands and feet. Ecchymoses may develop from increased capillary fragility and decreased platelets.

Laboratory Evaluation

Serum T_4 and T_3 levels and resin T_3 uptake will be low in patients with myxedema coma. In primary hypothyroidism, TSH (thyroid-stimulating hormone) levels will be high. If hypothyroidism is the result of disease of the pituitary gland or hypothalamus (secondary and tertiary hypothyroidism), TSH levels will be inappropriately normal or low. However, as in patients with thyroid storm, if myxedema coma is suspected, treatment should not be delayed until these results are back to confirm the diagnosis.

Serum sodium levels may be low owing to impaired water excretion and resultant water retention. Impaired water excretion is the result of the inappropriate antidiuretic hormone (ADH) secretion and cortisol deficiency that frequently accompany hypothyroidism. The patient should be monitored for signs and symptoms related to hyponatremia such as weakness, muscle twitching, seizures, and coma.

Hypoglycemia is uncommon unless hypothyroidism is related to pituitary or hypophyseal disorders and/or coexists with adrenal insufficiency. Adrenal insufficiency may also result in serum cortisol levels inappropriately low for stress. The production and degradation of cortisol is decreased in myxedema coma, resulting in hypoglycemia.

Complete blood count (CBC) may show a normochromic normocytic anemia. Leukocytosis (elevated white count) is frequently absent despite stress or underlying illness.

The slowed metabolism will also cause elevated CPK, SGOT, LDH, cholesterol, and triglycerides. Elevated cholesterol and triglycerides predispose individuals with hypothyroidism to the development of atherosclerosis.

Laboratory manifestations of myxedema coma are summarized in Table 14–25.

Nursing Diagnoses

The nursing diagnoses which may apply to a patient in myxedema coma are based on assessment data and include:

1. Fluid volume excess related to impaired water excretion
2. Decreased cardiac output related to decreased contractility, decreased heart rate, decreased stroke volume, pericardial effusions, dysrhythmias
3. Hypothermia related to the inability of the body to retain heat
4. Sensory/perceptual alterations related to slowed metabolism, cerebration, hyponatremia
5. Ineffective breathing pattern related to hypoventilation, muscle weakness, decreased respiratory rate, ascites, pleural effusions
6. Potential for injury related to edema, decreased platelets
7. Activity intolerance related to muscle weakness, anemia
8. Altered nutrition; less than body requirements related to decreased appetite, decreased carbohydrate metabolism, hypoglycemia
9. Knowledge deficit related to disease process, therapeutic regimen, prevention of complications

Collaborative Management

Myxedema coma requires immediate intervention if the patient is to survive. The primary objectives in treatment of myxedema coma include identifying and treating the precipitating cause, providing thyroid replacement, restoring fluid and electrolyte balance, providing supportive care, and patient/family education.

Thyroid Replacement

The best method of thyroid replacement is controversial. Either liothyronine sodium (Cytomel; T_3) or levothyroxine sodium (Synthroid; T_4) may be used. Remember that T_3 is more potent than T_4 and most of T_3 comes from peripheral conversion of T_4 to T_3. Thus, liothyronine will require lower doses, and levothyroxine will ultimately provide the patient with both T_4 and T_3 replacement.

Levothyroxine sodium is the more commonly used drug. It has a smoother effect, longer activity, and a portion of it will be converted to T_3 in peripheral tissues. A dose of 500 to 700 μg IV is required to restore the patient in myxedema coma to a low-normal thyroid state. The preferred route is intravenous because absorption of oral or intramuscular levothyroxine is variable. The initial dose may be decreased if the patient has underlying factors such as angina, dysrhythmias, or other heart disease. These patients may receive only 300 μg initially. The initial bolus is followed by 50 to 100 μg IV, or 100 to 200 μg PO daily.

Liothyronine sodium has heightened metabolic effects, a more rapid onset (6 hours), and a shorter half-life (1 day) than levothyroxine. Intravenous preparations are not available, so it is given orally or via nasogastric tube. The optimal dose is not known and can range from 10 μg every 12 hours to 100 μg every 6 hours. An average dose is 12.5 μg every 8 hours. Because of its potency, liothyronine administration may be complicated by angina, myocardial infarction, and cardiac irritability, and thus is generally avoided in older populations and not used in myxedema coma.

The effects of levothyroxine are not as rapid as those of liothyronine but its cardiac toxicity is less. Serum levels of T_4 will reach normal in 1 to 2 days. Levels of TSH will begin to fall within 24 hours and return to normal in 7 to 10 days. Drugs used to treat myxedema coma are summarized in Table 14–29.

Restore Fluid and Electrolyte Balance

If the patient is hypotensive or in shock, thyroid replacement will usually correct this, but cautious volume expansion with saline will also help. Vasopressors should be used with extreme caution. Patients in myxedema coma will be unable to respond to vasopressors until they have adequate levels of thyroid hormone available. Simulta-

Table 14–29. DRUGS USED TO TREAT MYXEDEMA COMA

Levothyroxine Sodium (Synthroid)
Class
Thyroid hormone; T_4
Action
Same effects as thyroid hormone (see Table 14–22)
Dose
200–500 μg IV loading dose; then 50–100 μg/day IV
Side Effects
Symptoms of hyperthyroidism
Allergic skin reactions
Nursing Considerations
Monitor for signs and symptoms of hyperthyroidism
Monitor cardiac response closely

Liothyronine Sodium (Cytomel)
Class
Thyroid hormone; T_3
Action
Same effects as thyroid hormone (see Table 14–22)
Dose
12.5 μg PO every 8 hr
Side Effects
Same as levothyroxine plus
Angina, myocardial infarction, cardiac irritability
Nursing Considerations
Same as Synthroid

---

neous administration of vasopressors and thyroid hormone are associated with myocardial irritability.

Hyponatremia usually responds to thyroid replacement and water restriction; i.e., the patient will be able to get rid of free water once thyroid is replaced. If hyponatremia is severe (<110 mEq/L, or seizures), hypertonic saline with or without furosemide (Lasix) may be administered, but only until symptoms disappear or the sodium level is 120 mEq/L.

Glucose should be added to intravenous fluids to provide support to the patient with hypoglycemia and/or concomitant adrenal insufficiency. Hydrocortisone, 100 mg, is given initially followed by 50 to 100 mg every 6 hours in the first 24 hours. Subsequently, this dose is 50 to 100 mg every 8 hours for 7 to 10 days (Gavin, 1991). The adrenal abnormality may last several weeks after thyroid replacement is begun, so this support should be continued during that time.

Supportive Care

1. Hypothermia is treated by passive methods; i.e., blankets. A more active method of rewarming such as a heating blanket is dangerous. It can result in peripheral vasodilatation, circulatory collapse, and death. Thyroid replacement will slowly return the patient's temperature to normal.

2. Ventilatory support may range from oxygen supplementation to intubation and assisted ventilation. This will depend on the severity of hypoventilation, hypoxia, and hypercapnia.

3. Avoid narcotics and sedative drugs. All drugs need to be administered cautiously owing to the patient's hypometabolic state. As a result he/she will have delayed drug turnover and degradation.

Patient/Family Education

Education of patients and family/significant others is critical in identifying and preventing episodes of myxedema coma. Discharge goals include the patient/significant other will be able to

Describe the pathophysiology and therapeutic regimen for hypothyroidism
Identify the signs and symptoms associated with the development of hypothyroid crisis
List stressors that can produce a hypothyroid crisis
Describe situations that require notification of the physician
Describe rationale for and appropriate administration of drugs used in treatment
Identify signs and symptoms of side effects and toxic effects associated with thyroid replacement drugs (hyperthyroidism, angina)

The treatment of myxedema coma is summarized in Table 14–30.

Outcome Criteria

Outcomes for the patient with myxedema coma include:

1. Normal fluid volume
2. Normal hemodynamics and metabolic rate
3. Temperature within normal range
4. Return to baseline mentation and personality
5. Effective breathing pattern
6. Intact skin without edema or bleeding
7. Return to baseline activity level
8. Adequate nutrition and stable body weight

NURSING CARE PLAN FOR THE PATIENT IN MYXEDEMA COMA

Nursing Diagnosis	Outcome	Intervention
Fluid volume excess related to impaired water excretion	Normal fluid volume as indicated by: Urine output >30 ml/hr Blood pressure within 10 mm Hg patient baseline Weight close to patient baseline No edema No pericardial or pleural effusions	Maintain fluid restriction Monitor hourly I&O Daily weight on same scale at same time of day Monitor for signs and symptoms of hyponatremia Monitor for signs and symptoms of cardiac failure (see nursing diagnosis for decreased cardiac output below) Institute protective measures to prevent injury related to edema (see nursing diagnosis for potential for injury below) Monitor blood pressure every 1 hr Administer and monitor effects of thyroid drugs
Decreased cardiac output related to decreased contractility, decreased heart rate, decreased stroke volume, pericardial effusions, dysrhythmias	Normal hemodynamics and metabolic rate as evidenced by: Cardiac output 4–8 L/min; cardiac index 2.5–4.0 L/min/m^2 Pulmonary artery pressure, wedge pressure, and CVP within normal limits Blood pressure within 10 mm Hg of patient baseline Urine output >30 ml/hr Control of dysrhythmias No pericardial effusion	Assess and monitor patient for signs/symptoms of cardiovascular collapse Cardiac output, cardiac index, SVR Heart sounds: diminished, murmur, gallop BP every 1 hr Urine output every 1 hr Chest pain, signs of ischemia Heart rate and rhythm Institute treatment to control dysrhythmias Administer volume or pressors cautiously to maintain BP Administer and monitor effects of thyroid replacement drugs
Hypothermia related to inability of body to retain heat	Temperature 37°C, 98.6°F	Warm patient passively with blankets (no active warming) Monitor temperature every 1–2 hr or continuously with probe Control room temperature; avoid exposure to cold Administer and monitor effects of thyroid replacement drugs
Sensory/perceptual alterations related to slowed metabolism and cerebration, hyponatremia	Return to baseline mentation Normal personality pattern (per family member/significant other)	Protect patient if having seizures: padded side rails Provide simple, clear explanations of all activities, procedures and equipment Reorient as needed Minimize extraneous, meaningless stimuli Monitor serum sodium and signs of hyponatremia Administer and monitor effects of thyroid replacement drugs
Ineffective breathing pattern related to hypoventilation, muscle weakness, decreased respiratory rate, ascites, pleural effusions	Effective breathing pattern as evidenced by: Normal rate and depth of ventilation $PaCO_2$ 35–45 mm Hg, pH 7.35–7.45 Patient reports no dyspnea with activity	Assess effect of hypometabolism on breathing Rate, depth, and rhythm of respiration Breath sounds ABGs Pulmonary function tests: tidal volume, vital capacity Minimize physical activity Provide ventilatory support as needed: supplemental oxygen, airway, suctioning, intubation, mechanical ventilation Monitor tidal volume and vital capacity Draw ABGs as ordered and PRN Minimize water retention (see fluid volume excess) Monitor anemia Administer and monitor effects of thyroid replacement drugs
Potential for injury related to edema, decreased platelets	Intact skin without edema or bleeding	Provide frequent mouth care Keep skin warm, dry Turn patient every 2 hr Provide pressure relief measures: egg-crate mattress, air mattress, heel protectors

NURSING CARE PLAN FOR THE PATIENT IN MYXEDEMA COMA *Continued*		
Nursing Diagnosis	**Outcome**	**Intervention**
		Inspect skin every 2 hr for signs of reddening or breakdown Assess extent of edema Assess for signs of bleeding Monitor/minimize puncture sites for signs of bleeding, guaiac stools Assess gastric and pulmonary secretions and urine for signs of blood Assess for easy bruising
Activity intolerance related to muscle weakness	Patient will return to baseline activity level	During acute crisis, minimize physical activity Provide all daily cares for patient Maintain on bed rest Allow for adequate rest/sleep periods Minimize group interruptions Assess patients' normal sleep patterns/habits and try to accommodate them Maintain quiet, calm environment Provide adequate nutrition Increase activity gradually when patient able Administer and monitor effects of thyroid replacement drugs
Altered nutrition; less than body requirements related to decreased appetite, decreased carbohydrate metabolism, hypoglycemia	Body weight will stabilize at patient's normal level Adequate nutrition as evidenced by: Serum albumin: 3.5–5.5 gm/dl Serum glucose: 70–110 mg/dl	Assess effects of lack of thyroid hormone on GI system Bowel sounds Anorexia Constipation Normal vs current weight (i.e., recent weight gain) Serum albumin level Ascites Provide adequate nutrition and calories Provide low-calorie diet with increased protein and moderate sodium Monitor adequacy of patient's intake; take measures to supplement if necessary; i.e., tube feedings, TPN Weigh patient daily on same scale at same time of day Provide adequate glucose to support metabolism Provide adequate dextrose in intravenous fluids Administer hydrocortisone as ordered Monitor for signs and symptoms of hypoglycemia Monitor serum glucose levels Administer and monitor effects of thyroid replacement drugs
Knowledge deficit related to disease process, therapeutic regimen, prevention of complications	Patient/family member/significant other verbalizes understanding of disease, therapeutic regimen, and prevention of complications	Assess patient/significant others' level of knowledge and readiness to learn Design a teaching program that includes information on: Pathophysiology of hypothyroidism Therapeutic regimen prescribed for patient Signs and symptoms associated with development of hypothyroid crisis Stressors that can precipitate hypothyroid crisis Situations that require notification of the physician Rationale for and appropriate administration of drugs Signs and symptoms of side effects associated with thyroid-replacement drugs and toxicity (angina, hyperthyroidism) Provide written materials for all content taught; provide means for patient/family member/significant other to get questions answered after discharge Schedule follow-up session after discharge

Table 14–30. TREATMENT OF MYXEDEMA COMA

Identify and treat underlying disorder
Thyroid replacement: levothyroxine sodium 200–500 μg IV loading; 50–100 μg/day IV
Restore fluid and electrolyte balance
- Administer pressors cautiously
- Hyponatremia: <115 mEq/L hypertonic saline; >120 mEq/L fluid restriction
- Hypoglycemia
  - IV glucose
  - Adrenal hormone replacement: hydrocortisone 100 mg IV bolus; 50–100 mg every 6 hr over first 24 hr up to 500 mg; then 50–100 mg IV every 8 hr for 7–10 days

Supportive care
- Passive warming with blankets (don't actively warm)
- Ventilatory assistance
- Avoid narcotics and sedative drugs

Patient/family education

9. Patient/significant other verbalize understanding of disease, therapeutic regimen, and prevention of complications

See Nursing Care Plan for the patient in Myxedema Coma.

Recommended Reading

Alspach, J. G. (ed.) (1991): *Core Curriculum for Critical Care Nursing.* 4th ed. Philadelphia: W. B. Saunders.

Boehm, T. (1983): Hyperglycemia in critical care medicine. *Critical Care Quarterly* 6(3):43–60.

Burman, K. D. (1983): Interpretation of thyroid function tests in systemically ill patients. *Critical Care Quarterly* 6(3): 1–10.

Doenges, M. E., Jeffries, M. F., and Moorhouse, M. F. (1984): *Nursing Care Plans: Nursing Diagnosis in Planning Patient Care.* Philadelphia: F. A. Davis.

Felig, P., Baxter, J., Broadus, A., and Frohmna, L. (1987): *Endocrinology and Metabolism.* New York: McGraw-Hill.

Fisher, K., Lees, J., and Newmann, J. (1986): Hypoglycemia in hospitalized patients. *New England Journal of Medicine* 315:1245–1250.

Goodman, J. M. (1988): *Basic Medical Endocrinology.* New York: Raven Press.

Gotch, P. (1983): Hyperglycemic crisis: A standard plan of care. *Dimensions of Critical Care Nursing* 2:262–270.

Hadley, M. E. (1988): Endocrinology. 2nd ed. Englewood Cliffs, NJ: Prentice-Hall.

Havlin, C., and Cryer, P. (1988): Hypoglycemia: The limiting factor in the management of insulin-dependent diabetes mellitus. *Diabetes Education* 14:407–411.

Hellman, R. (1980): The evaluation and management of hyperthyroid crises. *Critical Care Quarterly* 3(2):77–92.

Hoffenberg, R. (1980): Thyroid emergencies. *Clinics in Endocrinology and Metabolism* 9(3):503–512.

Johnston, J. (1985): Management of diabetic ketoacidosis. *Clinical Diabetes* 3:121–123.

Karch, A., and Boyd, E. (1989): *Handbook of Drugs and the Nursing Process.* Philadelphia: J. B. Lippincott.

Kitabchi, A., and Murphy, M. B. (1988): Diabetic ketoacidosis and hyperosmolar hyperglycemic nonketotic coma. *Medical Clinics of North America* 72:1545–1563.

Klein, I. L., and Levey, G. S. (1984): Thyroid emergencies: Thyroid storm and myxedema coma. *Topics in Emergency Medicine* 5(4):33–39.

Matz, T. R. (1988): Hyperosmolar nonacidotic uncontrolled diabetes: Not a rare event. *Clinical Diabetes* 6:25–30.

Moorhouse, M. F., Geissler, A. C., and Doenges, M. E. (1987): *Critical Care Plans: Guidelines for Advanced Medical-Surgical Care.* Philadelphia: F. A. Davis.

Morris, L. R., Murphy, M. B., and Kitabchi, A. E. (1986): Bicarbonate therapy in severe diabetic ketoacidosis. *Annals of Internal Medicine* 105:836–840.

Niedringhaus, L. (1983): Acute adrenal crisis. *Focus on Critical Care* 10(1):30–36.

Pope, D. W., and Dnasky, D. (1989): Hyperosmolar hyperglycemic nonketotic coma. *Emergency Medical Clinics of North America* 7:849–856.

Roberts, S. L. (1987): *Nursing Diagnosis and the Critically Ill Patient.* Norwalk, CT: Appleton & Lange.

Robinson, A. G. (1984): Acute adrenal insufficiency: Addisonian crisis. *Topics in Emergency Medicine* 5(4):40–44.

Rush, D. R., and Hamburger, S. C. (1980): Drugs used in endocrine metabolic emergencies. *Critical Care Quarterly* 3(2):1–10.

Sanford, S. J. (1988): Endocrine crises and patient care. In: M. G. Kinney, D. R. Packa, and S. B. Dunbar (eds.). *AACN'S Clinical Reference for Critical Care Nursing.* 2nd ed. St Louis: McGraw-Hill, pp. 1088–1110.

Shafrir, S., Bergman, M., and Felig, P. (1987): The endocrine pancreas. Diabetes mellitus. In: P. Felig, J. D. Baxter, A. E. Broadus, and L. A. Frohman (eds.). *Endocrinology and Metabolism.* New York: McGraw-Hill.

Vernoski, G., and Chernow, B. (1983): Steroids: Use and abuse. *Critical Care Quarterly* 6(3):28–38.

Vick, R. L. (1984): *Contemporary Medical Physiology.* Menlo Park, CA: Addison-Wesley.

Watts, N., Gebhart, S., Clark, R., and Phillips, L. (1987): Postoperative management of diabetes mellitus: Steady-state glucose control with bedside algorithm for insulin adjustment. *Diabetes Care* 10:722–728.

References

Bagdade, J. D. (1986): Endocrine emergencies. *Medical Clinics of North America* 70(5):1111–1128.

Butts, D. (1987): Fluid and electrolyte disorders associated with diabetic ketoacidosis and hyperglycemic hyperosmolar nonketotic coma. *Nursing Clinics of North America* 22:827–836.

Gavin, L. A. (1991): Thyroid crisis. *Medical Clinics of North America* 75(1):179–192.

Graves, L. (1990): Diabetic ketoacidosis and hyperosmolar hyperglycemic nonketotic coma. *Critical Care Nursing Quarterly* 13(3):49–61.

Hamburger, S., Rush, D. R., and Bosker, G. (1984): *Endo-*

crine and Metabolic Emergencies. Bowie, MD: Robert J. Brady.

Isley, W. L.: (1990): Thyroid disorders. *Critical Care Nursing Quarterly* 13(3):39–49.

Johnson, D. (1983): Pathophysiology of thyroid storm: Nursing implications. *Critical Care Nurse* 3(6):80–86.

Knowlton, A. I. (1989): Adrenal insufficiency in the critical care setting. *Journal of Intensive Care Medicine* 5(4):35–45.

McChance, K. L., and Huether, S. E. (1990): *Pathophysiology: The Etiologic Basis for Disease in Adults and Children.* St. Louis: C. V. Mosby.

Meek, J. C. (1980): Myxedema coma. *Critical Care Quarterly* 3(2):131–137.

Reasner, C. A. (1990): Adrenal disorders. *Critical Care Nursing Quarterly* 13(3):67–73.

Chapter 15

Nancy C. Molter, R.N., M.N., CCRN
Deborah J. Duncan, R.N., M.S.N., CCRN
Charlotte L. DePew, R.N., M.S.N., CCRN

Burns

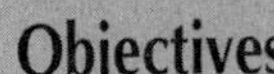

Objectives

- Review anatomy and physiology of the integumentary system.
- Discuss the pathophysiology of burns.
- Compare types of burn injuries.
- Identify assessment during resuscitation and acute phases of burn management.
- Relate nursing diagnoses, outcomes, and interventions for the burned patient.
- Formulate a plan of care for the patient with a burn injury.

Historically, burn injuries have been one of the most lethal forms of trauma. Despite the major advances in burn therapy that have occurred, a patient who is admitted with burn wounds covering more than 50% of the body surface remains at considerable risk. It is estimated that over 500,000 emergency department visits and 70,000 inpatient admissions for burn injuries occur each year in the United States. Approximately 20,000 of the admissions are to hospitals with special capabilities to care for extensive burn injuries ("Hospital," 1990).

The tissue damage that results from a major burn injury elicits a biphasic multiorgan response of early hypofunction followed by later hyperfunction. All organ systems manifest changes in proportion to the extent of injury that are characteristic responses to any severe trauma. Thus, the burn patient can be viewed as the universal trauma model (Pruitt, 1984). Care of such patients requires a team representing a number of disciplines to maximize favorable patient outcomes.

Traditionally, there are three treatment phases of burn care. The resuscitative phase is approximately 48 hours in length, and is the most crucial period for the patient. The primary goal is to prevent shock secondary to changes in capillary dynamics and fluid shifts.

With the onset of diuresis, approximately 48 hours postburn, the acute phase begins, and lasts until wound closure has occurred. This phase may continue for weeks or months. Nursing care focuses on interactions to promote wound healing and prevent complications.

Although the critical care nurse is rarely involved in the rehabilitative phase, the care given

---

The opinions or assertions contained herein are the private views of the authors and are not to be construed as official or as reflecting the views of the U.S. Department of the Army or the U.S. Department of Defense.

in the first two phases is instrumental in the final outcomes achieved with rehabilitation. The primary goal in this phase is to restore the patient's ability to function in society and return to an established family role and vocation.

There is no greater challenge in critical care nursing than to care for a severely burned patient. Even with the expanded network of burn facilities, most patients are seen first in the community hospital. Therefore, it becomes crucial that emergency department and critical care nurses gain the skills necessary to provide resuscitative care to burn-injured patients.

Pathophysiology

ANATOMY AND PHYSIOLOGY OF THE SKIN

The skin is composed of two layers, the epidermis and dermis, with the outer epidermal layer being the thinner of the two (Fig. 15–1). The dermis contains the sweat glands, hair follicles, sebaceous glands, and sensory fibers for pain, pressure, touch, and temperature. The underlying subcutaneous tissue is a layer of connective tissue and fat deposits. The skin (or integumentary system) is the largest organ of the body and is crucial because of its many functions.

There are many physiological and psychological alterations that place the patient in jeopardy when an extensive amount of skin is damaged because of injury. Such alterations in function include loss of body heat, fluids, and thermoregulatory control; loss of protective barriers against infection and sensory contact with the environment; and loss of presentable cosmetic appearance.

DEPTH OF INJURY

The severity of burn injury is dependent on the duration of contact with the injuring agent, the temperature of the agent, the amount of tissue exposed, and the ability of the agent and tissue to dissipate the thermal energy. Although injuries have traditionally been classified as first, second, or third degree, currently they are described as partial-thickness or full-thickness injury.

Partial-thickness injury is subdivided into superficial and deep injury. Superficial partial-thickness injury may only involve the epidermis, such as occurs with a sunburn (first-degree injury), or it may involve a variable portion of the dermis (often termed second-degree injury). A sunburn typically heals in 3 to 5 days. Those burn injuries that cause only erythema and do not involve the dermis are not included for calculation of fluid requirements. Superficial partial-thickness injuries that involve the epidermis and a limited portion of the dermis usually heal within 21 days. Deeper partial-thickness injury involves destruction of the epidermis and most of the dermis, with only the epidermal cells lining

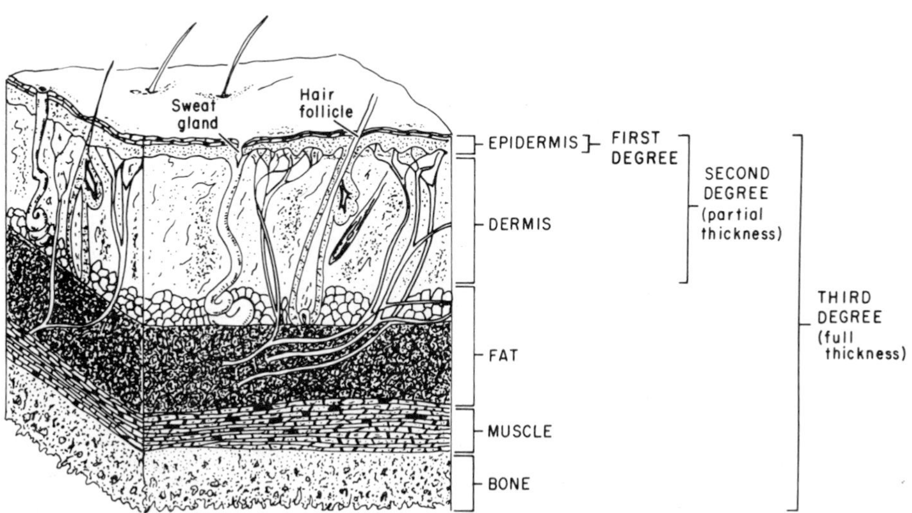

Figure 15–1. Depth of burn injury determines whether a burn will heal or require skin grafting. First- and second-degree burns will heal because they are partial thickness; thus, the elements necessary to generate new skin remain. Full-thickness injury destroys all dermal appendages and requires skin grafting to achieve coverage. (From Kravitz, M.: Thermal injuries. In Cardona, V.D., et al.: Trauma Nursing: From Resuscitation Through Rehabilitation. Philadelphia: W.B. Saunders, 1988, Fig. 28–1, p. 709.)

hair follicles and sweat glands remaining intact. Although such wounds can heal spontaneously within 3 to 6 weeks, they are most often excised and grafted to achieve better functional and cosmetic results, and to decrease the length of healing time and hospitalization.

Destruction of all layers of the skin down to or past the subcutaneous fat, fascia, muscles, and/or bone is defined as a full-thickness injury. The nerves are destroyed, resulting in a painless wound. These injuries always require skin grafting for permanent wound closure. Initially it may be difficult to differentiate partial-thickness from full-thickness injuries particularly in the elderly or in children. Table 15-1 describes the characteristics of partial-thickness and full-thickness burn injuries.

Three zones of thermal injury are used to describe the relationship of tissue effects to severity of injury and ultimate viability of the injured tissue (Fig. 15-2). The greatest area of tissue necrosis is central in the wound. Peripheral to this area is a zone of stasis where vascular damage and potentially reversible tissue injury have occurred. Without adequate resuscitation, this area may progress to tissue death. The area of minimal injury is termed the zone of hyperemia, and is similar to a superficial partial-thickness burn.

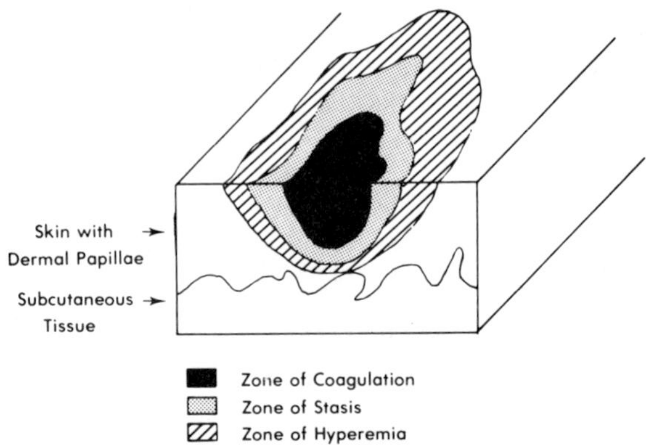

Figure 15-2. Zones of thermal injury. The zone of coagulation is the site of irreversible skin death. The zone of hyperemia is the site of minimal cell involvement and early spontaneous recovery. In the zone of stasis, infection or drying of the wound results in conversion of this potentially salvageable area to full-thickness skin destruction with irreversible cell death. (Modified from Zawacki, B.: *Ann. Surg.* 180:98, 1974.)

PHYSIOLOGICAL ALTERATIONS

Local Response

Significant hemodynamic, metabolic, and immunological effects occur locally and systemically as a result of cellular injury by heat. The release of cellular enzymes and vasoactive substances, as well as the activation of complement, result in altered vascular permeability. There is a significant shift of protein molecules, fluid, and electrolytes at the capillary level from the intravascular space to the extravascular space owing to the increased membrane permeability of the vessels. Cellular swelling may also occur secondary to a decrease in cell transmembrane potential with a shift of extracellular sodium and water into the cell (Demling, 1987). In addition, the leaking of serum proteins eventually decreases or ceases the lymph flow as a result of blockage of the lymphatic vessels (Pruitt, 1984; Pruitt and Goodwin, 1987).

In extensive burn injury (>25% total body surface area, TBSA), the edema occurs in both burned and unburned areas from the increase in capillary permeability and hypoproteinemia (Arturson, 1961), and/or as a result of the volume and oncotic pressure effects of the large fluid re-

Table 15-1. DEPTH OF BURN INJURY

Degree of Injury	Morphology	Healing Time	Characteristics of Wound
Superficial Partial-Thickness (First Degree)	Epidermal destruction only	Approximately 5 days	Red, dry, painful; blisters rarely present
Superficial Partial-Thickness (Second Degree)	Destruction of epidermis and some dermis	Within 21 days	Moist pink or mottled red, painful, blisters
Deep Partial-Thickness (Second Degree)	Destruction of epidermis and dermis; some skin appendages remain	Within 3-6 weeks	Pale, mottled, pearly white, mostly dry; often insensate; difficult to differentiate from full-thickness injury
Full-Thickness Injury (Third Degree)	Destruction of epidermis, dermis, and underlying subcutaneous tissue	Requires skin grafting	Thick, leathery eschar; white, cherry-red, or brown-black in color; insensate; blood vessels thrombosed; dry

suscitation volumes required (Mason, 1980). The magnitude of the response is proportionate to the extent of injury. Maximum edema is seen 18 to 24 hours postburn, and with adequate resuscitation, the transmembrane potential is restored within 24 to 36 hours (Pruitt, 1984; Pruitt and Goodwin, 1987).

Systemic Response

All organ systems are affected in burn injury with the response manifested by a biphasic hypofunction-hyperfunction pattern. The degree of physiological change is proportionate to the extent of burn and reaches a maximum response in patients with burns over 50% TBSA. When the wound heals or is closed, organ function returns to normal (Pruitt and Goodwin, 1987). Specific organ system response is summarized as follows.

Cardiovascular Response. Redistribution of blood flow occurs early in the postburn period to perfuse essential viscera in association with a decreased cardiac output and increased peripheral resistance. Arterial blood pressure is maintained by the catecholamine-induced vasoconstrictive response producing the increased peripheral resistance. With adequate fluid resuscitation, cardiac output is normalized toward the end of the first 24 hours postburn and becomes supranormal thereafter until the burn is closed (Pruitt and Goodwin, 1987).

Host Defense Mechanisms. With the loss of skin, the primary barrier to microorganisms is gone. The mechanism for many of the immune defects that occur with extensive burn injury remains unclear. However, most authorities suggest that complex interactions of several factors that include nutrition, hypermetabolism, and immunological alterations may be caused by either an altered host environment or an injury-induced host deficiency state or both. The end result is overstimulation of suppressor T cells, complement activation, and a depression of other components such as T-helper cell and T-killer cell activity and polymorphonuclear leukocyte activity (Warden, 1987).

Pulmonary Response. With any major burn, there is an initial transient pulmonary hypertension that may be associated with a modest decrease in oxygen tension and lung compliance resulting from the release of vasoconstrictive agents (Pruitt and Goodwin, 1987). Lung injury, secondary to the inhalation of smoke and products of incomplete combustion, causes an age- and burn size-related increase in mortality above that due to burn injury alone (Shirani et al., 1987). Inhalation injury is classified as (1) injury from carbon monoxide, (2) injury above the glottis, and (3) injury below the glottis (Nebraska Burn Institute, 1989). Table 15-2 summarizes characteristics of each type of injury. Inhalation injury may be the cause of admission to a burn unit even when there are no surface burns.

Renal Response. The biphasic renal response manifests as an initial oliguria secondary to a decreased plasma flow and glomerular filtration rate, followed by a diuresis secondary to an increase in cardiac output. The diuresis may be modest because of the slow mobilization of edema fluid and the increased evaporative water loss that occurs with the loss of skin (Pruitt and Goodwin, 1987).

Gastrointestinal Response. An ileus usually occurs secondary to hypovolemia and the neurological/endocrine responses to injury. Mucosal erosion and eventual ulceration may occur if the gastric mucosa is not protected with antacids and/or H_2 histamine receptor antagonists (Pruitt and Goodwin, 1987).

Metabolic Response. Hypermetabolism begins as resuscitation is completed, and is one of the most significant alterations after burn injury. The rapid metabolic rate is probably mediated by the secretion of catecholamines, and is required to support wound healing. Peak hypermetabolic rates are reached between the sixth and tenth postburn days. The amount of protein wasting and weight loss that occurs is affected by several factors: percent body surface burned, age, sex, preburn nutritional status, other health problems,

Table 15–2. TYPES OF SMOKE INHALATION INJURY

Type of Injury	Pathology
Carbon Monoxide Poisoning	Carbon monoxide binds to hemoglobin molecules more rapidly than oxygen molecules; tissue hypoxia results
Inhalation Injury Above the Glottis	Most often a thermal injury. Most heat absorption and damage occurs in the pharynx and larynx; may cause obstruction after resuscitation is initiated
Inhalation Injury Below the Glottis	Usually a chemical injury that produces impaired ciliary activity, erythema, hypersecretion, edema, ulceration of mucosa, increased blood flow, and spasm of bronchi/bronchioles

Compiled from material from the Advanced Burn Life Support course manual. Nebraska Burn Institute, Lincoln, NE, 1989.

and nutrient intake. When the wound is closed, oxygen consumption, protein mass, and weight begin to return to normal (Wilmore, 1987).

TYPES OF BURN INJURIES

A variety of injuries involving thermal trauma can result from heat, cold, electric current, and/or chemical agents. The focus of this chapter is on injuries resulting from heat to include electric and chemical burns. A limited discussion of care required for patients with toxic epidermal necrolysis is included since the extensive loss of skin that can occur with this condition may necessitate admission to a burn unit for specialized wound care.

Thermal Injuries

A heat source of less than 44°C (111.2°F) will not cause a burn regardless of the length of exposure. The extent of damage increases with temperatures above this level in direct proportion to the duration of exposure. Full-thickness injury occurs when sufficient heat is applied to cause protein coagulation and cell death (Pruitt and Goodwin, 1987). Exposure to temperatures of 140°F (60°C) (which is the common setting of home water heaters) will cause tissue destruction in as little as 3 to 5 seconds. Children and the elderly may be at greater risk for thermal injury from lower temperatures owing to their thinner skin and decreased agility in moving to avoid harm.

Chemical Injuries

Although chemical injuries account for only a small percentage of admissions to burn centers, they can be severe, causing both local and systemic effects. The severity of injury is related to the type of agent, concentration of agent, duration of contact, and volume of agent. Chemical agents are part of our lifestyle, thus the potential for injury from exposure is great. Unlike flame or scald injuries, tissue damage continues until the chemical is completely removed or neutralized. There are three categories of chemical agents: alkalies, acids, and organic compounds.

Commonly found in cleaning products used in the home and industry, alkalies produce liquefaction necrosis with loosening of tissue, allowing the chemical to diffuse more deeply into the tissue. Therefore, this category of chemical agents can produce far more damage than acids.

Acids are also found in many household and industrial products such as bathroom cleansers, rust removers, and acidifiers for home swimming pools. Acids cause coagulation necrosis of tissue with precipitation of protein.

Organic compounds such as phenols and petroleum products can produce chemical burns as well as systemic effects. Phenols cause severe coagulation necrosis. In addition, systemic effects such as central nervous system depression, hypothermia, hypotension, pulmonary edema, and intravascular hemolysis may be severe and can lead to shock and death. The solvent properties of hydrocarbons such as gasoline promote cell membrane injury and dissolution of lipids with resulting skin necrosis. Chemical pneumonitis and bronchitis may occur as a result of hydrocarbon excretion from the lungs. Other complications observed with gasoline inhalation include hepatic and renal damage and sudden death (Mozingo, et al., 1988; Nebraska Burn Institute, 1989).

Electrical Injury

Electrical injury is caused by contact with such varied sources as household current, car batteries, electrosurgical devices, high-tension electric lines, or lightning. Injuries are arbitrarily classified as high voltage (>1000 volts) or low voltage (<1000 volts) (Nebraska Burn Institute, 1989; Pruitt, 1988).

Tissue damage is the result of the electrical energy being converted into heat. Many factors can affect the degree of injury to include type of current, pathway of current, duration of contact, environmental conditions, and resistance offered by body tissues. The least resistance is in nerve tissue and the greatest is in bone tissue. Current density, and thus the greatest heat, is at the point of entry or exit, which is often on the extremities. Injuries of the trunk are not as frequent. Although alternating and direct currents are both dangerous, alternating current has a greater probability of producing cardiopulmonary arrest, and has a tetanic effect which may "lock" the patient to the source of electricity. As high-voltage current ceases, the superficial tissues begin to cool more rapidly than the deeper tissues. Therefore, it is not unusual to see deep tissue necrosis beneath viable more superficial tissue. All patients with electrical injury should be monitored closely for cardiac dysrhythmias. There are many other severe complications related to electrical injury, which are summarized in Table 15-3 (Pruitt, 1988; Pruitt and Goodwin, 1987).

The mechanism of lightning injury is by a direct strike or side flash causing a flow of current between the person and a close object struck by lightning (Nebraska Burn Institute, 1989). Often cutaneous injury is superficial since the current travels on the surface of the body rather than through it. Lightning injuries frequently result in cardiopulmonary arrest as well as transient but severe central nervous system deficits (Nebraska Burn Institute, 1989; Pruitt, 1988; Pruitt and Goodwin, 1987).

Nonburn Injuries

Toxic Epidermal Necrolysis (TEN). This is an exfoliative dermatitis usually associated with mucosal involvement of conjunctival, oral, and/or urogenital areas. The most common etiology is a reaction to drugs, particularly sulfa, phenobarbital, and phenytoin (Heimbach et al., 1987). In some cases there is no apparent etiologic agent.

Staphylococcal Scalded Skin. This is caused by a reaction to staphylococcal toxin, and often presents with a clinical picture similar to TEN. There is a low mortality (5%), with skin slough occurring as a result of intraepidermal "splitting." In contrast, TEN is associated with a high mortality (25-50%), with the epidermal "split" occurring at the dermal/epidermal junction. The differential and/or definitive diagnosis is made by microscopic examination of the denuded skin to determine the level of skin separation (Pruitt, 1987a).

Although the massive fluid shifts seen in thermal injury do not occur with TEN, immune suppression does occur and contributes to the life-threatening complications of sepsis and pneumonia (Pruitt, 1987a). Patients present with fever and flulike symptoms, with the development of erythema and blisters occurring within 24 to 96 hours. As large bullae develop, the skin and mucous membranes slough, often resulting in significant and painful partial-thickness injury. Admission to a burn unit is advisable to ensure proper wound management (Heimbach et al., 1987).

Table 15-3. COMPLICATIONS OF ELECTRIC INJURY

Complication	Cause
Early Death	Cardiopulmonary arrest
Oliguria	Inadequate fluid resuscitation based on small surface injury
Acute Renal Failure	Hemochromogens in small volume of urine
Hyperkalemia	Muscle destruction
Deep Tissue Necrosis	Direct effect of electric current
Neurologic Deficits	Direct or delayed effect of current
Cataract Formation	Immediate or delayed effect of current
Cholelithiasis	Unknown

Adapted from Pruitt, B. A., Jr., and Goodwin, C. W., Jr.: Burn injury. *In:* Moore, E. F. (ed.): *Early Care of the Injured Patient.* 4th ed. St. Louis: C. V. Mosby, 1990, p. 301.

Assessment

The critical care nurse must assess indices of essential organ function to prevent complications in patients with major thermal injury. Initially, monitoring occurs frequently to evaluate changes in the patient's condition that may occur rapidly during fluid resuscitation. Assessment in the resuscitative and acute care phases must focus on early detection or prevention of the following problems.

RESUSCITATIVE PHASE

Respiratory. Upper and lower airway edema; pulmonary insufficiency; decreased lung compliance.

Cardiovascular. Decreased cardiac output in first 24 hours; low central venous pressure and pulmonary artery wedge pressure; significant alterations in vital signs reflective of hypovolemia and the neuroendocrine response to injury; absence of peripheral pulses in extremities with circumferential burns.

Neurological. Decreased level of consciousness reflective of hypoxemia and/or hypovolemia.

Blood, Fluid, and Electrolytes. Loss of plasma volume; hyponatremia; hyperkalemia; hemoconcentration (typically blood hematocrit values are in a range of 50 to 55%); hypoproteinemia; hyperglycemia (except in children who do not have adequate glycogen stores and may become hypoglycemic).

Renal. Oliguria (without adequate resuscitation.)

Gastrointestinal. Absent bowel sounds—ileus.

Integumentary. Edema in burned and nonburned tissue.

Psychosocial. Extreme patient/family anxiety, combative behavior, severe pain (with partial-thickness injury).

ACUTE PHASE

Respiratory. Tachypnea, dyspnea, abnormal breath sounds, purulent secretions.

Cardiovascular. Dysrhythmias, hypertension or hypotension.

Neurological. Restlessness, confusion, lethargy.

Blood, Fluid, and Electrolytes. Hyponatremia (usually resolves in 1 week); hypernatremia (most commonly due to inadequate replacement of evaporative water loss); hypokalemia; hypoproteinemia; negative nitrogen balance; metabolic acidosis; leukopenia (usually from silver sulfadiazine); hyperchloremic metabolic acidosis (from mafenide acetate); hyperglycemia (from infection or excessive carbohydrate loading); increase in white blood cells (from infection); prolonged coagulation times and fall in platelet count (from infection).

Renal. Excessive diuresis (postburn diuresis should be moderate); glycosuria (sign of early sepsis or preclinical diabetes).

Gastrointestinal. Stress ulcers; inability to maintain gastric pH levels above 5 (sign of impending sepsis).

Integumentary. Temperature should be between 99 and 101°F—hyperthermia or hypothermia may indicate sepsis or extensive loss of heat from open wounds or those in wet dressings; wound biopsies indicative of bacterial or fungal invasion.

Psychosocial. Manipulation, regression, sleep deprivation, pain and pruritus, inability of patient to cope, family inability to cope and provide patient support.

■ Nursing Diagnoses

RESUSCITATIVE PHASE

1. Ineffective airway clearance related to tracheal edema secondary to inhalation injury.
2. Impaired gas exchange related to interstitial edema manifested by hypoxemia and hypercapnia.
3. Fluid volume deficit secondary to fluid shifts to the interstitium and evaporative loss of fluids from the injured skin.
4. Disturbance in acid-base balance related to anaerobic metabolism secondary to decreased tissue perfusion.
5. Tissue injury related to impaired vascular perfusion in extremities with circumferential burns manifested by decreased or absent peripheral pulses.
6. Potential for infection related to loss of integument and invasive therapy. (Continues into acute care phase until wounds are closed.)
7. Disturbance in bowel motility related to decreased perfusion secondary to hypovolemia.
8. Potential for hypothermia related to injury of skin and external cooling. (Continues into acute care phase.)
9. Disturbance in comfort: Acute pain related to burn trauma. (Continues into acute care phase.)
10. Potential for injury related to stress response manifested by GI hemorrhage and hyperglycemia. (Must begin monitoring and prophylaxis treatment in resuscitative phase; continues in acute care phase.)
11. Potential for ineffective individual/family coping related to acute stress of injury and potential life-threatening crisis. (Continues in acute care phase.)

ACUTE CARE PHASE

12. Alteration in fluid and electrolyte balance related to diuresis and/or evaporative water loss.
13. Increased metabolic rate related to elevated catecholamine levels associated with catabolism and weight loss.
14. Impaired skin integrity related to burn wound and potential impairment due to immobility required to promote graft adherence.
15. Potential nutritional deficit related to increased metabolic demands secondary to wound healing.
16. Impaired physical mobility and self-care deficit related to therapeutic splinting and/or contractures.
17. Alteration in family processes related to acute illness and potential lifestyle/family role changes.
18. Knowledge deficit related to discharge goals.

Interventions: Resuscitative and Acute Care Phases

PREHOSPITAL INTERVENTION

The first priority of care in the prehospital setting is to stop the burning process, while preventing further injury to the patient and injury to self (Nebraska Burn Institute, 1989; Pruitt and Goodwin, 1990). Flame burns may be extinguished by rolling the patient on the ground, smothering the flames with a blanket or other cover, or dousing the flames with water. The patient should be kept in a supine position as flames may otherwise spread to the upper parts of the body causing more extensive injury. Scald burns and tar/asphalt burns should be treated by immediate cooling with water if available, and/or immediate removal of the saturated clothing. Clothing that is burned into the skin should not be removed, as increased tissue damage and bleeding may occur. No attempt should be made to remove the tar at the scene.

Chemical injuries differ from thermal injuries in that the burning process continues as long as the chemical is in contact with the skin. All clothing, including gloves and shoes, should immediately be removed from the patient and water lavage should be instituted prior to and during transport. Powdered chemicals should first be brushed from the clothing and skin prior to lavage. Chemical burns of the eye should be initially irrigated with water or physiologic saline at the scene of injury with lavage continuing during transport to the emergency department. Cross contamination of the opposite eye should be avoided during lavage. When neutralizing agents come in contact with chemicals, the increased heat production that occurs could further increase the depth of injury. Therefore, no attempt should be made to use such agents.

Immediate treatment for electrical injuries involves prompt removal of the patient from the electrical source while protecting the rescuer. Thermal injury can also occur if clothing is ignited.

As with any other type of trauma, the next priority at the scene of injury is to complete a primary survey of the ABCs of patient management (airway, breathing, circulation, and C-spine) (Nebraska Burn Institute, 1989; Pruitt and Goodwin, 1990) (Fig. 15–3). After a burn injury, patients are normally alert. If they become confused or combative, some degree of hypoxia may be the etiology. Hypoxia occurs with inhalation injuries, or may occur after an electrical injury secondary to tetanic contractions of the respiratory muscles. Table 15–4 summarizes specific clinical findings that may be indicative of respiratory injury. All patients with suspected smoke inhalation should be treated at the scene with 100% humidified oxygen delivered by face mask. If the patient exhibits respiratory stridor indicative of airway obstruction, endotracheal intubation should occur at the scene.

Burn injury rarely results in hypovolemic shock in the early prehospital phase. If evidence of shock is present, then associated internal or external injury must be suspected. Cardiac arrest is a common complication of high-voltage electrical injury, necessitating the institution of cardiopulmonary resuscitation. Peripheral pulses should be assessed, especially in circumferential burns of the extremities, to confirm adequate circulation. All restrictive clothing and jewelry should be removed and secured to prevent constriction and possible ischemia to distal extremities secondary to edema formation during resuscitation.

Potential spinal injury should be evaluated at the scene prior to moving the patient. Patients with electrical injuries are at especially high risk for compression fractures due to tetanic contractions of the paravertebral muscles, or fractures as a result of falls. Transport of the patient should occur only after placement on a back board with cervical collar applied.

A rapid head-to-toe assessment should be completed as part of the secondary survey to rule out any additional trauma (Fig. 15–4). An accurate history of the events that led to the burn injury should be obtained, to include date and time of injury, source of burns, and any events leading to the injury. Often the patient is the most alert during this postinjury period; therefore, obtaining a brief medical history, including allergies, current medical problems and medications taken, past surgeries and/or trauma, time of last meal, history of tetanus immunization, and current weight, is beneficial (Nebraska Burn Institute, 1989).

In preparation for transport, the burned patient should be covered with a clean, dry sheet and blankets to prevent further contamination of the wounds and prevent hypothermia. Heat loss occurs very rapidly in a major burn injury as the

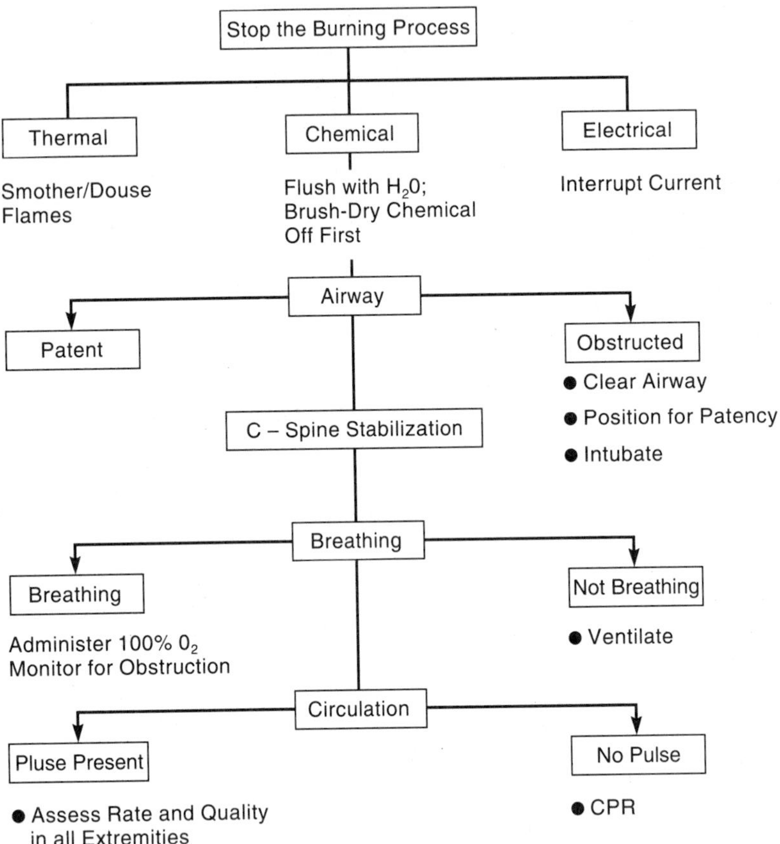

Figure 15-3. Major burn injury—primary survey.

protective covering of skin is lost, allowing heat to escape. Ice should never be applied to the wounds, since further tissue damage may occur as a result of vasoconstriction and hypothermia. Intravenous therapy is not required unless the patient is greater than 45 minutes from the emergency department, or unless other associated injuries resulting in hemorrhage are present. Narcotics should be avoided during prehospital treatment because they may decrease the blood pressure, depress respirations, and prevent the accurate assessment of level of consciousness. The patient should remain NPO prior to and during transport to prevent vomiting and aspiration. Vital signs should be monitored enroute to the nearest appropriate hospital (Pruitt and Goodwin, 1990).

Table 15-4. RESPIRATORY INJURY: CLINICAL INDICATORS IN BURN PATIENTS

Facial burns
Presence of soot around mouth, nose, and in sputum, singed nasal hairs
Signs of hypoxemia (tachycardia, dysrhythmias, anxiety, lethargy)
Signs of respiratory difficulty (change in respiratory rate, use of acessory muscles for breathing, intercostal or sternal retractions, stridor, hoarseness)
Abnormal breath sounds
Abnormal blood gas values

EMERGENCY DEPARTMENT INTERVENTION—RESUSCITATIVE PHASE

Upon arrival at the emergency department, the ABCs of patient management should be reassessed. If the patient is already intubated, check for accurate tube position. Ensure that the endotracheal tube is securely tied in place with umbilical or tracheostomy cloth ties to prevent accidental extubation (Gordon, 1987a) (Fig. 15-5). This is especially important with young children,

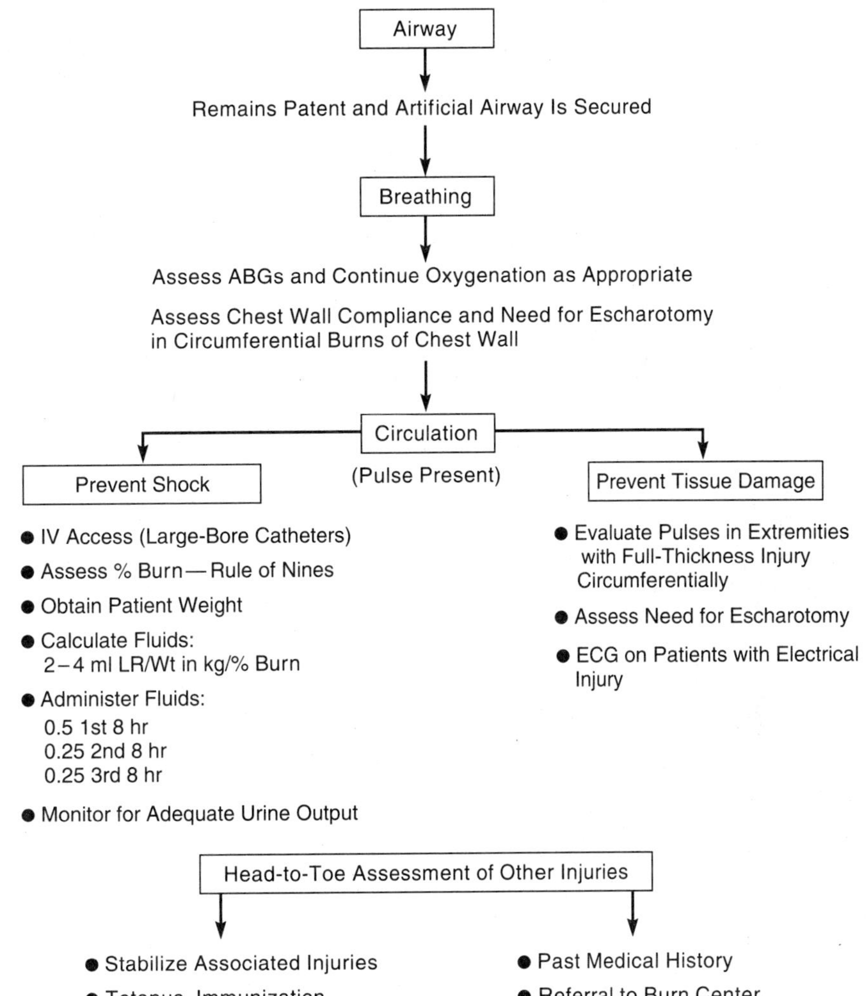

Figure 15–4. Major burn injury—secondary survey.

who often require the use of uncuffed endotracheal tubes. If the patient has a circumferential full-thickness burn of the thorax, assess for adequate ventilatory effort because edema may inhibit chest wall expansion. Young children with a more pliable thoracic wall are more prone to this complication and an immediate chest wall escharotomy may be indicated to facilitate breathing.

Special attention should be given to circumferential full-thickness burns of the extremities. Pressure from the edema that develops as resuscitation proceeds may impair blood flow to underlying and distal tissue. Peripheral pulses should be palpated or auscultated with an ultrasonic flow meter (doppler) every hour, and upper extremities should be elevated above the level of the heart. Preparation should be made for an escharotomy to relieve the pressure if pulses are absent or progressively decrease on serial examination. A fasciotomy may be indicated for deep electrical burns or when severe muscle damage has occurred. If not yet removed, it is imperative that all jewelry and constrictive clothing be removed and secured to prevent further injury as edema develops.

In determining fluid resuscitation requirements, the depth and extent of injury must be estimated. The quickest method to initially calculate the extent of injury is by using the Rule of Nines (Fig. 15–6), which recognizes that in the adult the surface area of various anatomical parts represents 9%, or a multiple thereof, of the total body surface area. The Rule of Nines varies between adult and pediatric patients owing to the

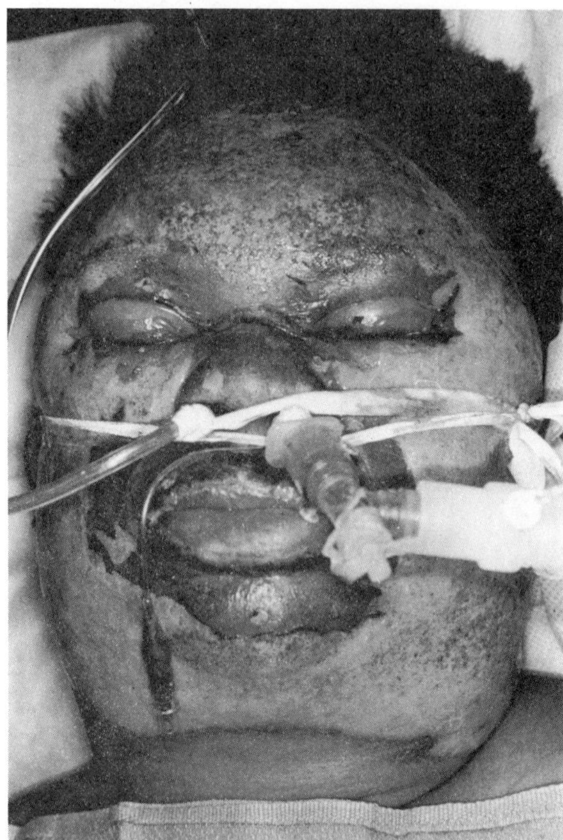

Figure 15-5. Facial edema. The massive edema that develops during fluid resuscitation in a major burn victim can lead to potential complications unless closely monitored by the critical care nurse. All facial tubes such as endotracheal and nasogastric tubes should be secured with the use of cloth ties to prevent dislodgement. Care must be taken to prevent ties from placing pressure on burned ear.

significant difference in the proportion of surface area of the head in children compared to adults. In evaluating the extent of injury in small, isolated burns, the Rule of the Palm may be used, whereby the size of the patient's palm equals 1% of his or her total body surface area. A surface area chart, such as the Lund and Browder with Berkow formula (Fig. 15-7), correlates body surface area with age, providing a more accurate determination of the extent of burn injury.

If the patient has a burn injury greater than 20% of the body surface area, at least one, and preferably two, large-bore (#16 or #18 gauge) intravenous catheters should be inserted peripherally in an unburned area of the extremities if possible. They must be well secured. Ensure that the catheters are not placed distal to circumferential burns. Central lines should not be used unless other options are not available, and should be placed in a femoral vein if required. Infuse Ringer's lactate at 500 ml/hr initially (Pruitt and Goodwin, 1987). Number all solution containers sequentially and begin recording intake and output as soon as possible. An indwelling urethral catheter should be inserted to monitor hourly urinary output. Baseline laboratory studies to include a CBC, serum electrolytes, creatinine, glucose, blood urea nitrogen (BUN), arterial blood gas values (ABGs), carboxyhemoglobin level (if inhalation injury is suspected), and urinalysis should be obtained.

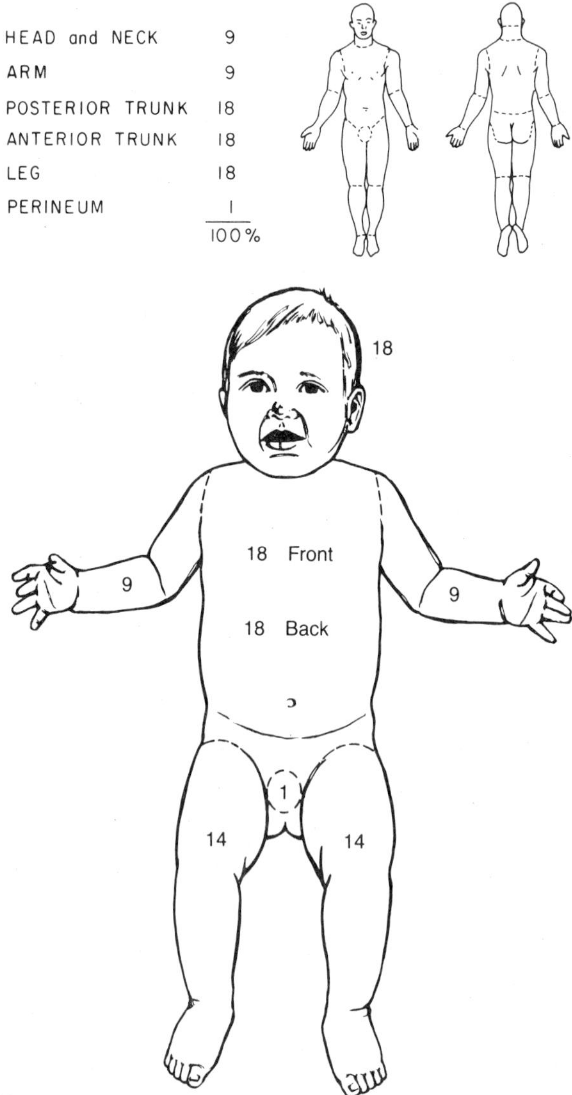

Figure 15-6. The Rule of Nines is a commonly used assessment tool that permits rapid estimation of the size of extent of burn injury. Small children and infants have a proportionately larger head size related to lower extremities, therefore an adjusted Rule of Nines is required.

BURN ESTIMATE AND DIAGRAM

AGE vs. AREA

AREA	Birth 1 yr	1 – 4 yr	5 – 9 yr	10 – 14 yr	15 yr	Adult	2°	3°	Total	Donor Areas
Head	19	17	13	11	9	7				
Neck	2	2	2	2	2	2				
Ant. Trunk	13	13	13	13	13	13				
Post. Trunk	13	13	13	13	13	13				
R. Buttock	2½	2½	2½	2½	2½	2½				
L. Buttock	2½	2½	2½	2½	2½	2½				
Genitalia	1	1	1	1	1	1				
R.U. Arm	4	4	4	4	4	4				
L.U. Arm	4	4	4	4	4	4				
R.L. Arm	3	3	3	3	3	3				
L.L. Arm	3	3	3	3	3	3				
R. Hand	2½	2½	2½	2½	2½	2½				
L. Hand	2½	2½	2½	2½	2½	2½				
R. Thigh	5½	6½	8	8½	9	9½				
L. Thigh	5½	6½	8	8½	9	9½				
R. Leg	5	5	5½	6	6½	7				
L. Leg	5	5	5½	6	6½	7				
R. Foot	3½	3½	3½	3½	3½	3½				
L. Foot	3½	3½	3½	3½	3½	3½				
						TOTAL				

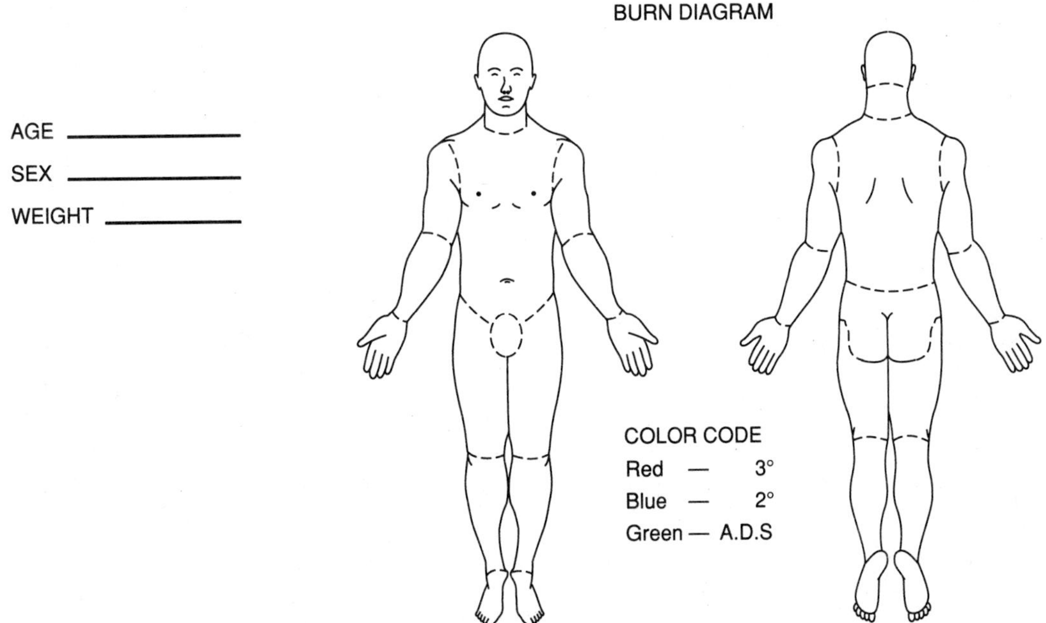

Figure 15-7. Burn estimate and diagram. The form depicted was developed and is used by the US Army Institute of Surgical Research. Based on the Lund and Browder chart with Berkow formula, it allows for more accurate assessment of extent of burn injury based on age and depth of injury.

Appropriate fluid resuscitation requirements for burned patients are estimated according to body weight in kilograms, percentage of total body surface area (TBSA) burned, and age. The Consensus Fluid Formula outlined in Table 15–5 specifies the fluid requirements for adults and children during the initial 24 hours postburn (Nebraska Burn Institute, 1989). One-half of the calculated amount is given over the first 8 hours postinjury, and the second half is given over the next 16 hours. The estimated fluid requirements serve only as a guide to start resuscitation. Actual infusion rates will be titrated to ensure a urinary output of 30 to 50 ml/hr in adults and 1 ml/kg body weight/hr in children less than 30 kg. Children require relatively more resuscitation fluid because they have a greater body surface area to mass ratio than adults. They also may require additional maintenance fluid, which will be calculated by the physician (Nebraska Burn Institute, 1989; Pruitt and Goodwin, 1990).

Patients with high-voltage electrical burns or crush injuries may require larger volumes of resuscitation fluids owing to the hemochromogens released as a result of severe deep tissue damage, which often is not apparent. Urinary output for these patients should be maintained at 75 to 100 ml/hr (Nebraska Burn Institute, 1989; Pruitt, 1988; Pruitt and Goodwin, 1990). After the initial 24 hr postburn, as capillary permeability returns to normal, the fluid requirements change and colloids are commonly administered.

A chest film should be obtained upon admission to the emergency department, and other x-rays will be ordered as indicated by the patient's condition. Spinal precautions are continued until all seven cervical vertebrae are clearly visualized on x-ray with no evidence of injury. An electrocardiogram is done on admission with serial evaluations ordered for patients with electrical injuries (Nebraska Burn Institute, 1989).

Because patients with a major burn injury generally develop an ileus, a nasogastric tube is inserted and connected to low suction to prevent aspiration. The medical history and history of the injury should be conveyed to the medical team, and the patient should receive tetanus immunization if indicated. A short-acting narcotic such as morphine sulfate may be administered by an intravenous route only for pain relief. No intramuscular medications should be given during the resuscitative phase because of poor perfusion of edematous tissues. As fluid is later mobilized, medication poorly absorbed from edematous tissue may reenter the blood stream and lead to an overdose (Pruitt and Goodwin, 1987, 1990).

Table 15–5. FLUID RESUSCITATION FOR BURN PATIENTS

First 24 Hours

- Consensus Formula
  - Adults: 2–4 ml LR/kg wt/% burn
  - Children: 3 ml LR/kg wt/% burn
- 1st 8 hr postburn: administer 0.5 of total fluids
- 2nd 8 hr: administer 0.25 of total fluids
- 3rd 8 hr: administer 0.25 of total fluids
- Use glucose-containing fluid if child develops hypoglycemia. Titrate fluids to maintain urine output of 30–50 ml/hr in adults and 1 ml/kg/hr in children weighing <30 kg
- EXAMPLE: (Using 2 ml value; 50% burn; 70 g: 2 ml × 50 × 70 = 7000 ml of LR in 24 hours. Administer 3500 ml in first 8 hr postburn.

Second 24 Hours Postburn

- Albumin diluted to physiologic concentration in saline: 0.3–0.5 ml/kg/% Burn
- Adults: administer electrolyte free water to meet metabolic needs and maintain urinary output.
- Children: administer 5% glucose in half-normal saline to meet metabolic needs, maintain urinary output, and prevent hypoglycemia.

PREPARATION FOR TRANSFER TO A BURN CENTER

Caring for a patient who has sustained a major burn injury requires the availability and expertise of a specially trained multidisciplinary health care team. Factors such as the patient's age, health status, extent and depth of burn, and body part burned will significantly influence the severity of the injury. Small hospitals may not have the personnel or medical supplies needed to provide the specialized care that these patients require. The American Burn Association has developed guidelines to determine which burn injury patients should be referred to a specialized burn center

Table 15–6. GUIDELINES FOR BURN CENTER REFERRAL

- >5% total body surface area (TBSA) of full-thickness injury
- Partial-thickness and full-thickness burns involving:
  - 10% TBSA: <10 years of age or >50 years of age
  - 20% TBSA: All other ages
- Burns involving: face, hands/feet, genitalia, perineum, major joints
- Electric and chemical burns
- Presence of inhalation injury
- Preexisting chronic disease
- Associated trauma

after initial stabilization has occurred ("Hospital," 1990; Nebraska Burn Institute, 1989) (Table 15–6).

Once the patient is examined and transfer to a burn center is considered, the attending physician must make direct contact with a burn center physician. The burn center physician will determine the mode of transportation and treatment necessary to stabilize the patient for transport (Treat et al., 1980). Accurate and timely communication between the staff at both facilities is essential and can be facilitated with the use of a patient transfer information sheet (Fig. 15–8).

Safety is the prime concern during any type of transport. In either ground or aeromedical transport, environmental noise, vibration, poor lighting, limited space, and poor temperature control make emergency procedures, control of changes in patient condition, and management of supportive equipment difficult. To minimize risks, the following safeguards should be considered:

- Transfer should be expedited as soon as physiological stability has occurred to reduce hazards of complications that may surface later in postinjury management (Pruitt and Goodwin, 1990; Treat et al., 1980).
- Pulmonary and cardiac insufficiency, significant gastrointestinal bleeding, and hyperthermia exceeding 39.4°C are all con-

U. S. ARMY INSTITUTE OF SURGICAL RESEARCH

PATIENT TRANSFER INFORMATION SHEET

Date and time of call ______
Referring MD ______ Telephone ______
Hospital ______ City ______ State ______

PATIENT INFORMATION

Name ______ SSN ______ Status: Active Duty ______
Retired ______
Age ______ Sex ______ Pre-Burn Weight ______ Dependent ______
VAB/BEC ______
Date of burn ______ Cause ______ PHS ______
Civilian ______
Extent of burn ______ 3rd Degree ______
Areas burned ______
Inhalation Injury ______ Allergies ______
Association injury ______
Pre-existing diseases ______

TREATMENT CHECK-LIST

Resuscitation: Calculated need (2ml/Kg/% TBS) ______
Fluid in ______ Urine Output ______
Airway ______ Blood gases ______ E-T tube ______
Medication: Analgesics or sedatives ______ Tetanus ______
Antibiotics ______ Other Meds ______
Escharotomies: Arms ______ Legs ______ Chest ______
Wound Care: Wash and debride ______ Topical Agent ______
Lab tests: HCT ______ Electrolytes ______ BS ______ BUN ______
Request: Insert NG tube- Avoid general anesthesia or IM meds - Keep I&)

INFORMATION FOR FLIGHT PLAN

Burn Team ______ Family to accompany patient ______
Location of nearest airport with jet traffic ______
Transportation for team at destination ______

Figure 15–8. U.S. Army Institute of Surgical Research Transfer Information Form. The use of a transfer information form to summarize information concerning a burn patient's status promotes good communication between the referring and receiving facilities and ensures continuity of care.

traindications to transport and should be controlled or corrected before the patient is moved (Pruitt and Goodwin, 1990).

- Trained personnel with essential equipment for safe transport should be available to adequately monitor and manage resuscitation enroute (Pruitt and Goodwin, 1990; Treat et al., 1980).

To minimize complications during transport, the nurse has a vital role in assessing the patient based on the following guidelines prior to transport:

1. A secure, patent airway is present, with adequate gas exchange occurring. The endotracheal tube must be secured. If the tracheostomy tape is tied with a bow knot, it can be adjusted to accommodate facial edema. Chest x-rays are done to rule out pulmonary disease and pneumothorax and to ensure proper tube placement (Pruitt and Goodwin, 1990). A Heimlich valve is attached to a chest tube replacing the water seal drainage bottle. The ABGs are within acceptable limits on supplemental oxygen therapy. Suction and ventilation equipment are available at all times.
2. Adequate circulatory support is established. Administration of resuscitation fluids and monitoring of response must continue during transport. Intravenous lines are secured by sutures with connections taped. Only plastic solution containers are used. The indwelling urethral catheter is anchored to prevent accidental displacement. Strong pulses must be present in all extremities with circumferential burns, with or without escharotomies.
3. Mechanisms to prevent aspiration are initiated. The patient with a major burn is at significant risk for emesis and aspiration during transport. Correct nasogastric tube placement should be ensured and the patient should not receive any oral intake.
4. Thermoregulation is monitored. If the patient is transported within the first 12 hours postburn, the burn wounds should not be cleansed and covered with a topical antimicrobial agent. Wounds are covered with a clean dry sheet or wrapped with a nonconstrictive gauze dressing. To minimize heat loss, wrap the patient in blankets and remove during transport if hyperthermia develops. Adequate absorbent padding is needed under the patient to accommodate large volume plasma leakage from the burn wounds and prevent pressure breakdown of skin.
5. Maintain comfort with adequate pain control. Morphine sulfate can cause nausea; therefore, careful evaluation is necessary during transport. If the patient is properly wrapped and kept warm, pain is minimized.
6. Stabilize all associated injuries and transport with appropriate splinting devices in place. Ensure that tetanus prophylaxis is given and documented.
7. Providing patient and family support is necessary. Both the patient and family must be kept informed on the details of the transfer. A brief assessment of family demographics can help the health care team determine special needs, especially for long-distance transfers.
8. Ensure that all records are complete and accurate. Ensure that an accurate summary of events of injury, treatment given, and patient monitoring and response accompanies the patient.

With careful anticipatory planning and appropriate preparation, the severely burned patient can be safely transported by ground or air to a burn center. Transport should occur early in the postburn period, based on guidelines provided by the receiving burn center.

ACUTE CARE INTERVENTIONS—CRITICAL CARE BURN UNIT

Monitoring Parameters

Once the patient has arrived in the burn critical care unit, the primary and secondary assessments are once again performed. Critical indices are monitored at least once an hour to include blood pressure, pulse, respiration, temperature, peripheral pulses, and urinary output. In addition, urine specific gravity, sugar and acetone levels, and gastric pH and guaiac testing are evaluated every 2 hours. All intravenous catheters are usually replaced and the patient is weighed. Weights continue once or twice daily until preburn weight is obtained after diuresis. Thereafter they are obtained daily except during the immobilization period after skin grafting. It is important to document all parameters, including hourly intake and output for careful analysis of trends.

Massive edema formation is an anticipated response to fluid resuscitation in an extensively burned patient. The upper extremities should be elevated above the level of the heart to increase perfusion. Active or passive range of motion may be performed for 5 minutes every hour to increase venous return and minimize edema. The patient's sensorium must be evaluated hourly, as increased agitation or confusion may be an indication of hypovolemia or hypoxemia. The head of the bed should be elevated 30 degrees, especially in children under age 2, who are susceptible to cerebral edema from resuscitation fluid. Blood pressure measurements, and to some extent heart rate, are not reliable indicators of fluid resuscitation in burn patients. The burn patient often has a higher baseline heart rate of 100 to 120 beats/min, and blood pressure readings (arterial or cuff measurements) may be altered by peripheral edema or vasoconstriction. Initially, urinary output is the only reliable indicator of adequate resuscitation. Titration of calculated fluid requirements according to hourly urine output is an essential function of the nurse during resuscitation. For patients with cardiopulmonary disease, or those who require excessive volumes of fluid, pulmonary artery pressure monitoring may be indicated with frequent measurements of pulmonary capillary wedge pressures (Demling, 1987; Pruitt and Goodwin, 1987).

Serum electrolytes should be obtained at least two to four times a day during the resuscitative phase and as dictated by the patient's status during the acute care phase. Serum sodium levels typically approach the level of the resuscitation fluid being administered. Serum potassium levels may be elevated owing to release from injured tissue. Blood urea nitrogen may also be elevated when excessive protein catabolism occurs, and hyperglycemia may be noted as a result of catecholamine release. Arterial blood gas values should be evaluated frequently as metabolic acidosis may be indicative of inadequate tissue perfusion. A daily chest x-ray is required during the first week for patients with extensive burns or with inhalation injury.

Patients with suspected inhalation injuries who are not already intubated must be monitored frequently for hoarseness, stridor, or wheezing. These symptoms may not be apparent until after fluid resuscitation has been initiated. Carboxyhemoglobin levels are indicated when carbon monoxide poisoning is suspected. Injury above the glottis may be diagnosed by identification of edema of the oropharynx. Fiberoptic bronchoscopy or xenon 133 lung scan may be indicated in order to provide a definitive diagnosis of injury below the glottis (Nebraska Burn Institute, 1989; Pruitt and Goodwin, 1987). All patients with inhalation injuries should be assisted with coughing, deep breathing, and repositioning at least every 2 hours. Humidified oxygen should be administered via a face tent or oxygen mask, and the patient is monitored for respiratory distress. If nasotracheal intubation is indicated, the patient should be suctioned at least every 2 hours or as indicated. Oximetric monitoring of oxygen saturation and monitoring of end-tidal carbon dioxide levels should occur continuously as appropriate.

Patients with burns greater than 20 to 25% of the body surface area should have a nasogastric tube inserted. Acid content of the gastric secretions should be buffered with prophylactic antacid, and/or H_2 histamine receptor antagonists should be administered to maintain a pH of >5. Bowel sounds should be assessed frequently for return of gastric motility in order that enteral or oral feeding may be initiated.

Hypothermia is a potential problem for patients with major burns. Wound therapy such as bathing and application of dressings may potentiate heat loss. Patients must be kept warm with external heat lamps or radiant heat shields. Temperatures should be monitored closely until all burn wounds are closed.

Pain Control in Resuscitative and Acute Care Phases

The level of pain experienced in the resuscitative and acute care phases is related to the extent of partial-thickness injury and the amount of anxiety the patient experiences. Although full-thickness burns are insensate because cutaneous nerve endings have been destroyed, it is unusual for a patient not to have a mixture of both full- and partial-thickness burns. In addition, there are many painful procedures that are necessary in order to facilitate the resuscitation process. The entire experience usually produces much anxiety, which in turn can increase the perception of pain intensity.

Pain control in the resuscitative phase is best achieved with the use of small doses of narcotics given intravenously at frequent intervals. For an adult, morphine, 3 to 5 mg, or meperidine, 30 to 50 mg, are drugs of choice given at intervals established on the basis of the patient's physiological condition (Pruitt and Goodwin, 1990). A continuous infusion of morphine may be useful in maintaining a consistent level of analgesia. However, continuous infusions require close monitoring of the patient's response and are used most safely in patients requiring mechanical ventilation (Wolman, 1988). Subcutaneous or intramuscular injections are ineffective in this phase because of impaired circulation in soft tissue. If given, the potential for narcotic overdose is high as absorption increases with restored circulation during fluid resuscitation (Pruitt and Goodwin, 1990). Anxiety is generally lessened, and pain relief from analgesics enhanced, by simple techniques such as explaining all nursing care activities prior to performing them, talking in a quiet calm voice, or using simple relaxation and guided imagery techniques (Kenner and Achterberg, 1983; McCaffery and Beebe, 1989). Anxiolytics may be required. If the patient is alert, patient controlled analgesia may be helpful in maintaining a consistent level of analgesia and by providing the patient some control over pain relief, possibly reducing anxiety (Choiniere et al., 1990; Cram and Kealey, 1990).

There are many aspects of burn treatment in the acute phase that produce pain: hydrotherapy, debridement, the application of mafenide acetate, and physical therapy. Patient descriptions of perceived intensity of pain vary little despite differences in extent of burn, ethnicity, age, and socioeconomic status (Perry et al., 1981). When the patient is hemodynamically stable and the ileus is resolved, analgesic medications can be given safely by the intravenous, intramuscular, or oral route.

Although pain is reduced as the wounds heal or are covered with either temporary dressings or autograft skin, frequent surgeries and wound care procedures produce episodic periods of pain and anxiety until permanent wound closure/healing is completed. Despite the acute intermittent nature of the pain, the intensity of procedural pain, and the mild to moderate pain that occurs with movement contribute to an overall perception of constant pain (Perry et al., 1981). Itching also becomes a major problem that contributes to the patient's overall discomfort. Several medications, as well as soothing lotions, can assist in controlling pruritus.

The elimination of most of the pain of burn injury has been shown to have a significant impact in obtaining a positive outcome for the patient (Ehleben and Still, 1985). However, there is a necessity for a compromise between the patient's pain perception, the pain state, and safe medical practice in managing severe burn pain (Loeser, 1987). The major paradox of burn pain management is that the nurses inflict pain and then must relieve it. It becomes a challenge for the critical care nurse to develop a pain management program that implements safe pharmacological therapy in combination with nonpharmacological pain-control techniques.

Infection Control

One of the most important nursing interventions in caring for burn patients is control of infection. With improved formulas for fluid resuscitation, the use of topical antimicrobial agents, new antibiotics, improvements in nutrition, and more aggressive wound closure techniques, the survival of burn patients has significantly increased (Pruitt, 1987b). However, infection (primarily pulmonary) still remains the leading cause of morbidity and mortality in the burn population (Herndon, 1987; Pruitt, 1987b; Shirani et al., 1987). The immunosuppressive effects of burn injury, along with environmental and therapeutic factors, must be considered in developing an infection control policy. Burn patients are at high risk not only for invasive burn wound infection, but for septic phlebitis secondary to intravenous therapy, urinary tract infections related to long-term catheterization, pneumonia, and septicemia (Waymack and Pruitt, 1990).

Burn eschar is normally colonized with a variety of microorganisms. If these microorganisms invade underlying viable tissue, an invasive burn wound infection develops. Burn wound surface cultures should be performed upon admission and several times a week to monitor changes in wound colonization, but a burn wound biopsy is the only definitive means of identifying an invasive burn wound infection (Waymack and Pruitt, 1990). Once invasion is diagnosed, appropriate local and/or systemic antibiotic therapy must be initiated.

Infection control policies differ among burn units, but all stress reverse isolation techniques, strict adherence to dress code policies, and handwashing as environmental priorities in preventing infection (Gordon, 1987b,c; McManus, et al., 1987).

Wound Management

Prior to healing or excision and grafting of the burn wound, nursing care must focus on prevention of burn wound infection. All wounds should be cleansed at least once a day with a surgical detergent disinfectant and rinsed with warm saline or sterile/tap water. This is best accomplished in the shower or Hubbard tank, but bed baths may also be employed for hemodynamically unstable patients. The patient should not be immersed in water as there is a significant potential for cross contamination of wounds on patients with significant body surface area injury,

Burn Wound Assessment Documentation Tool

Code wounds on body figure according to legend below:

- Eschar (E)
- Granulation Tissue
- Epithelial Tissue

- Meshed Grafts (MG)
- Sheet Grafts (SG)
- Donor Sites (DS)
- Healed Skin (HS)

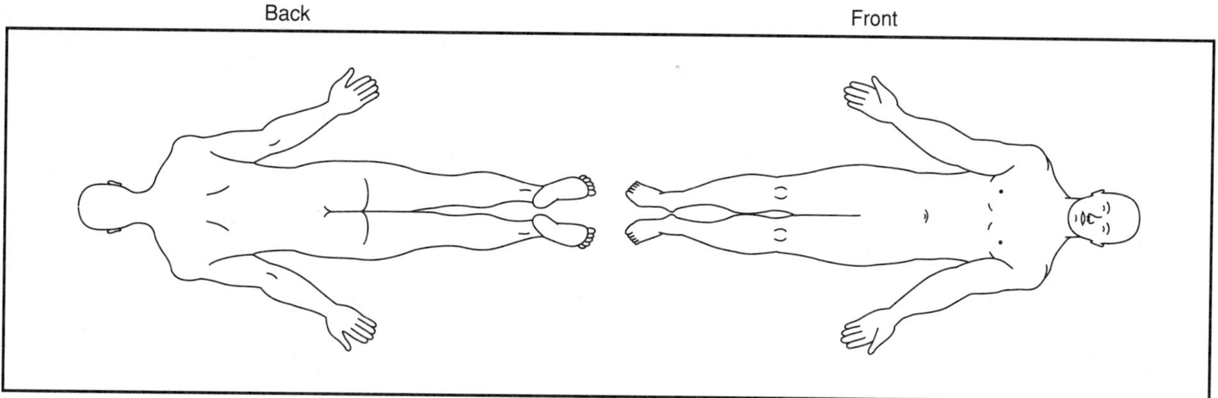

Check appropriate wound descriptor in adjacent box under body part selected. Line out any unused boxes.

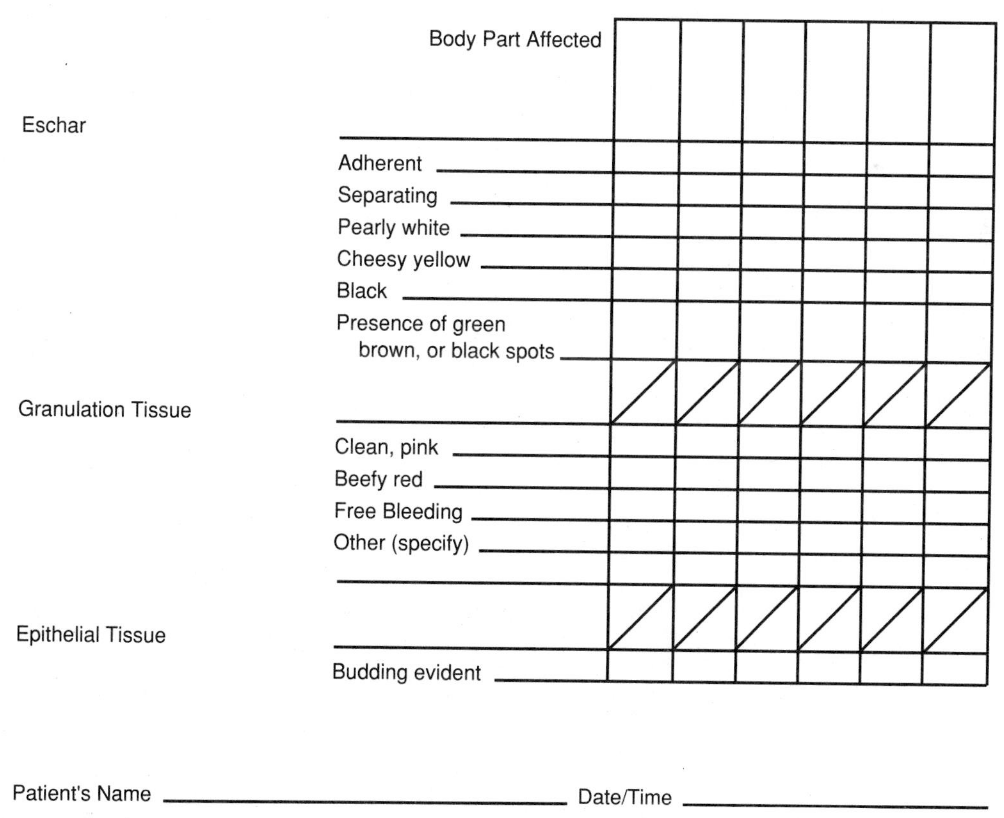

	Body Part Affected						
Eschar							
	Adherent						
	Separating						
	Pearly white						
	Cheesy yellow						
	Black						
	Presence of green brown, or black spots						
Granulation Tissue							
	Clean, pink						
	Beefy red						
	Free Bleeding						
	Other (specify)						
Epithelial Tissue							
	Budding evident						

Patient's Name ______________________ Date/Time ______________

Figure 15-9. Burn Wound Assessment Documentation Tool. Documentation of daily burn wound assessment facilitates evaluation of wound condition and early detection of complications. (Wound assessment tool developed by Blinn Bolcar, RN, MSN, with assistance by the staff at the U.S. Army Institute of Surgical Research.)

		Body Part Affected					
Ears							
	Clean & Dry						
	Purulent drainage						
	Edematous						
	Erythematous						
Grafts (meshed) Up to 72 hours							
	Dressings damp						
Dressing change	1st Post op						
	2nd Post op						
	Adherent						
	Interstices filling in						
	% Graft take (____)						
	Staples present						
	Staples removed						
Open to air							
	Skin intact						
	Dry, Scaly						
	Blisters						
	Open areas						
Grafts (sheet) Drainage							
	Serosanguinous						
	Sanguinous						
	Purulent						
	Amount (Lg, Mod, Sm)						
Appearance							
	Intact & Adherent						
	Vesicles present						
	Vesicles absent						
Donor Sites To 7th POD							
	Moist						
	Drying						
	Soupy						
	Red						
	Brown						
	Whitish						
To 13th POD	Dry						
	Healed						
	Problems (specify)						

Additional Remarks:

Signature/Title ______________________________

Figure 15-9 *Continued.*

and hypothermia is more difficult to control. It is important to remove all necrotic tissue, exudates, and fibrous debris from the wound bed to control bacterial proliferation and promote healing. Loose eschar and wound debris should be removed with gauze sponges or debrided with scissors and forceps during the bathing session (Gordon, 1989). Hair should be shaved three to four inches out from the wound margin. Wet-to-wet or wet-to-dry dressings may also be employed to aid in the debridement process in order to prepare the wound bed for grafting. All wounds should be inspected closely and their appearance carefully documented so that changes across time can be readily noted (Gordon, 1988a) (Fig. 15–9).

After each hydrotherapy session, the unhealed or unexcised burn wound should be covered with an antimicrobial topical agent or dressing (Fig. 15–10). Table 15–7 describes the most commonly used topical antimicrobial agents and nursing considerations. The topical agent will not only assist in controlling infection, but will also prevent wound desiccation, which impedes the reepithelialization process.

Two common methods of treatment used for care of burn wounds are the open and occlusive methods. When using the open method, the burn wounds are left open to air after the antimicrobial agent is applied. The occlusive method involves covering the wound with gauze dressings that have been saturated with a topical antimicrobial agent, or placing a thin layer of gauze over agent applied directly to the wounds. The dressings are then covered with a net bandage to hold the gauze in place. Each method has advantages and disadvantages, and specific protocols differ among burn units.

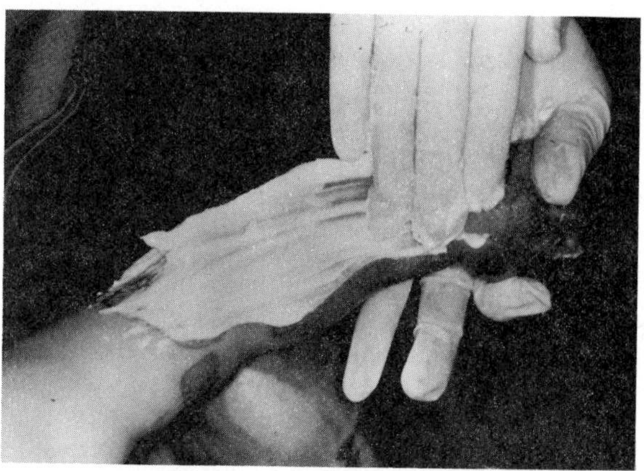

Figure 15–10. Application of a topical agent to a burn wound. A sterile gloved hand is used to apply a topical antimicrobial agent to the burn wound.

Any deep partial- or full-thickness burn wound that will require more than 3 weeks for healing to occur is a candidate for application of autograft skin. At present, autograft skin is the only permanent means of covering a burn wound. Biological or biosynthetic dressings are commonly used as temporary wound coverings

Table 15–7. TOPICAL ANTIMICROBIAL AGENTS FOR BURN WOUND MANAGEMENT

Agent	Indications	Nursing Considerations
Clotrimazole Cream	Fungal colonization of wounds	Apply thin coat of agent to wound and wait 20 min before applying any dressings. Must use an antibacterial agent in addition to antifungal agent. Painless; may cause skin irritation and blistering
Mafenide Acetate (Sulfamylon)	Active against most gram-positive and gram-negative wound pathogens; drug of choice for electrical and ear burns	Apply once or twice daily with sterile glove; do not use dressings that reduce effectiveness and cause maceration; monitor respiratory rate, electrolyte values, and arterial pH for evidence of metabolic acidosis; painful on application to partial-thickness burns for about 30 min
Silver Nitrate	Effective against wide spectrum of common wound pathogens and fungal infections; used in patients with sulfa allergy or toxic epidermal necrolysis. Poor penetration of eschar	Apply 0.5% solution wet dressings twice or three times a day; ensure that dressings remain moist by wetting every 2 hr. Preserve solution in a light-resistant container. Protect walls, floors, etc., with plastic to prevent black staining that occurs. Monitor for hyponatremia and hypochloremia
Silver Sulfadiazine (Silvadene)	Active against a wide spectrum of microbial pathogens; use with caution in patients with impaired renal or hepatic function	Apply once or twice a day with sterile gloved hand. Leave wounds exposed or wrap lightly with gauze dressings. Painless

for freshly excised burn wounds until autograft skin is available. They may also be used as a dressing for partial-thickness burns, meshed autograft skin, or donor sites to promote healing. Table 15–8 provides descriptions of the most common types and uses of biological/biosynthetic dressings (Gordon, 1988c).

Currently, research is being conducted related to the use of cultured epidermal sheets for permanent wound closure. The layered sheets of human epidermal cells (grown in the laboratory using tissue culture techniques to expand keratinocytes derived from a small full-thickness skin biopsy) provide hope for early wound coverage in extensively burned patients with limited donor sites (Waymack and Pruitt, 1990).

Priority areas for autograft skin application include the face, hands, feet, and over joints.

Table 15–8. BIOLOGICAL/SYNTHETIC DRESSINGS

Type of Dressing	Definition
Biological Dressing	Temporary wound cover of human or animal species tissue
Allograft (Homograft) Skin	Temporary wound cover composed of a graft of skin transplanted from another human, living or dead
Xenograft (Heterograft) Skin	Used as a temporary wound cover to promote healing. A graft of skin, usually pigskin, transplanted between animals of different species
Biosynthetic Dressing	A wound covering composed of both biological and synthetic materials
Biobrane	A bilaminate wound dressing composed of nylon mesh enclosed in a collagen derivative with a silicon rubber outer membrane. It is permeable to some antibiotic ointments
Integra—"Artificial Skin"	A wound dressing composed of two layers: (1) a "dermal" layer made of animal collagen that interfaces with an open wound surface; (2) an "epidermal" layer made of Silastic that controls water loss from the dermis and acts as a bacterial barrier. The dermal layer biodegrades within several months and is resorbed. The epidermal layer may be removed and replaced with autograft skin when appropriate

When preparing a wound for grafting, two approaches may be used. Early eschar excision and application of autograft skin is the more common treatment. Usually excision and grafting is initiated within the first week postburn, when the patient becomes hemodynamically stable. Advantages include earlier wound coverage, early return of function, a decrease in scar formation, and a decrease in length of hospitalization. The conservative approach involves wound treatment with antimicrobial agents, hydrotherapy, and debridement until partial-thickness burns are healed and full-thickness injury is ready for skin grafting. With the conservative approach, there is less blood loss and potential risk of complications associated with blood replacement therapy (McManus et al., 1989).

Autograft skin is applied to the recipient bed dermal side down, and secured with staples, surgical tape, fibrin glue, or sutures (Gordon, 1988b). Table 15–9 summarizes the types of skin grafts used with nursing care requirements. Splinting of graft sites may be indicated to prevent movement and shearing of the grafts until healing is complete. Upper extremities should be elevated to prevent pooling of blood, leading to increased pressure and thus potential graft loss (Waymack and Pruitt, 1990). Figure 15–11 represents a method of documenting wound treatment that facilitates communication of care requirements from day to day.

Nursing interventions must also focus on the care of donor sites (Gordon, 1986a). Once donor skin is harvested, the site must be covered with a dressing until healing occurs. Many types of dressings can be used (Table 15–10), but all should promote healing of the donor site within 8 to 14 days (Waymack and Pruitt, 1990).

Inherent in all wound care management is the necessity to improve and maintain function. Occupational and physical therapists are essential members of the burn team and should be consulted from the day of admission. Often the position of comfort for the patients is one that can lead to dysfunction or deformity. Specialized splints and exercises are required to prevent future complications (Malick and Carr, 1982). Although the critical care nurse may not actually develop the plan for such therapy, knowledge of and compliance with the plan are essential for positive patient outcomes.

Burn Wound Care for Special Anatomical Areas
(Pruitt, 1979; Pruitt & Goodwin, 1987)

Table 15–9. AUTOGRAFT SKIN: NURSING IMPLICATIONS

Type	Definition	Nursing Implications
Split-Thickness Sheet Skin Graft	Sheet of skin composed of the epidermis and a variable portion of the dermis that is split at a predetermined thickness allowing for transplantation to another area of the body	Grafted area must be immobilized. Pockets of serous fluid must be evacuated by needle aspiration or rolling of the fluid with a cotton tip applicator toward the skin edges. If fluid is not evacuated, graft adherence will be compromised
Split-Thickness Meshed Skin Graft	Split-Thickness sheet graft placed in a mesh dermatome that expands the graft from 1.5 to 9.0 times its original size before being placed on a recipient bed of granulation tissue	Grafted area is immobilized, often in splints. Skin graft is covered with fine mesh gauze then coarse mesh gauze and wrapped with absorbent gauze roll prior to being placed in a splint. Dressings must be kept moist with an antimicrobial solution, but not saturated, to prevent desiccation and promote epithelization of the interstices of the meshed skin. The first dressing change will be in 3–5 days
Full-Thickness Skin Graft	A skin graft that contains the full thickness of the skin down to the subcutaneous tissue	Requires the same care as a sheet skin graft
Cultured Epidermal Sheets	Layered sheets of human epidermal cells grown in the laboratory using tissue culture techniques to expand keratinocytes derived from a small full-thickness skin biopsy; Allows for the potential of covering extensive wound areas more quickly without having to wait for healing of limited donor site skin surfaces	In the first 7–10 days postsurgery, daily dressing changes involve only the outer layer of fluffy gauze. The underlying coarse mesh gauze and petrolatum gauze, which are sutured over the graft, are not to be disturbed. Unlike caring for meshed autograft skin, the outer dressing must remain dry. Many topical antimicrobial agents are toxic to the cultured epithelial autograft skin, and should not come in contact with the graft dressings. Once the petrolatum gauze is loose (7–10 days), it can be removed and wet saline dressings are used until approximately 21 days postgrafting when the skin graft is usually well adherent. Gentle passive ROM can begin once the petrolatum gauze is removed

Facial Burns

Facial burns can lead to significant complications, thus they require hospitalization in a burn unit. The presence of facial burns may signal inhalation injury, and massive facial edema may lead to a compromised airway. Close monitoring of the patient's respiratory status is essential. The head of the bed should be elevated to facilitate respiratory exchange and edema reabsorption. Special care must be taken in cleansing facial burns to prevent excessive bleeding and damage to new tissue growth. All hair should be shaved from the wound each day. Once cleaned and debrided, a topical antimicrobial agent should be applied per unit protocol. Owing to the rich blood supply in the face, partial-thickness burns will usually heal quickly as long as infection is prevented. Good oral hygiene is essential.

Burns of the Ears

The ears are especially prone to inflammation and infection (chondritis) that could lead to complete loss of the ear cartilage. It is important to treat ear burns with a topical antimicrobial agent and to prevent application of any pressure to the ears. Dressings should be avoided and cloth ties used to secure tubes to the face should not put pressure on the top of the ears. Pillows should not be used; a donut of foam with a hole for the ear to rest in while the patient is in a lateral position should be substituted.

Burns of the Eyes

Immediate examination of the eyes is necessary upon arrival at the hospital as eyelid edema forms rapidly. Contact lenses should be removed

Burn Wound Treatment Documentation Tool

Body figure: Code treatments on the body figure according to legend below:

- Topical Agents
- Dressings

- Physiologic Wound coverings (Indicate with letter code)
- Open to Air

Front

Back

Special Bed Required (Circle Yes/No)

Low Air Loss: Yes No

Air fluidized: Yes No

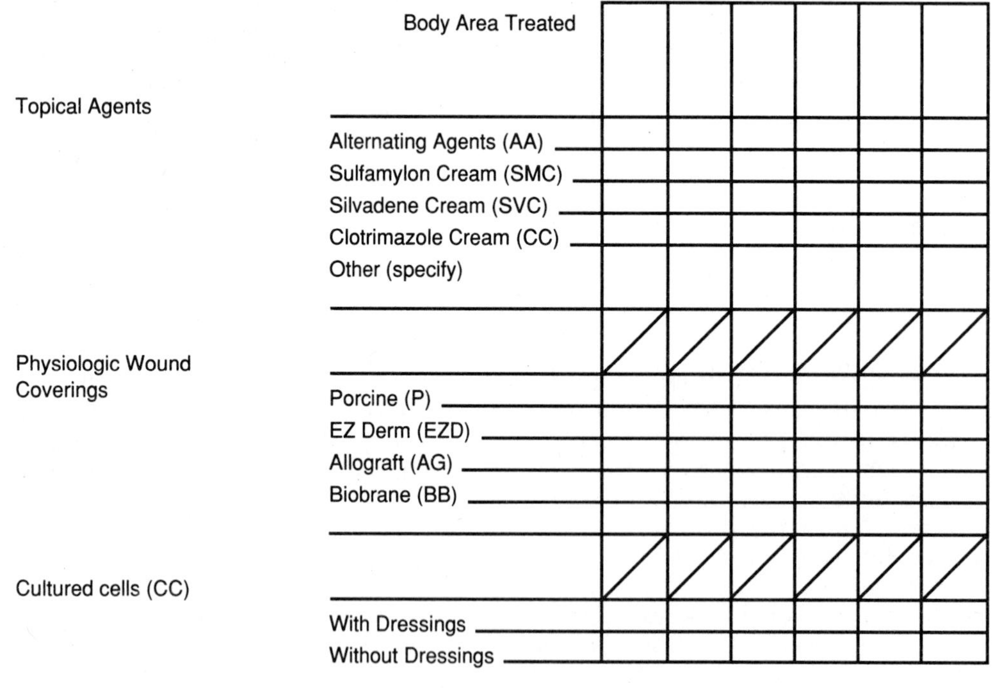

	Body Area Treated						
Topical Agents							
	Alternating Agents (AA)						
	Sulfamylon Cream (SMC)						
	Silvadene Cream (SVC)						
	Clotrimazole Cream (CC)						
	Other (specify)						
Physiologic Wound Coverings							
	Porcine (P)						
	EZ Derm (EZD)						
	Allograft (AG)						
	Biobrane (BB)						
Cultured cells (CC)							
	With Dressings						
	Without Dressings						

Patient's Identification ______________________ Date/Time ______________________

Figure 15-11. Burn Wound Treatment Documentation Tool provides a concise and comprehensive method for communicating treatment protocols between shifts of nursing personnel. The use of a body diagram minimizes potential errors in treatment. (Developed by Blinn Bolcar, RN, MSN, with assistance by the staff at the US Army Institute of Surgical Research.)

	Body Area Treated						
Dressings							
Type	Graft wet down						
	Graft dressing change						
	Wet-to-wet						
	Wet-to-dry						
	Dry						
Materials	Fine mesh gauze (FMG)						
	Course mesh gauze (CMG)						
	Kerlix (K)						
	Surgiflex (SF)						
	Exu-dry (ED)						
Solutions							
	5% Sulfa Solution (SS)						
	Normal Saline (NS)						
	1/4 Dakin's (DS)						
	Silver Nitrate (AgNO3)						
	Triple Antibiotic (TA)						
	Other (specify)						
Graft Care							
	Staples present						
	Staples removed						
	Crusts debrided						
	Edges debrided						
	Sheet grafts rolled						
Donor Site Care							
Heat lamps required: Yes or No							
	Biobrane						
	FMG intact						
	FMG replaced						
	FMG removed						
	Staples intact						
	Staples removed						
Devices Present							
	Slings						
	Splints: Continuous						
	Splints: Night						
	Cushioning pads						
	Net cradle						
	Other (specify)						

Additional Remarks:

Signature/Title ______________________

Figure 15–11 *Continued.*

Table 15-10. TYPES OF DONOR SITE DRESSINGS

Dressing	Description
Fine mesh gauze	Cotton gauze is placed directly on a donor site. A crust or "scab" is formed as the gauze dries and epithelialization of the wound occurs under the dressing. The gauze peels away easily as the wound heals
Fine mesh gauze impregnated with scarlet red	Cotton gauze is impregnated with a blend of lanolin, olive oil, petrolatum, and the red dye Scarlet Red. Healing occurs as with fine mesh gauze dressing
Xeroform	Fine mesh gauze containing 3% bismuth tribromophenate in a petrolatum blend. Promotes healing as with other mesh gauze dressings
Op-site	A thin elastic film that is occlusive, waterproof, and permeable to moisture, vapor, and air. Fluid under dressing may need to be evacuated
DuoDerm	A hydrocolloid dressing that interacts with moisture on skin creating a bond that makes it adhere.
N-Terface	A translucent, nonabsorbent, and nonreactive surface material used between burn wound and outer dressing.
Vigilon	A colloidal suspension on a polyethylene mesh support which provides a moist environment and is permeable to gases and water vapor.

if present. The eyes should be stained with fluorescein to rule out corneal injury, and irrigated with copious amounts of physiologic saline if injury is confirmed. A thorough examination by an ophthalmologist is mandatory for serious injuries. Once eyelid edema resolves, the cornea may become exposed as the eyelid retracts. Careful observation of eyelashes is also necessary as they may invert and scratch the cornea. Nursing care involves the frequent application of ophthalmic ointment or artificial tears to protect the cornea and conjunctiva from drying.

Burns of the Hands or Feet

Extensive burns of the hands and feet may cause permanent disability, necessitating a long convalescence. Nursing care is directed at preservation of function. Burned hands should be elevated above the level of the heart on slings or wedges to reduce edema formation (Fig. 15–12). Although range-of-motion exercises may be painful, they must be initiated as soon as possible after injury and performed frequently throughout each day. Active range-of-motion will prevent muscle atrophy, reduce or prevent the shortening of ligaments, and reduce edema. Passive range of motion is indicated if patients are unable to move their extremities actively. Splinting may be required to maintain function and prevent deformities of the affected part. An elastic bandage

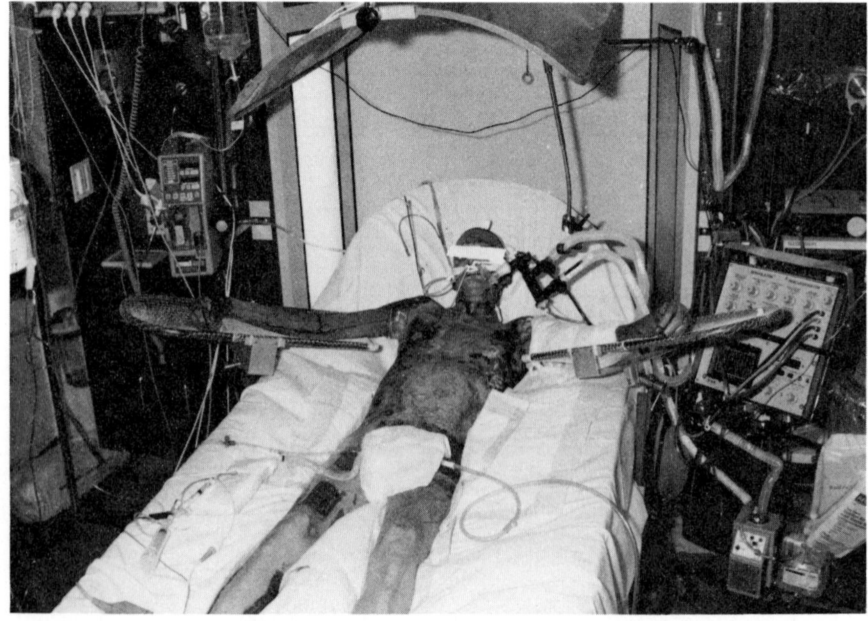

Figure 15–12. Slings used to elevate burned extremities. Slings can be devised to support and elevate burned extremities. The mesh on the slings pictured provides for air circulation that prevents wound maceration.

should be applied over burn wounds of the feet and legs when ambulating or sitting to prevent pooling of blood, but should be removed when the feet are elevated. In establishing a nursing plan of care, it is important to remember that patients with bilateral burned hands are totally dependent on nursing personnel for all of their physical needs.

Burns of the Genitalia and Perineum

Patients with perineal burns often require hospitalization for observation of urinary tract obstruction caused from edema formation, and meticulous wound management to prevent infection. Insertion of an indwelling urethral catheter may be indicated in order to maintain urethral patency until the wounds are healed or grafted. Meticulous wound cleansing is essential owing to the potential for fecal contamination. Perineal hair must be shaved as required. Scrotal edema is common, and the scrotum should be elevated on towels. Antimicrobial topical agents are applied to prevent infection.

Nutritional Considerations

Adequate nutrition plays a critical role in the survival of extensively burned patients. For optimal wound healing to occur, the burn patient must be in a state of positive nitrogen balance. Owing to the tendency toward catabolism mediated by the patient's hypermetabolic state, supplemental calories are essential to meet energy demands, and additional nitrogen is needed to replenish body protein stores. Inadequate nutrition may lead to significant body weight loss, delayed wound healing or skin graft loss, impaired immunological responsiveness, sepsis, or even death (Pruitt and Goodwin, 1983; Wachtel, 1987).

Caloric needs should be determined for each burn patient with a major burn by metabolic studies, taking into consideration the percent body surface area burned, preburn nutritional status, and the presence of other complicating factors such as inhalation injury. Coordination of the nutritional plan should be done by a registered dietitian according to requirements delineated by the physician. The dietitian and the nursing staff should provide vigorous nutritional support as soon as possible through the most appropriate method available. Enteral nutrition is the preferred route for any patient with a functioning gastrointestinal tract. Care must be taken to prevent aspiration if tube feedings are necessary. Parenteral nutrition is only indicated for patients whose clinical status precludes the use of enteric feedings.

Nursing assessment and intervention in assisting patients to meet nutritional requirements include accurate monitoring of daily weights, accurate intake and output measurements to include bowel movements, and careful evaluation

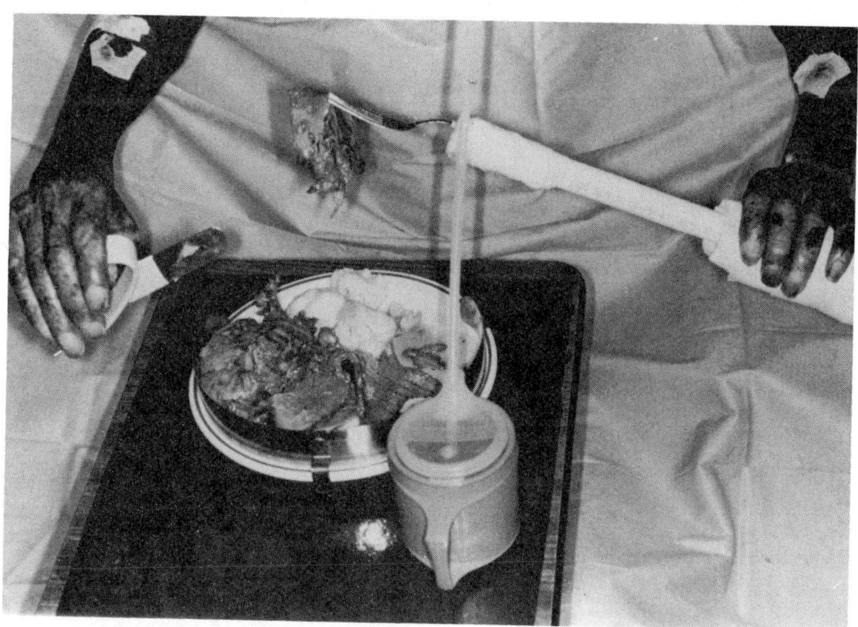

Figure 15-13. Adaptive devices to facilitate self-feeding are provided to assist the patient to eat, thus promoting independence.

of the nasogastric or enteric tube to ensure proper placement and patency. Nurses can play an important role in ensuring that devices to facilitate self-feeding are available and that mealtimes are planned around other therapeutic requirements to provide a relaxed, pain-free environment (Fig. 15–13). Allowing family members to visit at mealtimes and assist with feedings may also be beneficial to the patient as well as therapeutic for the family (Gordon, 1986b).

Psychosocial Considerations

Burn injury is one of the most psychologically devastating injuries to patients and their families. Not only is there a very real threat to survival, but the psychological and physical pain experienced, fear of disfigurement, and uncertainty of the long-term effect of the injury on future lifestyle and plans can precipitate a crisis situation for the patient and family. There are many stages of psychological adaptation that the patient may experience before appropriate functioning occurs (Table 15–11). Not all patients experience manifestations of all stages, but support and therapy are necessary for any patient and family experiencing a major burn injury. The critical care nurse needs to assess the patient/family to determine if adequate support systems are available and if appropriate coping mechanisms are being used. Interventions based on individual assessments are the most beneficial and may require consulting support personnel such as chaplains, clinical nurse specialists, psychiatrists, and social workers. As the patient moves out of the intensive care unit, support mechanisms need to continue to ensure continuity of care.

Table 15–11. STAGES OF POSTBURN PSYCHOLOGICAL ADAPTATION

Survival Anxiety

Often manifested by lack of concentration, easy startle response, tearfulness, social withdrawal, inappropriate behavior. Instructions need repeating, and the patient has to be allowed time to verbalize concerns and fears. Increased reports of pain are frequently associated with high levels of anxiety.

The Search for Meaning

During this phase the patient repeatedly recounts the events leading to the injury, trying to determine a logical explanation that is emotionally acceptable. It is important to avoid judging the patient's reasoning and to listen actively and participate in the discussions with the patient.

Investment in Recuperation

This is a period of increased cooperation with the treatment regimen. The patient is motivated to be independent and takes pride in small accomplishments. The nurse should educate the patient concerning discharge goals and involve the patient/family in planning for a program of increased self-care. The patient requires much praise and verbal encouragement in this phase.

Investment in Rehabilitation

As self-confidence increases, the patient is focused on achieving as much preburn function as possible. Depression may occur as new losses in function are realized. Staff support is limited in this phase, which usually occurs after the patient is discharged from the hospital and undergoing outpatient rehabilitation. Praise, support, and continued information are beneficial strategies.

Reintegration of Identity

The patient accepts losses and recognizes that changes have occurred. Adaptation is completed and staff involvement is terminated.

Adapted from Watkins, P., Cook, E., May, S., and Ehleben, C. Psychological stages in adaptation following burn injury: A method for facilitating psychological recovery of burn victims. *Journal of Burn Care and Rehabilitation* 9(4):376–384, 1988.

Discharge Planning

Discharge planning for critically ill burned patients must begin on the day of admission. Assessments should be made regarding patient survival, potential/actual short- or long-term functional disabilities secondary to the burn injury, financial resources available, family roles and expectations, and psychological support systems. Patient and family education is essential in preparing for eventual discharge and for transfer from the intensive care unit. Patients/families returning home must understand how to care for their physical needs, as well as their psychological and social needs. Nurses play an important role in multidisciplinary discharge planning by providing guidance for patient/family education, and in evaluating the need for additional resources to plan for patient rehabilitative and home care requirements.

■ Outcomes

With appropriate interventions, expected patient outcomes include the following:

PULMONARY

1. Patent airway with clear breath sounds on auscultation, after pulmonary hygiene
2. Normal arterial blood gas values and oxygen saturation

3. Decreased dyspnea and work of breathing with appropriate positioning
4. Ability to cough effectively and produce clear secretions

FLUID AND ELECTROLYTES

1. Appropriate weight gain in first 48 hours, with diuresis occurring over next 8 to 10 days at a weight loss rate of no more than 10% of weight gain per day
2. Urine output in first 48 hours of 30 to 50 ml/hr (75 to 100 ml/hr with electrical injuries) or 1 ml/kg/hr for children <30 kg in weight
3. Urine specific gravity that normalizes to 1.010 to 1.020 after diuresis; normal urinary sugar and acetone levels
4. Electrolytes within normal limits after adequate replacement therapy

CARDIOVASCULAR

1. A pulse ranging from 80 to 120 beats/min
2. A blood pressure adequate in relation to pulse and urinary output
3. A cardiac output and pulmonary capillary wedge pressure that are low the first 6 to 12 hours, followed by a normal or supranormal cardiac output with normal capillary wedge pressure until wound closure
4. Strong, palpable pulses in all extremities with good capillary refill

PAIN

1. Adequate respirations and hemodynamic stability after administration of narcotic analgesia
2. A decrease in perceived pain level based on a subjective scale or change in physiological parameters
3. Able to identify factors that contribute to pain

INFECTION AND NORMOTHERMIA

1. Body temperature between 99 and 101°F
2. Negative sputum, blood, and urine cultures
3. Absence of wound biopsy evidence of burn wound infection
4. Acceptable white blood cell and platelet counts, coagulation times, and serum glucose
5. Absence of purulence, erythema, and/or pain around invasive catheter sites
6. Adherence of allograft or autograft skin to granulation tissue

TISSUE INTEGRITY

1. Intact skin in nonburned areas
2. Wound closure within an appropriate time frame after burn injury or donor skin harvesting

GASTROINTESTINAL AND STRESS RESPONSE

1. Absence of aspiration
2. Gastric pH >5
3. Guaiac-negative stools and gastric contents
4. Presence of formed stools

NUTRITION

1. Positive nitrogen balance
2. Consumption of daily requirement of nutrients, based on formulas for appropriate caloric calculations

PHYSICAL MOBILITY

1. Range-of-motion of all joints equal to the preburn level unless there is dysfunction secondary to associated trauma at the time of injury

PATIENT AND FAMILY COPING

1. Ability to verbally describe goals of the treatment regimen
2. Demonstrates knowledge of the support systems that are available
3. Expresses concerns and/or fears

Summary

The physiological response to a major burn injury is one of a biphasic pattern of multiorgan system hypofunction followed by hyperfunction. A major goal of resuscitative care is to prevent burn shock. The critical care nurse's observations of the patient's responses are crucial to prevent complications related to the increased capillary permeability and massive fluid therapy required. In the acute phase, therapeutic goals include prevention of further tissue loss, maintenance of function, prevention of infection, and wound closure. As the patient progresses through various stages of wound care management, the nurse

NURSING CARE PLAN FOR THE RESUSCITATIVE AND ACUTE CARE PHASES OF THE PATIENT WITH MAJOR BURN INJURY

Nursing Diagnosis	Outcome	Intervention
Ineffective airway clearance/impaired gas enchange related to tracheal edema or interstitial edema secondary to inhalation injury and manifested by hypoxemia and hypercapnia	$Po_2 > 90$ mm Hg, $Pco_2 < 40$ mm Hg, O_2 saturation >95% Respirations 16–20/min Clear mentation Ability to mobilize secretions Clear to white secretions Absence of dyspnea and increased work of breathing with appropriate positioning	Assess respiratory rate and character every 1 hr, breath sounds every 4 hr, LOC every 1 hr; evaluate need for chest escharotomy during fluid resuscitation If not intubated, assess for stridor, hoarseness every 1 hr Monitor oxygen saturation every 1 hr, obtain and evaluate ABGs PRN Administer humidified oxygen as ordered Cough, deep breathe every 1 hr while awake Suction every 1–2 hr or PRN, monitor sputum characteristics and amount Elevate HOB to facilitate lung expansion Schedule activities to avoid fatigue, dyspnea Turn every 2 hr to mobilize secretions Assist with obtaining chest x-ray as ordered
Fluid volume deficit secondary to fluid shifts to the interstitium and evaporative loss of fluids from the injured skin	Weight gain based on volume of fluids administered in first 48 hr followed by moderate diuresis over next 8–10 days with a weight loss rate of no more than 10–12% of weight gain per day Hourly urine output: 30–50 ml/hr; 1 ml/kg/hr—children <30 kg body wt; 75–100 ml/hr—electric injury Normal specific gravity except during diuresis, when it may be slightly decreased; negative urine sugar and acetone Heart rate = 80–120 beats/min, BP adequate in relation to pulse and urine output Clear sensorium Laboratory values: Na^+ = approaches that of resuscitation fluid initially then returns to normal with diuresis; K^+ initially high, HCT 50–55% until adequate resuscitation established; all other values WNL	Titrate calculated fluid requirements in first 48 hr to maintain acceptable urinary output. Obtain and evaluate urine specific gravity and sugar and acetone every 2 hr Monitor vital signs every 1 hr until hemodynamically stable Monitor mental status every 1 hr for at least 48 hr Obtain and record daily or BID weights Record hourly intake and output measurements and evaluate trends Monitor electrolytes, HCT, serum glucose, BUN, creatinine at least BID for first 48 hr and then as required by patient status
Potential for impaired vascular perfusion in extremities with circumferential burns manifested by decreased or absent peripheral pulses	Absence of tissue injury in extremities secondary to inadequate perfusion related to vascular compression from edema	Check peripheral pulses every 1 hr for 72 hr by palpation and/or ultrasonic flowmeter; evaluate sensation of pain and capillary refill in extremities Notify physician of changes in pulses, capillary refill, or pain sensation; be prepared to assist with escharotomy or fasciotomy Elevate upper extremities
Alteration in comfort: acute pain related to burn trauma	Able to identify factors that contribute to pain Verbalizes improved comfort level Physiological parameters return to normal Adequate respirations and hemodynamic stability after administration of narcotic analgesia	Medicate prior to bathing, dressing changes, major procedures, PRN Reduce anxiety: explain all activities prior to initiating them; talk to patient while performing activities; assess need for analgesic and/or anxiolytic medication; use nonpharmacological pain-reducing methods as appropriate Monitor and document response to analgesics or other interventions

NURSING CARE PLAN FOR THE RESUSCITATIVE AND ACUTE CARE PHASES OF THE PATIENT WITH MAJOR BURN INJURY *Continued*

Nursing Diagnosis	Outcome	Intervention
Potential for infection related to loss of skin, impaired imune response, invasive therapies	Absence of inflamed burn wound margins Negative sputum, blood, and urine cultures. Absence of wound biopsy evidence of burn wound invasion Body temperature between 99 and 101°F Absence of glycosuria, vomiting, ileus, and/or change in mentation Aceptable white blood cell and platelet counts, coagulation times, and serum glucose level Clean dry invasive catheter sites with normal skin color and temperature Autograft or allograft skin adherence to granulation tissue	Assess burn wound and invasive catheter sites BID Assess and document characteristics of urine and sputum every 8 hr Obtain wound, sputum, urine, and blood cultures as ordered Assess and record temperature and vital signs every 1–4 hr as appropriate Provide protective isolation appropriate to method of wound care Adhere to CDC guidelines for invasive catheter care Provide wound care with antimicrobial topical agents as ordered
Impaired skin integrity related to burn wound, and/or consequences of immobility	No evidence of decubitus ulcers or other injury in unburned skin No evidence of progressive burn wound/donor site injury Burn wound/donor site healing, skin graft adherence occurs within appropriate time frames	Assess BID and document: skin over pressure areas, burn wounds, donor sites, pressure points under splints, dependent areas of unburned skin Pad pressure areas: heels, elbows, sacrum, scapulas, and burned ears Assess need for special beds such as low-air-loss and air-fluidized beds; at a minimum, provide extra padding to mattress Remove BP cuff from areas of burned skin after each reading Check circulation distal to restraints every 1 hr; check circulation of digits in splinted extremities Loosen securing devices for facial tube to accommodate changes occurring with edema; ensure that devices do not put pressure on ears Promote drying of donor sites as appropriate; keep heat lamps at a safe distance to prevent injury Immobilize skin graft sites for 5–7 days postgrafting to promote graft adherence Moisten meshed graft dressings as ordered or roll sheet grafts as ordered to promote skin graft adherence
Potential nutritional deficit related to increased metabolic demands secondary to wound healing	Consumption of daily requirement of nutrients, based on formulas for appropriate calorie calculation Positive nitrogen balance Progressive wound healing occurs	Monitor weights every day or biweekly Assess abdomen, bowel sounds every 8 hr Record all oral intake Activate enteral, parenteral feeding protocol as appropriate PRN Provide adaptive devices to facilitate self-feeding Have family assist at mealtime
Impaired mobility and self-care deficit related to therapeutic splinting and post–skin graft immobilization requirements	No evidence of permanent decreased joint function from preburn status unless directly related to trauma Return to vocation without functional limitations or adjustment to new vocation based on functional limitations	Perform ROM to all extremities every 4 hr Progress patient's activity as tolerated Promote the use of adaptive devices to decrease dependency Provide pain relief measures prior to physical therapy

continued

NURSING CARE PLAN FOR THE RESUSCITATIVE AND ACUTE CARE PHASES OF THE PATIENT WITH MAJOR BURN INJURY *Continued*

Nursing Diagnosis	Outcome	Intervention
Potential for hypothermia related to loss of skin and/or external cooling	Rectal/core temperature is 99–101°F	Monitor and document rectal/core temperature every 1–2 hr For temperature <99°F: warm with heat lamps or shield; warm solutions used for dressing changes; cover patient with foil blanket or other substance to conserve heat
Potential for ineffective patient/family coping related to acute stress of critical injury and potential life-threatening crisis; alteration in family processes related to critical injury	Patient and/or family verbalize goals of treatment regimen Patient and/or family demonstrate knowledge of support systems that are available Patient/family are able to express concerns and fears Patient/family coping is functional and realistic for phase of hospitalization; family processes are at precrisis level	Support adaptive/functional coping mechanisms Use interventions to reduce patient fatigue and pain Promote use of group support sessions for patients and families Orient patient and family to unit and support services and reinforce information frequently Involve patient and family in treatment goals and plan of care

must not only provide the skilled care, but monitor the patient's and family's response to the treatment experience. Psychosocial support is integral to the entire process to ensure an optimum outcome.

Although providing care to the burned patient is a team effort, it is the critical care nurse who is with the patient 24 hours a day. The support and skill of the nurse will truly make the critical difference in the patient outcome.

See the Nursing Care Plan for the Resuscitative and Acute Phases of the Patient with Major Burn Injury.

References

Arturson, G. (1961): Capillary permeability in burned and nonburned areas in dogs. *Acta Chirurgica Scandinavica* 274 (Suppl.):55–65.

Choiniere, M., Paquette, C., Grenier, R., and Paquin, M. J. (1990): A double blind study to determine the efficacy of patient controlled analgesia in burn patients. *Proceedings of the American Burn Association Meeting* 22:207 (Abstract).

Cram, E., and Kealey, G. P. (1990): Patient control analgesia: A strategy for controlling acute burn pain. *Proceedings of the American Burn Association Meeting* 22:208 (Abstract).

Demling, R. H. (1987): Fluid replacement in burned patients. *Surgical Clinics of North America* 67(1):15–30.

Ehleben, C., and Still, J. (1985): Psychological morbidity and pain. *Proceedings of the American Burn Association Meeting* 17:104 (Abstract).

Gordon, M. D. (ed.) (1986a): Burn care protocols—donor site care. *Journal of Burn Care and Rehabilitation* 7(2):154–159.

Gordon, M. D. (ed.) (1986b): Burn care protocols—nutritional support. *Journal of Burn Care and Rehabilitation* 7(4):351–356.

Gordon, M. D. (ed.) (1987a): Burn care protocols—anchoring endotubes on patients with facial burns. *Journal of Burn Care and Rehabilitation* 8(3):233–237.

Gordon, M. D. (ed.) (1987b): Burn care protocols—infection control in the burn unit. *Journal of Burn Care and Rehabilitation* 8(1):67–71.

Gordon, M. D. (ed.) (1987c): Burn care protocols—monitoring burn wounds for infection. *Journal of Burn Care and Rehabilitation* 8(6):568–572.

Gordon, M. D. (ed.) (1988a): Burn care protocols—documenting. *Journal of Burn Care and Rehabilitation* 7(3):266–267.

Gordon, M. D. (ed.) (1988b): Burn care protocols—surgical fixation of skin grafts. *Journal of Burn Care and Rehabilitation* 9(5):516–519.

Gordon, M. D. (ed.) (1988c): Burn care protocols—synthetic and biosynthetic skin substitutes. *Journal of Burn Care and Rehabilitation* 9(2):209–215.

Gordon, M. D. (ed.) (1989): Burn care protocols—mechanical debridement. *Journal of Burn Care and Rehabilitation* 10(3):271–275.

Heimbach, D. M., Engrav, L. H., Marvin, J. A., Harnar, T. J., and Grube, B. J. (1987): Toxic epidermal necrolysis: A step forward in treatment. *Journal of the American Medical Association* 257:2171–2175.

Herndon, D. H., Lingner, F., Thompson, P., Linares, H. A., Stein, M., and Traber, H. L. (1987): Pulmonary injury in burned patients. *Surgical Clinics of North America* 67(2):31–46.

Hospital and prehospital resources for optimal care of patients with burn injury: Guidelines for development and operation of burn centers. (1990). *Journal of Burn Care and Rehabilitation* 11:97–104.

Kenner, C., and Achterberg, J. (1983): Non-pharmaceutical pain relief of burn patients. *Proceedings of the American Burn Association Meeting* 15:99 (Abstract).

Loeser, J. (1987): Conceptual framework for pain management. *Journal of Burn Care and Rehabilitation* 8(4):309–312.

Malick, M. H., and Carr, J. A. (1982): *Manual on Management of the Burn Patient.* Pittsburg, PA: Harmarville Rehabilitation Center.

Mason, A. D., Jr. (1980): The mathematics of resuscitation. *Journal of Trauma* 20:1015–1020.

Mason, A. D., Jr., McManus, A. T., and Pruitt, B. A., Jr. (1986): Association of burn mortality and bacteremia. *Archives of Surgery* 121:1027–1031.

McCaffery, M., and Beebe, A. (1989): *Pain-Clinical Manual for Nursing Practice.* St. Louis: C. V. Mosby.

McManus, A. T., McManus, W. F., Mason, A. D., Jr., Aitcheson, A. R., and Pruitt, B. A., Jr. (1987): Microbial colonization in a new intensive care burn unit. *Archives of Surgery* 120:217–223.

McManus, W. F., Mason, A. D., Jr., and Pruitt, B. A., Jr. (1989): Excision of the burn wound in patients with large burns. *Archives of Surgery* 124:718–720.

Mozingo, J. W., Smith, A. A., McManus, W. F., Pruitt, B. A., Jr., and Mason, A. D., Jr. (1988): Chemical burns. *Journal of Trauma* 28(5):642–647.

Nebraska Burn Institute (1989): *Advanced Burn Life Support Course Manual.* Lincoln, NE: Nebraska Burn Institute.

Perry, S., Heidrich, G., and Ramos, E. (1981): Assessment of pain by burn patients. *Journal of Burn Care and Rehabilitation* 2(6):322–326.

Pruitt, B. A., Jr. (1979): The burn patient II: Later care and complications of thermal injury. *Current Problems in Surgery* 16(5):10–62.

Pruitt, B. A., Jr. (1984): The universal trauma model. *Bulletin of the American College of Surgeons* 70(10):2–13.

Pruitt, B. A., Jr. (1987a): Burn treatment for the unburned. *Journal of the American Medical Association* 257:2207–2208.

Pruitt, B. A., Jr. (1987b): Sepsis and survival in burn patients. *Journal of Intensive Care Medicine* 2:294–296.

Pruitt, B. A., Jr. (1988): Electric injury. In Wyngaarden, J., and Smith, L. (eds.): *Cecil Textbook of Medicine.* 18th ed. Philadelphia: W. B. Saunders, pp. 2380–2382.

Pruitt, B. A., Jr., and Goodwin, C. W., Jr. (1983): Nutritional management of the seriously ill burned patient. *In:* R. W. Winter (ed.). *Nutritional Support of the Seriously Ill Patient.* New York: Academic Press, pp. 63–84.

Pruitt, B. A., Jr., and Goodwin, C. W., Jr. (1987): Thermal injuries. *In:* J. H. Davis, W. R. Drucker, R. S. Foster, Jr., R. L. Gamelli, D. S. Gann, B. A. Pruitt, Jr., and G. F. Sheldon (eds.). *Clinical Surgery.* St. Louis: C. V. Mosby, pp. 2848–2902.

Pruitt, B. A., Jr., and Goodwin, C. W., Jr. (1990): Burn injury. *In:* E. F. Moore (ed.). *Early Care of the Injured Patient.* 4th ed. St. Louis: C. V. Mosby, pp. 286–306.

Shirani, K. Z., Pruitt, B. A., Jr., and Mason, A. D., Jr. (1987): The influence of inhalation injury and pneumonia on burn mortality. *Annals of Surgery* 205(1):82–87.

Treat, R. C., Sirinek, K. R., Levine, B. A., and Pruitt, B. A., Jr. (1980): Air evacuation of thermally injured patients: Principles of treatment and results. *Journal of Trauma* 20:275–279.

Wachtel, T. L. (1987): Nutritional support of the burn patient. *In:* J. A. Boswick, Jr. (ed.). *The Art and Science of Burn Care.* Rockville, MD: Aspen, pp. 203–217.

Warden, G. D. (1987): Immunologic response to burn injury. *In:* J. A. Boswick, Jr. (ed.). *The Art and Science of Burn Care.* Rockville, MD: Aspen, pp. 113–121.

Waymack, J. P., and Pruitt, B. A., Jr. (1990): Burn wound care. *Advances in Surgery* 23:261–290.

Wilmore, D. W. (1987): Metabolic changes after thermal injury. *In:* J. A. Boswick, Jr. (ed.). *The Art and Science of Burn Care.* Rockville, MD: Aspen, pp. 137–144.

Wolman, R. (1988, March): *Concepts in Pain Management.* Paper presented at the 20th annual meeting of the American Burn Association, Seattle, WA.

Recommended Readings

Cooper, D. (1988): Wound healing: A nursing responsibility. *In:* M. Kinney, et al. (eds.). *AACN Clinical Reference.* New York: McGraw-Hill, pp. 1460–1479.

Duncan, D. J. (ed.) (1991): Burn management. *Critical Care Nursing Clinics of North America* 3(2):165–267.

Gordon, M. D. (ed.) (1988): Burn care protocols—discharge planning and teaching protocols. *Journal of Burn Care and Rehabilitation.* 9(4):414.

Molter, N. C. (1991) Pain in the burn patient. *In:* K. Punctillo (ed.). *Nursing Management of Pain in the Critical Care Environment.* Rockville, MD: Aspen, pp. 193–209.

Pruitt, B. A., Jr., and Goodwin, C. W., Jr. (1990): Burn injury. *In:* E. F. Moore (ed.). *Early Care of the Injured Patient.* 4th ed. American College of Surgeons. St. Louis: C. V. Mosby, distributor, p. 286.

Watkins, P. N., Cook, E. L., May, S. R., Ehleben, C. M. (1988): Psychological stages in adaptation following burn injury: A method for facilitating psychological recovery of burn victims. *Journal of Burn Care and Rehabilitation* 9(4):376.

Index

Note: Page numbers in *italic* indicate figures; those followed by t indicate tables.